WHAT PEOPLE

TOXIC WORLD, TOXIC PEOPLE

An incisive examination of the many ills which afflict the modern world, full of wise advice, helping to lay down the path to a saner, more harmonious world.
Steve Taylor, best-selling author of *Waking from Sleep* and *Back to Sanity*

Everyone should read this book if they intend on living a long and healthy life. Anna has compounded sound information on everything we need to know about the ever-present toxic lifestyle we are leading and how we can avoid it and effectively rehabilitate ourselves. Her emotional and physical journey brings a compassionate, personal edge to the very real dangers we face every day and how we blindly proceed through life unaware of how the items we are exposed to are slowly destroying us. Anna has broken down the barriers, myths and misconceptions of everything from cosmetics to vaccinations, to food and our general state of mind. This guide is my go-to book for living a cleaner life. Every page is jam packed full of invaluable knowledge and is guaranteed to have you thinking twice or shaking in your boots about the toxic-filled life you lead
Laura Wells Australian Plus Size Supermodel, Greenpeace Activist & Environmental Scientist

An excellent guide book to ridding ourselves of the hidden toxicity that exists in everything from the food we eat to the consumer products we use daily, complete with a practical list of natural alternatives we can start using right away. This book is a great resource for anyone wanting to reach the next level of natural, vibrant health through lifestyle, habits and attitude – and most importantly, how to pass this on to their children for a lifetime of good health.
Ethan Evers, author of *The Eden Prescription*

This is an essential book for those looking to make conscious life choices for a cleaner, healthier way of living in this age of toxicity. Anna has combined the latest research to provide a comprehensive guide that covers a wealth of topics from toxic heavy metals and the nasty chemicals that lurk in everything from our food and drink to cosmetics and cleaning products, and how using natural foods, treatments and exercise can detoxify the mind, body and our environment. Anna also focuses on concepts such as contentment, forgiveness and affirmations to improve our happiness and wellbeing, and the latest parenting skills and techniques for bringing up happy and healthy children. Highly recommended.

Martin Gill, assistant editor, *Yoga Magazine*

Anna has poured years of life experience and deep research into this generous, compassionate and immensely helpful book. If you are raising children and want to look after their wellbeing, if you're trying to figure out how to stay healthy with food, water, and home and beauty products, or if you just want to hear the candid experiences of someone who suffered for making toxic choices – and learned how to fix them – then you'll benefit from hearing Anna's story and learning through her eyes and experience. She's been there and has done the research ahead of many of us, and shares it with the kindness and deep sense of compassion that is her trademark. I hope this is a sign of things to come – that home and beauty products look to people like Anna Rodgers for their inspiration, instead of selling the cheapest, most toxic stuff they can produce, and spending millions on ads to cover up their putrid toxicity. The beauty that Anna shares starts from inside your cells with good food, clean water, and a clean home and emotional environment, and extends outward. It's a well-researched, helpful, warm and compassionate book, and one I think every mother and daughter would enjoy sharing.

Liam Scheff, author of *Official Stories*

Anna is not only a wealth of information; she writes everything in such an inspiring and easy-to-follow way. This book is an immensely valuable resource for the eco-conscious and for anyone looking to lead even a slightly more ethical and natural life. Thank you, Anna. I know I'll refer to this for years to come (especially when I have kids).

Denise Duffield-Thomas, author of *Lucky Bitch* and *Get Rich, Lucky Bitch*

Toxic World, Toxic People is an inspiring, comprehensive step-by-step guide, through the toxic world we live in today. By using her own personal life experiences, Anna has managed to take us on a unique and informative journey to a healthier way of life.This book is not only interesting; it is factual, well-researched and well written. It is a must read for anyone wishing to live a toxic free, healthier and happier lifestyle.

Christina England, author, research journalist and Regional Director of the Natural Solutions Foundation for the European Union.

This book is so needed. I repeat, SO NEEDED. The first time I read it, I remember thinking 'Woah... this is way too heavy for me', but it wasn't; I just wasn't ready to hear the truths that this book reveals. Reading it is like having Anna on speed-dial. She shares her own personal journey about how she got sick and what she did to get well again, alongside amazing wisdom about the food we eat, toxic chemicals, natural beauty and how to be a fully aware parent. Anna is my number one go-to girl for busting myths about the health industry and providing real insight into conscious living, and this book is a game changer.

Lisa Clark, author of *SASSY: The Go-for-it Girl's Guide to Becoming Mistress of Your Destiny* www.sassyology.com

Having spent a great deal of my life pioneering Natural Health, organic skincare, conscious living and a global wellness company, I often get asked to endorse books, and have to politely decline. Not so with this gem! Anna's book shines her light with a must-have read & reference for anyone wanting to avoid a toxic world, for themselves, for their children, and for the planet. Contemporary solutions delivered with genuine love and care, excellent research, and inspired writing.

Paul Loveday, managing director, Organic Love System and Australian Bush Flower Essences

Toxic World, Toxic People will make a wonderful contribution to your health and wellness. Anna shows us the way to physical, mental, emotional and spiritual health benefits through a deep understanding of the basic principles fundamental to achieving the health, happiness and environmental standards we so desire.

From beginning to end, this book is a total labor of love. Anna's thorough investigation into the toxicity we are experiencing today leads to numerous positive solutions, such as building immunity, how to empower our lives and improve our personal as well as planetary environments. I was impressed with the book's vastness of scope, from taking charge of our own health through knowledge of nutrition and personal care products, to attachment parenting, to an extensive section on vaccination, to building loving relationships for adults and children, to the power of attraction, and so much more. There is absolutely no topic regarding physiological and psychological health left untouched in this powerful book, so essential for today.

Karen Ranzi MA, author of *Creating Healthy Children* and *Raw Food Fun for Families*

Anna Rodgers is a true trailblazer. Her mission? To transform how you look after your mind, body and how you raise your children. Packed with life-changing information, *Toxic World, Toxic People* uncovers the truth about what you are really facing when it comes to reclaiming your health and wellbeing. If you're ready to open your eyes and discover what is really going on, read this book!

Dr. Christy Fergusson aka The Food Psychologist and author of *Hot, Healthy, Happy*

Toxic World, Toxic People is not only a fantastic read, but is quite literally a must-have resource for a healthier life. This easy-to-read, well-researched book is full of helpful and comprehensive information and advice. The lists of health and eco-friendly companies make it easy to implement the toxin-free strategies needed to not only address acute and chronic health challenges, but also to lead a well and happy long life.

Dr. Rebecca Harwin, author of *Conquer Your Polycystic Ovary Syndrome Naturally*

Toxic World, Toxic People

The Essential Guide to Health, Happiness, Parenting and Conscious Living

Toxic World, Toxic People

The Essential Guide to Health, Happiness, Parenting and Conscious Living

Anna Rodgers

Winchester, UK
Washington, USA

First published by Soul Rocks Books, 2014
Soul Rocks Books is an imprint of John Hunt Publishing Ltd., Laurel House, Station Approach,
Alresford, Hants, SO24 9JH, UK
office1@jhpbooks.net
www.johnhuntpublishing.com
www.soulrocks-books.com

For distributor details and how to order please visit the 'Ordering' section on our website.

Text copyright: Anna Rodgers 2013

ISBN: 978 1 78099 471 0

All rights reserved. Except for brief quotations in critical articles or reviews, no part of this
book may be reproduced in any manner without prior written permission from the publishers.

The rights of Anna Rodgers as author have been asserted in accordance with the Copyright,
Designs and Patents Act 1988.

A CIP catalogue record for this book is available from the British Library.

Design: Stuart Davies
www.stuartdaviesart.com

Before you read this book, I must give you the following FDA-mandated
warning and disclaimer:

My statements regarding alternative treatments and health advice have not been
evaluated by the FDA.

Disclaimer: Information presented here is for information, personal opinion and
educational purposes only, and is not intended to diagnose, treat, cure or prevent any condition
or disease; nor is it to be relied upon as a substitute for your own research or independent
advice. You should always speak with a healthcare practitioner or a specialist in the subject
matter before taking any action. No responsibility is accepted for any errors, omissions, or
misleading statements on these pages or any site to which these pages connect. You should be
practicing always under the personal guidance of a qualified and experienced teacher.

Printed and bound by CPI Group (UK) Ltd, Croydon, CR0 4YY

We operate a distinctive and ethical publishing philosophy in all
areas of our business, from our global network of authors to
production and worldwide distribution.

CONTENTS

Dedicated to my beautiful daughter Lola
This book is for you and all the other precious children who have
to grow up in our toxic world

Extra Special Thanks

To my husband and best friend Nathan, thank you for setting me on my journey that allowed me to heal. To my brother and sister, Jim and Alice – thank you for giving me so much support and encouragement. I am so grateful you both already have an interest in natural health. To Mum and Dad, I hope this book helps you both to become healthier and happier too.

To Laurena, thank you for all our many hours of deep and enlightening discussions. Thank you for always being there for me. You are truly an amazing person. I couldn't think of someone more perfect than you to be our daughter's godmother. And thank you from the bottom of my heart for introducing me to Dr. Kucera; my health and I won't ever forget it.

Dr. Kucera, you gave me my life - and my sanity back, which is truly incredible seeing how sick I was and that most had signed me off as 'incurable'. I wish the entire world had access to your supplements, genius and advice. Hopefully they will soon.

To Ethan Evers, not only have you written one of the best books I have ever read, you were also kind enough to help me edit my book. Your suggestions and support were wonderful. Thank you!

To Star Khechara for being a wonderful example of walking your talk and helping others to be healthy. You are a genius with homemade beauty recipes and sensible health advice. Thank you so much for writing my foreword.

To Frank Arrigazzi, thank you for always bringing light and joy to my life – you are a very dear friend to me and one I admire so much. Your constant motivation to help people is incredible – I don't think I know anyone more kind than you are. I've learnt a lot from knowing you and I know I will continue to learn more. The world needs more people like you.

To Andra Mihut for always being there for me, supporting and encouraging me to never ever give up. You're *exactly* what a best friend really means. I'm so lucky to have met you all those years ago. Thank you for all of your encouragement and praise for my book – it means so much!

Thank you to Savannah Alalia, what a blessing it is to have you as a friend and a mentor. You are truly inspiring, kind, so caring, beautiful inside *and* out! The world needs to know about you.

To a special friend, Natalie Southgate, thank you for always giving me so much encouragement, understanding and inspiration.

A big thank-you to Kate Magic who helped suggest other wonderful products, books, movies, food and health info, and was just so kind to take time to encourage me on how to make my book better. You are an inspiration to me and so many people.

To my personal heroes, Dr. Joseph Mercola, Dr. Jayne Donegan, Christina England, Mike Adams and Dr. Andrew Wakefield – your dedication, guts and bravery to go against the tide, to speak the truth despite the ridicule is a huge reason why I have taken this journey. You are all so brave. Because of you, I realized I was not alone in thinking the way I do about health and the madness behind what has happened to our world.

To Alice Grist, and all at John Hunt Publishing, thank you for giving a girl like me a chance – a *huge* dream has come true because of you.

Foreword

When I found out that the gorgeous Anna Rodgers (aka Miss Eco Glam) was writing a book on how to live a healthy and beautiful eco-life, I thought 'YES!' and knew that Anna would mix in just the right amount of knowledge, experience and insight, flourished with personal touches, to make this a guide that anyone could pick up, easily understand and apply to their own lives to get results.

In this very toxic world we now found ourselves in, Anna has created the perfect manual to follow in order to detox our lives and create an abundance of health and happiness. Holistically aligned for seekers of genuine Natural Health, this book is the no-nonsense guide to non-toxic living in these dysfunctional times.

Anna has been influencing the health and beauty scene with Miss Eco Glam for a few years now and what has stood out the most is her utter dedication for sticking to her ethics of only promoting/reviewing products that were 100% animal and planet friendly.

Many on this path have allowed their ethics to be up for sale as they learned to make a quick buck by promoting more mainstream companies – not Anna! She truly is a shining example of how to lead a holistic yet sophisticated lifestyle.

With Anna you can be gorgeous, compassionate and elegant, yet still be an 'eco-warrioress', protecting the environment and inspiring people to improve their health. Genuine health and natural beauty in a plastic world does not have to be an ugly compromise. This book is easy to read and offers lots of useful information on a wide variety of lifestyle, health and beauty issues. Anna even divulges personal information about her toxic past and how she overcame many health issues by following the advice she now offers to you, with this book.

Even a seasoned holistic-lifestyler like myself learned plenty of new information, especially the very important parenting section, so if you are new (or old) to natural living this book will be an absolute gold mine and a 'must-have'.

From tampons to tanning, and how to bring up your children to ensure they have a fighting chance to be happy in this world, Anna gives everything in the average household a run for its money, which is why I recommend every house has a copy of her book, like a Bible (but without the preaching) for wannabe eco-chicks and eco-dudes.

What is truly unique about this book is that Anna is bringing awareness not only to the very real health dangers of toxicity, but also to the fact that most relationships between family members and loved ones are very toxic too, which also impacts society detrimentally. These two problems go hand in hand and it's been fascinating to read how someone can improve their family ties, if they decrease the levels of toxicity in their body, and therefore improve their brain health.

So if you want a beetle-free glitzy eyeshadow or that salon-quality hair color but without the salon toxins and you want to improve your *entire* life, then READ THIS BOOK and revel in the gorgeous new-and-improved, healthier, wealthier, happier you.

Star Khechara
Star is known as the 'The Facelift Food Coach' – she inspires people to improve their looks by incorporating a high raw-food diet into their lifestyle. Star is a trained nutritionist, holistic cosmetology teacher and regularly writes for various national publications.
www.starkhechara.com
www.FruitForBeauty.com

Introduction

If I told you that on average, each one of us comes into contact with over at least *80,000* toxic - and mostly untested for safety - chemicals each *year*, would you a) *believe* me? b) If yes, what implications would you perhaps think this may have on human health? Would you think that this exorbitant number may mean we now have an epidemic on our hands causing so much of the sickness, disease and death of today? Or would you think that the human body can simply cope with this assault and that it's nothing to worry about? Well, this is *exactly* what *Toxic World, Toxic People* is all about. I'm going to explain to you, with facts, figures *and* proof, just how this astronomical number has come to be undeniably true - and I am also going to explain what it's doing not just to your body's health but also to your *mind's* health.

This book is probably going to be perhaps one of the most alarming ones you've read, and some of it may even leave you feeling shocked, outraged and *really* concerned (good!), but it's also got huge potential to help you avoid many of these problems that are being caused by this massive exposure to toxicity.

If you have ever read the Bible, you may remember the story we are always told about Adam and Eve, who were said to be the first humans on earth. They lived in a beautiful and magical paradise. They were depicted as perfectly healthy (with fit and 'ideal weight' bodies) and seemed perfectly happy. They were surrounded by the most beautiful forests, with all the fresh (organic!) food they could ever want. Didn't this sound like *bliss* and what we are led to believe heaven is like? And for many of us, isn't it actually what we *wish* our life could be like right here on earth today? But sadly, this picture of perfect human health and a perfect planet, and the ability to live surrounded by purity, is almost now completely *impossible* to find.

A very long time ago, the entire earth used to be pure and in balance, back when Nature was in sync and humans were respectful, knowledgable and in tune with themselves, and the planet.

Fast forward millions of years later, and sadly, life nowadays is a *very* different story. Paradise only seems fit to describe just a few areas left on earth and even those are now vastly different to what they were originally like, or what they should *still* be like. We have literally ravaged most of the beautiful areas on earth, and still are, purely just for financial gain, with no thought about what it means for our future generations. And in regards to the places that are, what we think - still relatively untouched by mankind - as you will soon discover, they too, are victims of very harmful toxicity levels too.

'We the People' have become 'The Little People' who have had to suffer the serious consequences of irresponsible actions from Big Pharma, Big Government, Big Agriculture, Big Banking and all the other Big Corporations who seem to have absolutely no conscience or desire to do genuine good.

One of the most pressing issues today, which is not being discussed *anywhere* nearly enough, is that of *toxic exposure* and the deadly accumulative effects it's having on humans. These deadly effects are endangering our children in more ways than we even truly know. We are surrounded by disease-causing pollution, living in huge, bursting-at-the-seams cities with far too many people. Our buildings are built with toxic materials and are literally a health hazard to live and work in. Our food has become so unnatural and downright poisonous, causing countless types of cancers, heart disease, early death and other avoidable diseases.

Pure drinking water is exceptionally rare to find and instead, we are generally consuming highly toxic water full of many heavy metals, pesticides and more worryingly, high levels of many types of *pharmaceutical* medications. This alone is causing *massive* problems for not only our health but also the environments. Whatever we drink, we will therefore have in our bodies, and small amounts from each person, through urination and bathing, ends up *back* in the waterways, leading to large amounts. And all of this is damage that's been done mainly in the last 100 years. We've been here on earth, for so long, but we have managed to mess so much up in a relatively short amount of time.

Toxic chemicals are showing up in *all* corners of the earth, and in places you wouldn't normally think of. In the North Pole some male polar bears are now being born with *both* sets of reproductive genitalia. In alligators which inhabit Florida's Lake Apoka, many are now being found to have such small penises that they cannot reproduce. Whilst to some this may seem insignificant, when you understand the importance of a balanced animal food chain, it should set off alarm bells that these quirks in nature may actually harbor dire consequences for us. Since the 1980s when DDT (a very dangerous insecticide once classed as 'perfectly safe') was introduced, the alligators have been exposed to soaring concentrations of this toxic chemical, which effects mimics the production of estrogen.

If animals are being so deeply affected by just *one* toxic chemical, then *what* is happening to humans who are exposed to *thousands* more? For example in a scary echo of this, we see that young girls are developing bodies of women, growing breasts far earlier than is normal, due to the chemicals they are absorbing. And I will show you all of the many ways how we are doing this.

In the Himalayan plateaus, a place known for its beauty, tranquility, high peaks and 'fresh' air which can make a person feel like they are on 'the top of the world,' scientists have carried out studies on the soil. Whilst these plateaus are a very long way from any factory, chemicals have still impregnated the soil - very toxic things like mercury, lead and cadmium which have been carried in the air by pollution from factories far away, and settled down onto the soil. Soil always has some level of heavy metals in it, but when particles from air (or rain) *also* drop down, it causes the ratio to become really out of whack. This is happening in *all* of the pristine areas on earth. When scientists were researching the arctic to see what impact Global Warming was having on this part of the world, they were alarmed to see just how many toxic chemicals had settled into the ice, in particular the high levels of lead.

And with Eskimo women, native to areas like Greenland, who eat traditional foods such as raw whale meat and other fish, their breastmilk is becoming so toxic through the absoption of chemicals from the oceans, it's now very dangerous for their children to be fed like this. Mother's milk has become mother's *poison* to the children of the arctic.

Why is this happening, and why has it happened so quickly? Are we all to blame? It is mainly due to the large corporations and the far too easily 'bought off' governments who are really at fault, as they do not control chemicals and their products anywhere as much as they should, nor do they test them sufficiently *first,* for their safety. We as individuals are also very much to blame, although the biggest mistake we have made is to always assume that things are safe and not question what we are told. Now we need to realise that we actually have most of the power because if we refuse to buy certain products, the companies will have *no* way of making money. It is our cash (and the tacit approval it affords) that aids and abets them to continue to do what they are doing.

Some of the super wealthy are also to blame for many of our problems because they are the ones who can afford to buy several huge homes - which use so much water, consume many families' worth of electricity and gas and use more of our precious natural materials in general. The rich and famous buy countless cars, sail massive boats and fly private planes, which pollute the air *and* water, and they rarely seem to care about the footprint they are leaving on the earth. They are emulated by the rest of us, as having 'perfect' lives; their glitz and glamor lifestyle makes millions of people aspire to be like them, but blinds us all into forgetting about what's actually important in life: Health *and* Happiness!

With this huge mess on each of our doorsteps, the rest of us now have to try and comprehend *what* we are going to do to sort these enormous problems out, and how to wake others up so that they too, care about what is happening around them. We are leaving so much for our children and their children to have to deal with, and more worryingly, to *suffer* from. If nothing changes, would life in the future even be worth living?

Due to the soaring rise in population, massive technology boom and, last but not least, the chemical industry, we now have a *completely* different world. These so-called 'advances' bring with them the good, the bad and the *very* ugly. And I am not just talking about the superficial appearance of the earth either. What is most alarming of all the changes since time began, is the amount of toxins that are now found in our air, water, food, personal care products, environment, and now also found, in *all* of us. As you will discover, most babies, if not *all,* are being born with hundreds of unsafe industrial chemicals inside their bodies. This is *not* good enough and *not* how it's supposed to be. We've *got* to all do something about it. We've all got to know

I wrote this book - which initially was going to be a small ebook I gave away on my website - because people need to understand just how *serious* this all is, and how these toxins affect *all* of us, every single day. My book has become quite lengthy because the problem is *big* and requires lots of detail. It was impossible to tell you about all of these pressing issues with just a few pages.

More often than not, despite that people have heard of toxins, they still don't *really* get just how big a problem it is for their own health, their children's and their entire families. They think (and this is sadly still only a very small percentage of the population) that the only chemicals to perhaps worry about are what's in their food and beauty products, when it's actually *so* much more than that. Or they think because they have no current symptoms or because they don't feel ill that there really isn't something to be concerned with now. But the truth is, toxins, for all of us are a ticking time bomb. They *do* affect all of us because there are simply too many floating around for us to avoid. Once I share the facts about them with you, you will clearly see, the real urgency of this threat to all of us.

Toxic chemicals are making us fat, infertile, unhappy, angry, sick, violent, depressed, and are causing countless other types of disease and cancers, in men, women *and* infants too. They are even affecting the health of our pets and many other animals, like that of the alligators. Everything that is a living and breathing creature is suffering from chemical accumulation.

I mention the word *toxins* a lot throughout this book, but really, the best way to picture the word toxin is to think of '*poison*' when you read it, for that is exactly what toxins are. Toxins *poison* us, sometimes very suddenly - just say if you were to come into contact with a large amount of pesticides for example - but most of the time they cause ill health very *slowly*, over many years of constant exposure and gradual *accumulation*. This picture of accumulation, is *exactly* what I want you to think of throughout this book, because this is where the problem lies, that with each new day, as more chemicals are ingested, inhaled and absorbed into your body, they are most likely not going to be excreted in the way that they should be - which only spells disaster for your health.

Years ago, before the industrial and chemical revolution, your body most likely would have been able to detox most of these chemicals quite easily, for that's what it's designed to do. But when exposure happens far too quickly and from far too many different types of chemicals, even Superman would have trouble staying fit, healthy and happy.

Before we begin on this journey, I want you to know, this knowledge I am sharing with you, is *not* about turning everyone into paranoid beings, who are scared of living, it's simply about being *aware* of what you can do to *limit* your exposure as much as possible. Luckily, it is actually quite easy, once you know how. That's where this book comes in handy, as I am going to share with you how you can make sure you keep (or achieve) long-term good health.

As cheesy as this may sound, I also want to help you become as *happy* as you are meant to be. The majority of people today would admit they rarely feel truly happy and if anything, are maybe suffering from some level of depression even right now, or have at least gone through it a few times in their lives. They may even be likely to suffer with it on and off *forever*, if they don't sort out the root cause. Toxicity from chemicals is causing many of these problems with unhappiness too - because many are neurotoxins which damage the nerves and affect brain function - but it's also coming from many other aspects of our society. We will talk about this too.

Throughout my journey, where I have spent many years delving into this subject matter, it became apparent to me that not only are we toxic health wise, a large percentage of us, are also toxic *relationship* wise. We have difficult problems relating to our parents, our partners, our own children, our work colleagues and sometimes, even our own friends. We may argue often, feel upset regularly and for some, it can cause almost daily anguish. These sorts of problems may even bring deep unhappiness to one's entire life, where they never feel at peace with the people around them, or with themselves. And this lifetime of unhappiness and the behaviours developed because of this, may even affect many generations to come. We can pass on many things to our children. We *must* change our own lives for the sake of our children. The other *huge* epidemic in society today is unhappy children who more often than not, go on to become deeply unhappy and depressed adults, who feel and often are not able to contribute to society in a positive way, or in the best way possible. They simply do not know their purpose or what they are meant to do with their lives and this leaves them feeling empty and sad. You only have to read about the alarming statistics of people taking antidepressants to know that this is true. Antidepressant use has skyrocketed at a rate which is almost unbelievable. In just 20 years, it has risen by a whopping 400%. Back in the early 90s, approximately only 2% of patients were taking antidepressants and now it's reported to be *one in ten* people over the age of twelve. And many of these patients remain on them over many years, without ever really sorting out the *root* cause. We have simply become a world of pill addicts, at times even demanding them from our doctors. We are not only *not* educated to find out *why* we are depressed, nor are we ever encouraged to do something about our mental health for the *long* term. We are looking for quick fixes that aren't actually truly fixing our problems.

We are not looked at in a holistic way by the majority of our doctors, instead due to very short appointments, we are often seen as a number (and sometimes not even remembered by our name) and our lifestyle is not generally taken into consideration. We present with this or that symptom and are typically sent off with a prescription. And many times the drugs are useless, and worse, areeven dangerous. If our doctors had the time and the *training* to look at us *holistically*, we could, most of the time, stop our symptoms from reoccurring or from getting far worse. And we would not need prescription after prescription, year after year. With holistic treatment, the root cause would be discovered, treated successfully and *safely*, and our health and happiness would be improved for the better. Then we would be contributing to society so much more productively.

Today, pharmaceutical medications are being prescribed far too easily. And many of them are much more unsafe than what you might think and can also be seriously ineffective, and quite often, can actually make the problem much *worse*, or leave you with other side effects which may require another pill. *Real* health is your body functioning well on it's *own*, with healthy food, regular exercise, sun exposure and perhaps a few effective supplements. It's common-sense stuff really. The body should *not* need to be on countless medications. *This* is what we need from our doctors and healthcare advisors - to truly know just how to get the body to work optimally. Speaking from personal experience, I relied on medications for decades, and was given them far too easily. I was *never* encouraged to look at my life in a holistic way, so my health and life did not get much better for me at all, only far worse. Over twenty long and excruciatingly painful years I was severely depressed and took many types of drugs for various different 'ailments' which never actually worked. They never helped my depression, they never helped with my desperately low energy levels, nor with my constant sickness and only added more to the already concerning levels of toxins in my body. To wean myself off some of these medications was actually one of the *hardest* things I ever did, and still remains so to this day. Giving birth was far easier!

Alarmingly, none of the doctors who prescribed me these medications, even *warned* me of what it would be like to get off the drugs, and that it would be very difficult to cope with the withdrawal effects. Not one of the doctors read the side effects out to me, or told me to read them before taking. None of them knew it would literally take me a few years to feel that I was not still suffering from any side effects from these drugs. I look back on that time in my life as a period of utter despair and agony. I would *not* wish it upon anyone. Yet, worryingly, it's happening to *lots* of people, right now - and some won't cope at all well with the withdrawal effects as we will discover in Part 2.

I really only discovered much later, that the combination of toxic accumulation from the many different forms and also from the stress caused by a very unhappy childhood, made me *very* sick. Stress, whether it's from emotions or toxins, or both, is detrimentally damaging to the body *and* brain. I now see that my own story of ill health and unhappiness is also now extremely *common* for countless other people I have met along the way. Chronic Fatigue and other 'mystery illnesses' are happening to so many people at a truly alarming rate. Even most doctors are baffled as to what is causing this huge increase. They just aren't making the connection yet, to toxicity. But its only a matter of time before they do.

Most of our problems to do with unhappiness, come straight from our experiences in childhood, where certain emotional, and even physical needs were not met. Whilst it's impossible for anyone to have a 'perfect' childhood, as no parent can ever get it 100% right, it does seem that we have very much lost our way with knowing what and how to *teach* our children. We don't even really know *how* to love them, or the best way to feed, what's the best treatment for when they are sick, and also how to *treat* them, so that they have a good chance at growing up feeling confident, happy and secure within themselves.

I do believe though that there is much we can do to break the cycle of one's own past so as not to pass on the same toxic relationship problems to our new generations. In part 3 I share valuable tips and advice on how you can try and ensure your own children stand a much greater chance of turning out happy and healthy, so that they in the future, when it's their time, will attract loving partners, develop healthy relationships and will in turn bring up successful children together for many generations to come. Creating strong family ties is one of the most important issues we must do something about. If you don't have children now or perhaps won't in the future, don't worry, this book can still be life changing for you. I don't think there is anyone that wouldn't be helped by what is in this book.

You would think that it would be so easy to find out this kind of vital information to improve ourselves, and the planet. But it's not taught in most of our schools. There are many reasons why powerful people and industries do not want us to be in true control of our own lives. The media is used to manipulate and to distract us from the real truth. They can make up other stories to cover up much more important ones so that certain events get played down or even covered up. The media is also tied financially to many powerful organizations, and only a small group of people own most of the media outlets in the world, which makes it *very* easy for them to put out what they want and keep to themselves what they don't want getting out. People that own newspapers also sit on the board, or own many shares in pharmaceutical companies. Government members will go through a 'revolving door' system where they will go from one corporate company back to government again, being seriously embedded in massive conflicts of interest. And there's no laws in place to stop this from happening.

We have *allowed* the media and it's big-spending advertisers to massively increase our superficiality, to dictate how we should live our lives, what products we should buy, what we should believe in and what we should eat. And we've trusted what they are telling us without questioning. This of course, would be great if it was from ethical, healthy and sensible sources, but when you have big profits involved, and with the twisted connections between governments, oil companies and Big Pharma, then it's always going to be a different story. It's better for them if we are sick, fat, miserable and broke. We just have to *read* between the lines because these corporations, the media and our own governments, are making nothing but *cash cows* out of us. They are taking away our truth, our rights and our health and happiness.

The most important thing we must deal with right now, is our physical wellbeing and emotional happiness, as a society and, as a planet. The healthier and happier and more balanced *we* are, the more caring we are, which means only then will we truly understand what life is really about. We will then want to actively help improve society rather than being confused, unsure, and blind as to what we can do.

The book is divided into four parts. Part 1 is about toxins, what they are, where they come from, what they do to us and how we can reduce exposure. We will cover toxins in food, beauty products, in our homes, our water supplies and in our environment. We will also discuss how pharmacetucials are being massively overprescribed and how we all have far too many 'legal drugs' and you will also discover how to effectively and safely detox your body.

Part 2 is about unhappiness, what are the real root causes, how the answer may not be turning to medications such as antidepressants, and in fact that *they* may be the real problem. You will find advice on how to go about becoming a happy and healthy person with tips on supplements, healthy sun exposure, a healthy diet (with some simple but very tasty recipes included) and what you can do to find peace inside yourself so that your life is one of more joy and contentment.

Part 3 is about encouraging you to consider new ways of thinking and behaving in regards to parenting – from breastfeeding, to education, to building healthy self-esteem (for you and your children), to choosing the right sort of food, to teaching kids to have a better relationship with money, and ways to treat and improve their health *without* harming their very important immune system. And I encourage parents to look into the safety aspects of vaccinations and having much more of a fully informed choice.

Part 4 is on the environment and what we can do to play our part in caring for the planet. In this section I've included fun and helpful recipes for making inexpensive homemade beauty and cleaning products. There is also some helpful information on gardening at home, even in small spaces and about sharing things with the people around you. At the back of the book you will find many references to articles/books/websites and documentaries and I hope you will find them as helpful as I did. In this book, I will show you how you can spend your money *wisely*, not only to help you and your family, but to be as light as possible on the environment.

If you have purchased this guide for yourself then it means that you do care or at least, are *curious* about your own health, happiness, and wellbeing. And if someone has given it to you, that means *they* care about your health and wellbeing too. And if you have bought it to help with being a better parent, then that already makes this for me, so worthwhile. *Nothing* is more important than our children's future.

This is a book that I hope you will want to dip back into often over the years and will feel urged to give a copy to your friends and loved ones. We have to get more people to understand how they can take their own health and happiness into their own hands.

Anyway, sit back and get comfortable – we do have lots of work to do, but it's work that will help change your life, your children's and our chances of survival as a planet for the better.

Anna Rodgers

The most alarming of all man's assaults upon the environment is the contamination of air, earth, rivers, and sea with dangerous and even lethal materials. This pollution is for the most part irrecoverable; the chain of evil it initiates not only in the world that must support life but in living tissues is for the most part irreversible. In this now universal contamination of the environment, chemicals are the sinister and little recognized partners of radiation in changing the very nature of the world – the very nature of its life. Strontium 90, released through nuclear explosions into the air, comes to earth in rain or drifts down as fallout, lodges in soil, enters into the grass or corn or wheat grown there, and in time takes up its abode in the bones of a human being, there to remain until his death. Similarly, chemicals sprayed on croplands, or forests or gardens lie long in soil, entering into living organisisms passing from one to another in a chain of poisoning until death. Or they pass mysteriously by underground streams until they emerge and, through the alchemy of air and sunlight, combine into new forms that kill vegetation, sicken cattle, and work unknown harm on those who drink from once-pure wells. As Albert Schweitzer has said, "Man can hardly even recgonize the devils of his own creation."

Rachel Carson, Author of the groundbreaking & bestselling book *'Silent Spring'* first published in 1962

PART 1

TOXINS AND THE WORLD WE LIVE IN

Chapter 1

My Own Journey into Chronic Sadness, Sickness and Back to Health Again

I remember when I was about 6 or 7 I stayed at a motel by the beach while on holiday with my family in my home country, Australia. For some strange reason my newly found friend and I decided to paint ourselves with thick white house paint which we had found lying around in half-used old tins by side of the motel. We applied it all over our body, including our arms and legs, pretending we were Aborigines who were doing a traditional dancing ceremony. We were behaving like typical kids, being silly, and using our imaginations to have fun. It all sounded harmless enough, didn't it?

Well, back then, in the 1970s all house paint still contained high levels of lead. As children, we simply had no idea what we had just done that day, and it wasn't until not long after that we realized we couldn't simply wash off the paint with water. We knew we had perhaps made a big mistake. And we weren't even worried about what was *in* the paint – we were far too young to understand about the dangers of chemicals back then but we were more worried about getting into trouble from our parents, or the motel owners. We had no idea that the lead that was in that paint was in fact so poisonous it could (and in my case, *would*) do serious harm to our health. And for me in particular it would be the start of ill health that lasted decades.

Lead is one of the most *dangerous* metals we can have in our body. Having traces of it in our bodies can mean that it may affect the red blood cells as it limits the ability to supply the tissues and organs with enough oxygen. And it also affects our bones by rendering them less able to absorb calcium, thereby causing them to become much weaker. While studying for this book, I gasped when I read this, because I have broken *five* different bones since I was a young girl.

More than just being 'clumsy', it appeared that my bone density, compared to that of my friends, meant that I spent quite a few times during my childhood with a plaster cast on some part of my body. It seemed that on average every 4 years I would fall and break something. And I wasn't even a very active child.

The shocking amount of lead that still exists in our atmosphere today, (despite it not being used anywhere near as much as it was back in the early 20th century), is hardly mentioned these days, but it is still around us in such high levels in the atmosphere. If people really knew this they would be wearing face masks all the time like many Japanese and Chinese people already do. It is extremely harmful for us to breathe it in, day in and day out, and the effects are not going away anytime soon. According to author Bill Bryson, lead stays in the environment for years and years:

> Even though lead was widely known to be dangerous, by the early years of the twentieth century it could be found in all manner of consumer products. Food came in cans sealed with lead solder. Water was often stored in lead-lined tanks. Lead arsenate was sprayed onto fruit as a pesticide. Lead even came as part of the composition of toothpaste tubes. Hardly a product existed that didn't bring a little lead into consumers' lives. However, nothing gave it a greater and more lasting intimacy than its addition to motor fuel. Lead is a neurotoxin. Get too much of it and you can irreparably damage the brain and the central nervous system.
>
> Bill Bryson, author of *A Short History of Nearly Everything*[1]

It boggles the mind to know that although the harmful effects of lead were widely known previously for a *very* long time, lead solder was not actually removed from American food containers right up until as recently as 1993. Those that raised their concerns about lead, all those years ago, were told that it was not true; it was 'completely safe' for everyone. Because of lucrative financial interest in the production of lead-containing products, the real dangers of lead poisoning were kept very quiet for a long time. And those that did speak out were vilified. Very much like what still happens today when people try and bring attention to all of the other problems in the world today.

Found in the blood of Americans today, there is about 625 *times* more lead than there was a century ago. That's a pretty frightening statistic. But despite lead now being banned from many items, its effects are still something we definitely have to worry about, in particular for our children.

When we think of a recently banned chemical, unfortunately we cannot think of it as: 'It's gone – now the problem is solved!' These sorts of chemicals hang around, literally and sometimes for centuries, or in worst-case scenarios such as lead, for life or hundreds, if not *thousands* of years. And it is thought that the toxic effects of lead are getting worse because not all of the industries have stopped producing lead-based products. Some countries still produce them as there hasn't been a worldwide ban on certain things. There is more information about lead and its harmful physical and mental effects coming up in Chapter 3.

After I painted myself with this lead-based paint, I did not tell a soul, not only for fear of getting into big trouble, but because I didn't think it was even worth telling anyone. I had no idea of the dangers I had just inflicted on my health, I was far too young to understand. When we found out what we could use to remove the paint, we applied *another* very toxic chemical to our bodies - mineral turpentine. I remember the big sponges we soaked in this very smelly liquid. It left our skin red and raw but afterwards we jumped straight into the motel's swimming pool and were pleased to quickly forget about what we had just done.

I now believe my body and also my mind, began to show problems relating to that episode shortly after. I was always tired and moody, a real 'bratty' and demanding child, who had plenty of outbursts and tantrums and subsequently became very difficult to look after. I never liked any physical exercise and preferred to stay indoors. After that day, I thought nothing of what had just happened; in fact I didn't really make the connection until only a few years ago, after researching for this book.

I'm certain that day with the paint was what started most of my health, energy and mood problems. And, because it was combined over many years with the effects from a very poor high-sugar diet, much emotional stress, the use of toxic beauty products and eventual drug use (both pharmaceutical *and* recreational), I got to an extremely low point. I had developed severe depression, suffered from terrible and at times, violent mood swings, and ended up being so exhausted that I was eventually diagnosed with chronic fatigue. Basically, my life and health were in an absolute mess.

From the very young age of 13, *I didn't even want to be alive.* I was so depressed that suicide was constantly on my mind, and rather obsessively too; I even attempted it quite a few times. A couple of the instances were actually quite serious and I easily could have died. On one occasion I was found in my bedroom passed out from an overdose and another occasion I also ended up having to stay in the local psychiatric hospital. That stay, in itself was a blessing because I got to see what goes on in those sorts of places, and it's *not* always good.

For 20 long years, I always felt so tired, couldn't concentrate very well - I would often forget vital information and at times would not even remember what I was saying mid sentence – and I was deeply unhappy, felt constantly sick and just exhausted most of the time. I got *tired* of being tired. Being constantly miserable and unbalanced created many problems with all of my relationships, with my family, my boyfriends, with my friends and also with my employment because I was always too sick and depressed and unable to function properly. I had many sick days off school and countless off work. I wasn't able to bring any sort of stability whatsoever to my life. I attracted lots of drama and would worry about every little thing. I was never able to think of the consequences of my actions. I would react to things before thinking them through. My brain was highly erratic and I found it very hard to even feel *normal*. I knew I was *not* ok. Because I was very suicidal from a young age, I spent most of my childhood years in my room, away from the world, wishing I had not been born. The constant and painful roller coaster I was on was so taxing on my fragile mind and on my health. I couldn't get away from how I felt and I always knew that I had serious problems. I had lots of paranoid thoughts, but I felt I couldn't tell anyone for fear of being sent off to a hospital. I had no idea that I would ever be able to feel happy and well. In my mind, I saw that I had been given a life sentence of hell, which involved being constantly unwell and constantly unhappy. I just had no hope.

Now, after what seems like a miraculous recovery, my experience has led me to believe this: having too many toxins in the body, and therefore too many toxins in the brain, *changes* who you are meant to be. It can distort *every emotional ability* that a human has. It can make you feel so happy and hyperactive that you can't sleep, and it can also make you feel so low, you just can't get out of bed. Too many toxins in the brain can make you become very angry and they can also bring on episodes of chronic sadness, triggering subsequent bouts of intense crying that can happen at the drop of a hat, causing the sufferer to feel like they are on a roller coaster. Too many toxins affect your hormones, which also affects the way your brain behaves and the way your body functions.

Despite the psychiatric industry saying that mental illness stems from a *chemical* imbalance, most of these doctors do *not* actually think to look at the amounts of chemicals, heavy metals and common toxins people actually have in their brains! As we will cover later in Chapter 15, modern psychiatry is not at all helping nearly enough people, and more are suffering from depression than ever before. In fact, certain medications are making many people's mental conditions even *worse*, not only increasing the risk of them but causing actual suicides and even causing some people to commit violent crimes, of which they never showed any behavior like this previously.

We will also touch on briefly how there is little *solid evidence* to prove that depression even stems from low serotonin levels, and therefore making it even more clear to see why anti-depresssants really just *don't* work they way they are said to. This chapter is particularly shocking and I hope will cause you to rethink mental illness, the way it's treated.

Chemicals that we inadvertently eat, put on our skin and breathe in cause us to have thoughts and trigger certain feelings (e.g. sugar can create a rush of energy and a short burst of happiness) and if these chemicals which are floating around the brain are actually toxic, then you aren't exactly going to be thinking happy thoughts. This overload can cause you to be constantly moody, erratic and angry, which is actually not really the true you. Healthy-bodied people are meant to be *happy-brained* too!

I have seen this happen to myself, after being a very angry and incredibly moody person for most of my life; my behavior made me feel, and quite often act, like I was a monster. I would have countless arguments with loved ones where I would lash out and say the most dreadful things, only to forget what I had said minutes later. I hurt many people's feelings as well as my own self-esteem. To behave like this day in and day out, and see that many people would not even want to be around me, was truly awful, yet it was also very difficult to change my behavior. I was trapped inside my own mind and literally thought I was born like that and would never be able to be 'normal'. The future, to me, was *very* scary indeed. I pictured either one day eventually ending my life, or suffering a long life of unhappiness. Unhappiness and mental torture was *exactly* what I got for two decades.

Now that I have healed and removed the most dangerous toxins from my body and brain, the difference in my mood and ability to concentrate is truly incredible. Because of this personal experience and what I have discovered through many years of research, I now believe that many angry people are more than likely actually *highly toxic* and that if they *remove* the majority of those toxins, they then have a good chance of helping their brain return to being able to function *normally* and in a much more balanced way. If the majority of toxins are gone, then the body can now have a much better chance to *heal* properly. Hormones will start to balance and the brain will start to function in the way it should. These toxins simply won't be in the way anymore, causing disruptive stress, physical and mental disharmony.

It's common knowledge that children become aggressive and hyperactive due to too much sugar, so it makes sense that more serious chemicals can affect the brain in a much more *serious* manner. And the most worrying thing about life today is; children are being affected by dangerous industrial toxins, *before* they are even born.

Even though many of you, thankfully, won't be subjected to a large dose of chemicals in one sitting like I was, it does *not* mean that what happened to me can't happen to you, but in a different, less obvious way. The poisoning from chemicals is happening to countless people but very slowly, through accumulation, with the effects not showing themselves until much later in life.

Toxic exposure builds up inside of us *each and every day* over many years. It's why there are so many people with cancers and other serious illnessess in their 50s+ (and more tellingly, many younger people are now becoming afflicted with these too, more than ever before) and it's why so many people now have extremely low immune systems, always catching this virus or that virus.

Their bodies have been absorbing chemicals bit by bit every day, until it gets to a point where the body simply cannot remove them anymore; the liver just cannot cope and now leaves a person to develop a serious health concern. The effects can either cause someone to suffer from stress, or, too much stress causes the body's systems to wear down, thereby holding on to toxins.

What happened to me, at such a young age, *could* be what happens to you, but *gradually* over time, perhaps much later in life. But I will tell you this: by that time, you will have your own families and have built a life for yourself that you simply *won't* want to lose or cut way too short. And you *won't* want to have to spend those precious years having painful chemotherapy or radiation if you can help it.

As we get older, life seems *so* much more precious and travels by so fast. We have a whole lot more that matters to us, so it makes sense that we need to be as fit and healthy as possible to live a longer time to enjoy it all. This is my point that I want to drive home: *take care and do what you can now!* Don't leave the problem building up inside you until a major problem rears its ugly head. Start to make changes, no matter how small, *now*. Why end up suffering with sickness, pain and cancers when we can do lots, right now, to avoid it all?

We must remember, we can *never* go back in time – it's impossible unless someone invents a time machine that is – so lead a cleaner and healthy life *now* and you will have a much greater chance at changing the entire future for you *and* your family. How I recovered has everything to do with *educating* myself about the risks and real dangers in regards to toxins, taking their effects *seriously,* improving my lifestyle choices and to not ignoring what they were doing not only to my health, but to the environment as well. Even though my past has been very difficult, I do feel that I have been blessed because without this sickness and depression, I would never have been able to discover how and why it all happened.

I'm now going to share with you what I have discovered with the hope that it can also help *you* regain, or achieve the happiness and health which we all are *meant* and *designed* to have.

Over the past one hundred years, our species has been engaged in a vast and complicated chemistry experiment. Each and every one of us, along with our children, our parents and our grandparents, has been a guinea pig in this experiment which uses our bodies, our health, our wealth, and our goodwill to test the proposition that modern science can improve upon the foods and medicines of nature.

Randall Fitzgerald Author of *The Hundred Year Lie*

Chapter 2

What's the Big Deal about Toxins?

I can now very comfortably and definitively state to you that, in my opinion, based on the evidence, every single chronic insidious disease process is related to one word: toxicity. You cannot address the issues of aging unless you address detoxification. The more success we've had, the clearer it has become: all chronic disease is TOXICITY. You get rid of that toxicity and you put out the fire. You may need to rebuild afterward, but you must put the fire out. Conventional medicine is just covering your eyes so you don't see the fire.

Dr. Rashid Buttar, *Author of The 9 Steps to Keep the Doctor Away*

What are toxins?

A toxin is basically a chemical in the form of a small carbon-based molecule, protein or peptide that causes harm when it comes into contact with the cellular receptors and enzymes in the human body. Our body is equipped with amazing mechanisms to rid itself of these toxins by breaking them down in the liver, excreting them as solid or liquid waste or even exhaling them as gas. But when we continually load our bodies with toxins day in and day out, we eventually reach a tipping point at which our body can no longer handle the sheer quantity of poisons. We then start to experience 'toxic overload'. At that point, even while our detoxification systems are working overtime, excess toxins start to build up in our tissues (brain tissue included) because the body simply cannot handle them anymore. The more toxins our body is forced to store, the more detrimental it becomes for our long-term health. The body, with the enormous job it has to do keeping us alive, simply cannot cope with a heavy toxic overload. And this is how health problems begin.

Why are there so many toxins these days?

The chemical revolution began right back in 1906, after the US Congress enacted the *Pure Foods and Drugs act*, which was put in place to instill the public's assurance that all foods and drugs allowed on the market were safe, yet what no one knew, was that rarely were *any* of these chemicals used in the foods or drugs, ever (nor still are) tested for *safety* in regards to human, or environmental health. They even had a slogan 'Better Health through Chemistry' which was used heavily in the media. The food, chemical and pharmaceutical industries all began to produce whatever they wanted with absolute free reign, and people would buy without hestitation or would never stop to think '*what* are they were made with?' Because of this Pure Food and Drugs Act, they simply believed what they were told.

This type of trust is still held very strongly by many members of the public, the same today as it was in the early 1900s. We are *still* making the same dangerous mistake that we can trust whatever is sold, prescribed or eaten by us today.

For those that still think this way, this book is going to turn your world-view upside down. There are now literally tens of thousands, some reports are saying at between at least *95,000 to 120,000*, of different industrial chemicals that are used in producing our food, beauty products, water, homes, clothing, cars, offices, planes, medications, trains, industrires which affect us, our animals *and* the environment. We can often be exposed to at least *1000* different chemicals each and every day, and none that are guaranteed completely safe for the body. What is so concerning is that despite that these countless chemicals in use today, the majority have *not* been tested for safety, they are allowed to be in the food we eat, the beauty and skincare products we use, are approved and recommended for use in furniture, in the production of electrical goods, found in decorating and constructions items in our homes, buildings, cars, trains, planes *and* some are even added to the water that we drink and bathe in. There aren't even *any* special regulations when it comes to things manufactured for babies and children.

Basically, chemicals are everywhere.

And despite the public assuming that the FDA (Food and Drug Administration) does its job to protect us, we really cannot trust them at all. They still are not enforcing individual chemicals to be tested, nor are they requiring we carry out tests on on how they react with *other* common chemicals. In fact there is no agency that is enforcing any of this:

Randall Fitzgerald, author of *The Hundred year Lie* writes:

Many people want to believe that the US Food and Drug Administration protects them from anything dangerous in our drug or food supplies. The fact is that when the FDA approves a new drug for public use it has *not* studied that drug's safety. The agency relies upon safety information from the drug manfucturers to make its approval decisions. Nor does the FDA test the safety ingredients in cosmetics and personal-care products.

Even the EPA (Environmental Protection Agency) don't really offer us much 'protection'. Well known toxin expert Doris J. Rapp paints us an even more worrying picture about the blatant misuse of public trust:

The Toxic Substances Control Act of 1976 allows chemicals to be sold and used unless they are proven to be a risk. The EPA however, does not conduct it's own safety tests, but relies on research conducted by the manufacturers.

Talk about a *huge* conflict of interest here! Basically the chemical companies are their own bosses, with no one making them accountable for their actions. These chemicals have been developed by lucrative industries, then literally put out into the world for people to use, eat and unknowingly absorb. This basically means that *we are actually the safety test* - all of us humans are the *guinea pigs,* just waiting to find out what harm all of this is going to cause us, and our children long term – although many of us actually already inherently know. The harm is *cancer* and other serious diseases and sickness.

Cancer rates are on the rise and we *all* know this to be true. According to the documentary, *Cut, Poison, Burn,* 20,000 people die every day from some kind of cancer. That is *8 million* people each year. Each year 1 million people are diagnosed with cancer and 500,000 will die from cancer in America. Back In the 1900s, 1 in 20 died from cancer. In 1940 it was 1 in 16. By 1970 it was 1 in 10. By the year 2000 it was 1 in 3. Now in 2013, some are saying its now *1 in every 2 people.* For each person that goes through cancer treatments it costs on average US $50,000. $500 *billion* is spent on cancer treatments in the USA.

It's interesting to note that the chemical industrial revolution really took off in 1906, and as more chemicals were added to the environment through the production of them so too did our cancer rates increase. Despite us not talking enough about cancer, and in fact many of us ignore it and instead just *fear* it without doing anything active to try and stop it from happening, statistics show, that we are *all* going to be affected by it at some stage. Whether it's to our own health or to our parents or worse, our children – it's going to happen.

Cancer patients who have 'toxin aware' doctors are being found to have high levels of certain chemicals such as dioxins, plastics and heavy metals in their blood. Many scientists are now saying that most of *all* disease stems from toxic exposure. This statement certainly makes total sense to me. Our health collectively in the world has *never* been this sick before, despite our medical 'advances', yet what has changed over the years? The one answer that always pops up is… *chemicals!* We have never before in human history had to deal with living amongst so many toxic, dangerous and untested chemicals. Most people are oblivious to this bombardment because they can't smell most of the chemicals that are around them, (of which many have been cleverly designed not to smell by the way) so the concern does not even enter their thoughts. And again, they *trust* that if drugs, food and chemicals in general were 'that bad', they would never have been allowed to be put out into the public in the first place. And they are right, but only because they should never have been allowed to be put out into the public before being tested safe. Our governments are *supposed* to be protecting us. Why else do we pay them taxes?

Remember that the word 'toxin' also means *poison* and no one would recommend having various poisons at *any* level in our bodies, yet we do, and in large amounts and in countless combinations over our lifetime. Some scientists are estimating we may come into contact with as many as *120,000* different chemicals each and every year. Let's now discuss what this means for our health.

What is toxic overload?

I always try and explain toxic overload to people like this: imagine your entire body is just like an empty bottle. Each time you come into contact with a toxin, the liquid (toxins) goes into the bottle (your body). As time goes by, the liquid in your bottle gets higher and higher, and as it starts to reach the top of the bottle, the liquid has *no choice* but to spill out the top, which means there is no more space for any more toxins to be stored. What happens next can be serious illness such as the development of different types of cancer, or autoimmune problems because the body cannot cope any longer to control what is already in there, has *no* room for more and starts attacking its own tissues. It sends the body totally haywire. It cannot keep all of these chemicals floating around without a harmful reaction to the body. It then starts to use these chemicals in any way it can, which causes the body to basically *malfunction*. It becomes completely overwhelmed, exhausted and unable to function anymore with its natural detoxing processes. The liver becomes an overworked and almost useless organ.

And I am so sorry to tell you this, but you can't think that any of us on the planet are *not* affected like this. One of the scariest statistics I have ever read is that babies today are being born with over *287 industrial toxic chemicals*[3] in their bodies. Things like lead, and PCBs (polychlorinated biphenyl), VOCs (volatile organic compounds), petrochemicals, oil repellents, Teflon, mercury, parabens, phthalates, plus a whole lot more. At least *200* other chemicals. I have even read that the real number far exceeds much higher than this because testing for every chemical on earth is virtually impossible to do. Perhaps the number is really more likely to be in the *thousands*. About *180* of these detected chemicals are known to cause cancer in animal experiments. Due to the way the world is going and the fact that *more* chemicals are being released into our environment every day, as more are being created by industries, the more time goes by, the *higher* this already dreadful number is going to be.

Children's health is at an all-time low rate – which we will cover later in this book. Samples have been taken from the umbilical cords of newborns and it's now been undeniably proven that babies are absorbing toxins in utero from their mothers, who have absorbed chemicals through skincare products, food, water, houses, medication and the air. And the mothers would have absorbed toxins in utero from *their* mothers and they from their mothers.

We all are born into a chemical circle of life.

Knowing this has spurred me into desperately trying to help people to be aware of the health risks their children are facing from day one. These innocent, supposed-to-be-pure children are already affected by toxins before they have even had a chance to draw breath. So chances are, *you* were born with dangerous, untested toxins in your body, and if you have had children or are pregnant right now, you will have already passed those toxins onto your children, and chances are these chemicals may still be inside their bodies. It's no wonder that many children today are suffering with serious illness, allergies, eczema, regular immune problems, and even many types of cancers from such a young age.

Chemicals that disrupt the process of development can cause severe birth defects, learning or behavioral difficulties and possibly cancer or degenerative diseases later in life. The timing of exposure to a substance is as relevant as the amount a child is exposed to because the nature of the damage caused may depend on the stage of development of different organ systems when exposure took place. A 1989 report by the Natural Resources Defense Council (an environmental action group) surmised that 'More than 50% of a person's lifetime cancer risk from exposure to carcinogenic pesticides is typically incurred in the first years of life'.[4]

Dawn Mellowship, *Toxic Beauty: How Hidden Chemicals in Cosmetics Harm You*

The National Cancer Institute reported that, for infants less than one year old, the cancer rate increased from 197.9 cases per million infants during the years 1976–84 to 264 cases per million infants during the years 1986–94. This was a 36% increase. The greatest percentage increase occurred for germ cell cancers (increase of 124%), central nervous system cancers (increase of 57%), liver cancers (increase of 50%), and neuroblastoma (increase of 35%).[5]

Asthma is also so common these days, it's now almost seen as fairly normal for a child to suffer from it. In Canada, asthma has increased *fourfold* over the past 20 years and 1 in 10 children are now diagnosed with asthma. Breathing difficulties should *not* ever be seen as 'normal' in children.

And what about the shocking increase in learning disorders such as autism? In the USA 1% or at least 1 in every 88 children (some say 1 in 60) are now autistic.[6] That is a 600% increase in the past 20 years and a 57% increase just between 2002 and 2006. Autism is now linked to being triggered by various types of toxins, particularly that of mercury and aluminum. Some doctors and scientists like to say that autistic people were 'always there we've just got better at diagnosing them' but if you have seen or been around autistic children/adults, due to their unusual behaviour of flapping of the hands, loud noises and at times violent and upsetting outbursts, they are people that you *just don't forget*. I don't know about you, but I have zero memories of seeing any autistic people growing up.

Many personal skincare products contain toxic chemicals that affect the estrogen levels in our bodies. In Rotterdam, babies are being born with genital defects at a rate never seen before. And one of those types of birth defects has had a 200% increase in the USA. I'm sure that even after reading just these few pages, the idea of a chemical epidemic is now perhaps not so hard to understand.

So how will having too many toxins make us feel?

Well, the short answer is, for most of us, not great; but quite a few won't even know they are affected by them until illness manifests itself. Because toxins accumulate, quite often it's not until someone gets cancer that they really feel the effects. But for those that suffer with low energy, or regular viruses, I can assure you, toxins are most likely to blame.

Remember what life was like as a child? You woke up easily in the morning, happy, full of energy and expectation for an exciting day ahead – you knew you could handle anything that life was going to throw your way. You felt vibrant, happy, clear-headed and alive. Well, when was the *last* time the adult *you* felt like that? Can you not really even remember? I *never* felt like that actually, not until I was about aged 33 after I had sorted my health issues out.

For most people, as children, our bodies back then were still able to deal with toxins in our environment. But as we got older, the toxic overload set in and our energy just vanished. Many adults these days will relate to this; they are always run down, super-tired, get lots of colds, flus, have constant headaches, and just generally don't ever feel good. They need a large dose of caffeine in the morning just to feel 'awake', and then need continual shots of sugar from cakes and biscuits, energy drinks and even more caffeine during the day to keep their energy levels going – and this pattern only makes matters worse as the body cannot sustain this type of treatment and remain healthy and strong.

The truth is, we should *still* feel pretty great even when we are adults. And we should be living for many years, more than the average norm of today. Yes! That's true – we should be living to some of the ripe old ages of 100+. And no, I don't want you to picture someone old who can hardly walk or is on death's door; I want you to picture those people you read about who live in the 'blue zones' – a term coined for certain areas in the world where the local people live till on average 100 years, sometimes longer, and are still *working* on their crops in their fields. I have seen them myself in places like Morocco: elderly women carrying huge bales of hay on their backs with relative ease. We shouldn't be becoming decrepit and sick before our time is up. The way most people die today, sick with cancer and in a lot of pain, is not the way Nature intended us to go. We are meant to die peacefully in our sleep, yet this hardly happens to anyone these days.

A truly fit and healthy human being should be feeling pretty energetic and happy most of the time. *Seriously!* So while it seems common that the majority of people are tired and run down all day, every day, it is *not* normal. Life is indeed very busy for most of us these days, due to rising costs of living, and the stress of this makes people very tired and with little time and energy to look after their health, but we *should* be able to handle this.

Don't get me wrong here; we *are* supposed to get tired, but only after a busy day, not first thing in the morning, and not feeling *constantly* drained every single day for years on end, until we…die. *What sort of a life is that?* Not a good one at all or not one that is lived in the *best way* possible. Yet sadly, it's just so common, isn't it?

It's the same with viruses; we are meant to have perhaps a couple of colds each year, as they are our body's natural way of detoxing and to it becoming *stronger*, but we are not meant to have them every few months or, for some, even more often - every few weeks. If you have regular colds, or even none at all, then that is your body's way of saying, 'Hello! Something is not right here!'

Lots of people proudly say that they never get colds. I was one of them, thinking that this was a good thing. I now know it is not. It may mean that the immune system is suppressed and that the body does not have enough energy to be able to recognize even acute illness. These sorts of people are often highly toxic (as I certainly was) and in extreme cases may even drop dead of a heart attack or stroke or other serious illness later in life. Toxic chemicals really affect the way the heart functions too.

Of course, we now know that chronic toxic overload can trigger off cancer cells to produce tumors. In fact, lab rats used for cancer experiments are actually given certain toxins which doctors know will initiate cancer virtually 100% of the time, but rarely will you ever hear a doctor who diagnoses you like this; 'You have a brain tumor because of these toxins found in your food from all the pesticides there were used, and because your water is full of chemcials, and the pollution in the air and all of the junk used to make your beauty products'. Because they are not being trained *extensively* on the effects on human health from 'common' absorption through toxic chemicals, doctors tend to not be able to offer a decent explanation as to why people have become so ill. It's because they have not yet made the *connection* between; too many toxins = poor health and disease. This is highly worrying as it should be just *common sense.* Isn't it logical to you even now, after reading these few pages, that it's an enormous problem? We cannot expect to come into contact with thousands of untested chemicals and to continue to detox them naturally. There's just too many for the body to cope with, and especially in relation to children. Their body weight ratio is far smaller than ours so the effects are more harmful.

When the majority of doctors are asked about chemicals and if they are harmful, they tend to say the same things and rarely look at the bigger picture; instead they will only look at one part of it, and say, 'Oh, what you absorb from that "one thing" won't do any harm long term.' This is where they, too, massively *fail* to see that all of these small parts of this or that, plus thousands of other chemicals they don't even know about, make up to *one very big amount of a chemical cocktail in the body*. And not enough doctors really are aware of, or ever *study*, the effects toxins have on health. As found in the book, *The Hundred Year Lie*, Dr Ballie-Hamilton, spells out the glaring truth:

> Unfortunately our bodies were never designed to protect themselves against this chemical onslaught. As a result, our systems usually fail to process and remove most of these chemicals once they have entered our bodies, so their levels start building up inside us. Consquently, every single human on the face of this earth is now permanently contaminated with these modern synthetic chemicals

Without too many toxins our bodies can heal

To me this makes perfect sense: in a healthy body we are equipped with natural defenses that keep us free from chronic sickness and disease. That's what the liver does; it cleans and processes things so that we can remain healthy and strong – it fights for us. If toxins become too much of a problem for the liver to process, it seems really obvious that when sickness and chronic disease start to be evident in the body, then it was the toxins in the first place that knocked the body off its natural course to heal. Our bodies are like cars in a sense; we must give them the *right* fuel, not the wrong sort, and we need to *clean* our engines otherwise they (and us) will not work, and in fact, if we do not, then the entire engine may need rehauling.

Cancer cells begin to multiply because the body now cannot heal itself and cannot stop the tumours from growing. The body was not able to fight off the invaders because it was too busy being bombarded with other invaders – toxins. If we looked at cancer, and how it usually starts, in a completely different way, and that is that we need to regularly remove and decrease these toxins from our bodies, eat better food and do all the typical and sensible lifestyle changes, what would this mean for the future of the world's health?

It means that we could really solve a lot of these medical problems before they even had a chance to begin and before people had to suffer so much.

The chemical threat is the ultimate threat to mankind, worse than bombs and war. You cannot hide from it. It reaches everywhere in the world
 Greenlander Ingmar Egede

Chapter 3

Common Deadly Environmental Toxins

While there are literally hundreds and thousands of dangerous toxins, we unfortunately don't have enough information yet to prove what they are really doing to our health, and what the effects are when combined with *other* toxins. Scientists are not studying all of them, as it's pretty much impossible. How do you study, at length, hundreds and thousands of different chemicals, or even tens of thousands? How would you get the funding for that and how could you complete the work in your lifetime? It's a mammoth job and unfortunately no one is undertaking it in the entirety we need it to be, to prove undeniably what they are all capable of, so we may never even know the full picture.

In the book *Hormonal Chaos* author Sheldon Krimsky tried to calculate just how many years it would take to do safety tests on 1000 chemicals with three unique combinations of a single dose. He came to this shocking conclusion; that it would take *166 million different experiments* to cover *each* possbibility – and it would take over *1000* years! When we look at the fact that the number of chemicals in use today is more than *10 times* this number calculated - then I probably don't have to spell it out what this means for us – we will *never ever* know the full extent, nor can we ever have the proof as to how unsafe these chemicals truly are. It is in fact, quite chilling.

My aim within this book is of course to make you aware that toxicity is an *enormous* problem and that hopefully the information that we do have already is going to be more than enough to encourage you to try limit your exposure as much as you can, and to do something about the ones you already have in your body. Taking it seriously is key here because toxins are destroying the planet and our health (namely our *brain's* health) in more ways than one.

This next chapter is about some common yet deadly toxins that are causing great harm to all of us. I have only written about a small amount of them as I simply do not have enough room in my book to cover them all. It's a *huge* subject and one that requires much greater attention. I have however, selected some of the most common ones which I think pose some of the greatest risks to us all.

In our environment there are many abundant toxins that we are all exposed to, as they are found in concerning amounts in our air, water and in the earth's crust. Despite them being classed as a 'natural' substance in their raw form, we can't assume that they are safe for us. But don't blame Nature itself; it's the fault of *industries* that they have become such a toxic part of our lives, thereby causing such damage to human and environmental health.

If we had simply left these minerals alone, we wouldn't be facing so many problems now. Since their discovery, industries have seen this gold mine from natural resources and why wouldn't they? Hundreds and thousands of different chemicals and ingredients are made from dirt-cheap materials which can then be made into huge amounts of other things, which leads to huge profits. I can just imagine the manufacturers rubbing their hands together saying this: 'If we *refine* them like this, or if we add *another* chemical to that, we can now make something *new*!' A million and one ways to make many things from a few raw materials! How ingenious and what an easy way to make so much money.

It's clear to see that human nature has always been like this. What can we do to make money, *lots* of money? How can we do it in the cheapest way possible and who cares about what it does to the world and its people?

Sad, isn't it, but also undeniably true.

There is a limitless supply of these minerals, and because it's so cheap for industries to buy huge amounts of them (and therefore go on to make enormous profits), they have ended up as ingredients in products that we consume, are found in the air we breathe, in the water and other liquids we drink, what we apply to our skins and what we use to build things with. And, shockingly, as you will find out shortly, some are even added on *purpose* to many of our supposed 'life-saving' medications. Ingredients of toxic heavy metals are found in medicines that we are told will make us healthier? Hmm. Isn't this an oxymoron?

Many chemicals that are waste products from making other chemicals are not just automatically thrown away but instead are commonly used in other methods, and these methods can even involve adding them to our food, to water and also to our medications. It's far easier for industries to find other ways to use them rather than having to dispose of them safely. Dumping *correctly* means the company will need to spend money doing it the right way as required by law, so if they can reuse or sell something instead of disposing then it means yet another way to make even more money.

Because many of these raw materials have been around since the beginning of time, some of these metals have now actually been tested extensively for their effects on human and environmental health, and the findings are certainly *not* at all pretty. While researching for this book, I read so much shocking information that at times it literally took my breath away – because it all hit home for me. The problem affecting humanity, and namely our health, which I had initially known to be big, is actually *much* bigger than big – it's *massive*.

I now have zero doubt in my mind that most health problems are related *directly* to the toxicity from these metals, their by-products and all the other dangerous chemicals. We were never designed to cope with tens of thousands of chemicals, and we haven't had enough time for us to adapt to them. It's all happened way too fast.

I am now going to discuss in this chapter, albeit only very briefly, some of the most common metals that we all have in our lives and in our bodies, purely because they are everywhere.

Aluminum

In the earth's crust, aluminum (a silvery-white substance also known as aluminium) makes up 8.4–14% of it, which is quite a concerning amount, when we understand what it does to human health. Aluminum is the most abundant element after oxygen and silicon, and this means there is *loads* of it around. So much so, that it's invading many parts of our lives and impacting our health, and in ways that may surprise you.

Most people think that aluminum is mainly in deodorants and aluminum foil (as I did for a long time too) yet the truth about all the things which do contain aluminium, is really very frightening. And after you get through this section and see how heavy metals are so abundant around us, you too, like me, may not be surprised anymore as to why so many people have got, and *will* get, Alzheimer's disease. Aluminum exposure is not just linked to Alzheimer's; it is a *direct* cause of it.

What does aluminum do to the brain?

Before we get further into where we find aluminum, I want you to understand just how bad it is for our health, in particular the health of our brain. The main problem with aluminum is that it is a *selective neurotoxin*, which means it is a nerve cell poison and one that has a specific affinity for the brain. It just *loves* attacking the brain's nerves. So the more aluminum you ingest, breathe, apply to the skin, have injected into you via vaccines, and absorb in other ways, means the more cell deaths your brain will experience. And over time, your brain function will start to get worse and worse, which is why people that have Alzheimer's lose so many normal and basic functions and skills, quite often very suddenly.

Studies carried out on deceased patients who had Alzheimer's disease, usually show high amounts of aluminum in the brain. While what it actually does to the brain is highly complex, and the actual science of it is not something I will cover here in great detail (although I will direct you to a wonderful book that will tell you all you need to know), what I *do* know is that the toxicity from aluminum sets off a whole lot of other problems in the brain and in the body.

A study was also undertaken at the University of Toronto, by Donald R. McLachlan MD, who is a Professor of Physiology and Medicine. By injecting, just once, the tiniest amount of aluminum chloride (100 nano moles) into the subjects' (cats) hippocampic area of the brain, the *entire* typical sequence of Alzheimer's symptoms was triggered. The doctor and his research team all watched the cats closely for signs of behavioral changes. At first, they did not display anything too unusual, but by day 9, the cats could not find where their food was kept (although they had often seen previously where it was hidden). After 10 days, their short-term memory was *completely gone*. Tests performed on other animals in which they had aluminum injected into parts of the body (such as the stomach) also produced similar results. So it seems that you can cause dementia/Alzheimer's through more ways than one, not just by toxicity to the brain. Due to the stomach being directly connected to the brain (doctors and scientists are only just beginning to really know this), it's no wonder that what we eat directly affects our brain function too.

Aluminum also competes with calcium for absorption, so the more someone has in their body, the more chances they have of suffering bone density problems such as osteoporosis and osteopenia.

Doctors don't tend to think that we can cure or dramatically improve Alzheimer's, but when you understand that in most cases it was *first* triggered by toxicity, and not always genes, if we remove those toxins early enough (which we will cover how in Chapter 13, 'The Vital Importance of Detoxing'), it is quite possible to slow down its progress, or even *reverse* it, despite what the medical world tells us. Since they are not looking at toxicity in an intensive way (e.g. understanding about all the other chemicals and different ways we are absorbing things), they miss out on this crucial link and are completely looking elsewhere for the cause.

The brilliant book *Toxic Metal Syndrome: How Metal Poisonings Can*

Affect Your Brain is absolutely inspiring and provides hope that this reversal can be done. It was written by two doctors who developed their own groundbreaking protocol for reversing many cases of Alzheimer's and dementia. If you know anyone who is showing signs of Alzheimer's, or you are worried about it yourself, please read their book. The aim with *my* book however, is to educate you on how you can try and *avoid* problems like these happening in the first place.

How do we get aluminum into our bodies?

Aluminum invades through all of our pathways. We are not just breathing it in due to amounts found in air particles, but we are also drinking it, cooking with it, bathing in it, swallowing pills and other medicines (such as antidepressants, aspirin, vaccinations plus loads more) that are made with it, applying it to our skin through personal care items and makeup, *and* we are also unknowingly *eating* it. Some scientists have roughly estimated that every single person will eat 30–50 mg every single day. Many popular and common food items have aluminum in them or absorb it from its many derivatives. Food items such as baking powders, cake mixes, self-raising flours (found in most breads that we consume), pickling salts, food starches, anti-caking agents and processed cheeses all contain aluminum. The tin cans that we buy – containing food such as tomatoes – are made with aluminum, and anything acidic that goes into these cans will absorb much more aluminum, which you end up eating.

Worryingly, drinking lots of coffee also increases your body's ability to absorb aluminum into the bloodstream. What is *really* frightening is just how much aluminum is found in common medications. Take antacids, for example. These are used to neutralize hydrochloric acid in the stomach and are one of the most popular over-the-counter medications people take. In a bottle of the popular brand Gaviscon, there are 160 mg of aluminum in each standard dose. Mylanta has approximately 400 mg for each standard dose. And some people take this stuff 3–4 times a day, every day for *years*. As you will find out throughout this guide, stomach health is directly linked to brain health. So if someone is taking toxic medication for an already unwell stomach, it's not going to lead to anywhere positive for your brain's health. That niggly little stomach trouble can and does lead to other problems that are anything but 'niggly'.

Aluminum is also found in high levels in countless other medications, such as antidepressants and also aspirin. Because these common types of medications tend to be taken every day (aspirin is now recommended daily for some people, particularly the elderly, who are already the most likely candidates for Alzheimer's!) this is going to add to a person's toxic burden in quite a large way.

In *Toxic Metal Syndrome: How Metal Poisonings Can Affect Your Brain,* found on page after page, are common medications listed as containing having high levels of aluminum. There are far too many to single out here. And if *you* are on many medications (such as the elderly often are) and, are drinking lots of tea and/or coffee, then the amount per day that you are ingesting through pharmaceuticals alone is absolutely harmful for your entire body. I bet this is *not* what you imagined your 'doctor-recommended' 'health' products would be containing! The problem is, doctors don't often know themselves just what dangerous additives are found in the medications they are prescribing, because the drug companies don't tell them, or they think it's just a small amount and don't think about adding up all the dozens of other ways in your life that you will absorb toxins too.

Another very common way of ingesting aluminum is by drinking tea. Regular, common, popular black tea has concerning levels. And in a country like Britain where pretty much everyone drinks copious amounts of it, this is really worrying. In the majority of tea brands, researchers found that there were concentrations of 2–6 mg of aluminum per liter brewed. There are also differences in these levels depending on what sort of water is used, i.e. hard or soft water. All of these common ways of ingesting it means that none of us are immune to the problems aluminum is causing. But you will learn how to limit your exposure as much as possible throughout this book.

I recently became aware just how much aluminum is in bread, so now the only bread I try and eat is either one that I make myself, or one that is completely organic. As we will discuss in the breast-feeding chapter, there are also high levels of aluminum found in infant formulas, and yes, probably in the brand you have used or your mum used with you. It tends to be found in all of the cow's milk and soy-based formulas are even *far* worse for levels of aluminum. Considering that infant brains are developing crucially at this vitally important stage, it's absolutely *criminal* that these food items are allowed as they are, with no safety tests before they are put on the market.

In regard to the serious subject of vaccinations containing aluminum, its derivatives and other harmful toxins, we will be covering this in much greater detail in Chapter 36. However, I will say right now, it is extremely concerning that they too contain aluminum (and in amounts, far higher than even the FDA state is safe) because if we are already ingesting lots of this heavy metal through eating, infant formula, the water we drink, the air, through our beauty (found in mineral foundations/powders, eye shadows) and personal care products etc., then knowing that our small babies are getting it injected into their bodies (they may have up to *48* doses of vaccines containing aluminum by the time they are 4 years old) is very worrying indeed. And causes logical questioning: how could this be good for an immune system and one that is not yet fully functioning? Remember, there is *no* human health benefit for *any* amount of aluminum – it serves no beneficial purpose. And vaccines don't just have a tiny bit in there either as you will see below; it is often in high levels far exceeding what is recommended as safe:

A recent study by Lucija Tomljenovik and Chris Shaw found that a newborn receives a dose of aluminum that exceeds FDA safety limits (5mg/kg/day) for injected aluminum by *20-fold*, and at 6 months of age a dose that was *50-fold* higher than FDA safety limits.[7]

We will be discussing vaccine safety concerns further in part 3.

How you can avoid ingesting as much aluminum as possible

- Drink organic black tea and consume minimally, drink herbal teas instead
- Eat organic foods
- Prepare/buy organic bread yourself to avoid self-raising agents
- Use organic skincare/makeup
- Avoid using infant formulas or use a goat's milk based one
- Avoid buying tinned goods, in particular tinned tomatoes; purchase fresh food stuffs or glassed products
- Do not cook with aluminum cookwear
- Do not cover acidic foods with aluminum foil
- Don't use deodorants containing aluminum
- Check your water for levels of aluminum (and other chemicals) by using a water-testing kit (see Chapter 9 for where to purchase)
- Drink less coffee and choose organic brands
- Research vaccinations, their ingredients and safety studies
- Use plants in your homes to improve air quality

Lead

This next toxin as you are already aware is quite close to my heart, and not in a nice sense. Lead, which is also found in extreme abundance in our earth's crust, is classed as a soft malleable bright silvery metal. It has been used in so many aspects of our lives: in household goods, paint, lead-acid batteries, bullets, insecticides, pigments, chemicals, construction of buildings, and as a radiation shield, to name but a small few. It has been used throughout history for thousands of years.

Lead is an environmental toxin that never disappears. It's been found in the blood of New Guinea Aborigines who live as far away as possible from any man-made sources of lead. As I stated previously, in the Arctic regions lead is being found due to airborne particles making their way to these far corners of the earth. It is also still being mined in huge amounts each year. Large amounts of it were used in the fuel industry as most petrol contained it, and this is mainly why it's still found in our environment today despite it being long since removed from use in petrol.

What does lead do to the body and brain?

Lead ingestion, in any amount, even minute, is never safe for the body, and most worryingly, particularly for children. Levels above 10 micrograms per 100 ml of blood are extremely dangerous to adults, but children are at far greater risk. According to CDCP (Centers for Disease Control and Prevention) director Dr. William Roper, 'Lead poisoning is the number one environmental threat to children, but it's preventable.' Concerning levels of lead are found in an estimated 3 million American children. Lead is linked to behavioral problems and also to an early disposition to developing Alzheimer's disease later in life.

As you know I came into contact with a large dose of lead when I was very young. Until the late 1970s, lead was in most oil-based house paints, and despite it now being phased out of paint brands, millions of homes today still contain lead-based particles on the walls. Not only are young infants exposed to breathing in lead through fumes in their houses, children sometimes also have an odd yet common habit of eating the paint chippings from the walls. The lead in the paint tastes sweet, so it's appealing and something that they may do quite regularly. This type of early exposure may often not show up as a health problem till they are in their adult years, when symptoms may start to show around the age of 45+.

Small doses (e.g. 10 micrograms) of lead can even affect children's IQ by several points, which can often cause them to become slow-thinking adults (aka 'learning impaired – like I was') or even semi-retarded. Bump up the exposure to around 25 micrograms and a child may develop severe problems with their memory and motor coordination. Levels higher than 50 micrograms cause iron deficiencies and kidney problems, and levels around 100 micrograms cause death. Lead loves attacking the grey matter of the brain, and damages the nerves. Lead also affects the red blood cells by reducing them, which has a very serious effect on the entire body. It can also affect bone density and cause brittleness and breakages. Once absorbed, lead is found in the spleen, kidneys and liver.[8]

Lead was also used to solder down cans containing preserved foods. Millions of people over the years were ingesting lead in their food. While this has been phased out now, the damage from this has already been done. We see it in the elderly today who are suffering huge rates of dementia-type conditions. Of course, as we will see, we have so many toxins causing this as well, but the point is to see just how we are all bombarded with many dangerous ways of becoming sick later in life.

I don't know if I ate paint chippings but I do know that I had lead-based paint all over my body for at least 1 hour. Our skin is the body's largest organ, which meant that I absorbed whatever was in that paint – namely, lead. Considering that no amount of lead in the body is safe, there is no possible way that that episode did not harm my health.

Looking at how my life turned out – with years of illness, five different bone breakages, constant fatigue, depression and mental problems, a shockingly poor attention span, great difficulty concentrating and, later in life, extremely bad memory – I was most certainly displaying some of the symptoms of lead and other toxic poisoning.

All children today have some worrying level of lead in their blood; it's simply found in our environment too much and is now impossible to avoid.

How to reduce exposure to lead

- Check (test) your water supply for lead (from old pipes) and use a filter

- If you think you have lead pipes in your house, when using water in your home, do not use the 'first drawn' part; let it run for about 3 minutes
- Be very careful about the type of water you use if you are feeding your infant with formula
- Avoid moving into old homes where the paints used may contain lead
- Properly remove lead-based wall paint
- Have healthy-air plants in your home
- Be careful of letting your child inadvertently eat soil – our earth contains lead

If you are concerned about lead levels in yourself or your children, you can have hair analysis done or specified blood tests. In Chapter 13, I discuss effective and essential ways of helping to remove the toxins that are already in the body.

Mercury

If the news about aluminum and lead was bad enough, I've got some not-so-nice news for you. Mercury is even *worse*. In relation to the damaging effects it has on human health, it is said that mercury is the second most toxic heavy metal. Mercury is found in the earth, just like aluminum, in the form of ore (rocks). Cinnabar, which is one of mercury's raw forms, is actually a very beautiful-looking reddish crystal. You wouldn't think that such a beautiful rock could hurt humankind as much as it does. But as they always say, looks can be very deceiving. Mercury is found in air dust particles, due to the coal, gold, pig iron and steel plants, and now shows up in our waterways (in all of them: oceans, rivers, streams, creaks, dams) and is therefore in the fish that we consume. Mercury is found in vaccinations (under the name Thimerosal) and also in our dental fillings (which contain on average 50% pure mercury).

What does mercury to do the brain?

In large amounts, as in toxic poisoning, mercury literally sends people 'mad'. Minamata, a coastal town in Japan, showed the world exactly what happens when people become exposed to large amounts of mercury over time. Over a period of about 30 years, a local chemical company called Chisso was discharging a methyl mercury compound into the air and it ended up in the drinking-water supply. This also contaminated the surrounding coastal waters, where the local people caught and ate fish. Despite the company starting the pollution in 1932, they were not stopped until decades later, in 1968. The company and media tried to cover it up and, by then, so much damage had been done to the people and the town and also to the surrounding environment that it took about 30 years to clean it up and to be pronounced safe. Over that 30-year period since the company started, their output of this deadly methyl mercury toxin had shot up from 210 tons to 45,245 tons per year. Is it any wonder it devastated so many people and totally ruined the health of the surrounding coast?

Approximately 2265 people suffered with 'Minamata disease', and sadly 1784 died due to the poisoning. The neurological health problems that this mercury exposure produced were not pretty. Victims developed skeletomuscular deformities and often lost their ability to walk. A huge number also lost their vision and were not able to hear or speak normally. In severe cases, the poisoning expressed itself through patients with paralysis, 'insanity' and eventual coma and death, just weeks after the beginning of symptoms. Even the local cats and dogs were affected by this exposure.

Because of these cases, 'Minamata disease' became a new medical diagnosis. More than 40 years later, the Chisso chemical factory was ordered to pay over $86 million in compensation to many of the families affected by the poisoning. But it was of course - too little too late for thousands of people whom lost their lives, or had them completely ruined.

Minamata has since become quite an inspiring story. Because of their huge environmental disaster, the people have now turned their city into a recognized eco town. They are very much into recycling (they have 24 different categories waste can go into), and Chisso, the chemical factory responsible for the devastation, were ordered to clean up its act. The town has opened a museum about the disaster of Minamata where victims educate the public and speak about what happened, to spread awareness about environmental toxins. They hope to cut their greenhouse gas emissions by 50% by 2050.

While most of us don't have to worry about coming into contact with large amounts of mercury like those of Minamata, it's crucial to understand that *small* doses of mercury can still, and does, wreak a lot of damage. Mercury not only has disastrous effects on the brain; it is also equally destructive to the immune system. These days, hundreds and thousands of people get diagnosed with 'mysterious illnesses' such as MS, ME, CFS, fibromyalgia, to name but a few. In all of these cases, the immune system is attacking itself and doctors don't seem to understand why. When we look closer at what mercury does to the immune system, it seems blatantly obvious why these cases are skyrocketing. Mercury literally *kills* cells, by interfering in their ability to exchange nutrients, waste and oxygen products through the cell membrane. What happens inside the cell once mercury has penetrated it is very worrying indeed. Mercury destroys DNA, which is our genetic code, and once that's happened, the cell won't ever be able to *reproduce* again. So the more cells that go through this process, the more it means it's literally killing us. Mercury embeds into the cell membrane, which then gives that particular cell the appearance of being nothing like a cell and more like an 'invader'; hence it becomes a trigger for the immune system to destroy that cell. When you have mercury in your cell membranes, your immune system will start attacking your own tissues, leading to autoimmune diseases such as MS, scleroderma, lupus and diabetes.

The town of Minamata is something for us to learn from. Whilst we may not be exposed to massive amounts of mercury like they were for 30 years, we *are* exposed to it in concerning amounts, and through other ways, that are causing us similar problems but stretched out over many more years. When it comes to poisons, a 'little bit' is still *far* too much for our health.[8]

Dental fillings

This next section should cause much concern, simply because so many people have fillings in their mouth which may even include you. Fillings are set into the teeth in a seemingly 'solid' way, so people tend to think that there is no way anything from them could possbily leak into their body. They see them as 'just like concrete', and once concrete has set, it can't leak, can it? But because our chewing action is so strong, and we do it so often, each chew from the pressure produced actually causes the mercury to leak out like a gas, which you then end up absorbing and swallowing. And if what you are swallowing is concerning amounts of a neurotoxin, then it's not going to be at all good for your health. If this 'leaking' sounds too far fetched to believe and you would like to see if this *is* possible, you can go to YouTube and type in 'Smoking teeth - Toxic fillings' where a short video made by reasearches from the prestigious Oxford University in the United Kingdom will provide startling evidence to just how much gas comes out. And it's also been featured on the Dr Oz show, (who has been turned into a household name (by Oprah Winfrey), where he demonstrated on TV with a live audience showing how mercury gas is omitted when brushing the teeth. The levels were very concerning even when brushing just for a few seconds.

So, if it *is* true that these mercury-based fillings leak, (and its important to know that the average filling can contain up to 50% mercury) over time, and of course with further fillings, this regular toxic exposure may contribute to triggering what is called 'subclinical illness' which is an illness that is not immediately apparent. For example, arthritis, premature aging, cardiovascular disease, gastrointestinal problems, allergies, disrupted immune system function, and many other common illnesses which often get labeled as 'psychosomatic' or 'unknown' – problems like chronic fatigue or ME, MS – all fall under this category. The worst effect of too much mercury is, of course, dementia and Alzheimer's disease, which is occurring in such great numbers that we now need to worry about it as much as we worry about cancer.

In March 2013, after Dr Oz aired his show *Are Your Silver Fillings Making You Sick*, the American Dental Association released a statement saying they were severing ties with the Dr OZ cofounded consumer website called Sharecare. This is part of what they said:

"The decision was made after a March 28 episode of 'The Dr. Oz Show' provided misleading information on dental amalgam."

The ADA also went on to say that the segment 'erroneously' portrays dental amalgam as a health risk '*when in fact not one credible scientific study supports this position.*'

Yet according to Dr Mercola in the article *ADA Ends Relationship with Dr Oz Website*, studies *have* been perfomed and are cause for great concern:

However, researchers from the University of Illinois at Chicago School of Public Health recently concluded that mercury alternatives are less hazardous to both public health and the environment, when comparing mercury-based dental fillings with alternatives like resin composites and glass ionomer fillings.

They reported:

"Based on current evidence, the ultimate goal of a phase-out of virtually all usage of dental mercury is recommended." The 47 nations of the Council of Europe also passed a resolution calling on the nations to start "restricting or prohibiting the use of amalgams as dental fillings," explaining that "amalgams are the prime source of exposure to mercury for developed countries, also affecting embryos, fetuses (through the placenta) and children (through breastfeeding)."

Now, by using a *logical* mind, I am sure you will come to the conclusion that if there were no problems with mercury fillings, then *why* have 47 nations agreed to restrict or completely phase the use of them out?

Could it because the World Health Organisation released a report on dental amalgam, urging dentists to switch to non-amalgam materials?

Mercury is highly toxic and harmful to health. Approximately 80% of inhaled mercury vapor is absorbed in the blood through the lungs, causing damages to lungs, kidneys and the nervous, digestive, respiratory and immune systems. Health effects from excessive mercury exposure include tremors, impaired vision and hearing, paralysis, insomnia, emotional instability, developmental deficits during fetal development, and attention deficit and developmental delays during childhood

Now *why* would the ADA not want the public knowing how dangerous mercury fillings are? Could it be that they are trying to cover their conflict of interest and are covering their tails in general?

It's a little known fact but the ADA has been a *patent* holder for amalgam and of course, were the organisation who assured the public they were *safe* when first introduced. It's clear that this has perhaps *always* been a lie, and that it was never safe in the first place.

Many dentists - in fact some stastistics point to approximately 50% in the US -are now very much aware that mercury amalgam fillings are causing damage to humans and are suggesting people have them removed, and are not using them in their clinics.

However, it's really tragic to know that despite many people *wanting* to have them removed, they actually cannot. Because it's such a detailed process and therefore very expensive, that many patients simply cannot afford to have them out. They have a ticking time bomb sitting right next to their brain and they can't do anything about it. How utterly tragic.

Even though the blame should squarely fall on the heads of the ADA (American Dental Association), for deeming these poisonous treatments as safe, no one has been able to sue. And it's highly unlikely they ever will be able to as the government will protect them.

If you do have mercury-based fillings (any silver-looking ones are mercury-based) and want to get them out, it's important to note that this removal process can also be quite dangerous because, if not carried out correctly, the mercury gas can also leak, and more than what is a typical dose of ingesting through fillings already there. Mercury fillings are also still available in many countries and if yours has a 'free' dental care health system, be careful – those fillings they may offer you are most likely to be still made of mercury.

Fillings can also contain literally hundreds of other ingredients including other metals such as tin, copper, nickel, zinc and silver. Dr. Hal Huggins, who is a true pioneer in bringing attention to the dangers of mercury-based fillings, tested thousands of his own patients over many years after seeing so many people visit him with autoimmune disorders who reported that they did not have these problems until they had fillings put in their mouth. After years of study, he saw that, among the patients that had these types of fillings, *90%* of them had an autoimmune reaction to their mercury-based amalgams! This is *beyond* shocking! Statistically that's an epidemic problem! So, basically, if *you* have any mercury fillings then it's highly likely that your body is already showing some signs of toxicity and displaying an autoimmune reaction as well. You just might not feel it yet.

Something else very concerning is when you have several fillings next to each other. Because metals are used to make these fillings, they can create an electrical current, and when they sit in the mouth next to another metal-based filling; the electrical currents go back and forth in your mouth (and are so close to your brain), and the impulses can also cause the mercury vapor to be released into the mouth more quickly and, at higher levels.[9]

If you go to your dentist right now, concerned about these problems with mercury fillings, chances are he or she will tell you that this problem is nonsense. If this is so, *find another dentist ASAP.* This response is immediate proof that they do *not* know what they are talking about. At the end of this section, I have put up a website that you can contact to find a dentist who is well aware of the dangers of mercury fillings and also is trained in the correct way to remove them. If you are not in the USA, google 'holistic dentist' in your area to find someone close to you. Dr. Huggins' books are also worth reading and I have included these in the resource section at the back of the book.

Sadly, like so many treatments and toxins, mercury fillings were once deemed as completely safe, and for many years the real truth was kept in the dark. Germany and Switzerland already know that mercury is deadly and have banned its use from dentistry. But too many other countries still use it today and are showing no signs of banning it. In the USA alone, it is thought that approximately 235 million people have teeth containing any number of mercury fillings. Every time they eat, a deadly gas is floating into their brains through the microscopic particles that are produced through chewing. Chewing gum and having hot drinks make the vapors release more quickly

Dr. Huggins conducted an experiment on a university professor who had a mouth full of amalgam fillings. Dr. Huggins wanted to see if he could get a mercury vapor reading from them and thought he would be the perfect candidate. What he saw shocked him more than he could have ever thought. A tube was placed over one of the fillings and Dr. Huggins saw the needle of the machine within *seconds* go from 10 up to 50 micrograms (mcg) of mercury per cubic meter of air. Dr. Huggins could not believe his eyes. He knew that according to the Occupational Safety and Health Administration, the maximum safe level of exposure for 8 hours in a 24-hour period was 50 mcg. If there was even 1 mcg over, the facility would be closed and the offender would be fined US $10,000.

Here was a man sitting in front of him whose fillings ended up pushing *90 mcg* on his machine. *Every* time this professor opened his mouth, he was literally poisoning himself, and even those that were *around* him. After conducting further tests on other patients, Dr. Huggins found that people were capable of exhibiting readings of up to *300 mcg* after chewing gum for just 2 minutes!

It's vitally important to note here that your teeth are of course inside your *skull*, which is exceptionally *close* to your brain. So these little vapors that you are inhaling don't have too far to get to the most important part of the body.[10]

Check out the Toxic Teeth website for more information about this massive problem in the dental industry:

✓ toxicteeth.org

Much more can be said about amalgams and their disastrous affect on human health. If you have any, please, I urge you to look into it much more. Dr. Huggins has a helpful website where you can look at some of his books and also search for a safe dentist:

✓ hugginsappliedhealing.com

If you do have fillings but can't remove them due to finances then what I can suggest is to regularly take *Pure Body Zeolites* to help excrete the mercury and the other toxins they are made with. You can learn more about them Chatper 13, *The Vital Importance of Detoxing*.

It's ironic that most of us dislike going to the dentist so much, yet we are not looking after our teeth and gums anywhere near as we should. However, there is lots we can do to help our visits to the dentist be much more pleasant (where they have to do hardly anything to your teeth). The following short section can give you an idea of what foods to try and avoid, and foods to eat more of.

Avoiding these types of foods can really help keep cavities at bay:

- Dried fruits – these stick to your teeth and are very high in concentrated sugars. If you eat them, make sure they are organic and also brush your teeth afterwards.
- Blueberries – these can stain your teeth due to the deep pigments. If you do consume, use a toothpaste with an abrasive action to help remove the stains.
- Fruit Juice – juices are pure sugar and are often very acidic – always brush your teeth after you have one or, drink a glass of water.
- Wine – red wine obviously stains the teeth but alcohol in general is not at all good for the health of the mouth and teeth due to the fact it decreases saliva production. Saliva is vitally important for healthy teeth. After drinking, have a glass of water or clean your teeth immediately.
- Citrus fruits – eating oranges, pineapples and even lemons can cause your teeth enamel to erode from the high acid content found in the fruit. Drink water after or clean teeth.
- Dry Starchy foods – enzymes in the mouth turn certain ingredients/foods into sugars, as does the reaction when eating things like crackers/biscuits. Make sure you brush your teeth after eating them.
- Coffee - this might be one of the worst culprits for staining teeth. Coffee also interferes with your mouth's saliva production so can turn your mouth into a bacteria loving atmosphere. You can chew on xyltiol chewing gum to help improve the saliva production and be sure to keep drinking lots of water and brush your teeth more often.

The following foods can help protect your teeth:

- Water – whilst one might not automatically think of water as a 'food', it is a substance that really helps fight cavities. Staying hydrated is vitally important to keep your mouth and teeth in great condition. Water helps to wash away acidity and also residue from food, particularly from sugary foods.

- Appes – apples that are neutral in taste are less sugary and better for your teeth. Apples contain a lot of fibre so they help to wash away stains from other foods. Their high water content keeps your saliva production in good amounts. Not-so-sugary apples are one of the best fruits to give children.

- Nuts - clinical research on nuts and teeth health show eating them in small amounts, regularly, can help prevent gum disease because they are low in sugar and have fat content. They also contain good amounts of phosphourus and calcium, which can help strengthen teeth.

- Celery – celery won't stain the teeth and because it's full of water, this will help saliva flow in your mouth.

- Cheese – it may surprise some as it did me, that cheese is proven to be good for your teeth. It soaks up acidity and is said to restore the nautral PH of the mouth to a more alkaline level. Cheese is high in calcium and phosphorus, which are both crucial for healthy teeth. A tiny piece after a meal is sufficient.

- Salmon – wild, ethically sustained salmon is full of vitamin D. Salmon is high in protein and helps balance out sugars from a raw or vegan diet.

- Xylitol – xylitol is amazing because it's not just a truly healthy sugar substitute, but it's also very good for your teeth. In studies, it's shown to be quite effective at preventing cavities. Look for chewing gums sweetened with xylitol instead of things like aspartame and sorbitols.

Keep another toothbrush in your kitchen so that you will remind yourself to use it more often. Have one in your handbag/backpack too so that when you eat out, you can quickly brush your teeth after eating. From the suggested tips above, it's clear that brushing teeth with the recommended twice a day might not be enough to really keep cavities and gum disease at bay.

List courtesy of renegadehealth.com

If you would like some more information about what you can do to help protect your teeth from any further dental treatment the book *Cure Tooth Decay: Remineralize Cavities and Repair Your Teeth Naturally with Good Food* by DDS timothy Gallagher & Ramiel Nagel is excellent.

Don't like the sound of mercury in your body& brain? Stay away from eating fish!

There is an enormous amount of pollution in the environment today, and our oceans are now so toxic, that fish are highly dangerous to consume due to mercury levels (and also other persistent, troublesome toxins too). Because fish eat *other* fish that eat smaller fish etc., the bigger types of fish we commonly eat, such as tuna, now have worrying levels of mercury in their flesh due to *bioaccumulation*. The mercury levels increase up through the food chain. As sushi is so popular these days, we are eating more fish than ever. Pregnant women are told to minimize the amounts of fish in their diet, but I would advise *not* to have any at all. Developing fetuses are *very* sensitive to mercury, and there are links with ADHD-related disorders developing in children later in their life, so I would say, put it on your list of things you should just not eat while pregnant.

A study was done on newborns in Minnesota, USA, and 10% of the babies tested had mercury in their blood that exceeded the Environmental Protection Agency's reference dose. This is very concerning.

Due to the Academy Award winning documentary *The Cove*, the town of Taiji, Japan, now infamous - shocked the world by bringing to light its brutal dolphin slaughter, which happens every year from

September to April. Thousands of dolphins are speared to death for the purpose of selling their meat, while some are sold to theme parks for huge sums of money. We can often find these 'luckier' dolphins in places like SeaWorld. This disgusting 'tradition', which has been going on for years and years (and is proving very hard to stop, no matter how many protests take place around the world), also hid another dirty little secret. Local children were consuming the dolphin meat and eating it pretty much daily. The Japanese actually have one of the highest consumption rates of fish in the world, so there was a natural cause for concern regarding high levels of mercury found in the dolphin meat. Concerned about the mercury effects on the local population, and in particular the young children, the National Institute for Minamata Disease conducted some research on a group of people in Taiji. While it has not been found that anyone is suffering from severe mercury poisoning as such, they are continuing their studies into the effects on children.

I used to love fish and would have it a few times a week. Going out for sushi was one of my favorite things to do, now after what I have learnt, I just don't want to eat fish at all anymore. It's easier to control the health of farm animals such as chicken and cows, than it is fish in the sea. Yes, there are ways of purchasing fish known to have less mercury, for example from companies who farm fish in special netted areas away from the oceans, but the problem with this is that it's a) more cruel to the fish, as they are often in very small areas b) the fish could be getting fed with GMO feed, c) the fish may be swimming in waters with high doses of antibiotics so they don't catch any diseases, which means you end up eating those antibiotics too. I just can't bring myself to enjoy eating fish anymore; I see them as 'dirty' because their flesh contains so many toxins, in particular mercury, and I just don't want that in my body.

If you want to find out how much mercury you may be eating through fish, use the website below, which will help calculate the amount you may be consuming. In Chapter 10 I have a helpful list showing the fish that have different levels of mercury in them, to help you try and eliminate or at least reduce eating the most dangerous ones.

✓ Go to gotmercury.org for the calculator

What I want you to think about is this: we have government 'safety' recommendations in regards to eating fish. They strongly suggest that pregnant women limit their exposure to eating fish or completely avoid it. Yet as we will see below, there are *no* government recommendations to limit mercury from our medicines, which get *injected* into our bodies, as opposed to just eating it.

It is even proven that eating fish can harm unborn babies' development. This has been proven in many studies. However, the medical industry and the CDC (Centre for Disease Control) recommend that pregnant women should have injections containing a mercury derivative, Thimerosal, to 'protect' against the flu. I know what you are, or *should* be thinking. This is highly confusing, *hypocritical* and downright crazy! How can they recommend that?

Here is a thought really worth pondering before we go further: in regards to 'poisons', what do *you* think is a safer way of having them administered? Swallowing them, or having them *injected* into your body?

Mercury in vaccinations

This is the most controversial, yet without a doubt, is also the most worrying, way that many people receive mercury. I go into further detail about this enormous subject of safety of vaccinations in Chapter 36 but I will mention a little bit more about it here now, just to get you thinking already: is it really *OK* that we, and (more worryingly) our children, are receiving doses of mercury, a proven neurotoxin (Thimerosal), into our bodies at all?

I want to give you a little background history on how mercury got into our vaccines. Some of this information may shock you, as it *should*, but if it's too much to believe, you can easily go and see for yourself that the facts I am going to share are indeed true and should therefore ring alarm bells in your mind. Truthfully, I would rather this information *not* be true and I have discovered that generally, anyone speaking out about the dangers of vaccinations risks their reputation, career and in my case, a mass of negative reviews and horrible comments. But, I *can't* ignore what I know, and I don't want to keep it to myself. It's your kids I am worried about.

Thimerosal was discovered in the early 1920s by the pharmaceutical company Eli Lilly. Thimerosal contains 49.6% ethyl mercury by weight and is a proven neurotoxin known to be at least *100 times more lethal* to the tissues than lead. It has been used in most vaccinations as an antiseptic and anti-fungal agent. Knowing that vaccines contain animal cells and also have aborted fetal tissue in them (yes, it's totally true as you will find out later on), I am not surprised they needed to find something that would stop the vaccines from producing bacteria and fungus. But realizing just what sort of antiseptic agent they do use, seems *very* crazy.

A vaccination which was made without preservatives ended up being proven to have carried staphylococcus, a very dangerous bacteria, and in 1928, 12 children who were vaccinated with the diphtheria injection all became infected and died. Understandably, after this tragic medical disaster, it's no wonder preservatives had to be included in all future vaccinations to gain back the public's waning trust. But the question many are asking today is: just how *safe* are these preservatives? Where is the *proof* that they are truly safe? And in the case of Thimerosal, should it ever have been allowed into our vaccines in the first place?

Apart from *one* test carried out in the 1930s, to this day there have been *no* other tests performed regarding the safety of Thimerosal in humans. Knowing that this stuff has been in use for nearly 100 years, isn't it odd that there is no *proof* that it is completely safe for use in humans (and most worrying our babies and infants) through our injections?

The only study that has been performed was in 1930 in a hospital in Indiana, USA, involving 22 patients who were dying from meningitis. Here is where it gets *really* concerning. These patients, who were deathly sick, were injected with solutions containing Thimerosal. They all died typically only a few days later.[11] Because they had already been diagnosed with meningitis, the Thimerosal did not even enter the equation to have caused their death, or at the very least, to have sped it up. The study declared that Thimerosal was safe to use because there were 'no adverse reactions'. Bear in mind that meningitis itself is an inflammation of the protective membranes which cover the brain and spinal cord. Someone who has this kind of life-threatening problem, I think it's clear to see, should not be having *any* injections with neurotoxins when their brain is already under that kind of stress. And was it even ethical or very *humane* to perform tests like that on patients who were days away from death anyway?

Teething powders used to also contain Thimerosal, and this was linked to outbreaks of the fatal 'acrodynia', otherwise known as 'pink disease' and 'infantile mercury poisoning'. This showed itself in infants as a very weepy red rash, with peeling skin, sensitivity to light, and anemia. It was later to be known as 'mercury poisoning'. In 1947, after the link was too hard to deny, Thimerosal was removed from all teething products. Pink disease suddenly became quite rare. It's very odd they didn't think to remove it from all of the vaccinations in use. Due to today's huge rise in autism disorders, some experts are linking this to children's grandparents who may have suffered from pink disease in their youth and passed the toxins down through the genes. The possibility of this could be indeed quite true, but I think as you will soon see, it's more than likely from the other way we get exposed to this neurotoxin.

Thimerosal has since become a huge problem in many parents' and concerned doctors' eyes. Many children who developed autism, when tested for mercury, were found to have an usually high level of it in their blood. And when the parents tried to figure out where it came from, the only *logical* direction tended to come from the recommended childhood vaccines that their children had received. Due to this pressure on the medical industry and pharmaceutical companies, they say most vaccinations now do not contain the levels of Thimerosal that they once did. But this is not exactly true, nor does it mean that this problem has gone.

The FDA never actually made it 'law' to remove the Thimeresol, they merely only 'recommended' it, so it's still found in quite a lot of vaccines to this day. However, parents now mistakenly tend to think that vaccinations have suddenly become much safer, yet the truth is, there are many other *just as concerning* toxic ingredients in them – which you will discover in Chapter 36.

Most flu injections today *still* contain Thimerosal.[12]

A typical dose of Thimerosal-containing flu vaccine contains 25 micrograms of Thimerosal. According to the Environmental Protection Agency (EPA), the safe limit for human exposure to mercury is 0.1 mcg per kilo of weight per day. Since almost half of the Thimerosal is mercury, this means that each flu shot contains just over 12 mcg of mercury, which would be considered *unsafe* for anyone weighing less than 120 kilos, or just under 265 pounds.[13]

And in other countries which have not phased out the Thimerosal, it's still in most of their vaccinations and is still, as yet, *not* proven to be safe. It hasn't been eliminated in its entirety, not at all.

If you listen to your doctor, you will know that flu shots are recommended for pretty much everyone – pregnant women, the elderly, the 'immune compromised' and babies from age 6 months – and are advised to be given *every single year*. This, in my and many others' view, makes it far *worse* than previously because the childhood vaccinations stop around age of 4 . But if you (or your mother or father) listen to your doctor and always have the flu shot every year from the age of 6 months, then you could be having about 60 of them in your lifetime, receiving regular doses of this neuro-toxic Thimerosal every single year. And because aluminium is *also* widely used as an adjuvant in flu vaccines, you will be heading *much* faster towards the development of Alzheimers or just having pretty poor brain function in general.

There are many other common medications that also contain levels of Thimerosal, such as cold and flu nasal sprays, hemorrhoid ointments and opthalmic solutions. I was going to list them all here, but there were literally pages and pages of medications! Its just madness - no one denies that mercury and all the other forms of mercury (e.g. ethyl mercury and methyl mercury) are *neurotoxins* and that 'no amount is safe', yet they are found in so many medications.

After what I have learnt about mercury, I wouldn't want *any* amounts of it anywhere up my nose, in my veins, near my bottom or in my eyes, thank you very much.

How to reduce mercury exposure
- Eliminate or avoid eating fish, especially those that are known to have high levels
- Research in greater detail how vaccinations, and their ingredients, affect health
- Find out if the medication you are recommended to take contains Thimerosal before giving it to your children or yourself
- Do not buy energy-saving light bulbs which contain mercury
- Do not have fillings containing mercury (amalgam)
- Look into having your present fillings removed safely
- Avoid working in industries where you will be exposed to mercury
- Detox your body with a heavy metal chelator such as carnosine, Pure Body zeolites or other methods, as mentioned in Chapter 13 'The Vital Importance of Detoxing'
- Remember that in regards to toxicity, it's all about *accumulation*; this is the *main* message in my book I want to convey as chemical exposure happens from *all* angles and adds up

exponentially in the body. And guess what? We haven't even scratched the surface of just how prevalent these toxins are, and the other ways in which we absorb them.

Cadmium

This is the last heavy metal I am going to discuss in this chapter. As I have mentioned, there are *so* many to be concerned about but I simply cannot cover them all. In fact, if I were to cover absolutely every single vital piece of information concerning all the subjects I present in this book, I would need to probably spend the next 20 years writing and publishing volumes and volumes of separate books. I just want you to see the basic picture here and also to inspire you to go and find out more information yourself. The best way to understand and remember something is to find the facts yourself - it becomes much more meaningful and clear that way.

Cadmium is another toxic heavy metal, which according to some scientists, is becoming more of a worrying pollutant than lead. Cadmium is another mineral found in the earth's crust but at much lower levels compared to other heavy metals. It's used, among other things, to make metals, and due to its natural resistance to corrosion its purpose was generally to coat other metals such as steel and iron with its non-rust outer layer. Particles of cadmium have entered into the air, and due to environmental concerns, cadmium is now not produced nearly as much as it was 50 years ago. However, it's still causing massive health problems among humans.

Cadmium is found in black rubber, motor oil, pesticides, plastic tape, refined wheat, silver polish, soil, evaporated milk, ceramics, fungicides, pesticides, water supplies, rubber carpet backing, rustproof materials such as what's used in boats, jewelry, paint pigments, oysters and other seafoods, dental prosthetics – and the list goes on...

What does cadmium do to the body and brain?
A common way millions of people are ingesting cadmium is through

cigarettes. In tobacco, cadmium is the heavy metal found in highest amounts. It's sprayed on the tobacco as a pesticide. In every single cigarette there are approximately on average 1.4 micrograms of cadmium. And because cadmium is a heavy metal that doesn't tend to leave the body too easily (or at all), smoking is a quick and easy way to increase your levels of this dangerous toxin. Worryingly (and unfortunately, I am the wife of a smoker), in each pack of cigarettes smoked, the user will ingest 4 micrograms of cadmium, which is then deposited into the lungs. This amount is approximately 10 times the amount of cadmium a *healthy* body can assimilate in one day. Smokers, on average, will have 4–5 times the level of cadmium in their blood and 2–3 times higher levels found in their kidneys than non-smokers. The lungs tend to absorb cadmium much easier than the stomach does, so smokers are really doing a complete assault on their body's health[14]

Certain minerals, such as zinc, which are found in the body also, can help the body to assimilate cadmium better, but it depends on what you eat. For example, refined white flour contains ratios of cadmium to zinc in levels, which are worse than that of naturally whole wheat. This unstable zinc/cadmium ratio is also found in other refined foods such as white rice and white sugar.

There are traces of cadmium found on the following foods: shelled seeds, organ meats such as liver and kidney, cabbage, potato chips, peanut butter and peanuts, french fries, cookies, celery, cereals (wheat and bran) boiled potatoes (with skin on).

Cadmium has been found to weaken so many vital body functions. It causes the immune system to weaken, and things like parasites, fungi, worms and bacteria will grow, but most concern-ingly, it causes the growth of malignant tumors, i.e. cancer. It has no beneficial function in the body, so no amount is safe. It affects the kidneys, accumulating in them with age, causes high blood pressure, damages the liver, causes anemia and contributes to bone problems such as osteoporosis. Scientists are studying the link between cadmium exposure and breast cancer as it seems that women are more at risk of developing health problems related to this heavy metal. Cadmium is also showing up in testing of patients suffering from Alzheimer's.

Cadmium toxicity can reveal itself in conditions such as chronic fatigue syndrome, yellow staining of the teeth, calcium stones, pain in the lower legs and back, and problems with bones. Interestingly, people who are overweight tend to suffer with cadmium toxicity *less* than someone who is thinner. Fat stores toxins such as cadmium in its tissues and tends to keep them away from the organs. But don't let this make you think it's OK to be overweight, as that in itself leads to other health problems.

Pregnant women who have levels of cadmium in their bodies will often expose their unborn babies to this toxin, which can lead to the child being born with a low birth weight.

How you can limit your exposure to cadmium

- Avoid refined foods such as rice, sugar and wheat, non-organic potatoes, non-organic shelled seeds, organ meats, french fries, peanuts, cookies, celery and cabbage
- Do not smoke or instead smoke organic tobacco with raw unbleached papers (please note: this does not mean they are good for your health, just less toxic)
- Avoid breathing in second-hand smoke
- Avoid using pesticides or eating conventionally farmed foods
- Avoid or limit eating oysters and other fish
- Don't eat evaporated milk and what is usually made with it (e.g. caramel tarts)
- Check your water supply and install a filter – 'soft' water contains more cadmium than 'hard' water
- Detox with methods suggested in Chapter 13

Organic tobacco companies
✓ motherearthtobacco.com
✓ nascigs.com

✓ sfntc.com

Test kits for heavy metals
✓ novadetox.co.uk
✓ heavymetalstest.com
✓ osumex.com
✓ amazon.com
✓ amazon.co.uk

* * *

This chapter is just a *drop* in the ocean in regards to heavy metals, how abundant they are, how they are getting into the food chain and what they are doing to our bodies. I am sure you can already see why toxicity is perhaps the number one cause of disease and death.

For even more information on toxicity, please check out the video presentation on this website:

factsontoxicity.com

In 1940, we produced about one billion pounds of new synthetic chemicals. By 150, the figure had reached fifty billion pounds, and by the late 1980s, it became 500 billion pounds, including a wide range of toxic, carcinogenic, neurotixc and other chemicals. Most of these chemicals have never been tested for toxic, carcinogenic or environmental effects

Dr Samuel Epstein – Speaker at the 1994 Conference of The American Collage For The Advancement Of Medicine

Chapter 4

Are You Dying to Look Beautiful?
The Hidden Poisons in Your Cosmetics

Today, you can buy beauty products that will stay on for '24 hours', foundation that will cover up your pores, giving you 'perfect skin', fake tans that give the illusion that you have been on holiday – and oh yes, they can make you look 'thinner' too! There are mascaras that make you look like you have super-long eyelashes, hair dye that will give the appearance you are a natural blonde, facial treatments to refine your skin so that it will 'look like it did when you were young'. And there are thousands of other products, which are all seductively waved under your nose by the advertisers, who use sneaky and proven marketing techniques to make you want, or feel you *have*, to buy. But as appealing as all these products and promises are, at what cost to your health are you *really* paying for?

Back in 1996, I was living in my home country, Australia, and studying to be a beauty therapist. Ever since I was a young girl, I had always been interested in the skin and looking 'good'. I attended an Aveda course, which at the time was a company which pioneered natural beauty. I listened to the teacher educate us young and eager beauty trainees about the long list of chemicals that were in pretty much 90% of our skin and body care products, perfumes, makeup, and hair care items.

When I listened to the information about what these chemicals can do in their individual state (before they are mixed in with our ingredients), I was absolutely *horrified*. Many of the chemicals were used also as *industrial* cleaners, or came from petrol. These chemicals, when in their original containers and shipped from their factories, had to be marked with the poison symbol on them! Back at the factory, if there was an accidental spill of these chemicals, and a person was exposed, it would require the person to go straight to hospital for immediate medical care in case they had inhaled or absorbed (or been burnt by) the chemicals. I learnt that there had even been thousands of deaths from accidents or severe poisoning from over-exposure to these sorts of chemicals. I also heard that there were hundreds and thousands of dangerous chemicals.

Then we were told that these same types of chemicals were in all the common things we put on our face and body parts, including on our children. And that many of these typical products actually contain at least 10 different dangerous chemicals in them. In fact, some products have *nothing* safe or truly natural in them at all. Even the so-called 'natural' scents were most of the time fake, or from disgusting sources. After learning this, I went home that night, and looked at all my products in closer inspection. *Everything* I was using had all the worst chemicals – and I had bought the most commonly used brands; they were the trendy, fashionable brands I had read about in my magazines, and the ones all my friends were using. I threw pretty much everything out immediately, as it really made total sense to me to just get rid of it. I saw it as very serious to my health, and I didn't want that stuff on my skin any longer.

I already knew from my training that our skin is also an organ, in fact, our largest living breathing organ, and absorbs *everything* which is put onto it. It is also a carrier or entry-way into the body and transports chemicals to other organs and parts of the body. It does have its own natural protection shield, but it's nowhere near as strong as we think and, with regular use of poisonous products, it simply cannot keep things out.

I want to show you what these common chemicals found in beauty products have been proven to cause:

- Cancers
- Immunotoxicity / Immune suppression
- Allergies
- Neurotoxicity
- Endocrine (hormonal) disruption

- Developmental/reproductive toxicity
- Irritation (eyes, lungs)
- Enhanced skin absorption (some chemicals actually cause our skin to absorb even more chemicals)
- Toxicity to vital organs – liver, kidney etc
- Biochemical or cellular level changes

Not a nice list, is it? And there are probably quite a few other reactions I have not included. Who would think that such damage could be done just by putting things on our skin, hair and body? I now want to take you through each category of beauty products and why they are so harmful if containing harsh chemicals.

Cancer-causing cosmetics

Not many people are aware of this but there are currently *no* laws in place that require a cosmetics company to test the safety of their products before putting them onto the market. This means that they can pretty much put in whatever ingredients they like, without seeing if they're actually safe for humans to use. There are over a whopping 150 toxic cancer-causing ingredients currently used in common cosmetic products. According to federal law in the USA, products containing cancer-causing substances must carry a written warning. But the FDA does not enforce this with cosmetics or personal care products. 'FDA cannot require companies to do safety testing of their cosmetic products before marketing – FDA Office of Cosmetics and Colors (FDA 1995).'[15]

Considering that the skin and scalp are just like sponges, and absorb everything, this non-compliance with the law is very alarming. When makeup is formulated with harsh chemicals, it's particularly bad for our skin and health as it is usually applied every day. And, in a more superficial way, products with chemicals will also make your skin worse over time, causing it to prematurely age, often leaving a person with highly sensitive skin that they did not have when younger.

So the makeup that we use to make our skin 'look' better ends up doing us more harm than good and makes us need more makeup over the years because it deteriorates our skin. I think we all want to have good skin naturally and not just have to cover it up all the time.

What is interesting, and equally alarming, is to learn that makeup has always had toxic origins throughout the history of its creation. The wealthy ladies (and men too) in the Elizabethan age wore white face powder to cover up their skin, to make them look like an 'aristocrat' (ie posh and rich!). This powder contained high levels of lead and not only made their skin terrible (it was usually covered in rampant acne) but also later on would poison their brains as well, causing them to go mad. Ironically, the very poor, who could not afford to buy makeup, were luckily much better off; they were left with much healthier skin and had fewer health complaints generally, and were less 'mad' too.

In a way, not much has changed and we have *not* learnt from history. There are shocking ingredients used in makeup and some *still* contain levels of lead, with many big-name brands still using it in their formulas today. And this especially includes the expensive brands.

Makeup often contains other heavy metals such as arsenic, mercury, nickel, cadmium, selenium and beryllium. Many ingredients come from minerals from the ground which are basically crushed-up rocks. These rocks are full of heavy metals. All of these minerals are found in common concealers, bronzers, foundations, blushers, eye shadows, and lip products such as lipsticks and glosses. These last two items are the most worrying because we ingest anything that is on the lips.

Manufacturers of a good makeup brand will remove the heavy metals from their mineral powders and other items before they develop their cosmetics, allowing you to feel safe with what you are using. Heavy and soft metals are always in our bodies, but only minute amounts are considered safe. When their 'acceptable' ratio is disrupted, it is very dangerous for the body's natural function. And it's not just heavy metals we need to worry about in our makeup either; there are a huge amount of new and scientific 'next-generation' untested chemicals that are mixed into our cosmetic products.

Some companies bring out foundations that they claim can stay put on the skin for up to 24 hours. These are particularly toxic and not safe at all. For something to stay on that long and not rub off the skin (and also require a heavy-duty cleanser to remove), you can bet that something terribly nasty has been used to keep it from coming off your face.

Lots of companies also claim that they do not test on animals. Yet they fail to tell you that there are animal body parts in their makeup. I nearly fell over when I heard about the ingredient 'carmine'. Carmine is a very commonly used ingredient that is in many shimmery products like eye shadows, eyeliners and body powders. Carmine is an ingredient which is made from the backs of Mexican insects! Their shimmery backs are removed from their bodies and then crushed up into a powder and mixed in with colors so that you get a colorful and shiny eye shadow. Can you believe it? Your 'not tested on animals' eye shadow contains ingredients that come from an animal! So these companies are using half-truths to get you to think that their product is not harming any animals by lying and saying that they don't use animal testing! Isn't it funny how they change the name to sound more scientific when it really should be labeled as 'dried and crushed-up Mexican insects'.

Oh, the big fat lies these companies get away with is just shameful! And not only do the toxic products affect us; they also affect the workers who have to produce the products, and also the communities surrounding the factories because the waste ingredients usually go directly into the environment, through waterways and into the earth where they are dumped. So the makeup industry alone really is a massive problem. Much more than just being unsafe for the user, it is unsafe for the entire planet.

It must also be said that if you use a regular-brand body cream, then that is a very easy way to put loads of toxins into your body as you use much more body cream than you do when applying anything to your face. I know it's scary, but I would suggest you go and have a look at your own products right now and see what is in them. If you want to check exactly what each ingredient can do to your body long-term, and also how bad the product itself is in general, you can visit this very brilliant, helpful and in-depth website:

✓ ewg.org/skindeep

And for those that want to make sure they aren't buying anything that has been tested on animals, please check out these websites:

✓ uncaged.co.uk/crueltyfree.html
✓ buav.org

You will find some great organic and natural brands that don't test on animals!

It can be downright confusing to choose products that are totally natural. Sometimes even I get it wrong and with things like makeup and skincare ingredients it is almost impossible to get something completely organic. I believe the key is to find products that do a great job but are as minimal as possible in their chemical content. You want a company to clearly state how much of their product is natural and how much is organic. But the sad truth is, many companies don't offer this information and use pretty words to make you think that a product is from Nature.

The list below shows some of the worst and most common chemicals found in skincare products.

The top ten worst ingredients in beauty products
- Diazolidinyl urea
- Imidazolidinyl urea
- Diethanolamine (DEA)
- Triethanolamine(TEA)
- Parabens: ethyl, butyl, methyl, propyl, and parahydroxyben-

zoate
- Propylene glycol
- PVP/VA copolymer
- Sodium lauryl sulfate
- Sodium laureth sulfate
- Stearalkonium chloride
- Synthetic colors
- Mineral oils
- Synthetic fragrances

The following detailed list also shows other harmful chemicals which are commonly used in personal care products.

Direct carcinogens (directly cause cancer)
- Benzil acetate
- Butyl benzyphthalate
- Butylated hydroxyanisole (BHA)
- Butylated hydroxytoluene (BHT)
- 'Coal tar dyes' (and lakes) D & C Red 2, 3, 4, 8, 10, 17, 19 & 33, Green 5, Orange 17, FD & C Blue 1, 2 & 4, Green 3, Red 4 & 40, Yellow 5 & 6
- Crystalline silica
- Diaminophenol
- Diethanolamine (DEA)
- Doictyl adipate
- Disperse Blue 1, Disperse Yellow 3 (colorants)
- Fluoride
- Formaldehyde
- Glutaral
- Hydroquinone
- Methylene chloride
- Methylisothiazolinone and Methylchloroisothiazolinone
- Nitrophenylenediamine
- p-Phenylenediamine (following oxidation)

- Phenyl-p-phenylenediamine
- Saccharin
- Talc (only in loose form, particularly around genitalia)

Contaminants

These are hidden carcinogens contaminating other chemicals such as dioxane, a highly potent carcinogen.

- 1,4-Dioxane. In ethoxylated alcohols, including PEGs, oleths, polysorbates, nonoxynol.
- Arsenic and lead. In coal tar dyes, polyvinyl acetate, PEGs (polyethylene glycols).
- DDT and related pesticides. In lanolin, quarterniums.
- Diethanolamine (DEA). In DEA cocamide/ lauramide condensates, quarterniums.
- Ethylene oxide. In ethoxylated alcohols, including PEGs, oleths, polysorbates, nonoxynol.
- Formaldehyde. In polyoxymethylene urea.

Nitrosamine precursors

Nitrosamines are highly carcinogenic. Nitrosamine precursors interact with other chemicals in the product to form nitrosamines.

- Bromonitrodioxane
- 2-bromo-2-nitropropane-1,3-diol
- Diethanolamine (DEA)
- DEA-cocamide, lauramide and oleamide condensates
- DEA-MEA/Acetate
- DEA-sodium lauryl sulfate
- Metheneamine
- Morpholine
- Padimate-O
- Pyroglumatic Acid
- Triethanolamine (TEA)

- TEA-sodium lauryl sulfate

Formaldehyde precursors

Formaldehyde is highly toxic, neurotoxic, genotoxic and carcinogenic. Formaldehyde precursors react with other chemicals in the product to release formaldehyde (used to preserve dead bodies).

- 2-bromo-2-nitropropane-1,2-Diol
- Diazolidonyl urea
- DMDM-hydantoin
- Imidazolidinyl urea
- Metheneamine
- Quaternium-15
- Sodium hydroxymethylglycinate

Endocrine (hormonal) disruptors

- Parabens (methyl, ethyl, propyl, butyl, also known as hydroxy methyl benzoates). Three university studies have shown that parabens get absorbed into the bloodstream and disrupt the hormonal system. They may be associated with breast cancer.
- Benzophenone
- Butyl benzyl phthalate
- Butylated hydroxyanisole (BHA)
- Butylmethoxydibenzoylmethane (B-MDM)
- Dibutyl phthalate
- Diethyl phthalate
- Homosalate (HMS)
- Methyl-benzylidene camphor (4-MDC)
- Octyl-dimethyl-PABA (OD-PABA)
- Octyl-methoxycinnamate (OMC)
- Resorcinol

(This list is courtesy of Margo Marrone of the Organic Pharmacy)
✓ theorganicpharmacy.com

These chemicals alone can: disrupt your hormones, are linked to cancers, may damage your vital organs such as the liver and kidneys, are also linked to the huge rise in breast cancer and testicular cancers, as well as leading to fertility problems. Kind of worrying, right? All this risk, *just* from using makeup and beauty products?

If you want to find out about more dangerous skincare ingredients please check out this site too:

✓ equilibra.uk.com/dangerous.shtml

I now want to show you, on average, how many different toxic chemicals are in certain beauty products:

- Shampoo – 15
- Hairspray – 11
- Eye shadow – 26
- Lipstick – 33
- Nail varnish – 31
- Fake tan – 22
- Deodorant – 32
- Blush – 16
- Foundation – 24
- Perfume – *250* (!)
- Body lotion – 32

(List courtesy of drjones.tv)

Some brands actually have many more in them; the numbers above are just the 'averages'. Really concerning, isn't it? Your personal care products which you bought to make you 'look, feel and smell better' have *hundreds* of dangerous cancer-causing and other disease-causing chemicals in them. In these products, some of the ingredients that are used are linked to cancer, and linked to harming the development of babies. Scary.

So what products *can* you rely on then?

Below is a list of my favorite reliable skincare brands that I have tested, researched and still regularly use, with most of them selling everything you need, and some at a very affordable price, for your face and body as well as makeup items and things for your hair. Some brands are really organic and some have a smaller organic content (approx. 10%), but all are 100% natural. The brands also have different price points. I have looked for great products for purchase in the UK, Australia, Canada and the USA to help you choose, if you are from those countries. There is also a list of other brands, at the end of the section, that has been endorsed by Dr. Bronner.com whose company was a pioneer of authentic organic and ethical skincare.

Green People

UK-owned and made, this extensive range of products has items for men, women, children and teenagers, and offers highly organic products for hair, body, face and makeup. It's basically a brand for the entire family. Their products clearly state the organic and natural content and are of exceptional quality but without a high price tag. Their products do not contain parabens, phthalates, SLS and other harsh chemicals.

✓ Greenpeople.co.uk

Bare Skin Beauty

This 100% natural skincare range is impressive because it actually makes the skin remarkably better in a short amount of time. The brand's creator, Juliette Scarfe, says her 'skin food' products are original due to the unusual ingredients she blends into her skincare items. Low temperatures are used to mix the ingredients together, ensuring that the precious enzymes and active ingredients are still very much 'alive'. The range is highly organic and active. I get sent a lot of products to test out and this is by far the *best* natural beauty range I have ever tried. Bare Skin Beauty's ingredients are also sustainably and ethically sourced from suppliers who really care about the environment. The products are supplied in packaging that is fully recyclable or reusable and contributes towards a better planet. If I had to suggest that you try any natural brand, this is the one.

✓ bareskin-beauty.co.uk

Balm Balm

This range is very impressive due to the fact that each and every single product has a 100% organic content, as well as having Soil Association certification. They started out with a balm that became so popular that the range now includes products for bath and shower, face, hand and body care, as well as products for baby. They achieve this 100% organic status due to not using any water whatsoever in their products. Water can never be certified as organic so this reduces the organic content in many brands' products. Balm Balm also make beautiful organic perfumes.

✓ balmbalm.com

Essential Care

Another UK-owned and made company, mother-and-daughter team Margaret and Abi have created an extensive range of organic products for the entire body, as well as a makeup range. They have hair products and items for expecting mums and babies. Each product has the Soil Association certification on it and the content is clearly stated. Even the makeup range has been approved by the Soil Association and has fair trade ingredients. Their website also sells supplements for all types of concerns.

✓ essential-care-co.uk

Alva

German brand Alva is a 100% natural brand with approximately on average 10% organic content in all of their products. Their skincare is always of the highest quality. They also sell a highly effective acne range based on Rhassoul mud. Alva has an impressive range of natural deodorants and also sells makeup such as liquid foundations, lip glosses, lipsticks and mascaras. An affordable price tag makes this range even better for the customer.

✓ alvanaturalskincare.co.uk

Lavera

Another German brand, Lavera has one of the most extensive ranges I have seen. With literally hundreds of products to choose from, everything you could ever want has been created by Lavera. They sell products for all different skin types, all different price points, as well as all different ranges, depending on your needs. They are 100% natural and have an organic content around 10% on average. Their products really do work as well and I have regularly said that they are one of my favorite brands because the majority of products are very inexpensive and are available all over the world. Lavera and LAVERÉ products are: free from parabens, SLS and synthetic preservatives; free from fragrances, emulsifiers and petroleum-based ingredients; and are cruelty free, gluten free, and GMO free.

✓ pravera.co.uk/lavera-natural-cosmetics
✓ Lavera.com

Weleda

Another huge favorite of mine is the brand Weleda. In fact, this is one of the best, again for the price, the availability (sold worldwide) and for their ethics. Weleda was created decades ago (in 1921) and they always have used bio-dynamic organic farming methods. They only source the best plants and herbs and only use 100% natural ingredients. There are products for the whole family, including babies and children. I have tried many things from their ranges and have never been disappointed, only ever super-impressed. They even make supplements for children such as homeopathy remedies and healthy cough syrups for adults. You simply *cannot* go wrong with Weleda products.

✓ weleda.com

100 Percent Pure

This beautiful and super-cute brand consists of exactly what it says: 100% pure products with ingredients only from truly natural and organic sources. It's quickly becoming such a popular brand because the company have got their marketing and appeal spot-on. The packaging is beautiful and their website makes the products look good enough to eat. I find this brand exciting because it has the power to really become so well known through its appeal and many of the big-name magazines are writing about the products; because it's a celebrity-loved brand, they like to include these sorts of trendy ranges throughout their beauty features. The more readers that see these types of brands in 'those' sorts of magazines, the more likely it may be that new people will become converted to natural and organic brands. I love that they are very honest and upfront about what's in their products. 100% Pure products are truly 100% pure – no synthetic chemicals, chemical preservatives, artificial fragrances, artificial colors, harsh detergents or any other unhealthy toxins. The makeup range is truly special; they use fruit powders to obtain their colors and pigments, and due to the healing powers of fruits and vegetables the makeup is actually really good for your skin too. Everything smells so darn pretty and the makeup is truly exceptional. Such a great brand!

- ✓ 100percentpure.com
- ✓ 100percentpure.co.uk
- ✓ 100percentpure.com.au

Amakai

The UK really has some wonderful made and owned brands, and Amakai is another company who do the natural health world very proud. I have recently become a huge fan of their delectable skin creams that not only smell incredible but have simple and effective ingredients that are wonderful for dry and even sensitive skins. Their products are on average 80% organic and completely 100% natural. They also support fair trade charities, and their packaging is 100% recyclable and reusable.

✓ amakaiskincare.com

AESOS

This one-of-a-kind UK-owned and made brand have created an ingenious line of skincare that is so unique. Each product contains crushed-up rose and clear quartz crystals which are said to re-energize the skin. Each product contains the best organic herbs (with many that are bio-dynamic) and exquisite oils. This luxury brand has beautiful and luxurious products for face, body, bath, their own crystallized perfumes, and they also have a beautiful makeup range, also made with biodynamic ingredients.

✓ aeos.co.uk

Live Native

Live Native is another favorite range of mine, which is also highly unique. Their products contain nothing but the best organic and 'raw' ingredients – this means nothing heated above 45 degrees, and formulated with absolutely zero harsh chemicals. Their face and body products are just exquisite and skin responds really well to them. They have also created 'raw' deodorants which are unique to the market. Their 'Every Body Every Day Cream' is good enough to eat! A truly remarkable and original brand.

✓ Livenative.com

Jane Iredale Makeup

Jane Iredale is known as 'the skincare makeup' brand. The company's philosophy is to create only makeup that is good for the skin. Using many organic ingredients, each product goes through a strict cleaning process to remove most of the heavy metals that are commonly found in the minerals which originally come from the earth. Only natural preservatives are used. The products are truly phenomenal, innovative and long-lasting. They leave the skin looking truly flawless. Nothing will disappoint! It's my personal favorite makeup brand and I have tested much of their range.

✓ janeiredale.com

Terra D'Oc Makeup

This French brand also has EcoCert certification. Each product is from 100% natural origin and has on average 20% organic ingredients. The colors and effectiveness of the products are really incredible. This fantastic range rivals some of the top makeup brands. Their liquid foundation is divine.

✓ pravera.co.uk/terre-doc

Miessence

This Australian brand started out very small, but is now a global company. Miessence sells pure organic products for hair, body, skin, makeup, supplements, babies and men, as well as offering a stunning perfume range. And all are 100% certified food-grade organic ingredients, which is quite rare in the beauty world. This range is another one of my personal favorites.

You can find Miessence through my website:

✓ www.missecoglam.com

Benecos Cosmetics

This German-made range is *very* exciting, mainly because of its very low price point, yet contains high quality and safe ingredients. Natural and organic brands do usually tend to be more expensive than the common beauty brands, so can sometimes be out of people's budget -especially for teenagers. Benecos is a beauty brand that has an extensive makeup selection with all prices under £10.00. It is a range of 100% natural ingredients with many certified organic ingredients. The products therefore contain no:

- Paraffin
- Parabens
- Silicones

- PEG
- Synthetic Colour
- Synthetic Fragrance
- Synthetic Preservatives

I absolutely love this brand because of the price. I am very lucky and regularly get free products to test out for my site but when I do have to buy products, I am actually quite a cheapskate, I don't want to spend a lot on something I need to use all the time. At the time of writing, I have tested out their natural foundation and without a doubt, its one of the *best* I have ever tried. The texture is simply fantastic, provides the best coverage yet feels light on the skin. It also smells beautiful with a hint of lime. A little bit really goes a long way, which again, is great for people's wallets. Benecos unfortunately only have three shades on offer at the moment so the foundation won't suit all skins but those that can wear it will probably be as thrilled as I am. They also sell natural-based nail polishes too as well as stock mascaras, mineral powders, eyeshadows, lipsticks etc. Even if you can't wear the foundation, their other makeup products will suit your skin no matter what the colour. Prices on average are £6.99

✓ benecos.eu
✓ pravera.co.uk/benecos-natural-beauty

Intelligent Nutrients

This impressive range was developed by the founder of Aveda, who wanted to create a 100% safe range for his customers. So pure are his products, the organic ingredients are actually certified food-grade organic and no harsh chemicals are ever used. Not content with making products as good as these, scientists and chemists set about creating something very unique – plant stem cells. These are culti- vated in the purest lab conditions without soil; they are toxin-free and incubated in complete nutrition from the mother host: the plant. This is a world first, using and manipulating Nature in a way that is both revolutionary but still kind to Nature. This huge range has products for hair, skin, body, supplements, teas, chocolate, baby and pet care. A truly trustworthy and stunning brand.

✓ intelligentnutrients.com

The Honest Company

If you are looking for a range you can really trust *this* is it. Jessica Alba is a celebrity recognized all over the world for her acting abilities and of course, stunning looks. But she's soon to become a household name in the eco world too. Jessica's just authored her first book, *The Honest Life*, which educates and inspires people, parents in particular, to become more toxin aware. Like this book you are reading, she shares advice on how to eat better and how to find safer products to use.

After becoming pregnant with her first daughter, Honour, Jessica became very passionate about finding out how to give her child the best start in life. She was shocked as to how many chemicals there are in the world and how they are affecting all of our kids. Jessica realized it was hard to find truly 100% toxic free diapers, 100% safe cleaning products and proven completely skincare for children and adults. With the huge gaps in the market, Jessica formed the 'Honest Company' and now offers an impressive and inexpensive range of beautiful products that have been especially made just for her brand. So pure and effective are some of the formulas, that there are patents pending so it is top secret as to what makes them so good.

None of the Honest Products contain: phthalates (DEHP, BBP, DBP, DMP, DEP); PVC; formaldehyde; alkylphenols; benzene; TEA (Triethanolamine); MEA (Monoethanolamine); parabens; phosphates; chlorine; chlorinated or brominated solvents; ceteareth 20; polyethylene glycol (PEG); resorcinol; bronopol; quaternium 15; nanoparticles; triclosan; sulfur oxides; organohalides; hexavalent chromium; DMDM hydantoin; organophosphate pesticides; 1,4 - dioxane; SLS/SLES (sodium lauryl/laureth sulfates); optical brighteners; mineral oil; petrolatum; BPA (bisphenol-A); a-chlorotoluene

There are shower washes, baby (and adult) body products, toothpastes for kids, sunscreens, things to use in the kitchen and things to clean the bathroom, do your laundry with and there's even an eco-friendly bug spray. Even though I haven't been able to test them personally yet, from what I have read, the Honest diapers do sound absolutely amazing. Not only are they super cute to look at, with trendy patterns like skulls, peacocks and bright checks, they are quite possibly the best eco diapers on the planet due to the materials used. They have plant based inner and outer layers, are produced with no chlorine or harsh chemical bleaches and use natural citrus *and* chlorophyll odor-ihibitors. Corn and wheat is blended together and found in the absorbent core and they use sustainably harvested wood pulp. There are even diapers/nappies you can use for kids when they swim.

Parents can join up to get these beautiful diapers, skincare, supplements and cleaning products delivered on an 'autoship' basis so that you don't have to worry about re-ordering.

Theres even a small range of organic whole-food supplements for kids and pregnant mothers. They are GMO free and don't contain any synthetic fillers.

I'm hoping we can eventually buy them in the UK and other countries too. I have a feeling we will - Jessica is onto something pretty special with this company – it's one that you can completely trust because you realize that she uses all this stuff on her own kids and wouldn't allow anything less then the best. It's great to see a celebrity use their fame for so much good.

✓ honest.com

The Organic Pharmacy

Created in 2002, the Organic Pharmacy I think single-handedly made 'organic' appeal to the high-end customer; no longer was 'organic' a word associated only with hippies. Margo Marrone and her husband

Franco have been so successful that The Organic Pharmacy products are now sold globally and regularly featured in magazines such as *Vogue* and *Harper's Bazaar*. Margo is a trained homeopath and also studied pharmacy, specializing in herbal medicine and nutrition. The Organic Pharmacy has a huge range of products for men, teenagers, children, babies and women, and they really are as organic as they appear.

Most of their products are 99.9% organic – the only non-organic ingredient in these is non-organic vitamin E which is still naturally derived. Other products are over the 95% organic level and some of the very high-tech products are 85% organic but they always clearly state this in their packaging. In their stores, highest-quality homeopathic and herbal remedies are available and personally tailored to the customer. These are truly exquisite and trustworthy products.

✓ theorganicpharmacy.com

So Pure Skin Care

So Pure Skin Care is created by Geeta Sood who dreamt of making her own organic skincare range since she was a little girl. After completing intensive skincare training in the formulation of natural products, Geeta launched her own line in the UK in May 2013. Her products are all 100% natural and highly organic. They also smell absolutely divine. Her anti-aging Nutrient Elixir is just out of this world. Geeta's talent is that she uses unusual ingredients such as prickly pear, tomato, date seed oils and as well as brown seaweed, edelweiss flower, white lily, yeast collagen and Hyaluronic acid - both vegetable derived. This lady really knows her stuff and has created a truly special range. Look out for her orange scented cleansing balm, which is so wonderfully thick and rich and leaves the skin glowing.

✓ sopureskincare.co.uk

Alpha Dream Raw Creams by Raw Living

Over the years, I have been sent so many things to test out and these

Alpha Dream creams are absolutely *amazing*. Handmade with love and care, these 100% raw vegan unique creams are just delicious on the skin. The 'Alpha Dream Cream' smells good enough to eat (you actually *could* eat it, it's that natural – and yes, I did try!), and the 'Alpha Dream Supreme Cream' also has a slight touch of edible glitter in it so makes your skin sparkle in the light. It contains MSM, hemp oil, cacao butter, Monoi de Tahiti and coconut butter. There is even an 'Alpha Dream Dragon' cream for men (although you may end up stealing it for yourself). These creams are truly a joy to use.

✓ rawliving.eu

Dr. Bronner's Magic Soaps

This may well be one of the most ethical brands on the planet. Dr. Bronner was a very eccentric man who was always super-passionate about the planet and people's health. He created a liquid soap and on the bottles he also wrote very inspiring words and messages about how to keep the planet beautiful. He did this 60 years ago before being eco was cool, and was a true pioneer in the natural beauty world. Today his products are sold all over the globe and the company also employs fair trade farmers to produce their ingre-dients. Everything is organic, high quality, and the original messages are still on the bottles today – makes for a very enlightening read. The best-selling all-in-one soaps last for a very long time and have 18 uses, from washing your hair to cleaning your laundry.

Dr. Bronner passed away quite a few years ago now but his family still run the company and, despite it being worth many millions, the company have a rule whereby salaries are capped at approximately US $200,000 per year. Other employees annually receive 15% of their salary paid into a retirement/profit-sharing plan, up to 25% of salary as a bonus, and a no-deductible PPO health insurance plan for themselves and their families. The Dr. Bronner company is so passionate about being 100% ethical that they are making a stand when it comes to other not-so-fair companies – they have actually created the 'coming clean' organization, which is putting pressure on brands who call themselves organic when they really are not. This pressure (involving court cases) has encouraged many brands to change their formulations and/or marketing claims. Dr. Bronner's sells many other brilliant own-brand products as well.

✓ drbronners.com

Australian Bush Flower Essences 'Love System'

Just before my book went to print, I was sent a selection of products from this range which I had yet to test out. Ironically, it had taken me years to be led to this newly favorite brand which, like Miessence, another favorite of mine, is also Australian! I find it funny I had to travel halfway around the world to realize that the best skincare in the world was created right in Australia. Australian Bush Flower Essences and the Love System is now at the very top of my list for highly recommended skincare ranges that tick all the boxes. In fact, it does more than that – it surpasses all of my expectations. There is not another range on the planet that has had so much creativity, care and thought go into the products. I have a lot to tell you about the many wonderful qualities of this range.

Australian Bush Flower Essences was created many years ago, in fact over 25, by its founder, Ian White, who grew up in the outback of Australia. He came from a long line of healers and herbalists, and his grandmother was the first to show him about the little-understood yet extremely powerful effects that Australian plants, herbs and flowers had on the human skin, spirit and wellbeing. These exquisite essences are now loved by hundreds and thousands of mothers, fathers, healers and practitioners all around the globe. I am going to tell you more about their wonderful essences (used for mind, body and health) in Chapter 37, 'Natural Ways of Healing Your Child'.

The skincare line, aka the 'Love System', took creator Paul Loveday 7 years to create. Combining his skills from his background in pioneering natural medicine modalities (homeopathy, herbal medicine and natural skincare), the Love System products are a work of art. Combined, they contain over 110 naturopathic bespoke ingredients, ones that were specifically chosen for bringing vibrance to the skin, enjoyment from the beautiful scents and a self-acceptance to the soul. The Love System is the meaning of a truly holistic range.

Australia has the harshest climatic conditions in the world, so the flora has evolved to withstand yet still thrive in such extreme conditions (hardly any rain, extreme heat etc.), which is why the products are so profoundly effective for the user. The company even offers a guarantee that they will work on a superficial level and on a deeper, spiritual level.

I love every aspect of this range. I cannot find one thing that is not exceptional. On an appearance level, the packaging is bright and beautifully designed and looks wonderful in the bathroom. The lids and pumps are of the best quality so you won't find the product getting clogged. I love the way the essences are clearly marked on each product, making it easy for you to go and research them if you want to. And on closer inspection, you will see that there are inspirational words printed on the boxes (all ethically produced, by the way, with recycled paper and eco-friendly inks), such as 'Love Your Body, Love Your Soul, Love Who You Are'. And on the product itself the directions say: 'Gently apply to your beautiful face.' Seeing words like this every day may actually be quite *powerful* for the user, more than what you might initially think. How many of us do not feel this loving way about ourselves? Too many. The mind is very easily prone to messages that we see around us all the time, and most of the time it's the negative messages that get locked into our subconscious. People are now educating others to surround themselves with positive affirmations and to 'change their thoughts to change their life', to help turn their negative self-view into a much more positive one. Using products like the Love System, and seeing the beautiful inscriptions every day, truly does help you to start seeing more of those positive messages.

The high-quality packaging is certainly very impressive but more so is what is *inside* these gorgeous bottles and tubes. The delicate combinations of the very powerful Australian flora are comparable to no other range I have tried before. With cute-sounding essences such as 'Billy Goat Plum', 'Five Corners', 'Bottle Brush', 'Little Flannel Flower' and 'Fringed Violet', each product contains at least 6 combinations of essences from the 110 ingredients that have been researched and extensively tested by the company. The scent of each product is truly divine, with a different experience from one product to the next. No product is too heavy or too oily and the skin just seems to drink the creams, lotions and gels right in, but without still feeling like more is needed.

The company is famous for its 'emergency' range which has been loved worldwide for its immediately soothing and calming abilities. The oral spray in particular is a well-known 'must have' for natural-health enthusiasts and one that I regularly use on Lola when she is a bit unsettled due to teething or being overtired. It's truly amazing.

Some of the delicious scents I have never experienced before, due to the rareness of the ingredients used. Each product contains a very high percentage of organic and ethically sourced ingredients and this is clearly marked on each box/product. Products are at least 75% organic and most are around the 85–90% mark. Despite the Love System being such a high-quality product, its items are quite affordable yet the company have made sure they are still paying the farmers very fair prices. Part of the profits goes to the 'Love Trust', helping people in need around the world.

I am definitely a huge, huge fan and recommend this range to anyone. No wonder the company receive thousands of emails, letters, calls and countless testimonials from people all over the world, raving that their products not only improved their skin, but changed the way they feel about themselves on a much deeper level. No wonder it's expanding so fast and is found in 30 countries worldwide. More to come about this beautiful range for its medicinal purposes in Chapter 37

✓ ausflowers.com.au

Dr. Alkaitis

The story of this brand is quite amusing. Dr. Alkaitis is a highly acclaimed research scientist and an expert authority on organics, as well as being a molecular biologist, ethnopharmacologist (studying traditional ways of healing, mainly with plants), pharmacognosist (studying the medicinal properties of plants), *and* he has a PhD in physical chemistry. His wife used to bring home beauty products, show him and ask his opinion. Most of the time he would say, 'Nope, these are not good. I would *not* put that on my skin.' So, to get his wife using safe products, he made and developed his own range of products that are so safe, you can actually eat the products. Dr. Alkaitis uses certified organic, bio-dynamic and ethically wild-crafted ingredients in their raw state for the greatest effectiveness.

✓ alkaitis.org

* * *

The brands listed below are the companies which Dr. Bronner's have put pressure on to change their marketing claims and formulas. Till they do, it may be best to avoid them.

- Avalon 'Organics'
- Desert Essence 'Organics'
- Earth's Best 'Organic'
- Giovanni 'Organic'
- Goodstuff 'Organics'
- Head 'Organics'
- Kiss My Face 'Certified Organic Botanicals'
- Nature's Gate 'Organics'
- Physician's Formula 'Organic' Wear
- Stella McCartney '100% Organic'

(organicconsumers.org)

Yes! You can trust these certified organic products:

- Alteya Organics
- Baby Bear Shop
- Badger
- Brittanie's Thyme
- Bubble and Bee Organic
- Earth Mama Angel Baby
- Indian Meadow Herbals
- Kimberly Parry Organics
- Little Angel
- Mercola products
- Nature's Paradise
- Niko Cosmetics
- OGmama and OGbaby
- Organicare
- Organic Essence
- Origins Organics
- Purely Shea
- Rose Tattoo Aftercare
- Saint Francis Organics
- SoCal Cleanse
- Sensibility Soaps/Nourish
- Terressentials
- Trillium Organics
- Vermont Soap

Many of these brands I have told you about are sold over the world, so if something takes your fancy just google the name wherever you are in the world, and see if the range is available to you, or check the websites provided.

I also believe that there are some good products out there that, while they might not be 100% natural, or 100% organic, are OK due to missing the worst chemicals. If they are labeled in a way that is clear and they are not abusing the organic and natural claims, then they may still be worth purchasing. If you can find beauty products that are *without* the sorts of ingredients listed below, then you are still onto something that is far better than typical mainstream brands.

- Parabens
- Sulfates
- Propylene glycol
- Phthalates
- PABA
- Petrolatum
- Paraffin
- DEA

Of course, buying products as pure as possible is always best but it really depends also on how much you cut down the *entire* amount of toxins in other areas of life – that is what makes a huge difference. No one avoids cancer just because they stop using toxic beauty products; a big change has to be made *holistically*. Excluding toxins from beauty products is definitely a great way to start, but there are other changes, which are also very important. I will be discussing them throughout this book.

A little tip about organic products is that you will find they usually last you much longer than the typical supermarket and mainstream 'fashionable' products. This is because they are much more concentrated due to the natural ingredients. The big brands are usually cheaper, yes, but you tend to need to use lots more to do the 'job', so you end up buying more regularly, which in fact, costs you more in the long run. We also generally have much more respect for things that cost us more. We tend to not waste them whereas with a cheaper product we subconsciously squirt out a lot more as we think, 'Oh, it only cost me 3 quid' or 'a few bucks'.

Despite all of this scary news about ingredients in beauty products, there are some good changes happening in certain countries. The French government has now banned the inclusion of parabens in beauty products, so let's hope the rest of the world follows suit soon. Great step forward, but an enormously long way still to go. That's only one ingredient from a big list that's much longer than your arm.

There are so many fantastic brands these days that it's impossible to list them all here. I have most likely left out many great ones that I have not yet heard about. Sometimes there are great brands made by small companies who cannot afford to be officially credited with being 100% organic but may actually be in fact, very organic.

In relation to how they choose their products, some people follow this motto: 'Don't use anything on your skin that you wouldn't eat.' While it does make sense, and is a great way to choose your skincare, I do feel that, as previously mentioned, you have to limit your toxic exposure in as *many* aspects as your life as possible.

Hair to die for

Unfortunately hair dyes are probably the most *dangerous* products we can possibly use. I actually read a book on pregnancy in 2012 and they were saying that hair dyes are completely safe to use when pregnant! That nearly made me laugh out loud when I read it as I have it on good advice from a top scientist I personally know (who is a biochemist and knows how products are formulated as he makes his own) that hair dyes are *extremely* poisonous. I have been coloring my own hair every month or so since I was 12. I cringe when I think about how many times that is over the last 22 years. I used toxic hair colorants for most of that time too, until I knew better.

Coloring hair is so dangerous, not only because of the formulation, but because the products get applied directly to our scalp (which is even more easily penetrated by toxins than our skin is) and then washed off quite vigorously with hot water, again making the toxins more absorbable through the scalp. And for the raven-haired beauties out there, I have got bad news for you: the darker the coloring, the more dangerous it is toxin-wise.

The main nasty ingredients in hair colors are: ammonia, resor-cinol, parabens, and the most dangerous is p-Phenylenediamine. This last chemical has been banned in many countries but alarmingly is still allowed in products in the UK and has been directly linked to several cases this year of severe allergic reaction and, sadly, a few deaths.

Each year many women report these allergic reactions, some so serious that they have to be admitted to hospital. In a recent case in England, hair dye caused a lady to be put in the intensive care unit because she had such a severe reaction; it almost killed her. Within hours her face and scalp began to swell so badly that her eyes were almost shut and her scalp was weeping pus. She said it was the scariest experience of her life, and she literally thought she was going to die.

There was another case that happened literally 2 weeks after the one I just mentioned, which tragically caused a 17-year-old to lose her life. She had been coloring her hair for many years and finally her body had had enough of the chemicals, so she developed an immediate and violent allergy and died on her living room floor in front of her family. Her hair dye contained – wait for it – p-Phenylenediamine. And another case was reported in the paper today, again a near-fatal incident, directly related to p-Phenylenediamine.

Thankfully, many of us will not have a reaction like this to hair dyes, but that does not mean they cannot do us harm. We never see the chemicals that go into our body; they simply get absorbed, lying dormant, with the body unsure of how to deal with them.

While I can't say you must stop coloring your hair (most of us ladies are quite proud of our hair and would rather stay home than be seen with bad roots or grey hairs showing), I can suggest some excellent alternatives that are much, much safer for you to use.

Just to make you aware, p-Phenylenediamine sometimes shows up in so-called 'natural hair dyes'. So make sure you check the back of the label before you purchase. This is the most dangerous chemical used in hair colorants.

Daniel Field Mineral Water Colors

This company has a great selection of different colors that are made from pure minerals, and are mixed only with warm water to activate them. The product turns into a light foamy mousse so is very easy to apply. It is so gentle on the scalp and hair itself that it does not do one ounce of damage to your hair. The only problem is, these colors don't tend to last as long as the regular chemical-based ones. But they are quite inexpensive too so you will be able to afford to color your hair every 3 weeks if you need to. They do cover grey as well, but heat needs to be applied. A little tip is to use a hair dryer while the product is on to help activate the color.

Logona Naturkosmetik Colors

I only recently discovered these incredible colors from German company Logona, which are based on henna but have added softeners and shine enhancers which make the hair soft and shiny as well as changing the hair to the shade that is desired. These colors cannot lighten the hair, only darken or enhance, but they contain heavy-metal-free minerals from the earth. They use organic ingredients, are EcoCert approved and are completely 100% natural. If you have grey hair, give this brand a miss.

Henna

Another alternative is using henna, but you must try and get an organic brand as most hennas are full of heavy metals. Henna can be messy as you have to mix the mixture into a thick sandy paste, but the effect it gives to your hair is pretty amazing. It also covers grey very well. And the ingredients come from Nature, not from a laboratory.

Surya Henna Colors

These 100% natural henna-based colors cover stubborn greys from the first application. They contain no peroxides, ammonia, resor-cinol, PPD, parabens or heavy metals. You can purchase as a powder and add water to it, or purchase premixed so you can apply straight away to the hair. The colors contain essential oils of rose, ylang ylang, jasmine and sandalwood plus many other enriched plant extracts. They are semi-permanent colors and only last around 7 washes but are so kind to the hair. The formulas actually help with the condition of hair and also growth. They are so natural and non-harming that they can be used on people undergoing chemotherapy. They are sold worldwide so please google the brand name to find where you can buy closest to you. This brand is truly *amazing* – I personally won't be using any other hair coloring product apart from this one in the future.

* * *

For a fantastic organic salon in London, I thoroughly recommend Hair Organics in Notting Hill where they use the complete Daniel Field Range and other high-quality organic brands. I had a color there last year and it was probably the best I have ever had. My hair was slightly lightened with their seaweed-based product (I wanted to be more red) but there was *no* damage at all. They even now do a high-gloss treatment that lasts 6–8 weeks which is entirely natural.

Here are the websites for the products mentioned:
- ✓ danielfield.com (Mineral Semi Colors)
- ✓ suvarna.co.uk (Surya Henna and Logona)
- ✓ hairorganics.co.uk (London Salon)
- ✓ amazon.com and co.uk (Surya and Henna)

Hair styling products

Hairspray is *extremely* toxic and must be avoided as much as possible as it easily gets into the body. It's very hard not to breathe it in when it's sprayed on your hair. Sadly, hairdressers have statistically shorter lives (and increased risk of health problems) due to constantly being around hair colors, washing countless people's hair with toxic sulfate-based shampoos, and using massive amounts of styling products. They breathe in countless fumes from the products and they also absorb them through their skin.

What gives the 'hold' in hairsprays is the chemical formulation, which is like a glue, and comes from solvents and polymers. Don't they sound like they belong in paint, not in your hair product? You only have to smell them to know that these things aren't meant for your lungs to breathe in! And sometimes extracts from fish are used as well to make hairspray. Prawns in particular! Yuck!

The eco-friendly brand Lavera make a fabulous non-toxic hairspray and it's quite inexpensive too. It's sold in Whole Foods, Planet Organic and most health-food shops as well as online stores. You will find this brand worldwide. You can also check out Intelligent Nutrients, and Suncoat, who both make non-toxic hair products.

Personal hygiene products

Ladies, if there is one thing I feel so strongly about and beg you to take note, it is to change your ordinary tampons to organic ones. It might literally save your life.

Here is why: tampons and pads are made from cotton (as well as other chemicals too). Cotton is one of the most heavily sprayed crops, with countless pesticides and fungicides used. It literally is an extremely toxic and dirty crop. Throughout one growing cycle, sometimes up to 40 different chemicals are sprayed onto the cotton. Each and every chemical is labeled toxic and dangerous on the container that it comes in. When you take cotton products home, despite the workers washing the cotton during the process, these chemicals are still on whatever you buy. In fact, it could take countless washes to remove all of the toxins.

If you use non-organic cotton tampons and pads (tampons being the worst by far because they go right inside your body) for many years, then each time of the month, for those few days, you are literally sticking toxic poisons directly into your most private of parts! Your body is absorbing these chemicals, however minute the amount may be that day. Over time, they will more than likely build up to an amount (along with all the other chemicals in life) that is just not safe. Cotton products such as pads, tampons and toilet paper also contain dioxins which are used to make the product white. This is a form of bleach and very worrying as well.

If you continue to use these products for years and years, as well as the other typical cotton things, then I think it makes sense to assume that this is putting you at serious risk of problems.

Cervical cancer has been linked to sexual activity from a young age, but there is evidence suggesting that using these toxic sanitary products could be making that risk much, much higher.

Not only do we have to worry about the pesticides used in feminine products, but there is also another highly dangerous chemical used in the production process. Anything that is bleached in terms of paper and cotton contains dioxins, which are persistent environmental pollutants. According to the World Health Organization, they are extremely toxic and can cause reproductive and developmental problems, damage the immune system, interfere with hormones, and also cause cancer. Because dioxins are in the majority of feminine hygiene products and used from a very young age, their use really concerns me. And it's not just me that is trying to spread awareness about the hidden dangers of using bleached sanitary products. According to the Livestrong website:

House Resolution 373, named the tampon safety legislation, was introduced in Congress in January 2003 by Congresswoman Maloney of the 14th District of New York. This legislation directs the Institute of Health 'to research health risks to women – including endometriosis and cancers of the breast, ovaries, and cervix – from the presence of dioxin, synthetic fibers, and other additives in feminine products.' The Endometriosis Association in their report indicates, 'Until research addresses the risks, health experts recommend unbleached, organic cotton sanitary pads and tampons (without plastic applicators).'[16]

The concerning problem with dioxins is that they stick around in the environment, and in the body, for a very long time. When in the body, they are attracted to the fatty tissues which is where they will stay put as they have a life of 7–11 years. But logically, we will *always* have a certain level of them in our bodies because we absorb them every single day. Dioxins are now found in animals too, so if you eat meat or fish regularly you will be eating a higher concentration as the animals and fish would have eaten them in their food too. Dioxins are also found in dairy. They are in the soil and in the air due to manufacturing processes and from factory accidents.

I personally stopped using normal tampons years ago and have been buying Natracare or Organyc products ever since. They are both fantastic and, most importantly, completely safe to use. They do not irritate or cause you to itch like some sanitary items can.

✓ Natracare.com

✓ organyc.co.uk

You can also find ethical menstruation products such as 'moon times sea sponges'. These are natural sponges that you insert just like a tampon and can be washed and reused over and over again. They are non-irritating, comfortable, and can also be composted when they have started to degrade.

✓ moontimes.co.uk

Many people are also starting to use reusable pads made from organic cotton and bamboo; some are even backed with wool or felt. They can come in all different shapes, sizes and thicknesses. These are so soft to wear and much more comfortable than any disposable product can be.

✓ earthwisegirls.co.uk

Some women love using a 'moon cup' (known in the USA as MCUK) which is reusable and made from medical grade non-toxic silicone. You basically insert it like you would a tampon and remove it when you would normally change to a new one and wash the moon cup out with water, and replace. This is the most environmental way of dealing with your 'time of the month' because you do not throw anything away. Knowing that the average woman may use approximately 11,000 pads or tampons in their lifetime, this innovative little device is really wonderful.

mooncup.co.uk

Please think about at least changing to organic sanitary products or any of these other products ASAP, if not *today*. You just don't want harmful products in your body, or even next to your skin, let alone against your private parts.

Shocking facts about 'natural' cotton

- The California EPA reported that only 15 chemicals accounted for 77% of the pesticides used on cotton from 1989 to 1998 and that these were some of the most toxic chemicals in the world. Cal EPA and US EPA analyses illustrate that 7 of these 15 most-used cotton chemicals were probable cancer-causing pesticides, 8 caused tumors, and 5 caused mutations. Twelve of the top 15 cotton pesticides in California caused birth defects, 10 caused multiple birth defects, and 13 were toxic or very toxic to fish or birds or both.
- On average, 7 times as many pounds of toxic fertilizer are regularly used on cotton as are pesticides. Cotton fertilizers have fouled the air and polluted rivers, groundwater basins and aquifers wherever cotton is grown.
- Cotton fertilizers and pesticides have killed and injured millions of fish, birds and other wildlife as well as countless thousands of rural residents.
- 75% of the cotton and cottonseed in the USA is genetically modified.[17]

Cotton is really a terrible product and it's best to try and avoid buying it. I realize it's cheap and most clothes are made from it, but many times we don't really need anything new! Most of us have far too many clothes!

Not only is it better for us to avoid cotton, but it is safer for the poor farmers who are, more often than not, working in very harsh conditions, usually in very hot countries, with nothing to breathe in except for the dirty pesticides. Many people (sadly, young children included) have died from this exposure to the chemicals used on the crops. *How many?* An estimated minimum 1 million cases of pesticide poisoning occur every year, resulting in 20,000 reported deaths among agricultural workers and at least 1 million requiring hospitalization.[18]

Cotton farming is also causing a massive environmental impact. So much water is used, children are being used as slave labor to farm it, and of course the chemicals are going into the environment as well; and even more shocking, the chemicals from the clothes seep into our own skin. Most of our clothes are also derived from petrol and from plastic.

Wearing organic cotton or certified organic bamboo clothing is a much better alternative. Plenty of companies online are now offering these types of fabrics in their collections. Use Google to find out where.

I am a big fan of Asquith of London which is a brand that makes bamboo and organic cotton yoga and leisure wear:

✓ asquith-yoga-clothing.co.uk

For bamboo clothing you can shop online at BAM:

✓ bambooclothing.co.uk

Emma Nissin produces amazing fashionable clothing that is made with:

- 100% organic cotton
- 70% sustainably grown bamboo and 30% organic cotton
- Lenzing Tencel – made predominately from eucalyptus
- Lenzing MicroModal – made predominately from beech wood

✓ emmanissimshop.com

You can also purchase clothes made from hemp fibers; hemp is also a very skin-friendly and environmentally friendly fabric. Purchasing vintage clothing is a great way to make use of clothes that would otherwise be thrown away. Luckily it's also very 'cool' to wear vintage so, if you are into fashion, you may just love this type of clothing. Lots of vintage clothing is also made from synthetic fabrics so you really have to learn what is a natural fabric versus manmade. I personally love shopping for vintage; today's clothes don't have a patch on quality in comparison to well-made vintage.

Deodorants

Now we get back to personal care products. Regular use of an aluminum-based deodorant is a *disaster* waiting to happen to your health. This chemical alone has been directly linked to breast cancers[19] which are so prevalent in women today, more than ever before, and now that men are affected by these types of products as well, some are getting diagnosed with breast cancer too. Aluminum is what makes you stop sweating – 'keeps you dry' like the advertisements tell us. The problem is, stopping sweat itself is not natural for the body and is a health problem in itself. That area (and other areas with lymph glands) of the body is meant to sweat, for the purpose of detoxifying the body, and if it doesn't do its job, then how do the toxins get out? Well, they don't get out through there – that's for sure. And because we spray the deodorant directly onto the underarm gland, it means that the chemicals get transported into the body much more quickly than something applied to regular skin.

Thankfully, there are many non-toxic deodorants available these days and some are very inexpensive. I like the 'crystal' mineral deodorants which are completely natural. You can buy them in rock form, spray and a roll-on.

Products without aluminum do not stop you from sweating, but as I mentioned previously, it's a bad thing to stop the body from doing what it is meant to. We need to work with our bodies, not against them. It is also worth noting: if your body odor is not exactly pretty, that too can be a sign of an imbalance that is happening inside of you. Sweat should smell OK, not gross or too overpowering. Later on you will hear about my own story of smelling bad. Changing to a non-toxic deodorant is a must, so please do so today!

Check out the brands: Lavera, Weleda, Madara, Live Native, The Organic Pharmacy and Alva, for safe deodorants. These are my favorites. You can purchase most of these brands worldwide. There is also a fun recipe in the back of the book, in the DIY section, for how to make your own deodorant.

Fake tans

Oh goodness me, these products really, really are of great concern because they are used so much these days, even by very young girls. It's quite sad to see these beautiful young things with so much fake tan on that they look almost orange or like a clown. They are copying the celebrities they see on TV who have made this orange look 'fashionable'.

Not only is it so *not* attractive, these formulas are, more often than not, very heavily chemical-based. I used to use fake tans years ago and they would make my skin so dry and quite often itchy. This alone was enough to hint to me that the formula was not kind to the skin, and because it was sprayed, rubbed in and left on, this meant a huge amount of the body was covered by the product, up to 95% in fact. Also, information is now showing that for 24 hours after fake tan has been applied, your skin is much more susceptible to free-radical damage from the sun. The ironic thing is, in a survey conducted with women who use fake tan, most of them said they felt that their fake tan protected them from the sun and they would go out and not cover up.

What is concerning about salon spray tan procedures is that you breathe in the product as it's being sprayed on your body. It enters through your nose, mouth and also your eyes and of course through the skin, and if it's something you do regularly, well, you know what

I am going to say: it's not a good thing for your health long term. Many of the fake tanners contain parabens, among other things, and these ingredients harm the endocrine system, disrupting hormones, and if you are pregnant they can harm the baby's development. These can negatively affect even your weight, your energy and your moods. If you can't go without using fake tan, Lavera, Jane Iredale, The Organic Pharmacy and Green People all make wonderful self-tanning products that are natural, highly organic and are really lovely on the skin. And they won't give you that dreadful, yet sadly ridiculously popular oompa-loompa effect either!

- ✓ Janeiredale.com
- ✓ greenpeople.co.uk
- ✓ Lavera.co.uk
- ✓ theorganicpharmacy.com

Nail products

I am sure you can guess what I am about to say, and that is that nail polishes are just like house paint and are highly toxic. Yes, it's true. And because our nail beds on the fingers and toes are very porous, the chemicals get into the bloodstream very quickly. The toes are actually more porous than the fingernails as the nail itself is quite a lot thicker. I used to wear nail polish a lot when younger, but now I find that having short tidy nails which have been buffed to appear super-shiny is the best way to look after your nails. They look naturally healthy and also grow very fast due to the buffing action on the nail. It stimulates blood and brings fresh nutrients to the area. If you can't go without painting your toenails or fingernails, then I can recommend the following safer nail brands:

- ✓ Butterlondon.com
- ✓ Mavala.co.uk
- ✓ Suncoatproducts.com
- ✓ Theorganicpharmacy.com
- ✓ Scotchnaturals.com
- ✓ Kurebazaar.com

✓ Zoya.com

Is there a safe nail polish remover?

I never thought that there was until recently, but I have come across one made entirely with vegetable and fruit extracts which does a wonderful job of removing nail polish, even the toxic kind, and does not strip your nails and surrounding skin of vital oils. Eden, by Fresh Therapies, has created this unique lime-scented polish remover that is just brilliant.

✓ freshtherapies.com

False nails

And what about fake nails that are made with acrylic or gel? Don't even think that they could be good for you! The smell alone in the nail shops should tell you just how bad they are. It stinks to high heaven, and all of those fumes are not only breathed in by you as the nail technician applies them, but you absorb into your body whatever is stuck onto your nail! I remember being told this shocking story: a friend knew a lady who owned a popular nail salon, and she would quite often do home visits to clients. One hot summer's day, she left her nail products in her car while she went to get lunch. Guess what happened? The chemicals literally created a 'bomb', which blew her entire car up! Luckily no one was hurt, but it made the lady realize just how dangerous nail products were and she stopped doing them then and there.

And in any case, the amount of nail infections from a *fungus* that grows underneath the false nail is another reason why natural nails are always best. I used to apply false nails years ago when I worked as a beauty therapist and some of the fungal infections I saw were just gross. Bright green moss-type fungus would grow on the nails and was often quite hard to treat.

It's worth noting: if you can't grow your own nails well, then it could be a sign of a deficiency which can usually be addressed by healthy eating and, most importantly, removing toxins from your body. Our skin, hair and nails are mirrors of what is going on inside the body. They give you clues as to what you may need to add to your diet, or what else is maybe going on with your health.

If you love having colored nails but want another option besides polish, you may be interested in nail transfers – little stickers with patterns or different shades that you put over your nails and file at the edges. These are not eco-friendly at all but they do have fewer chemicals than nail polish does. Personally I don't wear them, but it is another option for you.

Essential oils

When you see these little bottles, you automatically think of them as 'healthy' and 'natural' because they smell nice and come from flowers, plants and herbs, right? Well, what you may not know is that unless they are 100% organic, they tend to be made completely synthetically in a lab and therefore may be highly toxic to the human body. So, if you are using these in facials or in body treatments and beauty products, these so-called healthy oils are actually doing the opposite to what you think they are. They can cause sensitivity on the outside and toxic harm on the inside! I was astounded when I discovered this.

Most beauty brands use the synthetic kind because they are dirt cheap and require no farming or land production to make them. These fake 'oils' make products smell nice, and when marketed using the word 'natural' they fool the customer into thinking that the ingredients really do come from Nature.

My most favorite and trusted organic essential oil brands are:

- NHR Oils
- Young Living
- Miessence

All three brands are of the highest quality I have found. They always smell incredible because they are super-concentrated. Young Living actually has a cancer clinic in South America where the organic essential oils are being taken internally – that is how pure they are.

- ✓ youngliving.com
- ✓ mionegroup.com
- ✓ nhrorganicoils.com
- ✓ tisserand.com
- ✓ nealsyardremedies.com

Perfumes

Perfumes make up a huge percentage of sales in the beauty market and they are absolutely everywhere – every single celebrity seems to be making their own signature scent these days. Whenever we go shopping in department stores, we get offered them to try and even sprayed near us as we walk past. While some may smell beautiful, the problem is, that smell is highly toxic. Perfumes are some of the *worst* products to use if you want to keep your health protected. Despite the expensive price tag, more often than not, these formulas are very cheap to make and it's only the bottle and packaging that has had money go into it. So not only are we getting duped into spending our money on something that appears to be luxurious; the real truth is, it's a toxic soup. And because per*fumes* (quite an ironic spelling, isn't it?) are sprayed into the air and on our body, they go straight into our bloodstream through the nose, the mouth, the eyes and the skin.

Really young girls are buying so much fragrance these days due to their favorite celebrities endorsing them. Because a perfume is generally something that is applied every day, it's adding more to their toxic burden. Perfumes and 'fragrance' are added to so many of our beauty products, in fact to most of them. If they don't smell appealing, who would buy them? Fake fragrance is even used in much of the food we eat too.

Perfumes are especially dangerous because they can contain anywhere between *50 and 200* different ingredients, with only about 2 or 3 being a 'natural' extract. Sometimes none of that content is natural. The rest is all garbage, stuff you wouldn't even want to clean your house with if you knew what it was in its raw form. Ninety-five percent of fragrances contain synthetic chemicals and are also petrolatum-based. Headaches and allergies can be triggered by these chemical concoctions. The fragrance industry uses more than 5000 different chemicals but only approximately 1300 have been tested and evaluated so far.[20]

I really worry about the ladies and men working in perfumeries or department stores, where they are in enclosed spaces, spraying all that stuff around, day in and day out. I don't think they realize that being exposed to those chemicals creates more of a chance of developing asthma, or neurological, cancer and nervous system problems. I absolutely hate walking through that section at the department store. If someone tries to spray me with a perfume, I back right away.

To see what health problems are linked with synthetic perfumes please visit this very informative site:

✓ naturalingredient.org/syntheticfragrances.htm

Thankfully, there are many natural and organic perfume brands that are creating beautiful scents that are non-harmful. My 4 favorites are:

Miessence Perfumes

These are 100% certified organic and oil-based; no alcohol at all is used. There are 6 stunning scents in the range.

✓ mionegroup.com

Intelligent Nutrients Aromatics

These certified organic aromatics were the first in the world to be made entirely from food-grade essential oils and flavors. They contain no petrochemicals, parabens, phthalates or artificial fragrance. Intelligent Nutrients was created by the founder of Aveda, Horst M. Rechelbacher, who wanted to create a range of skin and body products that were so safe you could eat them. The aromatics are exquisite and there are 7 in total.

✓ intelligentnutrients.com

Balm Balm Single Note Perfumes

These 100% organic perfumes are certified by the Soil Association and are highly unique. They are sold as 'single note', which means just one essential oil. There are 7 in total and each is so reasonably priced that you can buy 3 or 4 for the price of a regular mainstream brand and mix and match the scents as you wish. Balm Balm also sell little sample sizes of each of the perfumes so you can experiment with which combination suits you. Personally, I love them all and the fact that you can create a different scent every day if you wish. The company sends tips on combining them together, but really the fun is when you decide what to try.

✓ balmbalm.com

Organic Glam Fragrances by the Organic Pharmacy

These 5 signature luxury perfumes are each 100% natural and 85% organic, and are made from a combination of plants, resins, essential oils, ester and alcohol. These will far exceed any department store perfumes, and won't be damaging at all to your health.

✓ theorganicpharmacy.com

Salon beauty treatments

Having worked as a beauty therapist for almost a decade, I can tell you from experience that visiting a beauty salon is, most of the time, definitely *not* good for your health. If the salon does fake nails (or even manicures and pedicures) there are going to be some pretty nasty fumes in the air. Not only that, but 9 times out of 10, a beauty salon does not use organic and natural products. So when you spend all that money for a facial (or hair treatments at the hairdressers), you are walking away with creams and products used on your skin that will actually age and damage your skin (not to mention your organs internally too) due to the toxic chemicals in the products. We tend to see beauty salons as places of health and beauty, but the opposite is actually more true.

While I have seen some products make the skin 'look' better, it is only temporary due to the clever ingredients used. For sensitive skins, certain chemicals are used to calm the skin down, but it's not usually from a natural source; or if there is a natural source in there, it's only a minute amount. It's unfortunate that these so-called skin experts, the beauty therapists, really *don't know* what truly makes beautiful skin. They talk a lot about this product or that product and very *little* about diet. They, of course, have to talk 'up' whatever brand their salon owner has taken on board. When I was a therapist, I rarely sold anything and would quite often whisper to a client, 'No, don't buy that – it's not good for you.' I lost quite a few jobs due to not selling enough – how unsurprising.

If you do need to visit a beauty salon, try and search for one that uses organic and natural products and does not offer false nails. Talk to the beauty therapist about your concerns with toxins in their products/salon. The more people who mention these things, the more likely the industry may change.

Cosmeceutical beauty treatments

You only have to open a magazine to see the advertisements for Botox, fillers and facial peels, now aimed not only at teenagers and women but nowadays even aimed at men too. I see these ads on trains and buses now as well. These ads, just like for beauty products, are everywhere. While some of the cosmetic effects seem to be impressive, rarely has the skin been treated in a way that is actually good for it long term. And you often have to continue to do the treatments again and again to keep it looking 'good'. During my almost a decade of being in the beauty industry, I had many treatments done on my own skin. I always thought that the more of them I had, the better it would make my skin look. I occasionally would work in a salon where we had doctors practicing Botox and other cosmetic treatments. Once (regrettably), I was used as a guinea pig for the doctor to test out a treatment he was creating. It consisted of a microdermabrasion (a machine that literally sands away the skin!) treatment with some liquid vitamin C infused on the top. While it sounded like a great treatment, it gave me the worst rash I have ever seen, right smack bang all over my forehead. I had to come into work, as I of course wasn't sick – I just looked *really* frightful. The look on my clients' faces when they saw me was hilarious and they all asked immediately, 'What *ever* did you do to your face?' I had to assure them this treatment was not on our menu (but that it was probably on many other salons' menus).

The facial treatment I had was really not that toxic compared to most, but there are a few popular cosmeceutical treatments which are *very* toxic to the skin and body. A common one is a facial peel that uses 'TCA', which stands for trichloroacetic acid, and is one of the most dangerous you can have done. It does exactly as it sounds: it *burns* the skin from an acid reaction. It's used to 'even out pigmentation, improve acne scarring and just generally "refresh" the skin. Sounds like a great treatment, right? Well, not when you know how toxic the actual chemical is. It's acid. If you drank it you would most likely die, so why should we put it on our skin? You wouldn't pour acid onto any other organs, would you?

It's nuts we have actually thought that any type of burning to the skin is a good thing. TCA treatments used to be only carried about by doctors, but now beauty therapists can treat their clients themselves, and most worrying is the fact that pretty much *anyone* can purchase TCA kits off the internet. I know because years ago, I bought a big bottle of TCA liquid myself. I actually found it on Ebay and it was *dirt* cheap. I think it was £5, yet the doctors were charging up to £1000 for one TCA peel (and would recommend a course of several!). And they did the exact same routine as I did: cleanse the face, pat it dry, then apply the liquid, letting it sit on the skin for only a few minutes, wash it off and apply some sort of calming cream – except they made about £995 profit and spent about 10 minutes, all up, doing the treatment.

The chemical is so powerful it can penetrate very deeply into the skin within seconds, which means it also gets very deep into the bloodstream! I treated my face and also my arms *and* chest area. You basically cleanse the skin, dry it, then apply the liquid to the area and wait about 1 minute or so – if you *can*, that is, because it burns immediately and you have to have ice packs at the ready for when it comes off. And it doesn't just end there either: for a few days after the peel, you need to stay at home because your face will go bright red (think: worst sunburn ever!), and then it will peel off in what looks like brown sheets of skin! I shudder at the thought, now looking back, as I know that this peel definitely added to my already high toxic levels of dangerous things I had in my body. My vanity back then was more important to me at times than being careful, and to this day I *regret* doing those peels. My skin has *never* been the same (so sensitive and in some areas quite thick and rough-looking and, at the time of writing this section, just never looks healthy) and now I have to be so careful because I have exfoliated it way too much over the years.

While some of these treatments are held in high regard by plastic and cosmetic surgeons, the safety aspect has never been studied long term. Remember, there is little to no regulation of cosmetics, so at this stage we really *do not know* the harm these chemicals can do long term.

Also be very wary of AHA (alpha hydroxy acid) Peels, Phenol, Retinoic, Jessner and Beta Hydroxy Peels. I am also not too keen on microdermabrasion either, as I think it can be very harsh on the skin. If you do exfoliate, do it occasionally (say, once to twice a week, max) and use something very gentle.

However, if you are after something non-toxic which can help improve and change the texture and appearance of your skin, then you could consider trying the S5 brand, a first ever range of certified organic cosmeceuticals. S5 uses only 100% natural, active, and very powerful ingredients. It is even non-irritating on sensitive skins. All of the products are free of parabens, SLS/SLES, PEGS, DEA, mineral oil, silicon, propylene glycol, GMO and synthetic ingredients.

✓ s5skincare.com

If you do want to try a more intensive peel that won't harm your health, Sunshine Botanicals make a fantastic enzyme peel based on pumpkin. This is an at-home peel you can do yourself and has wonderful results on the skin. All of the products from this brand do not contain parabens, phthalates, propylene glycol, all sulfates, EDTA, synthetic fragrances, mineral oil, petroleum, triclosan, synthetic and artificial colors.

✓ sunshinebotanicals.com

The best skincare advice anyone can give

It has to be said that if you want to have truly beautiful skin, then it will more than likely come from your *diet* and not necessarily from products alone. Too many people spend lots of money on expensive beauty products but don't look after their health with the same respect. It would be much wiser to spend your hard-earned money on organic fruits and veggies and greens than it would be to spend lots on facials and beauty products. Obviously, if you can do all three, then it will increase the likelihood of having great skin even more, but the first area to start is always with your diet. Drinking fresh cold-pressed juices and green smoothies can help bring vitality to your skin. We will cover the subject of food in much more detail in Chapter 10.

Chapter 5

Why Are These Toxic Products Allowed on the Market?

Now *that's* a great question! Unfortunately the answer is fairly simple: it's typically down to money, irresponsible companies, and the fact that the industries themselves don't have any regulations to adhere to and often just regulate themselves, which means that many problems are arising due to them ignoring serious concerns. And because so many of these products and chemicals have been used for many years it's a problem that's been pushed under the carpet. No one of power is telling these companies to stop making them, or to make them safer. And the problem is, it's hard to get things banned in the first place and can often take decades. In regards to the entire subject of toxins causing cancer, it's very difficult to actually prove that just one product or one ingredient gives someone cancer. I know that contradicts everything I have been saying, but hear me out. Think about it like this: because chemicals are absolutely everywhere around us and we are being bombarded with hundreds of different chemicals each day, the finger cannot be pointed at any one thing. That's why it's very hard to prove that illness and cancer was caused by just one chemical.

So the governments can't (and rarely do) ban any of these products (or the ingredients) because it cannot be proven that the chemicals in, say, a suntan cream are actually the only reason why someone got cancer. And as there is little to no regulation, the manufacturers put whatever they want in their formulas without any consequences. This is another major problem because the toxic overload in the body comes from many chemicals being used over a very long time, *accumulating* in the body. So that's why you have to completely look at your entire lifestyle, what you are using and eating, in order to protect yourself.

If you have a typical beauty routine of using shampoo, conditioner, body lotion, body wash, face wash, hairspray, styling products, nail polishes, shaving cream, makeup, fake tan etc. that are all unsafe, then every day you are actually absorbing quite a few *hundred* different chemicals. And we haven't even talked about other ways of absorbing chemicals yet.

It's also worth mentioning that products that are designed to be left on the skin, such as a body cream, are obviously more damaging than the ones which are designed to be washed off. So a body lotion is going to be more reactive and damaging than a shower gel. If money is a problem for you and you can't go out and change everything at once, just change the most concerning products first: those that stay on your skin a longer time.

What is the media doing to educate people about toxins in products?

Great question! Well, unfortunately, not much at all. Even though magazines are starting to include organic products in their beauty pages, the majority of ads are still from the 'big guns' like L'Oreal, Revlon, Estee Lauder, Maybelline etc. which are seen as the most 'fashionable' and accessible brands in the world. If it wasn't for these advertisements, the magazines wouldn't be able to afford to continue their publication. These are multibillion-dollar companies which can afford to display their ads all over the planet. This means they are pretty much in every single country, and hardly anyone on the planet does not know who they are.

I know that you and I have seen them; these ads are in bus stations, trains, on billboards, on TV, shown before movies, and are in practically every fashion, health and beauty magazine. Most especially are found in all of the teenage magazines. So these brands get programmed into the minds of young people (and all of us) very early on. And we now even get their ads on the internet when we watch YouTube. You simply cannot easily get away from these ads and their subliminal messages (that you must use their products to be beautiful). Maybe if you moved to a cave then you would be able to shield yourself from them, but in real life they are absolutely everywhere. So for you, the shopper, who has been unaware of the toxins in these products, the brainwashing that you have received is because you have grown up with these brands, and now think that it's 'normal' and safe to go out and buy them.

The advertisements are so seductive and they are very clever at using suggestive wording so that your mind literally thinks it *needs* these products. And let's not forget: they do use amazing scientists to create these products, and the way they market them does make them sound very appealing. Having super-shiny soft and 'healthy' looking hair *is* very appealing! And to have perfect skin – well, who doesn't want that? Or who doesn't want their body looking like it's been on holiday with a lovely golden glow? And why wouldn't you want to look younger and not have any wrinkles at all?

That's the 'beauty' of advertising, it simply *makes* you want to have all those qualities it's telling you to have! And the thing is, their products really do appear to work. Due to the scientists working on a formula, sometimes for years and years, they do tend to deliver results, yet the problem is, it's at a *huge cost* also to your long-term health. And that's the scary part: we have been seduced by wanting to look good right *now*, at *any* cost, and are not being educated to care about how we will *end up* in the future. Trust me, if you are sick with cancer, the last thing you are going to think about is how pretty you look; you will just be praying that you can survive the disease.

The advertisers have also made you feel *safe* and that you can really *trust* their brand. And because they are usually really inexpensive products, pretty much everyone can afford them. Then we add *celebrities'* endorsements to the mix. 'They' all claim to use these products and all of the famous makeup artists for the catwalks apply them on the 'supermodels', who make us believe that if it's 'good enough for them' then it's so good enough for us! In fact, if we don't use them, we are really a nobody.

Hmm, do we really think an actress worth many millions would use a cheap cream that cost £3? Maybe some do, but I bet the majority don't; even the 'faces' of the brands would probably not use the products they themselves support. And when the companies are looking for a spokesperson for their brand, they don't ring around Hollywood and ask people, 'Hey, what popular famous celebrity uses our products?' No, they pick someone who is very popular at the time, who is 'beautiful', and then they approach them to be the 'face' of their products, all the while making them sign a contract that says they will state in interviews that they 'only' use their products, even though the chances of that are very slim!

See how we get conned! And we only have to look at the teenagers who are more obsessed with makeup and fashion than ever before and are starting to use these products at a much younger age. Whenever I see ads for mainstream beauty products, trying to make women think they need their products to be 'beautiful', I see them for what they truly are: that they pretty much glamorize toxins, use seductive words and images, and promote products made from dirt-cheap ingredients. The companies put most of their money towards making the ads themselves and do not have our best interests at heart. Only their bottom line, popularity and profit-share, is what manners to them.

A massive case of hypocrisy in the industry, which truly *infuriates* me is that of Estee Lauder and their 'pink ribbon' charity. Every year the Estee Lauder brand campaigns for breast cancer 'awareness'. The glamourous Liz Hurley has been the face of this campaign for many years and probably feels very proud of the 'awareness' she has brought to the issue of breast cancer. Yet what is sadly *so* ironic is that the products and brand she endorses, are full of parabens and other *cancer-causing* ingredients, that are linked directly to causing breast cancer. Yes, it's true. Don't you think it's totally hypocritical and disgusting? Liz probably herself doesn't even know, but I don't think the company would not know as they would be sent email after email from concerned people to ask them to change their formulas; they are just choosing to ignore it because they've probably been told 'it would be impossible to prove your products on their own cause cancer'.

So here lies one of the *biggest* problems in the beauty industry – accountability and the *lack* of wanting to change.

And while we are on the subject of this 'breast cancer awareness' and the 'think pink' campaigns, it's quite easy to see that for the majority of companies involved it's all just about making loads of money for them. In 2010, KFC released special-edition pink buckets of chicken during the month of October. In KFC chicken alone, there are several ingredients and processes which are linked to causing cancer. This is just one example of the hypocrisies that are obvious if people just looked hard enough.

Breast cancer has been transformed into a market-driven industry. It has become more about making money for corporate sponsors than funding innovative ways to treat breast cancer.
Health Studies researcher Samantha King, author of *Pink Ribbons Inc.*

To discover more about the breast cancer industry, please visit Natural News for a free report:

✓ naturalnews.com/Report_Breast_Cancer_Deception_0.html

Chapter 6

Labels and Lies – Which Ones Can We Trust?

We have all been duped into thinking that anything that says 'natural' or 'organic' means that the product or food item is automatically good. But like most things in the mainstream, the wording has been seriously misused. Because there are hardly any laws to do with labeling, a product can be labeled as 'natural' even if this is not quite true. Some natural-sounding products may only have a few ingredients in there that may be naturally derived but were still chemically synthesized before they ended up in your product. So in fact, they are *not* natural in the sense that you were made to believe. The word 'organic' is even worse; marketers know that people are buying more and more organic products these days, so they tend to try and use that word as a selling point. 'Organic' has become a very *fashionable* word and one that can also make a lot of money for companies.

Labels on products should make things easier for the consumer, right? But sadly, most customers get highly confused as to how to read if a product is safe or not. Sometimes even I can get fooled. Recently, I went on a trip to Greece. I left my usual body wash at home and had to get something from a pharmacy at the airport. I had seen ads on the TV for Sanex's '0% body wash', which I thought actually sounded quite good. It had only a small amount of ingredients and claimed to be biodegradable too. I assumed from the label it meant 0% chemical content, so purchased a bottle to take with me on our trip away. When using it in the shower that night, I had a chance to look at the ingredients. While it said that there were no parabens or colorants, the second ingredient was sodium laureth sulphate, which is its foaming agent. This ingredient also happens to be linked to cancer and is one of the main chemicals I urge people to avoid.

Does this sound like what '0%' should really mean? No! I felt really annoyed with myself for trusting the glossy advertisements – of all people I should have known better. It made me realise that you really have to have your wits about you when purchasing anything these days because too many companies are taking advantage of people's lack of knowledge.

I was recently sent some shampoo, conditioner and treatment that had the word 'organics' in the title. Guess how many ingredients were actually truly organic? Two – that's all! There were about 20 ingredients in each product and only two were from an organic source, yet the title gave the impression the entire product was completely organic. Very misleading and, really, downright lying if you ask me. And this happens all the time. As a shopper you really have to know your stuff to avoid being duped like this. The company that sent me these hair products, I'm sure really regretted it as I gave them a pretty nasty review, which they wholeheartedly deserved.

There are a few certifications labeled on products that can often help you figure out what is trustworthy and what is not. Bear in mind that hardly any brands are 100% organic and some still only have on average about 10% organic but I feel that if they are all naturally based (as in genuinely!) then it's still far better than using the regular brands. It's up to you how organic you want to be and how much you can afford. If the company is honest about what they do or do not have in their product, then they are still worth supporting.

I also try and encourage people that being genuinely healthy is a *holistic* thing too. Yes, you can really diminish your exposure to chemicals through buying safer products, but being able to keep on top of your total toxin exposure is about doing a whole bunch of other things of which I will cover later on throughout this book.

Soil Association

The seal of this UK organization means that each product must contain at least 95% organic ingredients, but also if more than 70% organic it is given to certain brands that clearly label the organic ingredients that can be proven organic by the Soil Association. It's very difficult for a product to get this approval; not only is it a costly process but many tests and strict requirements must be met to get this seal of approval.

USDA

The United States Department of Agriculture awards this seal to products whose total contents are 100% certified organic, or 95% certified organic where the remaining 5% of contents are drawn from a small, select number of ingredients that are not organically grown but pose no known risk to health or the environment.

EcoCERT

This French organic standard guarantees that:

- at least 95% of the total ingredients are from natural origin (water included)
- at least 10% of the total ingredients are from organic farming (water included)
- at least 95% of the total plant-based ingredients are organic.
- ✓ ecocert.com

CosmeBio

This label means that 95% of the vegetable ingredients result from organic agriculture and the ingredients must be of natural origin. Ten percent minimum of the finished product must be certified organic.

✓ cosmebio.org

ACO Australian Certified Organic Cosmetics

I'm proud to see such high standards from my home country, Australia.

Australian Certified Organic cosmetics and skincare products contain more than 95% certified organic ingredients. The remaining small percentage (maximum 5%) of non-organic ingredients must be naturally produced plant products and/or natural, non toxic preservatives/additives.

✓ bfa.com.au

NASSA (National Association for Sustainable Agriculture, Australia)
This also works on a 95% organic and 5% non organic standard
✓ nasaa.com.au

OFC (Organic Food Chain)
This is another Australian Cosmetics labelling certification. Again, they require a 95% organic content. Australia is really leading the way for genuinely organic standards.

✓ organicfoodchain.com.au

Canada Organic Biologique
Only products with organic content that is greater than or equal to 95% may be labelled as: "Organic" or bear the organic logo.

✓ organicguide.com

Natrue
The Natrue label guarantees that the products which have been accredited:

- contain only natural and organic ingredients
- use soft manufacturing processes
- use environmentally friendly practices.

And the products do not contain:

- synthetic fragrances and colors
- petroleum-derived products (paraffins, PEG, Propyl-Alkyls)

- silicone oils and derivatives
- GMO ingredients.

Also they are not irradiated or tested on animals.

✓ natrue.org

Demeter

This label means that bio-dynamic and organic farming principles have been used under strict methods and to the highest standard. 'Bio-dynamic' means that herbs, fruits and vegetables and other natural plants are grown in accordance with cycles of the moon, creating the highest quality known to humankind. This method was devised by the genius Rudolf Steiner back in 1924.

✓ demeter.net

* * *

Obviously, Soil Association, ACO, NASSA, Canada's Organic Biologique, and USDA certifications are far higher quality than EcoCert. In regards to choosing which product, it all depends on how chemical free you want to be. There are also labels that say if a product is vegan or has not been tested on animals; these labels are very easy to understand. Also, on the back of a product that claims to be organic, check the label for ingredients marked with an asterisk*. This will tell you how many ingredients of the entire product are organic. If it's only a few in a long list, but advertises itself in a way that sounds impressive, then you know it's a brand that is trying to pull the wool over your eyes.

In regards to organic products, European standards are much higher than the USDA standards, although we don't know if it will always remain like this.

Chapter 7

Home *Unsweet* Home! Something Else Adding to Your Toxic Overload

You're probably already feeling like you might just want to stay home and never leave, considering how many thousands of toxins are around us in the environment. But unfortunately, I can't tell you that our homes are always safe either. Our homes should certainly be a sanctuary for us, somewhere we can feel safe and comfortable. But unfortunately the truth is, they can also be making us sick in the long run![21] Indoor air pollution in many cases can be worse to breathe inthan being outside.

When a house is built, so many different toxic chemicals are used. Glues are used to stick down carpets and wallpaper, smelly varnish is used to coat the floorboards, chemical-based paints are used on all of the walls, and the furniture (and even more scarily, our mattresses) is sprayed with poisonous flame retardants which are often required by law.

All of these things together create a process that is called 'off-gassing', which means, as it sounds, that gasses are coming off items in the house and the things we have furnished it with. You won't be able to see them, just like you can't see air, but they are all around us. Indoor air has been reported to be *10 times more polluted* than outside air. So for this reason, I feel very strongly about urging people to think about what may be lurking in their own households.

If you live in a hot country, it is wise and easy to leave the windows open for as long as possible to air rooms out, but in the colder climates such as the UK and Canada, you just can't do this; so the reality is, you're living inside a completely enclosed environment (think of it like a box) each and every day. And night time, when your body is meant to be resting and rejuvenating, has actually become a time of stress for your body because you are breathing in all of these fumes, and it's trying to deal with them but just can't do the job it's designed to do – which is to rest and regenerate.

Another serious health problem in houses can be black mold. In the UK, because it's so cold, we have to keep our windows shut for most of the year, and with most of the houses being hundreds of years old, there are often water problems lurking underneath the floorboards and also behind the walls. I know this myself because the house that we moved into 4 years ago had a shocking amount of mold and we only discovered this after living here for 3 years. It makes total sense to me now because as soon as we moved in, I developed the worst bout of chronic fatigue I had ever had and knew it had something to do with this house. Black mold is a troubling concern because it turns into 'mycotoxins', which are said to be even more toxic than heavy metals due to their concentration. Mycotoxins affect the immune system and also other biological systems *more* so than that of exposure to pesticides *and* fungicides. And not only do these toxins affect your body; studies have proven they can also affect your brain.[22]

I also noticed that my own brain function in that house was the worst it had ever been so I personally think that the black mold in that house was indeed causing me to be very sick. Mold is linked to triggering chronic fatigue syndrome and other auto-immune disorders. It's interesting to know that in biblical times, if a house was affected by mold, they would completely rip down the house and build from scratch again.

In our own home's case, underneath the bathroom floor boards was a huge amount of toxic black mold, due to years and years of water leaking and not draining away. It took us 4 months of having a dehumidifier on 24/7 to get rid of the horrible smell and we had to replace the entire bathroom. Buckets and buckets of water were sucked out from the walls and floors, and all of that water would have had mold spores in it. Gross. No *wonder* I had been so sick. And, unfortunately, black mold found in homes is much more common than you may think. There are actually even more types of molds to be concerned about also. Some moulds are not even easily seen, so the problem can be right under your nose, except you won't actually be able to see it.

> Most people are not aware that harmful molds come in a variety of colors – they can be white, or orange, or blue, for instance. The color of a mold generally has to do with the spores it produces, and has no bearing on whether it is dangerous or not. There are some white molds that grow on walls and other surfaces that can be just as bad as the harmful black molds.
> (Sourced from Mold-Help.org)

This website is for helping people pinpoint what mold problem they may have in their house, and more importantly, how to treat it:

✓ mold-help.org

Now I know what you're probably thinking: 'What the heck can I do about my house - I can't afford to move!' If you rent, then it's up to the landlord to fix the problem so you might want to look into it and let them know what is going on. If your house smells and feels damp, then there is a high chance that mold is lurking somewhere. If you own your own house and insurance doesn't cover it, you could perhaps invest in a dehumidifier and an air-purifier; these can be quite expensive, but it is a great option for cleaning the air in the bedroom (and you can also move it to the living room during the day) if you can afford it. If you can, look into renting a dehumidifier if the problem is serious.

To improve the quality of oxygen in your home, what I can suggest, which is easy and affordable to do, is to put many 'healthy air' plants throughout most of your house with the majority being placed in your main living spaces such as your bedrooms and lounge room or wherever you spend the most time. Plants are designed by Mother Nature to filter our air, and without them doing this, well, we wouldn't even be here today! Having lots of plants in each room of the house (or the main rooms you use the most) can make a huge change to the air quality, allowing you to breathe healthily and also to sleep much better.

NASA conducted a study on the many benefits of plants on indoor air and released the findings in 1989: they discovered that houseplants were able to remove up to 87% of air toxins in just 24 hours.[23]

There are many types of amazing plants which are specifically beneficial for our living space. These plants actually thrive on absorbing toxic chemicals – how amazing is that?! And there is even a super-cool plant called 'Mother-in-Law's Tongue' that gives off oxygen at night, which means it's the perfect one to have in the bedroom.

For a large bedroom you may need 5–6 plants quite close to the bed for best results. You could have some either side of the bed where your head rests.

My top 5 favorite healthy plants are:

- Dracaena 'Janet Craig'
- Areca Palm
- ZZ plant
- Spathiphyllum (Peace Lily)
- Boston Fern

The *New Ecologist* also recommends the following 10 anti-pollutant houseplants that they rate the best:

- The Feston Rose plant
- Devil's Ivy
- Phalaenopsis
- English Ivy
- Parlor Ivy
- African Violets
- Christmas Cactus

- Yellow Goddess
- Garlic Vine
- Peace Lily

Below are 6 house plants which NASA has studied and found to dramatically improve air quality.

1 Bamboo Palm: According to NASA, it removes formaldehyde and is also said to act as a natural humidifier.

2 Snake Plant: Found by NASA to absorb nitrogen oxides and formaldehyde.

3 Areca Palm: One of the best air-purifying plants for general air cleanliness.

4 Spider Plant: Great indoor plant for removing carbon monoxide and other toxins or impurities. Spider plants are one of three plants NASA deems best at removing formaldehyde from the air.

5 Peace Lily: Peace lilies could be called the 'clean-all' plant. They're often placed in bathrooms or laundry rooms because they're known for removing mold spores. Also know to remove formaldehyde and trichloroethylene.

6 Gerbera Daisy: Not only do these gorgeous flowers remove benzene from the air, they're also known to improve sleep by absorbing carbon dioxide and giving off more oxygen over night.

Depending on the size of the room, if it has a high ceiling etc., you may need 3–5 large plants in a large area. If you can't immediately afford to buy all the types you need, just buy what you can at first and add more later on, and even ask for some as presents at Christmas and birthday times. You can even take cuttings from previously grown plants and repot them, making it much cheaper for you in the long run. And you can also purchase plants in their smaller size and repot them so that they will grow much larger.

Having a few plants in your house is way better than having none. And remember to give them some love with appropriate amounts of water, touching and wiping them occasionally. Plants have many magical qualities which we are only just beginning to understand.

I would suggest though that you learn to care about your plants properly because the soil can also become moldy if over-watered. I have killed a few plants due to not knowing how to care for them. My advice if you don't have green fingers is to get fern and/or peace lily plants as they seem to be very hardy and don't die easily.

If you work in an office, it would be wise to suggest to the managers to get a whole bunch of healthy-air plants – studies have also shown that flus and other viruses, which are quite common in the workplace, tend to be much less common when workers are surrounded by plants. And in schools, students report being much more alert and able to concentrate for longer.

I personally recommend the online shop 'House of Plants' in the UK to purchase beautiful plants from, but any nursery worldwide should be able to help you with these particular plants, or at least point you in the right direction.

✓ houseofplants.com

You can even purchase healthy plants through websites like Interflora. They often sell peace lilies and azaleas.

If you think you may have a problem with mold (and many houses in the UK and other cold countries do), it might be a good idea to test for it. Breathing Space sell mold test kits, which are very inexpensive.

✓ breathingspace.co.uk

The menace in the microwave

I haven't used a microwave in about 10 years and I am very glad I (literally!) threw ours away. Back when I did use them, I simply had no idea how harmful they were. Microwaving is thought to be one of the *worst* things you can do to your food and therefore to your health. Even though they are widely sold all over the world, the very clever and forward-thinking Russians actually knew years ago, when they were first being tested, that they were very dangerous, and microwaves have not been introduced as a normal household appliance in their country.

The waves that are created in these tiny machines heat the food from the inside out, which is a very *unnatural* method. It not only damages the structure of the food; it also basically irradiates most of the enzymes and nutrients, causing your food to become completely dead. Studies have shown it can destroy up to 97% of antioxidants in vegetables. And that means all the anti-cancer properties we eat the vegetables for!

In the November 2003 issue of *The Journal of the Science of Food and Agriculture*, which conducted a study on microwaving, it was reported that broccoli cooked in the microwave with a small amount of water lost up to 97% of the beneficial antioxidant chemicals it contains. In comparison, steamed broccoli lost just 11% or fewer of its antioxidants.

Perhaps the most concrete evidence of the dangers of microwaves comes from Dr. Hans Hertel,[24] a Swiss food scientist, who carried out a small but high-quality study on the effects of microwaved food on humans. His conclusions were clear and alarming: microwave cooking significantly altered the food's nutrients enough so that changes occurred in the participants' blood – changes that suggested deterioration. The changes included:

- Increased cholesterol levels
- More leukocytes, or white blood cells, which can suggest poisoning
- Decreased numbers of red blood cells
- Production of radiolytic compounds (compounds unknown in Nature)

- Decreased hemoglobin levels, which could indicate anemic tendencies

Dr. Hertel, shocked at what he had discovered, tried to alarm authorities, but subsequently lost his job and, worse than that, was issued with a court 'gag order' so that he would have to keep quiet, or face jail. He is still fighting to have this removed.

But as you will read below in other studies[25] from around the world, evidence is undeniable that food is completely left devoid of nutrients after it's been in the microwave:

- As mentioned above, a study published in the November 2003 issue of *The Journal of the Science of Food and Agriculture* found that broccoli 'zapped' in the microwave with a little water lost up to 97% of its beneficial antioxidants. By comparison, steamed broccoli lost 11% or fewer of its antioxidants. There were also reductions in phenolic compounds and glucosinolates, but mineral levels remained intact.
- A 1999 Scandinavian study of the cooking of asparagus spears found that microwaving caused a reduction in vitamin C.
- In a study of garlic, as little as 60 seconds of microwave heating was enough to inactivate its allinase, garlic's principle active ingredient against cancer.
- A Japanese study by Watanabe showed that just 6 minutes of microwave heating turned 30–40% of the B12 in milk into an inert (dead) form. This study has been cited by Dr. Andrew Weil as evidence supporting his concerns about the effects of microwaving. Dr. Weil wrote: 'There may be dangers associated with microwaving food ... there is a question as to whether microwaving alters protein chemistry in ways that might be harmful.'
- A recent Australian study showed that microwaves cause a higher degree of 'protein unfolding' than conventional heating.

- Microwaving can destroy the essential disease-fighting agents in breast milk that offer protection for your baby. In 1992, Quan found that microwaved breast milk lost lysozyme activity, antibodies, and fostered the growth of more potentially pathogenic bacteria

I recently read a very alarming story. As an experiment, a glass of water was heated up in the microwave on a typical high setting. That water was then cooled down, and poured into a pot plant. Within only 2 days, the plant was completely dead. If you are dubious about this, it might be worth experimenting yourself to see, although it would be a waste of a beautiful plant.

And here is another story that is sure to *shock* you as it did me.

In 1991, a lawsuit was in the works after a nurse at a hospital in Oklahoma assisted in performing a blood transfusion. The blood needed to be warmed to body temperature, but instead of using the usual method, the unsuspecting nurse put the bag of blood in the microwave, which then was injected into the patient.

Guess what happened? The patient *died* shortly after. The blood was simply not healthy or *normal* anymore. What does this say about what a microwave does? It says that the nutrients, all of the 'goodness', are completely destroyed and even dramatically changed. If that was not true, that blood would have been fine and the patient would have survived. A blood transfusion is a fairly simple procedure so deaths should not occur like this.

Also, when food is heated up in plastic containers or covered in cling film, you are making a recipe for disaster. Heat and plastic do not ever mix (well, they do but not in a good way in regards to food) and when the microwave is switched on, the intense heat and radiation cause the plastic to drop particles into the food. So, if you microwave your food in plastic containers or covered in cling film, you not only end up eating dead food with no nutrients; you end up eating bits of plastic particles as well.

I don't know about you, but that's definitely *not* the sort of meal I would want to eat.

It's also very worrying because every day we read articles about people becoming severely deficient in nutrients, and with so many people using microwaves, we can most certainly point the finger at this being one of the main causes. I don't think anyone who uses a microwave regularly could possibly be a picture of health. If we know food is a *form of medicine* due to the nutrient content, then cooking it in a way that destroys most of these nutrients, is not going to help provide the nourishment we need.

That says a heck of a lot for the safety of heating up food in general that way.

There is more info found below on the dangers of microwaves:

✓ halexandria.org/dward078.htm

Cookware that kills?

Another way to avoid dangerous toxins is to avoid using non-stick cookware. Even though it initially seemed to be one of the 'best' inventions over the past 50 years, it has actually become a huge health risk. 'Non-stick' is a coating called Teflon that was developed by a very powerful biotech company by the name of Dupont so that people could cook things like eggs and other typically hard-to-clean-after-use foods. It would allow the debris to slide off the pan easily, wiping out the hard work it typically took to clean the utensils.

Before we get into just how dangerous Teflon is, I want to give you a little background history of the company that is behind it, just so you know what sort of people are behind this product so that you can steer clear, even if it's only for the sake of a moral obligation and ethics.

Dupont is the third largest chemical company in the United States and has factories in 70 different countries. It produces agrochemicals, polymers, electronics, genetically modified seeds and safety materials. It began in 1802 and was started from money made by the purchase of gunpowder after the French Revolution. By

1811, Dupont was the largest supplier of gunpowder to the US Military. By the time the Civil War started, Dupont were big business. Between 1902 and 1912 Dupont began producing smokeless powder and dynamite. When World War 1 started, 40% of explosives used were supplied by Dupont. At this time the company realized its power and started purchasing smaller chemical companies. Dupont was taken to court after it was thought that they were creating a 'monopoly' as the company was taking over the explosives business. The court did not exactly do much to them and Dupont went on to create new chemical companies under a different name. It also founded the first two industrial labs and researched into improving military weapons. By 1914, Dupont also began to get involved in another lucrative business: the automobile industry. It created the first synthetic rubber, polyester, nylon and Teflon. During World War 2, Dupont was the largest producer of war supplies. The chemical company was also behind the creation of the first atomic bombs which were dropped on the Japanese cities of Nagasaki and Hiroshima. From the 1950s to the 1970s, Dupont went in another direction, developing new materials such as Lycra, Dacron and Mylar.

In 1999 Dupont quickly rose to become the largest seed company and was a producer of 'hybrid' seeds which are used for GMO corn and soy. Dupont is one of four bio-tech companies that produce 100% of GMO seeds and 60% of the world's pesticides. With so many people aware of the dangers of GMO and pesticides, Dupont is always using its money to lobby in Congress so that its policies get pushed through. One year, Dupont spent around $4.8 million.[26]

Teflon was first created in 1938 by a Dupont scientist by the name of Dr. Roy Plunkett.[27] He was working with different gases in the lab to come up with a better coolant gas. He left a gas overnight, and came back the next day to find that the gas had disappeared and in its place was a waxy solid, very slippery and impervious to all sorts of chemicals that are usually corrosive to most materials. He went on to name it 'tetrafluoroethylene' or PTFE for short. 'Teflon' is the nickname as most of us know it today. It wasn't until 1950 that Teflon began being used in cookwear. A Frenchman applied the Teflon to his wife's frying pan, with great success. After several years of selling 'Tefal' products, millions were being sold every year. Soon after, Tefal hit the US market – and the rest is history. Teflon is now one of the most popular cookwear products to have ever been created.

While it did seem like a great invention at the time, what people didn't realize then is that when these pots and pans were heated to high enough temperatures, it created at least *8 different chemicals* which go directly into your food. And these chemicals are *all carcinogens* which (I hope you know by now) means they cause cancer. One of the toxins released is hydrogen fluoride gas, which if inhaled actually turns into hydrofluoric acid in your lungs. This acid is known to be highly toxic and leaches calcium out of your bones. Take a look at the fine print on any non-stick pan you buy new. I once did – it told me not to use the pan in the same room as animals with 'sensitive respiratory systems' such as small birds. Well, what about *our own* respiratory systems? Is it OK to have yet one more dangerous toxin (or in this case 8 more) to deal with? No thanks.

There was also a study done where many people were reporting that their pet birds suddenly died, and it just so happens that the bird cage was in the kitchen when the owner was using non-stick cookwear.[28]

The biggest problem here is that non-stick coatings were *never* independently tested for safety and the FDA were given very flawed studies to allow them to be approved. The inventor of the product was actually taken to court by a group of pregnant workers who were passing the chemicals to their unborn children. The company was also dumping chemicals into the water and up to 12,000 people were affected. Not a company that you would want to support, right?

Dupont, to this day, still deny how toxic Teflon is. But I think the results speak for themselves. If you do own a non-stick pan, heat it up, and just have a smell of it while it gets hotter and hotter. It smells very odd, doesn't it? Very chemical and just strange. Why would you want to eat food that has been cooked off that?

For those that can't live without their non-stick cookwear, there is a company called Green Pan which make their coatings from a natural mineral called silica. They claim to be scratch resistant as well as heat resistant to 450°C and the safest coated cookware you can buy. I have a Green Pan – I wanted to get one to test before I recommended it to you. It's pretty good! You do have to be careful, though, that you don't heat even these up too high, but as long as you follow the instructions your meals cooked this way are much safer and more chemical-free. You can also use ceramic cook wear, such as the famous Le Creuset french brand.

- ✓ green-pan.co.uk
- ✓ green-pan.com (for USA)
- ✓ mercola.com also sells Dr. Mercola's own fantastic range of safe non-stick cookwear

How common household items 'off-gas' toxic poisons

Our electrical goods such as computers, stereo systems and TVs also give off toxic chemicals, which we breathe in. Remember when you sit inside a new car and you can smell that 'new car smell'? Well, that's *obvious* off-gassing. But in your home (and any buildings for that matter) there are lots of chemicals going into your nasal passages that you simply cannot smell, or have gotten so used to smelling it's now not obvious. It's actually more polluted *inside* your home than it is outside, which is pretty darn scary.

Computers omit a chemical called triphenyl phosphate which can cause allergic reactions. This chemical is a flame retardant that's added to many plastics. When the computer is turned on, the heat caused by the electricity will cause the chemicals to start evaporating around you, which of course, you will breathe in. This also goes for other electrical equipment such as TVs and kitchen goods too. If you can, try and move your computer near a window, which you can open often.

The dirtiest cleaning products

Well, I am sure you know that if beauty products are toxic to us, then our typical cleaning products sure as heck will be too! In fact, they are *way* worse. You only have to take the lid off your toilet cleaner to know that the body does not like it one bit at all. You can't even smell them for long because it can make you gag. Yet so many ignore this and continue using the products, because they *do* do a damn good job of making things clean.

Before I turned eco-minded, I used to always clean with the regular-brand cleaning products. I would get in the bath and shower with my bare feet and would clean them while standing in the water as it seemed the easiest way. A few days later I would notice that the skin on my feet would start to peel very badly. After a few times of this, I thought something wasn't right! If it was doing that on the outside, chances are it was doing something nasty to my insides, because I knew that the feet absorb so much, just like our scalps do.

When we spray our kitchens, bathrooms and floors with toxic chemicals, they will not only get in the air but will also be absorbed when you touch surfaces. Most worryingly, if you have a small child (and pets too) and they crawl all over the 'clean' floor, they are putting these chemicals into their bodies because of the child's natural response to put their hands in their mouth.

Here is a thought: perhaps when babies and children cry for no apparent reason, is it because they have tasted something very nasty or because they have a headache from the toxin they'd unknowingly put in their mouth which simply does not belong in their body? These types of cleaning chemicals have been found in the umbilical cords of new babies. Thirty-five different chemicals were tested for in one study and all of them were found in trace amounts.[29] These chemicals are found in everyday household products, such as sprays used to clean floors and onto surfaces, which children touch, such as high chairs.

And we must not forget that whatever we use in the house, cleaning-wise, will get washed down the sink into our waterways and will cause even more damage to the environment. Enormous amounts of toxic cleaners get flushed into our waterways, and some say they can cause more destruction to the environment than industrial pollution[30] – so this fact alone makes it so important to use safer cleaning products.

The best cleaning brand I have come across is Alma Win, a German brand that has created an impressive range of products for cleaning your kitchen, bathroom, floors, doing laundry, washing up, using the dishwasher... and they have even designed a delicious orange-based cleaner for polishing your furniture.

Every product is completely safe and does not harm the environment in any way, shape or form. Some of the 'eco' cleaning products claim to be very safe, yet what I have learnt is that they can be safe to humans, but not to the waterways. I love Alma Win because it is 100% safe for humans, animals and the planet.

If you or anyone in your family suffers with allergies, Alma Win products will not trigger allergies like most cleaning products can. For people with eczema, clothing can trigger outbreaks due to the chemicals from washing powders and detergents.

✓ Pravera.co.uk – UK
✓ almawin-usa.com – USA
✓ almawin.de – Europe and other countries

I also like these other brands:

Honest Company

Jessica Alba's cleaning product range is *so* impressive. I only just discovered it recently. Not only it is very affordable, with cute packaging the ingredients are so effective that there is a patent pending on some of the formulas. The range has things for all areas of the house and were tried and tested by Jessica and her own family before they settled on the perfect formulas. There are so many chemicals that the Honest company simply won't use, and some of them are found in eco-friendly formula's but they are still not proven 100% safe, so Honest, have left them out because they want to make certain that everything is proven safe. You can buy everything you need from Honest on a monthly order too so that you never run out. I hope that The Honest Company come to the UK!

  ✓ Honest.com

Mrsmeyers.com

All of their liquid products are biodegradable. Some of their powder products contain minerals that do not biodegrade, but do break down into non-harmful decomposition products and return to the earth as they left it.

- Products do not contain ammonia, chlorine, glycol solvents, parabens, phthalates, formaldehyde, artificial colorants, phosphates or petroleum distillates.
- Packaging is recyclable and they use 25% post-consumer plastic in their bottles.
- They do not test their products on animals, nor are the products made with animal-derived ingredients.

EcoEggonline.com

I recently was sent one of these amazing little devices. This egg-shaped object (yes, unfortunately made from plastic but it does last a very long time) is filled with balls of tourmaline and other cleaning pellets. The Eco Egg is placed into the barrel of your washing machine. The tourmaline weakens the adhesive force between the dirt and fabric. The white pellets naturally ionize the oxygen molecules in the water, which then penetrates into the material, taking away dirt and grime. This process does not damage the fibers, nor does it fade colors. The Eco Egg is great for sensitive skin and allergy sufferers too. And one of the best benefits is how much money it can save you. If you do 4–5 washes a week, this Eco Egg and its refills (which are supplied in the box) will last up to 3 *years*!

There are also no harmful chemicals in the Eco Egg so it's kind to the environment. Priced at £19.99.

Soap Nuts

These little beauties are just fantastic. And they are exactly what they sound like – little nut-like shells which are grown on trees in India. The shells contain saponins, and when they come into contact with water, they release mild suds and make the best environmentally friendly laundry detergent. They are also so inexpensive and can be used again and again. 1 kg of Soap Nuts can be used for approximately 100 loads of laundry. I have used these before and love them. They even make your laundry smell great! Google 'Soap Nuts' or visit the website below to find out more.

   ✓ salveo.co.uk

* * *

For other eco-cleaning products you may be interested in trying these brands:

- Green Shield Organics
- Earth Friendly
- Vermont Soap
- BioKleen
- Better Life
- Green Scents
- B_E_E
- Enviro Care Australia

If you do want to stick with your regular cleaning products (although I really do hope you will change them as it's so important for your health) then make sure you use them with windows wide open, wear protective gloves, and rinse all of the product away, carefully making sure that all of the residue has gone. Keeping windows open will help a little bit, but remember that anything that is in the air tends to stay there for quite a while. Even consider wearing a face mask.

At the end of this book, in the DIY section in Part 4, I have included some super-easy recipes for cleaning all areas of your house.

Scented candles

These yummy-smelling candles are unfortunately another health hazard. Mostly made with toxic ingredients, when lit, they produce poisons that are as bad as smoking, if not worse. If you burn them in a small room such as the bathroom, you will be unknowingly breathing these chemicals in. Usually these unsafe candles are made with paraffins which are a by-product of petroleum so are completely unnatural. If you have asthma, be aware, these candles could trigger an attack.

What is also concerning about the candles is that they usually contain synthetic essential oils to give them their pretty fragrance. Even though they may be marketed as having 'lemon' or other scents, they are not coming from Nature but instead coming from a laboratory, which means that, when burnt, it creates a chemical change through the smoke, which is not safe to breathe in.

Then there is the wick to think about! It too is not made safely (non-organic cotton and other chemicals) and when it starts to burn will create even more of a toxic smoke. So really, nothing about these candles is a good idea! And don't be fooled into thinking that once the candle is out, the air will be clear. In fact, it can take several hours to dissipate! Toxins in air can become very stagnant and often take a long time to go away. And if it's in a room with only small windows, then that time frame is going to be even longer.

So the only sensible thing to do is not to buy scented candles that have been made with unnatural ingredients. Many companies are now making soy or beeswax-based candles, combined with safe wicks and safe essential oils. These ones you can use in the bathroom with the windows and doors closed! They tend to last longer as well, even though they are a bit more expensive.

For luxury candles I absolutely love the brand NEOM. These organic candles are very long lasting, despite the expensive price tag, and all are exquisite scents. NEOM also sells skin and body care which has Soil Association approval. If you can't afford to buy NEOM, search online for non-toxic candles – use the words 'soy or plant-based candles' and 'beeswax' to make it easier to find.

Air fresheners

Another truly alarming product to saturate the consumer market is air fresheners. These are advertised to alleviate bad smells in the house, because of pets, damp and bathroom smells, or just because we should have a lovely-smelling house 24/7.

Nowadays, some products have been designed to plug into the wall and squirt out the spray according to how often it's set for. While these can smell very nice, they are highly toxic – in fact, purely chemical – and are said to be worse for you in regards to chemical exposure than being stuck in traffic in a highly polluted city with the windows down!

If you use air fresheners, this is happening right in your home.

Also, if you do not have the windows open, where are the chemicals going to go? Well, right into you and your loved ones, including your kids and pets! Anything that is in the air means that you and they breathe it in too (which I know you know by now!) and it will settle into the tissues, including your brain. Our nasal passages are protected with little hairs, but they can only do so much. They still let a lot of toxins pass through into the brain. In a minor reaction to these chemicals, it can often lead to migraines and headaches, but more alarmingly, yet again, this chemical concoction is being linked to cancers.

The types of chemicals in these products are really shocking and when you look at what each does individually, it's quite horrific.

Here is a list[31] of very scary-sounding ingredients commonly found in air fresheners:

- glycol ethers
- surfactant (quaternary ammonium salts)
- ethyl or isopropyl alcohol
- propellants
- petroleum distillates (6.0%)
- aluminum chlorhydrol
- bromsalicylanilide 2,3,4,5-BIS(2-butylene) tetrahydrofural
- metazene (4.0%)
- cellosolve acetate
- dichlorodifluoromethanol
- perfume
- ethanol
- fatty esters
- lauryl methacrylate
- methoxychlor
- zinc phenolsulfonate
- o-phenyl phenol
- methylene chloride
- p-dichlorobenzene
- pine oil (toxicity like turpentine)
- piperonyl butoxide
- pyrethrin
- synthetic surfactants
- trichloromonofluoromethane
- wax

Isn't it crazy that we can make ourselves sick just by trying to improve the scent of our homes? If you are going to use air fresheners, you can easily make your own out of water and organic essential oils by mixing 4–5 drops into a 500 ml spray bottle (which can be recycled from something you have bought previously), or you can purchase ones that are ready-made for you with similar ingredients. Making your own is so inexpensive and can even be fun. You could make them for friends or relatives as gifts. There really is no need to resort to buying unnatural air fresheners. They are total poison and need to be seen as such; they are not at all safe for you and your family, no matter how good and 'natural' they may smell.

Air purifiers

Another highly beneficial and safe way of cleaning the air around you in your home is with an air ionizer, sterilizer, or hepa filter. These machines remove allergens, impurities and airborne contamination. There are many types you can purchase and it's always best to get the right one depending on the size of the room you want treated and what concerns you the most. You can choose air purifiers that are designed specifically to remove pet dander from the air, tobacco smoke, dust mites, bacteria, fungus and cooking fumes. People that have asthma may really benefit from using one of these, and also hay fever sufferers. I particularly think that children need to have these in their rooms and especially newborn babies, as they are so sensitive and are already born with toxins in their bodies so it's a good idea to try and limit these as much as possible.

We moved again in late 2012 to a house with newly painted walls and new carpet. The average person might think, 'Oh great! A nice new "clean" house!' But to me, the immediate thought was: 'Eeek! New chemicals, and lots of them.' Luckily, we already have quite a few healthy-air plants, but I was concerned that it wouldn't be enough to absorb the majority of chemicals that would off-gas from this new update to the house. I started looking for an air purifier that would do the job better.

The best website I came across was Breathing Space; they have a huge range of different types of machines and were very knowledgeable and super-helpful in choosing the right filter for our home.

✓ breathingspace.co.uk

Moth balls

It's very common in colder climates for people to store their items with moth balls during the warmer seasons and put them away in cupboards or chests. Moth balls are used to keep the insects away so that they do not eat and damage the fabric. Moth balls do a great job of this, but the problem is, they are also *extremely* toxic to humans. I was on the train once and a dear old lady sat down next to me. Within seconds I could smell that she had stored her winter coat in moth balls. It smelt that bad, I actually had to move right away from her as I was feeling sick from the smell. I was 6 months pregnant at the time and my sense of smell was in overdrive, but I am pretty sure anyone else would have noticed it too. It's certainly a *very* unpleasant smell. I wrote a little blog post about moth balls a few years ago and discovered that the following ingredients are commonly used:

- naphthalene
- 1,4-dichlorobenzene

These two ingredients are *very* toxic pesticides and of course, this means they are also poisonous for humans. They might kill the moths, but when you wear clothes that have been in storage permeated by the scent, it will do you and the air around you much more harm than good. The chemicals you breathe in will harm your cells. Wearing clothes with that scent on it means that you will be breathing it in whether you like it or not. A natural and much healthier way to keep moths at bay is to make your own little scented pillows that you can hang in your wardrobe.

I have included some fun and inexpensive recipes found in Part 4 under the DIY section.

Dry cleaning

It probably won't surprise you to hear that dry cleaning is not a chemical-free process. Anyone that goes inside these shops can instantly notice that it stinks to the heavens and smells obviously of not so pleasant things. Over here in the UK we are always getting our winter coats cleaned, and when I have to go into the shop, I can immediately smell the fluid as soon as I open the door. I also have seen the boxes of cleaning fluid in the front of the shop, clearly marked with a *poison* sign. I am lucky – I can go in and out very quickly – but I feel *very* sorry for the workers there. Often they have hardly any ventilation and are around those chemicals sometimes up to 6 days a week. The staff never look healthy and always seem very tired and run down.

Not suprising. I imagine they more than likely also have huge energy problems and probably get headaches a lot. I wish I could say to them, 'Don't you realize how toxic this stuff is?' But most of them own the business and I doubt they could do anything to change their methods so they could avoid using these chemicals. I bet that if I came back in 20 years, they would all have serious health problems, or perhaps some would have had cancer or sadly some might even have passed away. Working in an environment like that is a perfect example of a health hazard. I find it very sad that people have to work in environments that may end up shortening their life span, all because we need to earn a living, and that we have no protection methods in place. . It's ironic that very wealthy peole who are fashion conscious, tend to purchase a lot of designer clothes made from delicate fabrics, and get everything dry cleaned. This means they are constantly wearing clothes permeated in dry cleaning fluids. Money can buy so much, but it doesn't always buy health and good sense that's for sure.

Tetrachloroethylene is the most common chemical found in dry cleaning fluids, and the International Agency for Research on Cancer has classed it as a carcinogen.[32] Tetrachloroethylene exposure can be evaluated by a breath test, similar to that of breath-alcohol measurements. Because it is stored in the fat cells of the body, and slowly released into the bloodstream, it can be detected in the breath for weeks following a heavy exposure. Tetrachloroethylene can also be detected in the bloodstream.

Can you wash 'dry clean only' items?

As I joyously discovered recently, yes! I did a little experiment on some of my winter coats, which normally cost quite a lot to get cleaned so I decided to see if I could wash one, knowing it could end in disaster, but if it didn't it could also save me money and help me to advise others on how to wash 'dry clean only' fabrics.

Here is what I did. All of my coats were 100% wool, so quite a risky fabric to begin with. Instead of washing on a full regular cycle in the machine, I soaked the coat overnight in a large bucket of cold water and some natural nappy san which I purchased from the laundry section at my health food shop. The next morning I put the coat into the machine and washed on a gentle wool cycle. After it was finished I hung it up with a coat hanger and left it to dry for a few days. The first coat I washed was a success and all the other ones since have been too! Some of them required ironing after they had dried to make the collar sit down properly, but all in all they turned out wonderfully and, for the first time ever, smelt good too! I used to despise having to get them dry cleaned as I knew how toxic it was to have against my skin.

I was absolutely thrilled to find out that I can continue to wash in this manner and can avoid the dry cleaners now! Even my hubby has started washing his wool suits and drying and ironing in the same way. So we are both saving money and avoiding using toxic chemicals. Now, I can't guarantee that yours will turn out like ours did, but after chatting to people on Facebook about it, I've found that many other people are having great results too! Just be careful and do one item at a time to see if it turns out OK.

What if you do use the dry cleaners?

Sometimes we do have to use dry cleaning as water can ruin certain fabrics. What I can suggest to you is, after they have been cleaned, *always* take the clothes outside, remove the plastic and let them air-dry for a while (maybe even up to a few days) so that you can get rid of the smell from the fluids as much as possible. Or hang them up near a healthy-air plant so that it can absorb the chemicals for you. I wouldn't even hold a child or infant when wearing any dry-cleaned clothing, because the chemicals will rub off onto their delicate skin.

Another option is to buy non dry-cleaning fabrics so that you never have to have your clothes cleaned at places like that. Sometimes a manufacturer will say 'dry clean only', yet really the fabric is safe to hand-wash – they are merely covering their backs in case something goes wrong. I have washed many 'dry clean only' dresses and found they washed beautifully. Sometimes you have to be so careful as what you think will wash can't, but it might be worth having a google to see what fabrics can really be hand-washed. Natural fibers don't need to be dry cleaned so look out for organic cotton, bamboo, hemp and ethically farmed silk.

Another alternative is to buy your own steam clothes cleaner. This just uses water, which will boil and create a steam so that you can remove underarm and other stains. Much safer to use and will save you money in the long run. There are also some 'green' dry cleaners being opened now, which don't use harsh chemicals. I am yet to find one in the UK but I know there are some in the USA. Just google 'green dry cleaners' and hopefully you will find something.

Chapter 8

Excess Stuff – Why it's not just cramping your house, it's cramping your mind

So now you have learnt about the many toxins found in your home, you may have even more nuisances lurking around. Another problem in many people's home is a large amount of unnecessary *'stuff'*! We are *so* addicted to it, due to the media constantly telling us we *need* this or that to be happy, and the magazines telling us we have to have the latest fashions to be accepted. This leads to not only an empty wallet but also a very full house, which can really only be doing something that is *very unhealthy* also for your mind.

I used to buy so much stuff. I come from generations of compulsive shoppers. My grandma adores shopping as does my mum and as did I. And we are not alone. You only have to go out to any high street, shopping centre or mall to see that the addiction to buying things has gotten way out of control. Some people purely live for shopping; it's their only enjoyable way to pass the day. Most people's houses are crammed full of stuff, yet they always still want to buy more. It's *never* enough; we never seem to have everything we want and always desire to have more. The TV and magazines tell us we aren't good enough the way we are, and that if we have this or that new item, then we will live a happy, fulfilled life!

I used to buy things all the time, to try and make myself happy. I would get quite stuck on wanting something, and when I actually had it, I would feel good for an hour or maybe for a few days, until the novelty of that item wore off – which it always did! Because of my addiction, I gradually began to have a wardrobe bursting at the seams, to the point where once I had opened the door, it stressed me out because it was far too jumbeled and crowded. I couldn't even get in to sort through the clothes, so I ended up wearing the same things – jeans and a plain T-shirt – despite having beautiful things, (as well as cheap frivolous items,) inside my wardrobe. I just couldn't stand looking inside the door; it would bother me so much that the only way to stop that stress was to shut the door and walk away. My whole house was in a pretty similar state as well.

My husband and I came over to the UK with only two suitcases, yet within a few years we had bought so much stuff, enough to fill a 2-bedroom flat! Most items were never used and were certainly not *important* purchases. What a total waste of money!

A cluttered house usually mirrors a cluttered mind, and for me that was *very* true. I had too much stuff going on with my thoughts (unhappiness, anxiousness and uncertainty) and when I saw the clutter, it would make me feel even worse, although at that stage I didn't make the connection – I simply thought I needed more of the 'right' things to feel happy. I always wanted more money to buy more things, but in reality, none of it was making me feel happier for long. I really think this quote below is very true:

> People with enormous amounts of money are, contrary to common folk wisdom, actually no happier than their less wealthy counterparts, and they are statistically more prone to depression and other forms of psychopatholgy.
> Psychologists Solomon, Greenberg, Pyszcynski

It's thought that in regards to weight, those that live in a cluttered house are more inclined to be overweight. According to Peter Walsh who is known as the 'Guru of Clutter':

> Your home is cluttered because you've lost control of it. And if your kitchen is out of control, it's highly likely your eating habits are as well. Because what you weigh isn't just about calorie counting or doing stomach crunches. What you weigh is about how you live.[33]

When I first began to declutter my home, I began with one room at a time. This is the easiest and the least overwhelming way, and it's what I can recommend you do, if your house is cluttered too. Just take small steps, as it's still a step in the right direction.

I cannot begin to tell you how *good* it felt to get rid of things that I never used or just weren't needed anymore. I gave lots of things to friends, neighbors, sold some on Ebay and donated some to charities who could do some good with it. What is someone else's trash can definitely be someone else's treasure, so nothing really has to ever go to waste.

What made me aware of this was when I watched the *Oprah Show* one day and saw an episode on house 'clutterers'. Although I was nowhere near as bad as the people on there (they had so much stuff they literally would fill a warehouse up with it all and were living amongst absolute filth), what Peter Walsh said made total sense. He explained that people who feel the need to buy so much stuff are trying to fill a hole to replace something that is missing inside themselves. And that thing was usually love or validation.

Have a think about this: perhaps, growing up, you didn't feel like your parents loved you, so you tried to find a type of love in having new things, or your parents shopped a lot when they wanted to be happy and gave you gifts when they wanted to show you their version of 'love'. You got a short burst of happiness after receiving gifts like this, which led to a lifetime of loving new 'stuff'. Don't worry – if this is you, you are most certainly not alone.

It's very common to have addictions such as buying things, because they, like drugs, are a quick fix, but without the obvious dangerous health effects. Despite it not really harming your health as such (ie. it's doubtful anyones been admitted to hospital because they spent too much money), it can certainly affect your life in general by causing more stress from the lack of space and tidiness, and it may also cause you to become constantly in debt. We often buy things to try and make us feel better, secure, and whole. Yet, can a pair of shoes or a diamond watch really make you feel that way long term? Nope, it's impossible. It's like filling a never-ending black hole – you simply will *never* fill it up. These things are not *connected* to us or a part of us; they are just *objects*. Sure, a special item of jewelry that someone you love has given to you is definitely special, but 99% of our personal items are not connected to real meaning. And who can you truly rely on to get the love you crave from? You, that's who. Only *you* can make you feel better, secure, and whole. Bestselling author & psychologist Steve Taylor shares with his readers in his book *Back To Sanity – Healing The Madness of Our Minds* this insight into our obsession with 'stuff':

Our mad materialism is partly related to our inner discontent. Because we feel uneasy and dissastified inside, we instinctively look to external things to try and alleviate our discontent. Materialism does give us a kind of happiness – the temporary thrill of buying something new and the ego-inflating thrill of owning it afterward. And we use this kind of happinesss to try to override – or compensate for – the fundamental unhappiness inside us.

In addition, our desire for wealth is a reaction to the sense o lack and vulnerability generated by ego-separation. This generates a desire to make ourselves more whole, more signif-icant and powerful. We try to bolster our fragile egos and make ourselves feel more complete accumulatin wealth and posses-sision.

It doesn't work, of course – or at least, it only works for a very short time. The happiness of buying or owning a new item rarely lasts longer than a couple of days. The sense of ego-inflation generated by wealth or expensive possessions can be more enduring, but it's very fragile too. Your happiness depends on comparing yourself to other people who aren't as well off as you, and evaporates if you compare yourself to someone who is wealthier. And no matter how much we try to complete or bolster our ego, our inner discontent and incompleteness always re-emerges, generating new desires. No matter how much we get, it's never enough. You thought a four-bedroom house would satisfy you, but now you'd like an even bigger one. You thought a six-figure salary would be more than enough to meet your needs, but after a couple of years your aiming to increase it even more. You thought your house was exactly as you wanted it, but soon you're itching to buy an unnecessary new carpet, a fashionable new type of fridge, or the latest type of hi-fi equipment. As Buddhism teaches, desires are inexhaustible. The satisfaction of one desire just creates new desires, like a cell multiplying.

I think most people can relate to this, I know I certainly can - it's how I operated for years and still can fall victim to at times.

Many people are just oblivious to *why* they buy so many things, yet it's also never enough. They don't sit and look around and think, 'Wow, I have all these things, but have they *actually* made my life truly better? Does it *really* mean anything important to me? Or is it actually ruining my life due to owing too much money or taking over too much space in my home?' Owning a designer pair of shoes or the latest fashionable dress is not something that you will remember as so important about your life, nor is it something you can even use to describe the real you. How you *feel* about yourself will be, and working on loving yourself, without all of that stuff, is the key to a truly happy and fulfilling life. Not the clothes you wear or the stuff in your house. There is no problem with wanting to be well-dressed and to have a lovely home, but it's important to put it all into perspective. Stuff does *not* make who you are - your heart and soul and kindness to others does that.

As you will see later in this book, love can be shown in a number of ways. For some, they find it easy to show their love by buying others gifts. This can also scew your *own* idea of love if that's all you got from your caregivers. If someone asks you, 'do you think your parents love you?' and your answer is 'yes - why? - Because they buy me nice things', then you really need to analyze that answer. Love is *not* only about *buying* people things, it's due to a whole list of other far more important actions too. For truly happy people who want to have healthy relationships you need to find out what people want in regards to love so that you both are getting and receiving what you want. Giving gifts is only *one* piece of the love puzzle.

I still like nice things, and that means yes, I do like to occasionally go shopping. And sometimes my shopping addiction tendancies even seem ready to rear their ugly head again but I always try and take a step back at how my life is at that stage and ask myself, 'am I a bit stressed right now? Am I not having enough "me" time, am I watching too much TV and not working on my spirituality enough? What hole could I be trying to fill?'

Television I particular is causing us to want more stuff due to reality type shows that show lives of the rich and famous which are more poplar than ever before. Steve Taylor discusses this in his book *Back To Sanity – Healing The Madness of Our Minds*:

> Another problem with TV – and the media in general – is that it provides an alternate reality that makes us less interested in the real world. It makes us less interested in our own lives, and less interested in making changes in them. If you eavesdrop a conversation in a shop, an office or a café, there's a good chance that, rather than talking about their own lives, people will be chatting about TV shows or media celebrities. And it's not so imperative to make our own lives more fulfilling or exciting when there's so much stimulation and excitement to be found in this unreal parallel world. But most of all, I dislike television because its primary function is to put us into a mental slumber, to blot out reality to take us out of ourselves, out of our environment, and out of the present, so that we don't have to face our psychological discord.

So TV can do far more harm than just putting ideas into your head about what will make you truly happy, it may even cause you to stop trying to improve your own life altogether by subconsciously thinking, 'Why bother? I will never have what they have.'

Now, when I do go shopping, I make sure I purchase either ethically produced or sourced things, or items that are going to last me a long time and that I will wear often so as not to be a waste Before I changed my shopping actions, I bought pretty much everything I could get my hands on. Useless things, that were poor quality, cheap and just a total waste of money. Most of the time I didn't even really like it that much at all. It was just a quick fix.

When it comes to clothing, I really liked the advice that Oprah Winfrey gave her audience. When she buys a new item of clothing, she removes one from her wardrobe (and gives it away to her staff/friends/charity) that hasn't been worn often so that she can keep the amounts of clothing in her wardrobe to a sensible level.

It's also worth noting: if you spend lots of time on the computer and if the computer itself is in a mess – as in, nothing is organized in it or you have lots of things on your desktop and everything is just chaotic – then it is well worth doing a big tidy-up. I am a victim (or perpetrator!) of 'computer chaos syndrome' and always have far too many emails so that my inbox is a complete mess, my photos are all over the place, my eBooks are in the wrong spot, and so forth. This, too, adds to clutter and also affects the mind. Always try and keep on top of the way your computer is organized. It can make a big difference to how you feel.

Peter Walsh has a very helpful website:

✓ Peterwalshdesign.com

Chapter 9

Water – Is It Healthy Anymore?

Every living organism on earth depends on water. Humans especially. Our brains are made up of at least 75% water, and as adults our bodies need at least 1.5–2 liters a day to remain healthy. Many people drink far less than that, or are having their liquid intake consist mainly of coffee, teas, soft drinks or sugary juices. I know some people who never drink a glass of water. To be functioning at a healthy and optimal level, pure clean water is *always* essential. Dehydration is a serious detriment to health and can cause a whole series of health problems.

Dr. Fereydoon Batmanghelidj (who once studied under the guidance of Sir Alexander Fleming, the discoverer of penicillin) is recognized worldwide for his contribution to the subject of water as a healing tool and how it affects human health. He has a truly incredible story.[34] Dr Batmanghelidj was born in Iran, and in 1979, when the Iranian Revolution broke out, he was jailed as a political prisoner for almost 3 years. During this time, he discovered the powerful healing ability of water. One night, a fellow prisoner was in immense pain from a peptic ulcer. Because there were no medications available, all that Dr. Batmanghelidj could do was to give him water. After the prisoner had two glasses of water, the doctor noticed that within just under 10 minutes, his pain had completely gone. So he instructed him to drink two glasses of water every 3 hours. His patient became completely pain-free during the rest of his 4-month prison stay. Dr. Batmanghelidj then went on to successfully treat 3000 other prisoners, who all suffered similar stress-induced ulcers, with just water alone.

During his own stay in prison Dr. Batmanghelidj documented his research into what was happening time and time again in his patients. He saw that water had an incredibly powerful and fast-acting medicinal affect and could prevent and relieve many painful degenerative problems. Due to his good behavior, Dr. Batmanghelidj was offered the chance to be released early but made the brave choice to stay in jail for 4 more months. He completed his research into the relationship between bleeding peptic ulcer disease and dehydration. These findings were published in the *Journal of Clinical Gastroenterology* and *The New York Times Science Watch* in June 1983.

The doctor has gone on to speak around the world on the subject of water and disease and has published the groundbreaking book *Your Body's Many Cries for Water: You're Not Sick, You are Thirsty! Don't Treat Thirst with Medications.* He writes that regular water intake may help the following:

- Asthma
- High blood pressure
- Adult-onset diabetes
- Heartburn
- Arthritis
- Back pain
- Angina
- Migraines
- Colitis
- Cholesterol
- Neurological and autoimmune disorders

While it's clear that water is so vital for our health, a huge problem that we are facing today is that our water *quality* is the worst it has ever been. And for water to have the health benefits it is capable of giving, the water has to be as pure as possible.

We tend to see water as pure, because it's a crystal-clear liquid with 'nothing' else in it, yet underneath a microscope there are typically so many horrible things lurking. And I am not just talking about bacteria either. One would think that water will always help our body flush out toxins and make us healthier, but sadly in many cases, water is only *adding* many more toxins into our bodies, some of which are *extremely* serious and are making us sick. What has been done to our water over the years is an *absolute crime*. Gone are the days when we could feel safe drinking water from our taps or having long hot showers and relaxing baths. Analysis all around the world shows high levels of toxins in our water supply, ranging from the poisonous fluoride to pharmaceutical medicines such as the contraceptive pill, painkillers and antidepressants. And most water supplies contain worrying levels of pesticides, insecticides, lead, and other heavy metals. Many water supplies have countless toxins found in them, yet nothing is done about it because the companies say that it's in 'trace levels'. But remember, a poison is a poison at any level and this entire book is based on the fact that the *accumulation* of toxic chemicals is what is actually killing people.

Water has to be processed so many times, with other chemicals added back in (and the precious minerals removed) so as to make it 'safe'. But the problem is, it's definitely *not* safe! Water nowadays generally contains more unsafe qualities than good ones and is linked to many health problems. The main culprits causing these health problems stemming from toxic water quality are the chemicals chlorine and fluoride.

Chlorine

Chlorine is a highly toxic and reactive halogen element that is used to kill bacteria in the water. It is responsible for more household poisonings than any other toxin, and it also detrimentally affects the ozone layer. In regards to the effect on human health, what scientists have discovered is quite worrying. When reacting with naturally decomposing plant and animal materials, chlorine creates by-products such as trihalomethanes and chlorinated hydrocarbons. This chemical reaction has been linked to certain types of cancers in humans. According to the President's Council on Environmental Quality, 'there is increased evidence for an association between rectal, colon and bladder cancer and the consumption of chlorinated drinking water'. Research also indicates that the incidence of certain cancers is 44% higher among those that are drinking chlorinated water.

Chlorine toxicity is also linked to other health problems such as heart attacks, and shockingly, also to cancers such as melanomas.[35] According to Dr. J.M. Price of the Saginaw Hospital, in Michigan, USA:

Chlorine is the greatest crippler and killer of modern times. While it prevented epidemics of one disease, it was creating another. Two decades ago, after the start of chlorinating our drinking water in 1904, the epidemic of heart trouble, cancer and senility began.

According to British Toxins expert Dr Paula Ballie-hamilton, chlorine seems like its more of a problem for the health of women:

Those who drink chlorinated water are at higher risk of developing breast cancer. It seems that chlorine reacts with some of the substances in the water to form trihalomethanes, compounds linked to breast cancer. This cancer-inducing effect has been demonstrated in a study performed on women drinking chlorinated tap water in Louisiana.

Let's have a think about how much water you come into contact with every day. When you have a shower, say, for 10 minutes (please note that most people usually have one for much longer), the chlorine you absorb is the equivalent of what you would absorb from drinking 10 liters of water. And if you have two showers a day, then do the math: that is a lot of chlorine. And if you go swimming in a chlorinated pool then, yikes, that's even way more. Of course, soaking in a hot bath for long periods of time is going to affect you even worse. And if you are drinking about 2–3 liters of water a day, which is the recommended amount, then it's quite easy to see just how serious this problem of accumulation of chlorine is for us. Unfortunately, because chlorine does do a great job of killing bacteria in the eyes of our water boards, it doesn't look like it will be removed from our water supplies anytime soon

If you are concerned when bathing, you can purchase 'Chlorine Balls' which you drop into your bath. These wonderful balls help to turn the chlorine into zinc chloride which, is completely harmless. Please google to find out where you can purchase them.

Let's now move on to the dangers of too much fluoride. I will warn you now: it gets *far* worse in regards to toxic water from here.

Fluoride

Most doctors and dentists think that the fluoride used in dentistry is very good for us, is necessary for strong teeth and is from a naturally occurring source. The *real* truth is far from good for us, and far from natural.

This is a little-known fact amongst our healthcare providers, but the fluoride used in our water, and in our toothpastes, is actually a *waste product* of the aluminum manufacturing process.[36] It is so *highly reactive* that when in contact with steel, glass, iron and most other substances, fluoride will actually eat right through it. Yet it's supposed to be good for our teeth and safe for our long-term health. How can it be, if that's what it does to steel?

It's undeniable now that lead is dangerous for our health, yet on the scale of toxicity, with lead being classed 3–4 as a 'moderate' toxin, *fluoride exceeds lead* as a 4 and is classed as 'very toxic'.

Fluoride seems to fit in with lead, mercury and other poisons that cause chemical brain drain. The effect of each toxicant may seem small but the combined damage on a population scale can be serious especially because the brain power for the next generation is crucial to all of us.[37]

Philippe Grandjean, Professor of Environmental Health, senior author of the Harvard Study

Chemically produced fluoride was first added to our water over 80 years ago with the purpose of helping reduce tooth decay. It was added to tap water with *zero* studies being performed. Nor was it ever approved by the FDA. Now that there *has* been lots of research, the results are generally being kept from the public. Probably because if governments come out now and say, 'Hang on, we made a huge mistake – this stuff is actually super-dangerous, has caused great harm and early death to many people', no one would ever take seriously anything else they say, currently or in the future. It's like a lie that has run so deep it's too late to turn back and tell the truth. If people do talk about how dangerous fluoride really is, they are classed as conspiracy theorists, and in many confirmed cases, people have been fired or threatened with firing from their job in certain government agencies.

Doctors and dentists also don't tend to know that when the first proposal was made (in 1939) to add fluoride to public water supplies, it was made by a scientist who was working for the *Aluminum Company of America*. Before 1945, the year that water fluoridation took effect, fluoride was in fact a known poison. The American Dental Association actually said it was classed as a toxin. An article in the 1 October 1944 issue of the *Journal of the American Dental Association* stated:

Drinking water containing as little as 1.2 ppm fluoride will cause developmental disturbances. We cannot run the risk of producing such serious systemic disturbances. The potentialities for harm outweigh those for good.[38]

A few brave people tried to get the government to stop adding fluoride to the water, but money and politics – surprise, surprise – got in the way. So it's now in many municipal water supplies worldwide. Luckily it's not found in huge doses in many of the towns and cities in the UK. In fact Europe is super-lucky: 92% of Europe does not have any added fluoride in its water supply, but

America and Australia do have particularly high levels. The reason fluoride is still in there today is because it was added over 80 years ago, and the proof that it is indeed a poison was, and still is, pushed right under the carpet. Despite many organizations kicking up a big fuss about it – and some towns indeed have managed to get the fluoride removed from their water supply, or have put a stop to it from being added in the first place – not enough people know about the dangers in their own current water supply.

Fluoride has an even *darker* history to its use. In many of the Nazi concentration camps, the prisoners drank fluoridated water. The Nazis knew it was a poison and wanted to see exactly what it would do to people:

In the 1930s, Hitler and the German Nazis envisioned a world to be dominated and controlled by a Nazi philosophy of pan-Germanism. The German chemists worked out a very ingenious and far-reaching plan of mass-control which was submitted to and adopted by the German General Staff. This plan was to control the population in any given area through mass medication of drinking water supplies. By this method they could control the population in whole areas, reduce population by water medication that would produce sterility in women, and so on. In this scheme of mass-control, sodium fluoride occupied a prominent place. I was told of this entire scheme by a German chemist who was an official of the great IG Farben chemical industries and was also prominent in the Nazi movement at the time. I say this with all the earnestness and sincerity of a scientist who has spent nearly 20 years' research into the chemistry, biochemistry, physiology and pathology of fluorine – any person who drinks artificially fluorinated water for a period of one year or more will never again be the same person mentally or physically.[39]

Charles E. Perkins, chemist, letter written 2 October 1954

Now, after reading all of this, (and I hope after a bit of your own research) I would be surprised if anyone still thought fluoride was OK and continued to feel safe drinking it. If not then you may indeed have been drinking fluoride for too long and it's affected your ability to think. Even though this is meant as a joke, it's actually serious too. In more than 500 peer-reviewed studies, the adverse effects of fluoride toxicity have been shown to cause birth defects *and* brain damage; it harms kidney function, is linked to osteoporosis, can increase hip fractures, causes thyroid disease and cardiovascular disease, and can cause certain types of cancer. In 1990, fluoride was found to be an undeniable carcinogen by the National Cancer Institute Toxicology Program.

Studies have been carried out in communities which have water supplies with high levels of fluoride as opposed to communities which have minimal amounts.[40] The results were astounding. The people living in the communities with the *higher* levels of fluoride in the drinking water showed a much greater incidence of 'mottled' teeth. And the people who lived in the less fluoridated areas had far less incidence of this problem. This mottled-teeth problem is now called 'fluorosis'.

NaturalNews.com recently exposed something truly shocking about the fluoride industry. After doing a simple web search on the well-known Chinese site Alibaba.com for wholesalers, they found various listings of bulk fluoride powders. What they discovered was quite alarming: this same fluoride, which is classed as an industrial chemical, and put into waterways all over the world, is also used in other industries such as these:

- as a bactericide and pesticide in agriculture
- as a UF 2 adsorbent in the nuclear industry
- as an anti-corrosion agent in the wood industry
- to fuse things together in the steel industry
- as a treatment of hides and skins in the leather industry

What is absolutely shocking is knowing this: If you have fluoride left over as a waste product, you are *not allowed to dump it into the ocean.* Yep, that's true. It's 100% illegal. Yet, for some crazy reason, it's allowed to be put into our drinking water! I know. Utter madness. But when you think about it, it makes sense that these companies find another way to get rid of this poison while making money out of it by selling it to another industry. Nice, huh?

What can too much fluoride do to you?

Here are some rather serious health problems which are linked to fluoride toxicity:

- Arthritis
- Gastrointestinal effects
- Bone fracture
- Hypersensitivity
- Brain effects
- Kidney disease
- Cancer
- Male infertility
- Cardiovascular disease
- Pineal gland problems
- Diabetes
- Skeletal fluorosis
- Endocrine disruption
- Thyroid disease

Facts about fluoride

- Toxic by inhalation
- Can cause increased porosity of enamel and staining of the teeth known as fluorosis – the CDC recently reported that 41% of American teenagers have some form of fluorosis. This is an increase of 400% since 60 years ago.

- Reduces infant IQ (concluded by Harvard Medical University Researchers) – 8,000 children were included in this study[41] and those that lived in areas where water contained high levels of fluoride had significantly lower IQs. Currently, 35 other studies have also shown that it reduces IQ. After reviewing 27 of these studies, Harvard scientists have stated that further research into this should be a high priority.
- Infants are much more at risk of being affected by fluoride due to their body weight – 400% more than adults per pound of body weight.
- Classed as a drug by the FDA: 'Sodium fluoride used for therapeutic effect would be a drug, not a mineral nutrient. Fluoride has not been determined essential to human health. A minimum daily requirement for sodium fluoride has not been established.'[42] (Source: Food and Drug Administration, 15 August 1963)
- The lethal dose of artificial fluoride is approximately 50 times that of natural fluoride.
- Fluoride has been used as a poison to kill rats (just like arsenic).

After knowing this, why would we want to drink water with fluoride every day? Why is it ok to drink water that is more like a drug? Why would we think it's OK to bathe and shower in it regularly? Why do our governments think this is OK for our health now that numerous studies are showing how *deadly* it actually is? Does it make sense to think our teeth will remain strong over years from using a highly toxic chemical which can eat through steel?

Recently, it was discovered that China has been openly selling fluoride to US companies who then put it in the water. These companies have clearly listed it on their website as a poison.

Some countries throughout the world have added fluoride into their water systems and others have not. Australia and USA are said to have fairly high levels (some cities and states are worse than others) while the UK has only 10% of local water with fluoride added to it. If you check Wikipedia and type in 'fluoridation' it will bring up some general information about worldwide use of this chemical.

Many people are becoming much more aware of how toxic and dangerous fluoride actually is and have demanded that their local water company remove fluoride from their community's water. If you are concerned, it's recommended to check with your local water company and ask for a report to see how much is in there. There are naturally occurring fluorides in the ground and in super-tiny amounts these are relatively harmless, but higher levels and the fluoride created industrially are the ones to be super-concerned about.

Something else which I really want to warn parents about is, using fluoridated water when mixing up formula for your children. In mothers' breast milk the trace amounts of fluoride is said to only be around 0.04% parts per million (ppm), so tiny that it does not cause any harm. Yet in infant formula, which is mixed with tap water treated with fluoride, the levels are about *240 times* higher than that. And since this crucial stage is when the brain is being formed, it's completely disgusting that more people do not know how dangerous fluoridated water is for their child's physical and mental development.

To avoid coming into contact with fluoride as much as you can, I recommend the following:

- Do not have fluoride treatments at the dentist – find a dentist that is more holistically trained
- Don't ever take fluoride tablets
- Avoid certain antidepressants as some contain fluoride (Prozac, for example)
- Do not use Teflon, or other brands of non-stick coated cookwear
- Breastfeed your child for as long as you can
- Do not use toothpastes containing fluoride. In a single use,

these can contain many more ppm (parts per million) than drinking fluoridated water. I have seen some dentist-prescribed toothpastes contain *5000 ppm* of fluoride. Look out for a homemade recipe for toothpaste in the DIY section, Part 4 in this book)

- Eat better-quality foods and fewer processed foods such as non organic chicken which can contain high levels of fluoride
- Do not ever use soy-based infant formulas
- Do not use fluoridated water to add to your children's food/drinks/formula
- Avoid drinking non-organic grape juice – grape juice contains high levels of fluoride
- Change the quality of your water supply at home (suggestions will be discussed in this section)
- Use a water filter that removes fluoride

You can also read more about the damaging effects from fluoride at:
- ✓ fluoridealert.org
- ✓ nofluoride.com

* * *

I'm sorry, but it doesn't stop here. Unfortunately chlorine and fluoride aren't the only chemicals lurking in our water. As reported by *New Scientist*, common chemicals from medications found in tap water can be any, and at times all, of these:[43]

- Atenolol, a beta-blocker for cardiovascular disease
- Atrazine, a herbicide banned in the European Union which has been shown to severely affect fish stocks. It is still in use in the USA
- Carbamazepine, a drug used to treat bipolar disorder
- Estrone, an estrogen hormone secreted by the ovaries and linked to causing gender changes in fish

- Meprobamate, a tranquilizer used in psychiatry
- Naproxen, anti-inflammatory and painkiller linked to increases in asthma
- Gemfibrozil, an anti-cholesterol drug
- Phenytoin, a drug used to treat epilepsy
- Sulfamethoxazole, an antibiotic
- TCEP, an agent used in molecular biology
- Trimethoprim, an antibiotic

Because so many people are on various medicines these days, they urinate them out, which means they go into the waterways, then back into our drinking water system again. It's just a constant cycle of chemicals that goes through us and back into the environment.

The waste water from our toilets, is even sometimes used by scientists so that they can find out how much of a certain medication is being consumed or flushed down the toilets. Researchers from the UK's Centre for Ecology and Hydrology made the discovery when they analyzed public sewage and waste water (from two UK towns with combined population of 214,000) over a period of 24 hours back between 2009-2010. They discovered that around *600,000* courses of Tamiflu, prescribed to treat swine flu were thrown down the toilet or not used at all, which some say costed the UK Tax Payer around £7.8 million in waste drugs. Because the drug only became active once consumed, the scientists were able to figure out, just how much Tamiflu had actually been taken. I don't know about you, but this really concerns me that tests can easily be done on the waste water to find out how much of a particular drug has been used. They were only testing for one drug, what if they tested for all commonly used in existence, and how much of these drugs are excreted then come *back* into our drinking water? As you can see from the list above, many are *already* showing up.

Let me tell you about the effects of just one of these chemicals in the above list. Atrazine is particularly dangerous because it is so prevalent in our world. And unfortunately it's also found in most of our water systems. Atrazine is a pesticide that has been shown to cause alarming defects in frogs, and not from exposure of a huge amount of the chemical either. Studies have shown that severe malformation is happening from just 0.1 parts per billion of atrazine. Frogs are developing several sets of *both* the testes and ovaries! And in some of the frogs, there are female eggs being discovered sitting in the sacks of the testes.

Other studies have shown that frogs born as a male have grown up and literally changed into a female! And some of them went on to have the ability to lay eggs, despite being born genetically a male! How does this happen? Well, atrazine is causing an immense disruption to hormones by affecting the natural production of testosterone. It turns on an enzyme called aromatase, which converts the testosterone to estrogen.

How does this relate to humans? Well, sadly, it does in a big way – and most especially to women. Breast cancer is the number one cancer found in women. Breast cancers are regulated in the body by estrogen and also by the enzyme aromatase. Aromatase will convert androgens into estrogens, which promote the growth of cancer cells, which will then turn into a tumor.

If this *one* chemical is causing such terrible effects to frogs, and is linked to breast cancers from just a small amount of this pesticide, what the heck is a whole mixture of other chemicals in our water going to do to us humans? It's quite clear to see how important it is to drink healthy water.

Not only do we need to worry about the levels of different drugs that are in our water, but we also need to ensure we have safer levels of things like lead, bacteria, iron, copper, sulfate, chloride, pesticides and a few more.

Some will argue that it is impossible to deliver healthy, clean water throughout big cities and this is the reason why water companies have to use the chemicals etc., but clearly, judging from the information above, how they 'clean' the water is not working. Highly dangerous chemicals are still in there and are directly affecting people's health. There are safe cleaning methods such as using UV lights to purify the water and this is used in many home water systems. It could easily be introduced by the big water companies.

The reason why the subject of tap water is so important is because, over time, the chemicals will of course add to all of the others already in your body and can go on to causing major health problems. Showering and bathing is the most worrying because you are exposed every day, as hot water seeps through the skin (and particularly through the scalp), drying it out superficially, while on the inside of your body the toxins are mixing in with all of the other chemicals that can't get out, and over time, can again add to your toxic overload. Many people think they have naturally dry hair but it's more than likely the constant washing with tap water that's causing this dryness. When I first used a shower filter, I noticed almost immediately how much better my hair was. My hair colour would not fade nearly as much and I didn't suffer with an itchy scalp like I normally did. The skin on my body was so much softer and I didn't get any itching, even in winter when hot water was a must.

When you look at the information and think logically, it makes perfect sense: our water quality is *seriously* harming our health. We swallow it, and whatever is in it goes directly into our cells and organs and brain tissues. *This is so worrying as our brains are 70% water.*

In more extreme cases, in some countries (not just Third World ones by the way) the water systems have been so polluted (illegally, I must add) due to industrial companies dumping toxic waste nearby. I am sure you all remember the movie *Erin Brokovich* – about the single mum who took on a huge civil action court case against Pacific Gas & Electric, and won? It not only gave Julia Roberts an Oscar; it also spurred Erin on to continue fighting for people's human rights in regards to environmental poisoning.

Right now she is involved in a case about Camp Lejeune, a military base in North Carolina where thousands of residents have been poisoned by the water, over a 30-year period, which was tainted with highly toxic cancer-causing chemicals. As many as 200,000 people have been affected – including children. Victims suffered leukemias, miscarriages, birth defects and terminal cancers. Over the 30-year period, nearly 1 million people drank this chemical water. Erin is fighting not just this case, but many others as well, such as investigating a Beverly Hills high school where it has been reported that up to 450 of the kids have developed cancers!

Toxic water pollution is not rare these days and is unfortunately becoming more and more common. In fact, I would doubt very much that any water supply anywhere is completely safe. How can it be with so many industries creating and spewing out these disease-causing chemicals? There are so many pollutants in the environment and companies are still being irresponsible and not disposing of their waste correctly – though we must ask ourselves: how can we dispose of something so toxic, *safely*? If we dump it in the ground we contaminate the ground, same with the sea, and if we burn it, it affects our air and atmosphere quality. We need to actually *stop* creating these kinds of chemicals in the first place. We rely far too much on man-made goods and services, and this will be (or should I say, is) our downfall.

Erin is working with Google to create a cancer 'cluster' map to show people where there is contaminated water supply. This lady is a true hero and if you want to check out what she is up to, please visit her website:

✓ brockovich.com

In 2011, Dupont, (who make the Teflon brand of non-stick cookwear,) were ordered to pay US $8.3 million due to polluting waterways close to their factory.[44] This contamination affected nearly *5000* homes in New Jersey where tests showed that the toxic industrial chemical perflurooctanoic acid (PFOA) was found in extraordinarily high levels. This was causing sickness among people who were unknowingly drinking this poisoned water. These dangerous endocrine inhibitors also take many years to disappear from the environment. The $8.3 million is going towards installing 5000 water filters in nearby residents' homes so that they can drink safer water.

What can you do about your own water?

With all this alarming knowledge about water just not being what we think it is anymore, you probably will want to stay away from absorbing and drinking unpurified tap water as much as you can. Because we need to drink lots of water each day and have regular baths and/or showers, the contact that we have with water is a heck of a lot, so it's highly recommended that you try and make the water that you come in contact with much safer for you and your family.

So, what can you do about having safer water throughout your home but not make it too expensive? I wish I could say that it's easy to get hold of spring water like we used to have hundreds of years ago, but unless you live near a spring (there are websites that can tell you if there is one nearby) it's very hard and pricey to have regular access to it. And most springs are contaminated with environmental chemicals anyway; if there are non-organic farms nearby then chances are the spring contains levels of pesticides in the water.

Luckily for the people of Iceland, they do not have to worry about this problem. Their tap water IS pure spring water. There are so many springs in Iceland that it's easier for them to use this natural source than to create a chemical-based one. And, not at all surprisingly, the people of Iceland are far healthier statistically than those of any Western countries. This *has* to be mainly due to the safe, pure water they drink.

In Monaco, it is reported that the water system is run through an ozone filter which removes all the bacteria and makes the water safe to drink. It's such a shame that you have to be a mega-multimillionaire to live there.

Thank goodness that for people like you and me, who don't live in these countries, there are plenty of excellent water devices on the market to help filter and clean the water.

Even though it's popular, I personally do not recommend using reverse-osmosis water filters, because the process actually causes the water to become 'dead' with no nutrients at all, and this type of water has been linked to osteoporosis (said to leach minerals such as calcium from the bones) and other problems. If you do get a RO water filter, find one that puts minerals *back* into the water.

After a few years of searching for something, I came across 'vortexed water'. A small pipe, made usually from copper, is unique because of how it has been designed on the inside. The way it has been made, with its grooves on the inner tube, allows a double 'vortex' to form, which, combined with pressure from the tap, causes the water to 'spin' just like it does in Nature. The spin is like that when you empty water out of a bath or sink and you see that it creates a tornado-like effect; this is what creates the vortex. The vortex puts energy back into the water as well as making unwanted chemicals 'implode' on the inside of the vortex. While it does not remove every single chemical, it is a really good substitution for having your water as clean as can be. Combined with another filter that can remove most of the chemicals, this sort of water is excellent for health.

According to Dr. Sergey Mjakin from the Radiant Research Centre in Russia, they recorded these findings:

Water revitalizer does result in certain changes in its structure, probably towards the formation of clusters. Furthermore and most interestingly, these changes are observed not only in the water directly treated in the WR but also in the remaining part of the water system previously being in contact with the portion passed through WR. The change in UV spectra of the samples passed through WR are the most significant and the values for the rest of aqueous system after WR treatment (e.g. liquid from the flask after a part of its content was treated by WR) are inter-mediate between those for the initial liquid before revitalizing and for the directly revitalized part. The most prominent evidence for this fact are obtained using very diluted solutions of benzoic acid since this substance is a highly sensitive indicator for those UV spectroscopy measurements (its solubility and consequently UV absorption/transmission performances strongly depend on the structure of the water in which benzoic acid is dissolved). Water is an intrinsically integrated object and revitalizing of even a small part of it results in a similar but certainly less strong effect in all of the water system being a whole before this procedure.

Vortex water apparently has 6 functions which tap water does not have:

- Hydrates the cells
- Supports the immune system
- Improves cellular communication
- Enhances waste removal from cells
- Enhances metabolic efficiency
- Helps transport nutrients to cells

Once installed in your home's water mains system, all of the water from your kitchen, laundry and bathroom will be vortexed and energized water, and the pipe lasts a lifetime and can be removed when you move house. You will notice a huge improvement immediately in your skin quality and hair, both being much softer, and the annoying winter itches are gone! Eczema and psoriasis sufferers will find this an absolute lifesaver! Even your laundry will wash better, your bathroom won't suffer from limescale buildup, and dishes come out of the dishwasher much cleaner.

These pipes can also be installed in schools, restaurants, hospitals, absolutely anywhere there is water. And using this water to fill your vases, and water your plants and veggie garden, will make things absolutely thrive!

Despite all of these findings, many people still are quite skeptical about vortexed water and if it really has any value for health. I believe, personally, that by having this pipe installed in our house, it made a *huge* improvement to our water quality. Whether or not it's completely purified to a 'perfect' level, I am still not sure, but I certainly think it's one of the best things we have spent our money on and I do feel safer bathing and showering in this water than I would with just untreated tap water. I do not always drink the water from the tap though, and instead collect water from a local spring near to us, and when I go out I try and purchase glass-bottled spring water just to be certain that I am drinking the safest water.

Many people who own a vortex pipe also have another filter attached to their kitchen sink which will purify the water after it's been through the vortex, to ensure that it is the best water possible you can have at home.

If you like the sound of the vortex pipe, yet it's a little out of your price range, another type is the CIR Vortex Energizer. Just like the pipe mentioned above, this copper-plated spiral device can be fitted to your mains system where it requires no future maintenance and will give your household's water a much healthier, more natural quality. It's also a lot more affordable than the vortex pipe.

- ✓ Available in the UK from mineralwaterfilter.co.uk
- ✓ Available for the USA from earthtransitions.com
- ✓ CIR Vortex Energizer from rawliving.eu
- ✓ Affordable whole house filters are available from uk-water-filters.co.uk

If you can't do anything to the mains system in your house if you are renting, or cannot afford it, then this next product for your bathroom is a great, less-expensive alternative. The 'Paragon' is a filter that also comes with a shower head which you can attach to pretty much any bathroom shower. You need to replace the filter inside every 6 months or so, possibly longer if you live on your own.

This filter removes up to 99% of chlorine and kills bacteria and fungi. This alone makes a big difference to your hair, skin and, more importantly, health. I had one of these for years before we bought the vortex pipe and it still gave us great results.

- ✓ Available in the UK from pureshowers.co.uk
- ✓ You can also purchase other types of water filters for bathing from:
- ✓ mineralwaterfilter.co.uk
- ✓ uk-water-filters.co.uk
- ✓ For similar filters available in the USA, go to mercola.com

For drinking water, this next product is really good, although a little pricey. The Vitalizer Plus is a jug that you fill with water, and when switched on, will create the vortex spin, adding oxygen and minerals to the water, therefore re-energizing the structure.

- ✓ Available in the UK from Aggressivehealthshop.com
- ✓ Available in the USA from vitalizerplus.net

I have heard great things about ozone water filters, and some people also swear by alkaline water filters. I am not personally a huge fan of drinking loads of alkaline water, but some of the testimonials I have read with dramatic health recoveries are worth looking into. I hear lots of great things about the Kanga water system.

Carbon filters, distillation systems and KDF water filters are all said to be very effective for cleaning water. You want water to be free of chemicals, but not too stripped that there are no beneficial minerals left in the water.

Bibo Water Filter

This compact machine, which looks just like a cute coffee machine, removes not only chlorine but also pesticides, heavy metals and other unwanted toxins that are usually in our water supply. It has a

UV filtration system that ensures the cleanest water possible. It sits on your kitchen bench and connects to your home water supply – it then boils and chills your water and is also very energy-efficient. It comes in a variety of cool colors and it also supplies chilled and hot water. You will need to replace the filters inside, a few times each year. For a small extra fee, the company sends over a qualified person to install your system in case you are not too sure how to connect it all up. This is one of the best at-home (or at-work) water filters I have seen.

✓ bibowater.co.uk

Eva Advanced Water Filtration System

This fantastic counter top water filter is said to eliminate over 98% of harmful substances such as lead, chlorine, copper, nitrate, aluminium, cadmium, arsenic, fluoride, bacteria & microbes. They claim to make the water so pure, it can be given to babies – either on its own or mixed in with formula.

It comes in a 7 or 12 litre size and filters need to be changed on average, every 9 months. This filter is one I am looking at buying.

Please google the name to find where you can buy it – is sold internationally.

For high quality and effective water filters in Australia, please visit nourishedlife.com.au

Bottled water

It should be no secret to you now that buying bottled water is a big fat no-no! Not only is it so bad for the environment as the plastic never breaks down (OK, it does break down, but it takes decades, if not hundreds of years!), but also the bottled water usually has a high dose of plastic particles floating around, which you end up drinking. These empty bottles usually end up in places like India (brought from other countries), just dumped there for years and years. Totally disgusting! When the bottles travel to their destination, they usually become exposed to intense heat, which causes the plastic to melt in a slight way; this is invisible to the naked eye but it happens nonetheless.

What this plastic does to you over time is pretty alarming: it causes havoc with your hormone levels, which in turn also affects brain function. And because of this hormone interference, it can also make you gain unwanted weight too.

If you are going to get bottled water, make sure it's in glass bottles, which can be recycled. Although plastic too can be recycled, it's more the plastic particles that concern me health-wise. I sometimes have to drink from plastic bottles if I can't get hold of glass-bottled ones, but make sure I take a dose of zeolites regularly to keep the plastic out of my body. I talk more about these in the chapter 'The Vital Importance of Detoxing'. I also think, if you live in the UK, make sure you buy spring water from springs in this country. The bottles are more likely to be transported in a cold environment which means that the leaching of plastic may be at a minimum.

The best spring water you can buy in the USA is said to be Mountain Valley. This company has been selling water for over 100 years and they are very open with what the water contains. It is sold in many different-sized beautiful glass bottles and the water is top-quality, true spring water.

✓ mountainvalleyspring.com

If you do buy plastic bottles, please try not to reuse them – you will notice on the bottle it will actually say: 'Use within three days.' So this means that they have proof that something happens to the bottle after it has been exposed to air. And that is, phthalates (a suspected endocrine disrupter) leach into the bottle and therefore the water after a few days. Many people refill their water bottles many times and some even leave them in a hot car; this is asking for double trouble as the warmth from the sun will make the chemicals leak into the water much faster, which you end up drinking.

When choosing any type of bottled water, check the nitrates level on the back. You do not want water with *any* nitrates in it if possible; the higher the level, the worse the water is for you. Nitrates come from pesticides from nearby local farming. When it rains these seep down into the springs and taint the water. Even relatively small doses can cause the water to be unfit for human consumption, yet the truth is, so many people are drinking what they think is healthy spring water that is actually heavily tainted with nitrates.

A really great brand of packaged water is from the highly ethical and compassionate company Aquapax. This beautiful mineral water is packaged in a non-leaching tetra pak so no plastic can taint the water. The water itself is sourced from deep below the earth, in fact 101 meters below ground, ensuring that it is as pure as can be.

✓ justdrinkingwater.com

If cost is a problem for you, then you can still help to make your drinking water much better quality. Even using a Britta Water Filter jug and adding a personal vortex energizer into the jug will help to restructure the water so that it is closer to its natural state.

You can also purchase tiny revitalizers which restructure liquids for when you travel. The Grander Water Technology Company, from Australia, offers customers the 'Penergizer' which is a pen-like tool you stir around in your liquid, such as water, juice, milk etc for about 20 times, then let it rest for a few minutes.

✓ grander.com.au

If you are interested in having the water you do drink tested, whether it's tap water, spring water, or mineral water, you can purchase kits off the internet which will allow you to test for a whole host of toxins such as bacteria, pesticides, lead, copper, arsenic, fluoride plus many more.

I tested our local spring water with a kit from Simplex Health. Even though I had a good feeling that the water was pretty good quality, I still wanted proof, so I ordered one of their kits off their website which tests for bacteria, nitrates (pesticides), lead, copper, iron and a few other things. I just wanted to make sure that it really was OK for my family to drink. The test kit arrived with several 'sticks' which you put in the water (just like when you do a pregnancy test) sampled from the spring. One of the tests, the bacteria one, took 48 hours to complete as the water needed to sit there for that long and see how much bacteria was detected. The other tests took only a few minutes to do. Luckily, everything came up as either negative or very minimal and therefore not a problem. While these simple tests can still not guarantee that the water is completely perfect (for example, it only tests for two types of pesticides and there are many in existence), it still gave me peace of mind that it was not testing up for anything too bad. Ideally I would put my spring water through some kind of filter to make sure it really was the best. And it's also important to remember that, with springs, the levels of minerals/toxins can change pretty quickly if there was something that happened nearby, such as if any local farmers started using new pesticides or something like Monsanto's Ready Roundup spray. It makes sense to test this kind of water quite often.

- ✓ simplexhealth.co.uk
- ✓ coleparmer.co.uk
- ✓ wagtech.co.uk

If you can't do anything at all about the water quality in your home, or you are concerned about other toxins your filter may not be able to remove, then please remember to make sure you regularly use Pure Body Zeolites by TouchStone Essentials to remove impurities from your body. This is a very inexpensive way to deal with toxic water.

You can find out what's in your water supply where you live by contacting your local government. You should be able to go onto a website and download the water reports. Or take matter into your own hands and test the water yourself. Bear in mind, though, that the tests will only test for a relatively small amount of chemicals and while the water may be, say, low in lead, it could be higher in other things.

Also, due to weather pollution, rainfall etc., your water could go from being OK one month to not so good the next. It really is best to get some sort of filter to ensure your water is safe at all times.

To find out what is in your water in the United States, please visit this website:

✓ ewg.org/tap-water/whats-in-yourwater

Here are some more tips on how to find safe drinking water:

✓ ewg.org/project/2009tapwater/EWG_safedrinkingwater.pdf

Chapter 10

Why Food Is One of Our Biggest Poisons of All

The modern diet is not providing enough vitamins. Malnourishment is going to make you more vulnerable to illnesses and less able to cope with them. The medical profession is only just beginning to take on board the implications of nutrition in patients.
Dr. Mike Stroud, author and world authority in human endurance and nutrition[45]

This is a *very* serious chapter because food alone is *killing* so many people all over the world, making them overweight, depressed, developing cancers, heart problems, diabetes and a whole bunch of other diet-related problems, more than ever before in the whole of human history. Most people right now are heading for a future that is going to be severely affected by poor health *just* from what they are eating.

You only have to look around you to see that this is true. It seems that it's more common to be very overweight these days than to fit within the healthy weight ranges. Overweight parents are having overweight kids, which means the kids think it's normal to be like this and are even less inclined to care about their own health. When you see others around you that look 'just like you', it's almost like it's 'safety in numbers' and you are more likely to feel like you fit in, rather than something is perhaps not right. Parents should be good examples in many ways, but sadly, this is a serious way where many are most certainly not. They don't know how to feed themselves and therefore do not know how to feed their children. With all of the blatant in-your-face advertising and cheap prices for junk foods, it seems easy to just do what the television and media are advising people to do. What is really shocking is this: junk food used to be *more expensive* than healthy food; 50 years ago, it was seen as a luxury and people really did have it only once in a while. Now the *opposite* is true: you may be able to buy several burgers as opposed to a decent amount of organic food. And with so many people struggling financially, the easy option for many, right now is to buy the junk food.

So many people now suffer with chronic stomach conditions and bowel problems such as IBS. This has also coincided with the rise in the 'invention' of processed foods and the chemicals used to sweeten and preserve them. They tend to take medication for this problem yet the way they eat, is generally the cause.

Food is very personal to all of us, and it is also one of the *toughest* ways to get people to change. We all know that eating too much of anything is not good and that it's all about balance, but what a lot of people don't realize is that even small amounts of certain foods can be terribly damaging to their health. Not to mention they can also be so very addictive. Some people will literally eat themselves to death and, when warned about the health implications by their doctor, and that a diet change is highly suggested, they simply just won't do it, and instead will eat themselves into an early grave. They just were so attached to their regular eating patterns; it was the 'one thing' that gave them a kind of joy, so they didn't feel they could change. *A change to a healthier diet makes some people prefer to die – isn't that absolutely crazy!*

But when we see just how many emotions are attached to food, then it's not so surprising. I grew up eating unhealthy foods pretty much *all* of the time. I was a fussy kid and always gravitated towards the foods that were just the worst kind for me. A typical day's worth of food for me was:

- A croissant with jam or butter for breakfast or a big bowl of Fruit Loops
- A packet of chips (crisps) with a can of coke for morning tea
- A meat pie with sauce for lunch followed by a cream bun or

donut
- Stir fry or casserole

Dinner was reasonably OK compared to rest because my mum would make something fairly balanced, but it was still not enough to make up for all of the bad food I ate earlier in the day. On the weekends I would eat more sugary things, lots of processed meats and also plenty of takeaways. The diet above is so typical – if anything it's better than a huge percentage of the population's eating habits. No wonder so many people are overweight and sick!

Looking back, the worst thing for me was the man-made chemicals that were in the food, and also the high sugar content. During school, I suffered with learning problems and could not concentrate, causing many teachers to think I was not trying or that I was perhaps just plain stupid. I certainly felt that way too, as I knew that my brain was just not doing what it should be. I was also constantly very angry and found it super-easy to get upset. I was always exhausted, and would have trouble keeping my eyes open in the class during the mornings. I was always getting into trouble for nodding off – of which I am sure is very common in classrooms today.

Given the state of my already fragile mental health, the sugar and chemicals were the *last* things I should have been eating. And you can bet that for *all* kids, this is detrimental to their development as well. Later in life, combined with constant periods of severe stress, the way I ate broke down my digestive system, in such a harsh way that when I did start to eat more healthily, my stomach could still not function. I couldn't absorb any nutrients from even the highest-quality organic food nor could I absorb any nutrients from high-quality vitamins. I had such severe nausea and a burning sensation, every day. If I hadn't sorted my health out, I have no doubt I would have gotten cancer or something else terrifying at a young age. My body was simply not being nourished properly and therefore my immune system was weak and unable to fend for itself. If cancer cells wanted to multiply, how could I possibly of been able to fight them?

Without the right type of nourishment, the body simply cannot keep toxins out or deal with processed chemical foods – in other words, it just can't remain healthy after too much stress!

I am the perfect example of what happens after a long period of eating terrible foods. In our youth, we think we can eat whatever we want because our metabolism is so fast. We rarely gain too much weight, our skin is still fairly good, so we think that whatever we are eating is fine. The truth is, the time we need healthy foods the most *is* when we are young because it sets us up for greater health later in life. We are still growing and need certain nutrients to be fit and strong, and they are essential for brain development and health. We need to realize we are actually *not* invincible, and over time, our seemingly perfect health that we are often blessed with during teenage years can quickly wear down. The body can only handle so much abuse. And abusing the body through food is just so intense and causes great stress.

These days, we have a huge amount of processed 'fake' foods in our supermarkets, which are made with toxic chemicals such as preservatives, colors, sweeteners, and are now often also genetically modified. All of these things are not anywhere near natural, and all give a negative chemical reaction inside the body. These additives are bad enough for us, but there are others that are far more troublesome. The sections below show the top main culprits for health problems related to food.

Monosodium glutamate or MSG – a salt of the amino acid, glutamic acid

MSG is something pretty much all of us have heard of and probably eaten quite a lot of. When people are questioned about MSG they think it's just in Chinese food but it's so not! It's everywhere! It's usually in the major fast-food products, and 'handy' supermarket items such as gravies, dipping sauces, Parmesan cheese products, soups, chicken and sausage items, soy sauce, fish sauce, cold meats and seasoning packets.

MSG is known as an 'excitotoxin' because it literally has the ability to to overstimulate cells to death.[46] It has not only triggered many asthma attacks in some people (causing deaths); it is now also linked to obesity, diabetes and high blood pressure. Whenever you buy food, check the labels, and if you go out to eat, always ask if the food contains MSG and avoid it if it does!

Here is a helpful list, courtesy of rense.com which will help you avoid buying MSG-laden foods:

Food Additives that ALWAYS contain MSG

Monosodium Glutamate
Hydrolyzed Vegetable Protein
Hydrolyzed Protein
Hydrolyzed Plant Protein
Plant Protein Extract
Sodium Caseinate
Calcium Caseinate
Yeast Extract
Textured Protein (Including TVP)
Autolyzed Yeast
Hydrolyzed Oat Flour
Corn Oil

Food Additives That FREQUENTLY Contain MSG

Malt Extract
Malt Flavoring
Bouillon
Broth
Stock
Flavoring

Natural Flavors/Flavoring

Natural Beef Or Chicken Flavoring

Seasoning

Spices

Food Additives That MAY Contain MSG Or Excitotoxins

Carrageenan

Enzymes

Soy Protein Concentrate

Soy Protein Isolate

Whey Protein Concentrate

If you are interested in learning more about MSG and other harmful excitotoxins, you can read the book by Dr. Russell Blaylock, *Excitotoxins: The Taste That Kills.*

HFCS

'HFCS' stands for High-Fructose Corn Syrup and is in pretty much every single unhealthy food there is. And it can be sneakily hidden in so-called healthy foods too. You really have to be on your toes to avoid this one.

HFCS is derived from corn and goes through an incredibly long processing method through heating, crushing, mixing, more heat and more crushing again, which leaves the once solid corn as a syrupy liquid that creates a very sweet taste. It, too, is also highly addictive and is in pretty much every can of soft drink, fast foods, and all of those so-not-freshly-made foods you see in supermarkets, 7/11 stores and petrol stations. Oh, it's also in cereals as well. Basically, it's everywhere. HFCS is linked not only to obesity, metabolic syndrome, and heart disease, but also to type-2 diabetes.[47]

In a can of soft drink there is 40 grams (8 teaspoons' worth!) of HFCS – in that one drink. Since many people drink nothing but soft drink these days, this alone is sending them to an early grave, not to mention how it affects the brain. Studies are showing that it's extremely addictive, hence why so many people are now addicted to junk foods. I wanted to include a helpful list for you here but it's very very long and would take up many pages.

Pesticides: herbicides, fungicides, insecticides – the common poisons on most of your food

These groups of chemicals have been used widely in the production of our food for over 50 years, which, ironically enough, is also when people's health started to rapidly decline. It's rampant use is also affecting our precious bees' health as well and they are rapidly dying, or going missing, because they keep feeding on plants and flowers that have been sprayed with chemicals.[48]

Years ago, farmers saw that there were problems with their crops dying by being eaten or infected with disease, so scientists set out on developing ways to keep insects, fungus and bugs off their plants. They invented harsh chemicals (most derived from petrol) which were sprayed directly onto the crops to keep the bugs and insects away. These certainly did work at keeping the bugs away, but they also contaminated the food in the worst possible way. It *boggles* my mind these were ever approved for use and are still in use today. Some chemicals are slowly being phased out, but it does not mean this problem is going to go away anytime soon. As you know, thousands of them have been created and it can take 10-15 years to get a chemical taken off a market (there are no worldwide bans of any chemicals as yet) so pesticides are causing huge problems all over the planet

What people do not realize, in regards to the production of food, is that it's not just a case of an apple getting sprayed with just one chemical. On average up to 48 different pesticides are used to keep that particular crop of apples surviving the season.[49] *Forty-eight different pesticides?!* That's crazy!

And if you have ever gone past a field where people are farming crops, when they are using chemicals they wear a top-to-toe completely covered-up protection outfit to keep them from getting poisoned! I was in Costa Rica in 2011 and it is one of the most lush and beautiful places in the world to grow food. However, I was horrified to drive past these stunning fields with men spraying the crops, covered in these protective suits, as I knew the chemicals would drift further away than just that field alone.

And it's even more horrifying when you see a plane flying over the crops with huge spray jets at the back, dousing the land and crops below. These chemicals not only go onto our food, but they also seriously harm the environment around us. It's getting into our air, our waterways, and seeping deep into the ground. And these chemicals stay in the ground for years. Just say you were a conventional farmer and you wanted to become an organic farmer. You owned a piece of land that had previously been farmed with chemicals. Well, to turn your land into an organic farm, you would need to wait for years to have that soil become as chemical-free as the certification bodies demand.

I meet a few people occasionally who say they do not think that non-organic foods are dangerous. I tell them to go and visit a conventional farm, get close to the person spraying and have a smell of the chemicals they are using. Or maybe even go and ask to be shown the container they originally came in and see all the warnings written on the side of the box. *Then* come back and tell me that they still want to eat food covered in all of this stuff! Or are they *still* happy to give their children this type of food? Eating foods every day with these chemicals on them is a very slow but pretty certain way to get sick.

Disturbing facts about pesticides*

- Every year, approximately 20,000 tones of pesticides are sprayed on UK farmland.
- Safety testing of pesticides assumes healthy adults. It does

not take into account vulnerable groups whose hormonal systems are rapidly changing: fetuses, babies, adolescents, the old and infirm.

- One teaspoon of agricultural pesticide poured down a drain could contaminate the drinking water of 200,000 people for a day.
- There are no limits to the number of pesticides in food. Maximum Residue Levels are set for food products but relate only to individual pesticides.
- Forty-nine hormone-disrupting pesticides ('Endocrine System Disrupters') have been identified by the European Union. Evidence of ESDs includes genital abnormalities, decreasing sperm counts and semen quality.
- Rainwater in part of Europe contains such high levels of dissolved pesticides that it would be illegal to supply it as drinking water.
- Studies have shown that 3 pesticides consumed together have 100 times the effect of any one chemical on its own.
- In 2008, 49% of European fruits, vegetables and cereals contained pesticides – the highest levels ever recorded.
- In a sample of 40 bottles of wine, 100% contained at least one pesticide, and one bottle contained 10 different pesticides.
- There are 442 apple pesticide products which are registered for use in the UK, containing over 70 active ingredients.
- There are 414 pesticide products for pears, with 61 active ingredients.
- Seals and cod in the Arctic Circle have pesticide residues as these chemicals are transported on wind, rain, and ocean currents from more southerly latitudes.
- Children's exposure to pesticides from all pathways (food, water, air, other) is likely to be higher, because they eat more food, drink more water, and breathe more air per pound of body weight.
- The World Health Organization believes that pesticides cause

772,000 new cases of disease each year.

- 40 pesticides used in the EU are toxic to bees. Certain pesticides have now been banned in some European countries because evidence has linked them to mass bee deaths. They are still permitted in the UK and other countries despite these findings.

Once thought safe, these pesticides are now banned

In 1986 after decades of rampant use, DDT, an insecticide, was finally banned. DDT is a toxic persistent organochlorine and probable carcinogen. It is also linked with polio-like (paralysis) reactions in people who came into contact with it. In 1988 Cyhexatin was banned after it was proven to cause birth defects. Aldrin was banned in 1991 and is also classed as a probable carcinogen. And in 2002, Lindane was banned as it was suspected to cause breast cancer. While it's great news that these are banned, in certain countries (mostly third world) they are *still* used widely. And many of these chemicals are still found our soil today, decades later. The question we must ask ourselves is: for how much longer will the rest be approved as safe, only to be banned later on, yet what damage will be done to us?

* For more information such as above please refer to pan-uk.org. They are known as The Pesticide Action Network. You can ask them to send an informative poster which covers this information plus more.

Why don't more people know about the harm these pesticides cause us?

Just like our beauty products, the amount of toxins one ingests over one day has never been proven to kill a person, so the companies can get away with still using these toxins. Also, sometimes the studies take years to complete, and the companies protest for as long as they can to avoid a chemical being banned. The government at times will also avoid banning it for as long as they can. But some studies *are* showing that over a long period of time, the effects are detrimental. Infertility, birth defects, stillbirths, miscarriages, learning disorders, breast cancer, prostate cancer and lymphatic cancers have *all* been linked to pesticides.

The subject of food today is *deadly* serious. Our food, 90% of the time, is now completely unnatural these days and is highly poisonous. No wonder there is so much sickness and disease. It really surprises me that most people still just don't make the connection that sickness is coming from all of our 'modern' advances (aka messing with Nature) and inventions.

Nitrates and nitrites

Nitrates and nitrites are chemicals which are used in fertilizers, rodenticides, and are also used as a food preservative.[50] These cancer-causing preservatives are found in meat, things like salamis, sausages, bacon and ham so that they last longer. Nitrates are said to be safe on their own but become deadly when heated, and since we never eat raw meat, they have always been heated to high temperatures and therefore become very toxic.

For people who regularly eat foods with nitrates, there is an increased risk of getting stomach cancer.[51] Look for nitrate-free products or avoid processed meat all together. Just this one change can reduce the risk of colon cancer.

Aspartame

This may be the *worst* food additive of the whole darn lot. Aspartame is one of the most deadly food ingredients that has ever been created. When it was first developed in 1975, the FDA (Food and Drug Administration) did not approve it for fears of safety because the tests on rats were showing unsafe results. Pretty much all of the rats developed brain tumors in a short amount of time. Many of the doctors who were involved in the testing agreed that they could not approve this sweetener. That was fine until Donald Rumsfeld joined the FDA.

He approved this previously proven deadly chemical within 2 weeks of being there (and would have fully known the outcome of these previous tests) and the rest is history – now aspartame is everywhere. Even in your children's 'no added sugar' 'healthier' cordial!

The pharmaceutical company Searle is responsible for the manufacturing and development of this fake sugar. And they now just happen to also make many drugs that will treat the side effects it causes.

It's more than sickening to see how it is all connected and how much money is made.

So what is aspartame?

Well, essentially it is a man-made sweetener to replace regular sugar. It allows big brands to say that their product is 'sugar free' or a 'diet' item and they market it (very successfully too) as a healthier food. The ironic thing is that aspartame can actually trigger your appetite even more, so your 'diet' food ends up making you *fatter*. You can find aspartame in pretty much everything, from cereals to breath mints, coffee drinks, frozen desserts, laxatives, milk drinks, soft drinks and pharmaceutical medicines, including ones for children! And this is just a small part of a very long list.

What they don't tell you is that aspartame is literally seen as a *poison* by the body and consumption has been linked to a whole list of problems such as:

- headaches/migraines
- dizziness
- seizures
- nausea
- numbness
- muscle spasms
- weight gain
- rashes
- depression

- fatigue/irritability
- tachycardia
- insomnia
- vision problems
- hearing loss
- heart palpitations
- breathing difficulties
- anxiety attacks
- slurred speech
- loss of taste
- tinnitus
- vertigo
- memory loss
- joint pain

According to researchers and physicians studying the adverse effects of aspartame, the following chronic illnesses can be triggered or worsened by the ingesting of aspartame: brain tumors, multiple sclerosis, epilepsy, chronic fatigue syndrome, Parkinson's disease, Alzheimer's, mental retardation, lymphoma, birth defects, fibromyalgia, and diabetes.

The FDA has received up to 92 different health complaints from people consuming aspartame-based foods.[52] Isn't this truly shocking? But the problem is, these kinds of foods are absolutely everywhere. Brands such as Nutrasweet® and Equal® are made from aspartame too. These manufacturers are very sneaky at hiding what is in their products by giving it a new-sounding name. To companies, aspartame is such a great money-making sweetener for them to use, because it is so very cheap to purchase.

Aspartame accounts for over 75% of the adverse reactions to food additives reported to the FDA. Monsanto purchased the G.D. Searle company in 1984, which means they now own aspartame and its other deadly products. More information on Monsanto is coming up below. If you have a sweet tooth it's always best to get sugars from natural sources such as raw honey, fruit, maple and brown-rice syrup and coconut sugar.

Do *not* ever eat anything with aspartame in it. Be smart and check all of the labels. And for your baby's sake, if pregnant *do not* ingest it! It could seriously harm your child's critical development!

For more info on aspartame please check out this website:

✓ sweetpoison.com

GMOs: Genetically Modified Organisms

Judging by the absence of published data in peer-reviewed scientific literature, apparently no human clinical trials with GM food have ever been conducted' Arpad Pusztai Ph D – Genetically Modified Foods: Potentential Human Health Effects 2003

When powerful biotech companies (who have been responsible for the development of things like DDT) start to recreate and manufacture foods in a laboratory, you know it's probably not going to turn out too well.

In studies carried out on 'Genetically Modified Organisms' (GMOs) and the effect they have on animal health, the results are coming up very dismal and quite terrifying indeed. The rats (and other animals used) usually die, or develop brain cancers, and their babies are being born deformed. A study that recently came from the French University of Caen, showing the actual photographs of the tumors on the rats after being fed GMO maize for a 2-year period, has sparked a huge outcry. These tumors were *enormous*, and undeniable proof that something is very wrong with GMOs.[53]

Yet governments are saying that GMOs *are* safe and are allowing them to be grown in their countries (even when there is a huge outcry of protest by the public) and sold in the form of food, animal farming included. Some scientists even like to say that the rats were given 'kgs' of the GMO's on purpose so as to force the negative result in the testing. So that the scientist carrying out the study, could get some kind of recognition and acclaim. I'd say in response to that, how does a tiny rat eat more than what it wants? How can it eat kilograms of food when it only weighs a tiny amount itself? And when a scientist goes against powerful companies who make billions, how can he get worldwide acclaim when he is David and the companies are Goliath? It's important to remember that even when something is clearly bad, PR teams are employed to make them look good.

Monsanto is at the forefront of creating GMOs. They also happen to be thought of as one of the most 'evil' companies in the world, causing many Third World farmers to go broke, where a huge number commit suicide or are resigned to being in debt for the rest of their lives. Not only that, but with their chemicals Monsanto have also polluted many areas in the world, and some humans have lost died due to this poisoning. And just to show you what sort of company Monsanto really are, they are also responsible for creating Agent Orange, which was used in the Vietnam War and is still wreaking havoc in people's lives today.

Here is something quite disturbing: Monsanto have also created 'terminator seeds' which they sell to poor countries. These seeds last only one planting, then become useless, making the often extremely poor farmer have to buy more seeds from Monsanto. This is enough information to show you that you do not want your food to come from companies like this.

Many animals when given GMO foods will simply not eat them, which is a big sign to me that we shouldn't be eating them either. Some animals, such as cows, are not exactly known to be super-intelligent, yet tend to they turn their noses up at GMO feed. Animals that have been fed GMO feed have died the very next day.

It is also very concerning and very unethical when you see the ties between Monsanto and the government. There are many people who have worked for Monsanto in high-power positions, and then gone on to work in Government at a high level, and vice versa. This allows massive conflicts of interest to happen and for the company to always get what it wants. There should be laws against this, but sadly there isn't.

We should all be able to freely choose what foods we purchase by the way they are labeled, right? Well, in the USA, GMO foods are required by law NOT to be labeled as GMO. How crazy is this? The companies simply do not want the public knowing what is in their food. It's an absolute disgrace. There was a huge campaign in the USA to label them and so many of the GMO companies paid huge amounts of money to support *not* labeling them. There was a vote carried out with many people saying it was completely rigged. They said that people voted YES to not labelling before the actual election was finished. They were never going to allow the NO vote to win. If GMO's are so good, then why can't we see them on the label? Why is it now law that they must NOT be labelled on our food. I think you will see, that this is just ridiculous.

Luckily in the UK we do have our food labeled with 'Non GMO', so conscious and savvy shoppers can find out what they are eating. It is important to know that GMO food does not just mean corn or soy products like it used to. GMO products have now been created for the following food items, of which certain ingredients are found in many infant formulas!

- Rapeseed
- Honey
- Cotton
- Rice
- Soybean
- Sugar cane
- Tomatoes
- Corn
- Sweet corn
- Canola potatoes
- Flax
- Papaya

- Squash
- Red-hearted chicory
- Cotton seed oil
- Tobacco
- Meat
- Peas
- Vegetable oil
- Sugar beets
- Dairy products
- Vitamins (ingredients like vitamin C ascorbic acid)

(Above list sourced from Disabled World – genetically modified foods information including list of GM foods with DNA changes and pros and cons of GM food: disabled-world.com)

Recently, President Obama said yes to GMO salmon entering into the food chain.[54] So if you eat salmon and live in North America and the USA, be very careful: what you think is a fish from Nature may be a fish that is anything *but* natural.

Most governments (particularly the USA) have direct ties to Monsanto, so before you think that they will stop this from happening, think again. They are all involved financially together. Ex-government workers now have lucrative jobs with Monsanto, and many ex-Monsanto staff are now working in government. What a clever way to make these ties tighter! Now knowing this information, hopefully you will realize the importance of buying local and organic food.

Hypocritically, the Obamas openly eat organic food and Michelle Obama has been photographed planting an organic garden at the White House,[55] yet Obama is showing support for the companies that make the GMOs that the rest of the world is eating. GMOs are not good enough for them to eat, yet it's fine for the rest of the world? And it's also well known that at Monsanto's headquarters, their own GMO grown food is NOT served in their cafeterias.

Please refer to this site for help with buying non-GMO brands:

✓ nongmoshoppingguide.com

For everything else you need to know about GMOs and Monsanto, please check out:

✓ bestmeal.info

For a brilliant documentary on GMOs please watch *Seeds of Destruction* which you can find online

So what *is* safe to eat then?

I bet you are seriously confused right now as to what to eat? I know – it can be very tough to completely rethink what you are used to buying. I am not going to bombard you with 'Try this diet or that diet' as many of them are fads and may not even suit you. There is just so much conflicting information around the 'right' way to eat that it can even cause massive arguments between followers of certain diets.

I have met many people who follow a certain type of diet to the tee; some seem fabulously healthy, energetic and rarely get ill, but some look very sick, seem very weak and you can tell that the way they are eating is *not* right for them. But at times, they hold so close their opinions or beliefs in the way that they eat, that they are missing the point, the *right* diet should make us healthy when it's truly right for us.

There will be people in the 'Paleo' camp (who eat animal products with every meal) who feel that we should all eat traditionally like they do, and it *can* be very convincing. Author Barry Groves of *Trick And Treat – How Healthy Eating is Making Us Ill* shares with his readers:

Our hunter-gatherer ancestors lived from one animal hunt, fishing expedition or egg-gathering foray to the next. There must have been times when food was scarce. That was our forebears' lives probably since the human species began. To tide them over these periods of famine, their bodies evolved the ability to store energy as fat. Indeed, for as long as *Homo Sapiens* has existed, our bodies' *preferred* soure of fuel has been its fat. That is precisely why our bodies store in that way. If a low-carb, high-fat diet were really as unhealthy for humans as we are constantly told, we simply wouldn't be here now. Those conditions existed for us 'civilised' people until only a relatively few generations ago, and many modern hunter-gatherers still live that way today. There really hasn't been enough time for any significant genetic changes in our digestive, biochemical and endrocine systems. Genetically, we are basically the same now as our distant ancestors. In other words, we should eat today what our paleolithic ancestors of 10,000 years ago ate.

But on the other side of the fence, in the vegan camp, they too, also have very convincing evidence to adopt a plant-based diet as the 'best' way to eat. In the very famous book *The China Study*, co-author Dr T Colin Campbell writes:

More commonly known as the China Study, this project eventually produced more than *8,000 statistically significant associations between various dietary factors and disease.*

What made this project especially remarkable is that, among the many associations that are relevant to diet and disease, so many pointed to the same finding: people who ate the most animal-based foods got the most chronic disease. Even relatively small intakes of animal-based food were associated with adverse effects. People who ate the most plant-based foods were the healthiest and tended to avoid chronic disease. These results could not be ignored. From the initial experimental animal studies on animal protein effects to this massive human study on dietary patterns, the findings proved to be consistent. The health implications of consuming either animal or plant-based nutrients were remarkably different.

Isn't it *confusing* to hear information from *both* of these sides that do seem very convincing? For this reason, I personally believe there is no diet on the earth that suits *all* of us - so I can't tell you what will suit you best. And if someone does say that a particular diet will suit you, '100% guaranteed' then they may not know enough about your own health like they actually should. Each of us has a different chemical makeup, and we are all from different corners of the earth. Some people will thrive being vegetarian, some will do very well being vegan, and some will say that they feel best on a high raw diet. But there will be some people who have tried them all and still do not feel good (or started to feel much worse) and feel they only got better when including some organic grass-fed animal products back into their diet. Vegans may not all agree with this, but if a person has tried everything and it doesn't seem to work for them, and their health is suffering, then surely we can't judge them for trying to find other ways that make them feel better. Scientific research tends to show positive and negative aspects to *all* kinds of diets. We actually do not know without a doubt, what is the best way to eat for all of us. It's completely individual.

And indeed, if diet was such an easy topic, we would all be able to eat the same things and all thrive in the same way. But we don't – we are all different and often need different types of ways to eat. And it's no wonder the diet book industry is worth billions!

However, I strongly believe, if I had to say which food item we all *do not* need, and one that does not help us in any way shape or form? And that is, refined sugars. A processed sugar-free diet is *the* only diet that is good for us. Regular white, heavily refined and processed sugar does not do *anything* of benefit to the human body, in fact, it can often leach much needed vital nutrients and minerals. The brain certainly does need sugar but you can get it from much better sources such as fruits and types of carbohydrates.

And it's worthwhile avoiding as much processed wheat as possible. It's simply *not* made the way it used to be many years ago. These new, highly processed types of wheat are so bad for most of us. Manufacturers often produce bread with nasty chemicals and use lots of water to make their bread appear soft and fluffy. As you may remember from previous chapters, wheat can often contain concerning levels of cadmium. I have had massive addictions to wheat in which I could tell through the lacklustre appearance of my skin that it was causing havoc on the inside. Wheat inflames the body and is highly allergenic for most people, yet is one of the most addictive foods on the planet.

> Wheat has 'gliadin' which is an addictive opiate that stimulates our appetite throughout the day and impairs our ability to say no to high carbohydrate foods. These exorphins cause food obsession and unbearable hunger.[56]

Wheat is also said to be one of the *main* causes of weight gain around the middle and it can also affect the function of the entire body. Author William David MD writes in his book *Wheat Belly: Lose weight, and Find Your Path Back to Health:*

> A wheat belly represents the accumulation of fat that results from years of consuming foods that trigger insulin, the hormone of fat storage. While some people store fat in their butocks, and thighs, most people collect ungainly fat around the middle. This 'central' or 'viseral' fat is unique: unlike fat in other body areas, it provokes inflammatory phenomena, distorts insulin responses, and issues abnormal metabolic signlas to the rest of the body. In the unwitting wheat-bellied male, visceral fat also produces estrogen, creating 'man brests;
>
> The consequences of wheat consumption, however, are not just manifested on the body's surface; wheat can also reach deep down into virtually every organ of the body, from the intestines, liver, heart and thyroid gland all the way up to the brain. In fact, there's hardly an organ that is not affected by wheat in some potentially damaging way. I definitely have a slight wheat belly

(and always have even when much younger) and after reading this, I'm definitely going to try and cut wheat right out of my diet, not only because of a superficial reason (I don't want a huge wheat belly!) but because I am very concerned at what the wheat may be doing to my general health. I'm also concerned at what it can do the brain.

If you are to continue eating bread (I agree, its *very* hard to give up) you can try and make your own organic breads. This allows you to have greater control and assurance of what's in it. There are many high-quality organic, wheat and gluten-free flours available these days and if you don't want to make by hand yourself, there are even bread machines which will allow you to have fresh wheat free breads daily, without too much effort. The german brand BEEM make very good non-stick bread machines (and waffle and toasted sandwhich irons too) that don't use a Teflon coating, instead use a safer kind, called 'Bio-lon Ceramic'. It must be said that having baked goods every day, even with good ingredients is still not a good idea for a truly healthy diet. Have them little and on occasion.

Some Sensible Diet Advice

The best advice I can give you in regards to what food to eat is this: it makes sense for *everyone* to eat lots of whole foods, avoid processed or packaged items and of course, consume the *least* toxic foods possible, with a 50% raw percentage. Food today is nowhere near as nutrient-dense as what it once was; our soils are very poor quality and this means that the vitamins and mineral levels are very low. And if you also cook a lot of your food then the nutrient content is even worse, almost becoming null and void. So if you can, eat lots of salads and fresh fruit and veggies that are raw, you will at least be able to provide your body with appropriate nutrient levels.

The best and most logical way to avoid all of the pesticides and other chemicals I have mentioned is to buy locally sourced and organic food as much as possible. Locally sourced is so important because it means its better for the environment, and it has not been affected by too much pollution from long travels. When humans fly, the radiation affects the body (especially the adrenal glands which control how you react to stress) so it makes sense that food that is flown in will also be affected in a negative way. So if you can, try and find locally sourced produce that is near you, or at least hasn't been flown in from other countries halfway across the world.

In the USA, food companies use radiation to 'purify' their food so that it doesn't break out with any food-contamination problems. This also harms the nutrient content in the food, causing people to eat even less nutrition, and this radiation is also linked to brain damage.[57] People rarely know, though, that the machine used is an actual nuclear radiation device that is incredibly dangerous and is marked with skull and crossbones on the side. I avoid buying all USA-imported food for this reason.

Is organic food always perfect?

It's also a bit disheartening to know that even the best organic food is going to have some traces of chemicals on it simply because the air alone is *full* of them. We also don't tend to know what sort of water is used on the organic produce either, which is where lots of the traces of chemicals come from, but compared to the quality of non-organic stuff, it's certainly *always, without a doubt* better! The best way to know how pure your food is, is to grow as much food as your own if you can. In Part 4 I give tips and suggestions for how to grow food even in small spaces, so don't worry – if you live in an apartment with no garden you can still grow something.

And another tip: it's also best to try to eat food that is *unprocessed* as much as possible. You want to eat foods that have required little to no preparation (or 'destruction' is another way to put it) before it gets to you. For example, you want to eat, most often, what are called 'whole foods' such as fruits and vegetables, and a small amounts of some nuts and seeds – if they digest well for you, that is. Your stomach will *tell* you what it likes; by signs of discomfort, bloating, gas etc. so you get advised by your own body whether to eat it or not!

It's worth noting, we never hear that organic fruits, vegetables and other healthy foods give someone cancer. It is simply not possible, that's why. These types of food heal the body, not harm it. So that fact alone is food for thought, isn't it?

How about, let's all eat the foods that aren't linked to cancers!

Eating animals

I could write another book about the horrors of animal farming, but I am not going to touch too much on this as I am pretty sure we all know by now what happens in these factory farms. Some people are very attached to eating lots of meat and, no matter what is said, they simply will not give it up. Meat and animal products are highly addictive to some types of people. If this is you, I would like to encourage you to look into cutting down on eating meat and other animal products and at least start buying only organic grass-fed animal products.

It's also important to realize that the amount of drugs that animals are pumped with these days is truly disgusting and whatever they have eaten or been medicated with ends up inside you too. And not only that – the amount of land used to farm animals is ridiculous. If the state of the planet concerns you, these facts will worry you. Many hundreds of football fields' worth of tree-covered land each and every day are being cut down. The world's most beautiful forests, such as the ones in Costa Rica, the Amazon, Brazil and other parts of the world, have had big parts of them cut down, and it's still going on. *Just* to produce meat. And mainly for the fast-food companies who sell the meat for dirt-cheap prices. In fact the meals are probably *cheaper* than buying actual dirt!

So, animal farming, on the level that it currently is, is one of the worst things for the environment, not just for losing the land space, but for the fact that our climate relies on trees to adjust the temperature. Trees act as lungs and they regulate the air, keeping the climate stable. If trees disappear (as is rapidly happening), then it means that the weather cannot behave in the normal, natural way. Just turn on the weather and news channels to have a look at what is happening all over the world. Major hurricanes and floods seem to have become normal over the past few years and they keep happening. But the destructive scale shows that they are certainly not normal. And methane coming from cows is also said to be harming the atmosphere.

Who is to blame?

If we can point the finger at any company or industry hugely respon-sible for such destruction to the planet, let's point that finger at the fast-food chains, for they are possibly the *worst* companies in the entire world for causing these problems. Combined, they have cut down so many forests, created so much waste, are incredibly cruel to animals (there is no way they can't be, no matter what they say, as they operate on such a huge and super-fast scale) and cause so much sickness in humans, such as obesity, that I personally think *they* are truly to blame and should have massive restrictions placed on them and have to pay very high taxes to the industries they're causing great harm to. Yet sadly, the governments are usually allies of them – and receive financial payments from lobbyists. And fast-food companies of course, are also supported by the most unconscious people who eat their food on a regular basis allowing this viscious cycle to continue. They also make some of the biggest profits throughout the world.

Eating a diet high in animal products is also linked to many cancers, bowel disease and heart attacks. Note that when a person is actually diagnosed with cancer, they are always recommended (by sensible healthcare advisers that is) to stop or at least cut down on eating red meat and animal products. The body does not see meat and animal products as a detox food, as they are also highly acidic inside the body. Many scientists say that cancer cannot grow in a more alkaline body.

People who drastically cut out meat and dairy products have been known to completely change their body's chemistry in a very short space of time, for example, in a few weeks. Those with diabetes, risk of heart attacks, cancers etc. can quite often make a huge turnaround in their health simply by *cutting* these things out. So if the cutting out of these things makes a huge improvement, then it's safe to say that these things in the diet were actually making people sick in the first place.

That alone says a heck of a lot.

And let us not ignore the fact that most farmed animals get treated so badly, and very often for their entire and *unnaturally* short lifespans. People seem to think that animals are incapable of having any feelings, but studies show that even fish can sense what is going on and feel fear too. Here is something to think about: 99% of factory farms are heavily guarded and locked up so that reporters (or the general public) can't look inside to see how the animals are being treated. If they were following the guidelines, then what are they hiding? Why don't they want us to see how they are treating their animals? Well, it's common sense to say: because they are treating them in disgusting ways. When undercover reporters do get a chance to take video footage, what they record is truly horrific and cruel. If we were there when it happened, witnessed what went on, and then someone served us a plate of steak, knowing what that animal had just been through, it would probably make us sick at the thought of eating it, wouldn't it? And so it should.

There is also a belief that whatever the animal feels, if it's intense fear and stress, we too end up eating, due to the chemical reaction that's left in the meat. When cows go inside the slaughterhouse, they can hear the cows in front of them while they are being killed, and knowing they are next, their bodies shoot out an enormous amount of adrenaline and cortisol which spreads through their flesh. So we end up eating those chemicals too. Some also say that eating meat also 'deadens' our ability to think compassionately and to connect with our spiritual side. Obviously this is something that is hard to prove, and I certainly know many kind people who still eat meat, but it could make much sense when you think about it. You could say that people who eat fast food regularly aren't at all compassionate because they don't care about what they are eating. Everyone knows junk food is bad for you, yet so many people just don't care.

In the recently released documentary *Vegucated* three hardcore meat-eaters were shown the horrors of the meat and dairy industry and, by the end, all three instantly became vegan. I'm not saying that you should become vegan by the way, but it is good to understand what is happening to animals on a large scale.

    ✓ Watch the trailer here: getvegucated.com

If you do eat meat, try to eat less and purchase grass-fed organic sources. Where I live is a biodynamic farm, Tablehurst, which produces biodynamically grown vegetables, fruits and herbs, chicken and various meats. Customers are allowed to look around the farm whenever they like to see how clean it is, and to see how the animals are treated. These are the sorts of farms that should be found everywhere.

Dirty fish

In regards to eating seafood, many have this thought – that because it comes from water, it means it's much cleaner, right? No! Another complete and utter tragedy is the health of our oceans. They are now *extremely toxic* too. Chemicals are still often (illegally) dumped in the oceans and now they have high levels of mercury (and other seriously harmful chemicals) due to all the boats that travel in the water. And people still throw garbage into the ocean – lots of it too. When I was in Costa Rica in 2011, I saw how much rubbish was washed onto the shore. I tried to pick up lots of it, but by the next morning the beach was covered again with bits of plastic and soft-drink cans. It was disgusting and so sad to see.

Everything that goes into the sea gets diluted and ends up in oceans and waterways at all corners of the earth. And after dreadful crimes against Nature, such as the truly horrific BP Horizon oil spill, which happened in 2010, our waters now have even more mercury (not forgetting lead and other serious chemicals) in them. Mercury and the other toxic pollutants travel a very long way due to the oceans' natural currents, moving everything around. And now we can also add lots more radiation to the mix of what's in our oceans because of the recent horrific situation in Japan. Over the next few years, we are going to hear reports from Japan and other countries close by of how their cancer rates are going even higher, and quite possibly babies will be born seriously deformed. There are already whispers that there are lots more miscarriages happening even in the USA due to the radiation traveling so far. I've even heard that the radiation is still continuing to leak every single day. We think the worst has happened, but really, it's not even started yet.

Scientists have carried out studies on fish all over the world and it seems it's almost impossible to find fish anywhere that have acceptable low levels of mercury (and unfortunately this applies to whales also).[58] And they are now discovering it's not just mercury that is in the water. Other serious chemicals, such as PCBs (fluids found in fuel) and POCs (persistent organic chemicals), are in our oceans as well, due to illegal dumping and from boats. Some of these chemicals were actually banned over 20 years ago but are still in our oceans – which shows us how anything that gets thrown in the water rarely disappears forever.

All waterways and oceans are sadly, said to be polluted. Even high-up beautiful mountain streams have tested positive for mercury and other chemicals. Enormous cruise ships fill our waters with human waste as well, which is quite worrying because the fish eat that too, so if someone has high levels of medication they are urinating and pooping out, the fish will be absorbing that, and when that fish is caught and served up as a meal – well, let's just say you are eating way more than just the flesh from fish.

I recently watched a documentary about the 'rubbish island'

which is off the coast of Hawaii and is said to be as big as the entire state of Texas in the USA. Like most people, I assumed that this 'island' was solid, with the bits of plastic all joining together. I naively thought, 'Well, can't we just go get a huge boat and pick it up and throw that big piece away?' The truth is, the majority of the pieces aren't joined together, but in fact are in bits – like a plastic soup – but it accumulates in one area of the ocean because of the way the oceans move around, creating a swirl. The rubbish dumps itself onto beaches every day, and when you see the amount of it that washes on shore, it is shocking. If you had a team of hundreds of people cleaning the beaches up, the next day the rubbish would be back again and just as bad. There is so much in the ocean that it is clear it will never ever disappear. Also, fish are attracted to the plastic, thinking it's food, in particular the red and orange pieces, so they eat this and it goes into their body. And if that fish is caught and eaten by a human, then you will be eating the plastic indirectly too. So always remember, whatever a fish has in its tissues (which is the part of the fish you eat, by the way) goes inside *you* when you eat it. A fish has a teeny tiny liver in comparison to us, so it won't be able to do a good job of processing those chemicals. It was never designed to do it in such an extreme way.

I think if we saw the ocean like a big dirty bathtub, we would never want to eat anything from it. It's such a *tragedy* to know that our water, from any source, is simply not clean anymore. But we have no one to blame but ourselves and the big corporations. I personally wish all of us would stop eating fish, right now, so that the oceans can thrive again. When a certain area is looked after through sustainable fishing methods, the fish count is up to 10 times more than it is in non-sustainable areas. Fish have a remarkable way of multiplying when looked after, but if it doesn't happen on a global scale in a big way, we are in big trouble.

If you still decide to eat fish, the list below shows the ones said to have the lowest amounts of mercury in them. Try to eat them *sparingly*, though, like as little as possible. Some are saying that it's only safe to have fish once a month, not 2–3 times a week like we were once told. Pregnant women should be even more cautious, and I think they should avoid it altogether.

Fish and seafood to avoid

- Atlantic halibut
- king mackerel
- oysters
- pike
- sea bass
- shark
- swordfish
- golden snapper
- tuna (steaks and canned albacore)

Tuna is also fast becoming extinct, as are some other species. It's really a good idea to consider not eating fish at all if you can. But if it's too hard for you to give up, then try and choose carefully what you eat.

Fish and seafood that is safer to eat

- shrimp/prawns
- crab
- salmon (be careful it's not GMO!)
- pollock
- catfish
- cod
- tilapia

Please *do not* eat anything that has been fished near the BP spill in the Gulf of Mexico. Fishing in this area is back on now in full swing after a few years of it being obviously contaminated. 'They' say the water is safe now but I find that very hard to believe. Petrol is very heavy and dense – remember the horrific photos showing how far the spill stretched to? There is *no way* that water is clean or safe today. The fishing industry from the Gulf of Mexico is worth millions and it took a real nosedive since this disaster so the fishing companies are desperate to make their money back ASAP.

In the documentary *The Big Fix*, the producers show viewers many clips of video footage which was meant to be kept hidden from the public. Whilst we all knew that Corexit, a very toxic chemical used to break up the oil was being heavily used, we really had *no* idea as to how much they were actually using. As captured in the documentary, authorities used planes and boats to spray and dump the chemical into the ocean *at night* when no one could see, making the public feel safe when they were told that the problem was all gone. What is shocking about this film is when you learn that there were other *much* safer methods companies can use to clean up oil spills. And in fact, Corexit is *banned* in use over near the UK because our officials declared it years ago, to be very unsafe. If you ask any of the locals around the Gulf if everything is OK, their answers are far from it. Not only have their livelihoods been completely ruined, with many people not yet receiving any financial help like they were promised, many are also very sick because of the chemicals found in the air. There has been so much corexit used, that when it rains, there are concerning levels detected in the rainfall. Even one of the movie's producers became ill after being exposed to it during filming. She developed an itchy and painful rash and had a bad chest cough.

I have no doubt that the water there is still highly contaminated. You might not be able to see the contamination, but it is showing up in water samples, and in the fish that are being eaten in huge amounts in this popular seafood-loving area of the USA.

Always ask where your fish/seafood came from before purchasing or eating.

Remember learning in school that there is a 'circle of life' that involves all animals on this planet? Well, I would like to coin a new term and that is the 'chemical circle of life'. Whatever we eat which has stored chemicals in it, we end up having that stored in our bodies too, which we then urinate out, back into the waterways, only to be consumed again.

Chemicals all have different reactions in the body: some will affect the kidneys, some will affect the skin or the heart, but the ones that are the most worrying are the chemicals that affect the brain. And guess what? As we know, mercury is linked directly to brain conditions such as memory loss (no wonder Alzheimer's is so prevalent these days), concentration problems, autism, and other learning disabilities. It basically makes your brain start to malfunction. The more mercury you add to the brain, the more your brain starts to suffer. And be very careful of taking fish oil supplements as the majority of them contain high levels of mercury. Look for the brands that have purified the oil through a strict cleaning process, or avoid using fish oils altogether. Touchstone Essentials make a very high-quality supplement called 'Wellspring'. It's made from vegetarian sources such as cold-pressed organic oils like coconut, flax, borage and pumpkin seed.

Fish that is farmed is even more worrying because they are penned in small enclosures, and the waters are filled with chemicals so that the fish do not spread diseases. But more often than not, they are fed GMO foods, which means you eat that too.

With some types of deep-sea fishing, huge nets are often used which drag along the bottom of the sea floor. This means not only that the sea bed gets incredibly damaged but also other species of animals are caught up in the nets. Fishermen fishing for prawns will also tend to catch lots of other types of fish and sometimes they even catch precious turtles and dolphins. If these are lucky enough to be thrown back in the water and are still alive, they may survive, but if not, they will die a completely wasted death. Fishing is a very selfish industry and the oceans are literally being pillaged with little to no regard for the consequences. And it's the Western countries which place such a high demand for fish to be served in our homes and our restaurants. It's up to us to say: *no more over-fishing.*

Without the oceans being able to sustain themselves in their natural cycle, the future existence of the whole of humanity is in dire straits. So even though shrimp (prawns) are listed above on the safer-to-eat list, I would still recommend trying to stop eating them or eating them very rarely.

For more information on mercury in fish please visit:

✓ epa.gov/waterscience/fishadvice

Organic food

OK, let's get back to the subject of organic food: I know for many people it is very hard, or out of their budget, to purchase everything organic. Unfortunately it usually is a lot more expensive than conventional food. In that case, I would recommend you spend your money on organic animal products first (if you decide to keep eating them) as these tend to contain the worst types of chemicals in them. Hormones, vaccines, antibiotics – that sort of really gross stuff. And because the animals are made to grow super-fast (highly unnatural) they have weakened immune systems and are susceptible to many diseases. Hence why they are pumped with so many medicines. There is evidence to support the idea that humans may be having trouble resisting disease and illness themselves due to the massive amounts of antibiotics consumed through meat.

Organic food is *always* better, and anyone that says it's not has not done their research properly, or used common sense. Recently, Dr. Oz, who was made famous by the *Oprah Winfrey Show*, landed himself in a huge spot of bother. On his TV show in late 2012 he was speaking highly about the organic-food industry and discussing the risks of eating foods with pesticides in them, in particular to children's health:

So you're being told organic food is no more nutritious than conventional and it's not worth your extra money. Well, I'm here to say that it is worth the investment. Why do I say that? Pesticides.

Dr. Oz, 19 October 2012

Fast forward to only a few short months later when Dr. Oz was interviewed by *Time Magazine* and quoted as saying that organic foods were only for the 'elitists and snobs':

> Nutritionally speaking, there is little difference between the farmer's-market bounty and the humble brick from the freezer case.
> Dr. Oz, *Time Magazine* interview, 'What to Eat Now'

Not *once* throughout this 5-page interview did Dr. Oz mention pesticides, yet several months before, he was filmed on a major TV station, on his *own* show, listing the real dangers of eating non-organic food. It seems Dr. Oz, in this instance has completely sold out to the powers that be. Disgraceful. It was heartwarming to see on Facebook, though, how many thousands of people stopped by his fan page to tell him exactly what they thought of this 'flip-flopping' that so many of our two faced and so easily bought politicians do these days. Thank god he didn't flip flop in regards to the dangers of mercury-based fillings!

If chemicals really are of a concern for you, just so you know, buying organic animal products does *not* mean the animal has not received any vaccines. They usually have, because it generally is required by law. So if it alarms you (as it should) that cattle vaccines contain many toxic additives such as what's on the list below, it might be another reason why you should at least cut down on eating meat. Here is what is used in treating cows in typical factory farms:

- Neomycin (antibiotic)
- 2-phenoxyethanol (2-PE) (preservative)
- Streptomycin (antibiotic)
- Polymyxin B (antibiotic)
- Mercury (heavy metal – proven neurotoxin)
- Aluminum (heavy metal – proven neurotoxin

- Monophosphoryl lipid A (MPL, ASO4) (adjuvant)
- MF59 –adjuvant
- Freund's (FCA) – adjuvant
- Sodium borate (used as a detergent and fire retardant in other industries – anti-fungal use in vaccines)
- QS-21 (adjuvant)

That tasty, juicy steak is suddenly not looking so good, is it? No wonder so many people today are having problems with antibiotics that are simply not doing their job anymore.

When you have any of your meals, try and make at least 50% of them with the addition of raw foods, such as salad, vegetables and fruit. This can help to keep the body functioning at an optimal level. If you like to lightly steam things, that is fine too, but always try and keep the heat and time to a minimum to help retain the nutrients. Raw foods are said to help break down the other foods you eat too, and your stomach will thank you for it as the valuable enzymes and natural probiotics will help keep it healthy.

Even though the raw movement is gaining huge popularity, you do not have to be 100% raw to be really healthy. It's something that can take a bit of time to adjust to, so it's best to do it little by little and learn to listen to what your body really needs. Personally, I tried 100% raw a few years back and it made me very sick because my digestion was in such a real mess. All the work it had to do to process all the things I was eating was very draining. The body really tells us immediately if something suits it or not. We just need to listen better to what it's saying.

Here is a little tip: try and eat your fruit before your meals or just early in the day, as this means that it will digest a whole lot better. There are some fruits and vegetables that, if non-organic, are still reasonably OK in terms of the pesticide levels. But, on the other hand, there are some that are not safe to consume.

The list below will help you choose what to buy and what to avoid.

Non-organic foods list

Fruit and veggies to be avoided (worst from the top):

1. celery
2. peaches
3. strawberries
4. apples
5. blueberries
6. nectarines
7. bell peppers
8. spinach
9. cherries
10. kale/collard/greens
11. potatoes
12. grapes

Safest non-organic foods:

1. onions
2. avocado
3. sweet corn
4. pineapple
5. mangoes
6. sweet peas
7. asparagus
8. kiwi
9. cabbage
10. eggplant
11. cantaloupe
12. watermelon
13. grapefruit
14. sweet potato
15. honeydew melon

The EWG (Environmental Working Group), which has supplied this list, also has a free phone-app where you can download this list to take shopping with you. Type in 'Dirty Dozen' to find the app.

I also want to mention that non-organic bananas are something it is best to avoid. Not because the inside is full of pesticides, but the actual skin is – and that's the part you touch. What is even worse is that most of the bananas are grown in tropical Third World countries where regulations are often ignored, or not even in place. The workers are paid awful low wages and are exposed to toxic chemicals, one of which in particular has been linked to many serious illnesses.

At least 5,000 agricultural workers from Nicaragua, Costa Rica, Guatemala, Honduras, and Panama have filed five lawsuits in the United States. The farmers claim that exposure in the 1970s to dibromochlorpropane (DBCP), a pesticide banned in the United States in 1979 for its reproductive toxicity, left them bereft of the pitter-patter of little feet.[59]

So I would recommend buying organic bananas (that are fair trade too), purely so you are not supporting unfair work practices, and you won't be exposing yourself to the dangers of DBCP. And if you keep buying regular bananas, or other tropical fruit for that matter, please don't let your children touch the skins.

Why Don't Our Doctors Know Much More About Herbs, Nutrition & Supplements?

One would assume that the first person to talk to about our diet, would automatically be our doctor, but apart from being told the standard 'eat less fat and sugar,' they don't *really* know much at all about what healthy eating involves, nor about the dangerous food additives we are commonly eating. They don't seem to discuss with their patients how eating foods grown with pesticides may increase your risk of cancer or other health problems. And despite that they know that most health problems come from lifestyle choices, they aren't really doing too much to really help their patients' health for the long term. It's because they aren't educated about it in detail, or at all. And they don't get taught about any herbal medicines in Medical school, despite the scientific evidence we have today that many of them are highly effective when used correctly.

As Ty Bollinger, co-author of *Work With Your Doctor* writes:

Rest assured, it is not your doctor's fault. When asked about natural medicine (by the rare patient who has the courage to ask), the most often heard response is, "I'm not sure if that stuff is any good" or something along those lines. Patients are often discouraged from using herbals, and indeed, sometimes even vitamin and mineral supplements. The fault lies not in the doctor, but in his **training**.

The modern medical industry is built on the foundation of treating the symptoms of disease, while doing virtually nothing to treat the actual cause of the disease or prevent it. It reminds me of an old Chinese proverb: "The superior doctor prevents sickness; the mediocre doctor attends to impending sickness; the inferior doctor treats actual sickness." However, the problem is not the doctors...it is the **system**.

The truth of the matter is that most physicians care and truly want to assist their patients in recovering from illness or pain. However, doctors work with the tools they learned in medical school. Unfortunately, medical schools are structured in a way that memorization takes the front seat while deductive reasoning falls far behind. This is due to the vast amount of data that has to be assimilated. In order for students to graduate and become MDs they have no choice but to learn what has become the AMA's "medicine of today."

And Ty continues:

The leaning of current medical schools is obvious when we look at a few facts. There are approximately 125 medical schools in the United States. Of those 125 schools, only 30 of them require a course in nutrition. During four years of medical school, the average training in nutrition received by U.S. physicians is 2.5 hours. When you consider the fact that the risk of death from a heart attack for the average American male is 50%, while the risk of death from a heart attack for an average American, vegetarian, male is 4%, the need for nutritional counseling for physicians is obvious. While vegetarians are not necessarily the healthiest people, this is most definitely a telling statistic.

From the book *Nature Cure*, written by Henry Lindlahr MD in the year 1914:

The diseases which we find most difficult to cure, even by the most radical application of natural methods, are cases of drug-poisoning. Substances which are foreign to the human organism, and especially the inorganic, mineral poisons, positively destroy tissues and organs and are much harder to eliminate from the system than the encumbrances of morbid materials and waste matter produced in the body by wrong habits of living only.

The obvious reason for this is that our organs of elimination are intended and constructed to excrete only such waste products as are formed in the organism in the processes of metabolism.

Tuberculosis or cancer may be caused in a scrofulous or psoric constitution by overloading the system with meat, coffee, alcohol, or tobacco; but as soon as these bad habits are discontinued, and the organs of elimination stimulated by natural methods, the encumbrances will be eliminated, and the much-dreaded symptoms will subside and disappear, often with surprising rapidity.

On the other hand, mercury, arsenic, quinine, strychnine, iodine, etc., accumulate in the brain, the spinal cord, and the cells and tissues of the vital organs, causing actual distraction and disintegration. The tissues thus affected are not easily rebuilt, and it is exceedingly difficult to stir up the destructive mineral poisons and to eliminate them from the system.

Therefore it is an indisputable fact that many of the most stubborn, socalled incurable diseases are drug diseases.

Chapter 11

The Alarming Misuse of Medicine – Why Drugs Should Never Be Your Only Answer

American medicine frequently causes more harm than good. It is evident that the American Medical System is the leading cause of death and injury in the United States. The number of people having adverse drug reactions in hospital to prescribed medicine is 2.2 million. Tens of millions of unnecessary antibiotics are prescribed annually for viral infections. 1 in 9 hospital patients develop a hospital-acquired infection. The incidence rate of medical harm occurring is estimated to be over 40,000 each and every day according to the Institute of Healthcare Improvement. An estimated 450,000 preventable medication related adverse reactions occur every year in the USA.[60]

Dr. Joseph Mercola

These alarming facts are often unfortunately very true for other Western countries also. You only have to turn on the TV to see how many advertisements there are for pain-relief tablets, diet pills, cold and flu medicines, and in America these ads are about 100 times more frequent and for many different types of drugs. Here in the UK, and in Australia too, there are strict rules about what can be advertised on the TV, so we never see ads for anxiety pills or antidepressants, but of course we still do see advertisements for cold and flu medications and common over-the-counter items.

The commercials in the USA or in magazines for pharmaceutical medicines are almost laughable because they depict healthy, happy, good-looking families saying how wonderful their life is because they use this or that antidepressant, painkiller or diet pill. But at the end of the commercial, they also say what the side effects are, and quite often, there are on average *about 15* of them, one of which is 'possible risk of death'. And just try looking at the full-page magazine ads for pharmaceuticals. The flip side of the nice, smiling and healthy-looking person is often a full page of warnings and side effects, written in the tiniest small print, so small it's hard to read and people rarely pay any attention to it. What does that say? That perhaps the pharmaceutical world doesn't want you to really know what can happen if you take their drugs? That's comforting, isn't it, for a medication that is *supposed* to make you well.

Now, before I go any further, if you are on medication, I am in *no way* saying to stop it right now, as that could be *very, very dangerous*, as you may legitimately need them and it could literally case you great harm to stop suddenly. But if you do reach for a headache pill all the time, use sleeping aids regularly, load up on cold and flu tablets because you are always getting sick, or you use painkillers often, then maybe it's *time* to think about *why* you need them so much and realize that this regular use, over time, is not going to help you remain healthy later in life. *All* medications have unwanted side affects.

It's therefore worth asking yourself: Are you getting colds because you are actually toxic and your liver and immune system is sluggish? Do you have back pain because you need to have your posture realigned or strengthened by doing yoga or other exercise techniques? Do you get headaches so often because you are actually dehydrated? Do you have sleeping difficulties and always reach for harsh medications because of stress, or is it because your hormones and /or adrenals are not balanced?

Our body gives us signs *all* the time when things are not right, but the regular use of most pharmaceutical medicines is like putting a sticking plaster over the problem. The symptoms may go after a while, but the *reason and cause* as to why you got the illness in the first place may still be there and won't go away anytime soon if you just keep pushing it under the carpet.

It must be said, though, that there have been some *incredible* and life-saving medical advances over the last 50 years. We *need* the medical world. Many people (perhaps even loved ones close to us) would not be here without particular procedures and certain medications. We really *do* need intervention at times of emergency or with certain diseases and disorders, so I do not want to sound like I am rubbishing medicine altogether, or to make you think that we don't need any of it. That's simply *not* where I am coming from. Lots of people in the natural health world make a mistake of coming across as saying that doctors should never be consulted – this is highly irresponsible advice. There are many doctors and procedures I actually really respect and marvel at, and some have personally helped me.

I recently gave birth, in February 2012. I thankfully had a natural and intervention-free labor, but when it was time for the placenta to come out, I was by then bleeding quite heavily. I had to have an injection to help the placenta to detach itself from the wall of the uterus, far more quickly than it would have done naturally. In the 'old days' or still in Third World countries today, a mother in my situation might have died if it was not for that quick procedure. So that little injection I had, pretty much saved my life, and left my daughter to still have her mother.

So I do not wish to come across as being against the entire medical industry. There are serious problems within the industry, yes, and far too many to mention here, but there is still lots of good. What I am saying, though, is that there are usually *other* ways of treating most people's health problems first, without having to resort to drastic operations and drugs which can leave toxic chemicals in the body, as well as harming major organs, not to mention increasing your risk at being one of the statistics of medical negligence as mentioned at the beginning of this chapter. We need a major overhaul of the medical world, and conventional medicine desperately needs to start working alongside natural medicine.

Seemingly innocent medicines can sometimes be the most harmful

Far too large a section of the treatment of disease is today controlled by the big manufacturing pharmacists, who have enslaved us in a plausible pseudo-science. The blind faith which some men have in medicines illustrates too often the greatest of all human capacities – the capacity for self-deception.[61]

Sir William Osler, speaking to the Ontario Medical Association, 1909

A very common medicine to take is paracetamol. It seems to be harmless enough because it's usually found in every household, right, and easy to purchase at the supermarket or pharmacy? Yet the truth is, chronic or even *regular* use of paracetamol has been linked to an alarmingly high rate of cancer, and also occasional use *raises* the already high risk of children developing asthma. This drug puts an enormous amount of stress on the liver. I know this from personal experience.

When I was about 16, and severely depressed, I overdosed on quite a few medications. The only one that the doctor was concerned about was the amount of paracetamol I had taken. I had swallowed about a whole card (12 tablets) and was told that any more than 6 taken at once was enough to shut my entire body down, meaning I could have died in severe pain over the course of a few horrific days... I was lucky and of course, thankfully survived. But it seems that this is the drug of choice to take for people wanting to attempt suicide, and because it's very easy to get hold of, and so cheap, young teenagers are especially susceptible to paracetamol overdoses. Found on the Random Acts of Reality blog [62] written by a London ambulance driver is this very sad story:

I'm driving on this particular shift; my crewmate is in the back dealing with the patient.

I'm grinding my teeth at the waste.

The patient is almost certainly going to die – he's taken an overdose. The tablets he's taken, and the way he's taken them, mean that parts of his body will start to fail over the next few days. His immediate future is a hospital bed, then an ITU bed, then either waiting for a transplant or death. It's too late for any treatment to work on him.

He's not in any pain, he doesn't feel weak, he has no symptoms.

He talks to my crewmate. The body language suggests that he is upset but not suicidally depressed.

It was one of those 'cry for help' things – asking why he did it gets the answer that he wanted to die, but now he doesn't. It's a common enough reason – that they change their mind and then phone us.

Everyone can get these pills – you can read the inference: how can they be that dangerous if you can buy them over the counter?

He lives in a nice house, has a family, had his future ahead of him.

I suspect that he thinks that he'll have a 'stomach pump', a chat with the psychiatrists and then come home. He doesn't realise the damage that he has done to his body.

We don't talk about the outcome to the patient – we'll leave that to the hospital after his blood tests show if he is telling the truth or not. We'll only see him for the ten minutes it takes us to drive him to hospital.

I'm hoping that the patient is lying, that he hasn't done what he says he has, but the empty pill packets speak for themselves.

I know I'll be thinking about him for the next few months long after I've forgotten his name.

His mother is travelling with him.

He's fourteen years old.

What a sad story and one that may be much more common than we may realize. After I was told that I had risked my life from taking just paracetamol, it was enough to make me understand just how dangerous it was. I thought that the other drugs I had taken were far worse, yet these common tablets that even small children take were what could have been responsible for my death.

Alarmingly, paracetamol-type medications are given to children these days and in some cases very often and unnessecary, so I will be discussing this in greater detail in Part 3, 'Rethinking the Way We Parent'. I must give you this warning: *never* ever drink any alcohol with paracetamol - this dangerous combination can prove deadly.

Drugs Companies and their Dangerous Deceptions

It seems not a day goes by that we don't hear about a massive lawsuit against a huge pharmaceutical company in the media. A pretty huge amount of money has been paid out to claimants who were victims of a serious drug interaction. According to the Public Health Citizens Research Group as seen in their report *Rapidly Increasing Criminal and Civil Monetary Penalities Against the Pharmacetuical Industry 1991-2010*:

Of the 165 settlements comprising $19.8 billion in penalties during this 20-year interval, 73 percent of the settlements (121) and 75 percent of the penalties ($14.8 billion) have occurred in just the past five years (2006-2010).

Four companies (GlaxoSmithKline, Pfizer, Eli Lilly, and Schering-Plough) accounted for more than half (53 percent or $10.5 billion) of all financial penalties imposed over the past two decades.

What an exhorbatant number this is – almost *$20 billion!* This is an undeniable indication that something (truthfully *many* things) is very wrong with our drug industry. It's a good idea to take note of the word *criminal* used in the above report, so we actually know what we are really dealing with. The dictionary helps us to see much clearer what criminal behavior means:

1. Of, involving, or having the nature of crime: *criminal abuse.*

2. Relating to the administration of penal law.

3.

a. Guilty of crime.

b. Characteristic of a criminal.

4. Shameful; disgraceful: *a criminal waste of talent.*

*n.*One that has committed or been legally convicted of a crime.

Now after you have seen the amount of money that has abeen paid out particularly in the last 5 years, due to *criminal* behavior at the hands of the pharmaceutical companies, this means nothing but possible dangers in regards to taking certain medications that have been either not tested for long enough, not proven to be safe or effective, or had their studies twisted to suit the outcome for the drug companies to benefit financially and *not*, you the patient, who puts your life in their hands.

Another type of danger from this criminial and unethical behaviour is that they have taken advantage of our trusting doctors who read the (poorly conducted studies) in their medical journals. They are trained to believe that what they see in these journals is what they should be recommending to their patients. Dr Maria Angell, ex-employee (spanning 20 years) of the New England Journal of Medicine and author of the New York Times Bestseller *The Truth About The Drug Companies – How They Deceive Us And What To Do About It* writes:

I witnessed firsthand the influence of the industry on medical research during my two decades at *The New England Journal Of Medicine.* The staple of the journal is research about causes of and treatments for disease. Increasingly, this work is sponsored by drug companies. I saw companies begin to exercise a level of control over the way reseach is done that was unheard of when I first came to the journal, and the aim was clearly to load the dice to make sure their drugs looked good. As an example, companies would require researchers to compare a new drug with a placebo (sugar pill) instead of with an older drug. That way, the new drug would look good even though it might actually worse than the older one. There are other ways to bias research, and not all of them can be spotted, even by experts. Obviously we rejected such papers when we recognized them, but often they would turn up in other jounrals. Sometimes companies don't allow researchers to publish their results at all if they are unfavourable to the companies' drugs. As I saw industry influence grow, I became increasingly troubled by the possibility that much published research is seriously flawed, leading doctors to believe that new drugs are generally more affective and safer than they actually are.

Drug Companies spend the most % of their money on marketing and advertising instead of on the much more important research and development (R & D), which is another perfect example that the public's best interests are *not* of utmost concern like they should be.

Dr Marcia Angell also shared with her readers:

According to Securities and Exchange Commission (SEC) and shareholder reports for 2001, the biggest drug companies spent on average about 35 percent of their revenues on 'marketing and administration' (called by slightly different names in different companies). That percentage was probably about the same for members of the Pharmaceutical Research and Manufactrurers of America (PhRMA) generally, and it had not changed much over the past decade. It is the largest single item in big pharma's budget, larger than manufacturing costs, and much larger than R & D. In 2002, for the top ten US companies, that percentage dropped slightly to about 31 percent of revenues. That's a heap of 'marketing and administration'. Many countries would love to have a gross domestic product as big as that.

And if you live in the USA, judging by the huge numbers of people taking medications, which is *more* than the total amount combined of Australia, Japan, Germany, UK, China, Brazil, Spain, Italy, France *and* Canada you are at the *most* risk of being harmed by Big Pharma's routine behaviour. As seen in the article **20 Signs That The Pharmaceutical Companies Are Running A 280 Billion Dollar Money Making Scam** by Michael Snyder reporting for prisonplanet.com:

#1 According to a study conducted by the Mayo Clinic, 70 percent of Americans are on at least one prescription drug. An astounding 20 percent of all Americans are on at least five prescription drugs.

#2 According to the CDC, approximately 9 out of every 10 Americans that are at least 60 years of age say that they have taken at least one prescription drug within the last month.

#3 The 11 largest pharmaceutical companies combined to rake inapproximately $85,000,000,000 in profits in 2012.

#4 During 2013, Americans will spend more than 280 billion dollars on prescription drugs.

#5 According to Alternet, last year "11 of the 12 new-to-market drugs approved by the Food and Drug Administration were priced above $100,000 per-patient per-year".

#6 The CDC says that spending on prescription drugs more than doubled between 1999 and 2008.

#7 Many prescription drugs cost about twice as much in the United States as they do in other countries.

#8 One study found that more than 20 percent of all American adults are taking at least one drug for "psychiatric" or "behavioral" disorders.

#9 The percentage of women taking antidepressants in America is higher than in any other country in the world.

#10 Children in the United States are three times more likely to be prescribed antidepressants than children in Europe are.

#11 A shocking Government Accountability Office report discovered thatapproximately one-third of all foster children in the United States are on at least one psychiatric drug. In fact, the report found that many states seem to be doping up foster children as a matter of course. Just check out these stunning statistics:

In Texas, foster children were 53 times more likely to be prescribed five or more psychiatric medications at the same time than non-foster children. In Massachusetts, they were 19 times more likely. In Michigan, the number was 15 times. It was 13 times in Oregon. And in Florida, foster children were nearly four times as likely to be given five or more psychotropic medications at the same time compared to non-foster children.

#12 In 2010, the average teen in the U.S. was taking 1.2 central nervous system drugs. Those are the kinds of drugs which treat conditions such as ADHD and depression.

#13 The total number of Americans taking anti-depressants doubled between 1996 and 2005.

#14 All of those antidepressants don't seem to be working too well. The suicide rate for Americans between the ages of 35 and 64 rose by close to 30 percent between 1999 and 2010. The number of Americans that are killed by suicide now exceeds the number of Americans that die as a result of car accidents.

#15 According to the National Household Survey on Drug Abuse, 36 million Americans have abused prescription drugs at some point in their lives.

#16 A survey conducted for the National Institute on Drug Abuse found that more than 15 percent of all U.S. high school seniors abuse prescription drugs.

#17 According to the CDC, approximately three quarters of a million people a year are rushed to emergency rooms in the United States because of adverse reactions to pharmaceutical drugs.

#18 According to the Los Angeles Times, drug deaths (mostly caused by prescription drugs) are climbing at an astounding rate....

Drug fatalities more than doubled among teens and young adults between 2000 and 2008, years for which more detailed data are available. Deaths more than tripled among people aged 50 to 69, the Times analysis found. In terms of sheer numbers, the death toll is highest among people in their 40s.

#19 In the United States today, prescription painkillers kill more Americans than heroin and cocaine combined.

#20 Each year, tens of billions of dollars is spent on pharmaceutical marketing in the United States alone.

And according to businessinsider.com, in 2010, Pfizer, who make hundreds of over-the-counter and prescription-only medications, most famously: Viagra, Provera, Premarin, Cisplatin, Depo-Provera, Efexor, Lipitor (they spend the most of their money advertising this drug for cholesterol), Mitrzapine and Zanax to name only a few, spent over *US $2.2 billion dollars* purely on advertising in the following media outlets:

TV: $831 million
Magazines: $333 million
Newspapers: $66 million
Internet: $46 million
Other: $847 million

This was just in one single *year*. And Pfizer is just *one* of the big pharmaceutical companies

According to Beth Synder Bulik author of the Pharmaceutical Marketing white paper found on gaia.adage.com, regulations for direct-to-consumer adverstising regulations have been drastically loosened over the last 15 years. The amount of money spent on marketing drugs has gone from 700 Million to a peak of *$5.4 billion* as of 2006.

And according to the article, *Direct-to-Consumer Pharmaceutical Advertising Therapeutic or Toxic?* **by C.Lee Ventola found on the** US *National Library of Medicine National Institutes of Health* **website, the increased spending on marketing began** *much* **earlier than 15 years ago:**

> For example, in 1980, total spending on DTCPA was $12 million; in 1990, it was $47 million; and in 1995, it was $340 million, representing a nearly 3,000% increase in expenditures during a 15-year period before broadcast ad regulations had even been relaxed.
>
> In 1997, after the FDA issued revised draft guidelines for broadcast DTCPA, the budgets for consumer drug advertising more than tripled to $1.2 billion in 1998 on DTCPA nearly quadrupled again during the following decade, topping $5 billion in 2006 and 2007, before dropping to $4.5 billion in 2009.
>
> In 2008, spending decreased because of the financial crisis and subsequent economic slowdown—this was the first substantial reduction in DTCPA since the late 1990s.

According to Dr Marcia Angell author of *The Truth About The Drug Companies – How They Deceive Us And What To Do About It,* doctors and other experts in their field receive lots of this money for marketing drugs, on perks and academic titles:

> Drug companies pay particular attention to wooing so-called thought leaders. These are prominent experts, usually on medical school faculties and teaching hospital staffs, who write papers, contribute to textbooks, and give talks at medical meetings – all of which greatly affect the use of drugs in their fields.
>
> Thought leaders have influence far beyond their numbers. Companies shower special favors on these doctors, offer them

honoraria as consultants and speakers, and often pay for them to attend annual conferences in posh resorts, ostensibly to seek their advice. In many drug-intensive medical specialties, it is virtually impossible to find and expert who is not receiving payments from one or more drug companies.

It would require much more information to really show you the true full scope of this blatant profit-before-patient-safety aspect in regards to the Pharmaceutical Industry. I simply don't have the room here, however, I have included many books in the resource section for you to investigate into further if you wish.

Wait a minute – drugs come from Nature too?

There are a lot of people today, most doctors included, who really rubbish Natural Health, saying it does not work. Yet drugs made by the pharmaceutical companies are generally synthesized forms of natural extracts like plants and herbs.[63] Yes, that's *100% true*. Even though the names of the drugs have nothing to do with plants or herbs and the packaging looks so scientific, it has been derived from *Nature*. Many scientists have been sent on behalf of pharmaceutical companies to places like the Amazon to source powerful herbs and plants, which have incredible medicinal qualities. They take these items back to the lab, and then begin to copy the effects, adding other things to them and turning them into drugs they can sell and patent.

Yet, unlike the natural form they came in, these drugs are created in a laboratory and have many other chemicals added to them (like mercury and aluminum!) to preserve them or to make them work more quickly or strongly. And these additives are always at least a little toxic to the body (and in many cases severely toxic), which is why they can give so many unwanted side effects, requiring the doctor to write yet another prescription for something that will treat those side effects. Talk about running in circles!

And let's not ignore the fact that many drugs were deemed as 'safe' and given to thousands of people but some have had disastrous consequences that have even ended in people's deaths due to inter-actions.

Here is Emma's story. She was prescribed the drug 'Tamiflu' which was the treatment for swine flu.

It was January 2010 and swine flu had been in the news for months now. Never in a million years did I think I would end up being diagnosed with the virus months later.

I started feeling unwell on Friday 8th January. I felt so tired and ached all over, like never before. I was shattered but couldn't sleep. My head was pounding and I had a fever but was also shivering cold, and by the Sunday night I developed chest pains that were getting worse and worse as the hours passed. I decided to make a phone call to my GP as it was the early hours of Monday morning by now, so I phoned the out-of-hours number. It went straight through to NHS Direct, so I spoke to this man who asked me to describe my symptoms to him. I explained to him how I had been feeling for the past few days, and right there and then, to my horror, he told me I had swine flu. I sat in fear and disbelief as people were dying with this illness – he assured me that once I had taken the course of antibiotics to treat swine flu, which was Tamiflu, I would be fit and healthy in less than a week and would be cured and back to myself.

That morning my husband went out to get me the tablets from the prescription that had been sent direct to our local pharmacy. We were given a code on the phone to release the drugs when we presented it to the pharmacist.

My husband returned with the tablets and on the packet it advised you to eat something before you took the Tamiflu – well, I had been completely off my food but I managed to force down a slice of toast and with that I swallowed the tablet.

By this point my husband was back at work and I was in the house alone. After taking the tablet I went back to bed, hoping to get some sleep. Well, I couldn't have been more wrong.

Forty-five minutes after taking the tablet, I was breaking out in a hot sweat, dripping, and was confused about where I was (I was actually lying in bed at home where I had been for the last past four days). I remember lying there thinking, 'Where is everyone?' – I was lying in pitch darkness and the light was coming through the blinds. I recall sitting up in bed and seeing stars. I went to get up out of bed and couldn't move my legs – all I could feel was this tingling sensation from the waist down. I could not get my legs to function and move.

'I have to get to the bathroom,' I thought, as I was feeling violently sick now by this point. I couldn't walk though. I had to physically crawl and drag my body, using my arms and hands, to the bathroom which was literally the room next door. I managed to get to the sink and pull myself up – I was holding on for dear life to the bath. I needed air and I wanted to try and cool myself down with cold water. I was starting to panic now as I honestly thought, 'This is it.' I wanted my husband and wanted my mum. For some strange reason I had taken my phone with me to the bathroom and was able to call my husband, but as I was trying to speak I was violently throwing up and just kept saying 'Mark!' down the phone – I did not have a clue what was going on. By this point I had hung up on Mark and he was trying to call me back but I was perched over the sink, holding on. The feeling in my legs was coming back but the tingling was still going strong; I still couldn't get my legs to move though. I was leaning over the sink with cold water running over my wrists trying to cool myself down. I remember thinking at this point I was in that film *Jurassic Park* with the dinosaurs and was being chased by the flying one – I was screaming and trying to hide from these creatures which I thought were real.

I woke up to my husband screaming my name as I had fallen on the floor and was curled up in a ball in the corner. When I woke up I was confused at what had happened; I remember thinking my mum had died and I was all alone. When in actual fact my mum was just at work and when I had called her she had just not answered and this was just all in my mind. And what I was seeing – everything was so vivid.

This was my reaction to Tamiflu and that was after taking just one tablet. Funnily enough, I never completed the whole course of Tamiflu and returned to my own GP on the Wednesday with the tablets in hand. I explained to her what had happened and her response was 'You must have had a bad reaction to it', advising me to complete the course.

'Yeah, right,' I thought, and left, leaving the tablets in the room.

Today I am left with panic and anxiety attacks that have affected my everyday life. I feel that Tamiflu is responsible for leaving me with these attacks as I have never experienced anything like them before and I dread to think what would have happened if I had taken the whole course of tablets and where I would be today.

Emma Hancock, UK
Age 25

Emma is certainly not the only one who had negative and horrible side effects and was affected neurologically after taking this particular drug.

There have been no reported deaths from Tamiflu in the United States, but in Japan, where the drug is much more widely used, at least 14 deaths have been reported. Five children under the age of 17 died after 'falling from windows or balconies or running into traffic', according to the FDA. According to Roche, two people under the age of 21 died from a brain infection, and seven deaths from neuropsychiatric symptoms have also been attributed to use of the drug by adults.[64]

Many of these types of drugs causing severe reactions went through all the 'proper' clinical testing yet ended up being withdrawn from the market (apart from Tamiflu which is *still* on the market despite these findings) after they made so many people sick or even die. I was going to write a whole list for you here but the truth is, it's a mile long! If you want to see this list yourself, please go to Wikipedia and type in 'drugs withdrawn from market'. You will be as shocked as I was.

Remember that these drugs were once promoted by doctors as safe, because the pharmaceutical companies said they were, so then doctors prescribed them to unsuspecting and trusting people who assumed that they were going to help them yet they ended up causing severe problems. In the case of the drug Vioxx, it killed at least 60,000 people.[65]

It's hard to remain trustful of the pharmaceutical companies after this knowledge, isn't it?

I worked for a few different doctors many years ago (that was an eye-opening experience, let me tell you) and I saw what medications most people were on. The elderly patients sometimes had up to 16 different types of medication. And they usually were on so many because they needed another pill to stop the side effects of another pill, and so forth. None of this stuff seemed to make them remarkably better; it just prolonged their life, which was in a pretty bad state, or made them deteriorate quickly. I never saw anyone glow with health, or bounce out of the doctor's surgery after being on such a lot of medication. And rarely did any of them receive any proper help with their diet either. Why would they, when doctors only get about 6 hours worth of nutrition training in their years at medical school?

One of the most common side effects of using so many pharmaceuticals is that the liver becomes sluggish and overworked to a point where it will then have to store many of the toxins. It simply cannot get rid of them effectively. Now, please again remember: I am *not* saying that all pharmaceutical medicine is bad; it's just generally being *misused* and handed out far too often. If I was in a car accident, there is no way that I would refuse to go to hospital or take their pain relief, nor would I say no to having an operation if I needed it. That would be silly and would lead to a terrible outcome. Some people do need to take medication to keep them alive. Remember, I am merely recommending that we try and avoid medications as much as possible and they should always be the last resort. There tend to be natural ways to help fix many symptoms and conditions, so I personally always try and use them first, with medical intervention a last resort. After all, plants and herbs were used as medicines long before pharmaceutical companies were started, and since time began.

Doctors aren't always to blame

In regards to the over-prescribing of drugs, it's *not* always the doctor's fault. Many patients are now *demanding* that their doctor give them this drug or that drug and often become quite upset if they don't get what they want. They usually go and visit doctor after doctor till they get the drug they think they need. They may have done some reading on the Internet or have seen an advertisement on the TV that makes them think they should have a certain medication.

Too many want a little pill to do something 'magically' whereas a change in lifestyle or diet is more than likely going to do it for them far more easily and safely. But due to the fact that it takes *effort*, some may just want to rely on swallowing a medication, rather than changing their diet or exercising more. Individuals need to take more control over their own health, rather than relying on doctors to prescribe things for them. And personally, if your doctor is not too easy to get prescriptions out of, they may actually be a good doctor! However, if your doctor automatically wants to always prescribe you something, it may be time to find a new one.

Chapter 12

'Legal' Drugs – Why They Are Not So Harmless After All

Millions of people reach for a big sugary strong coffee, cigarettes or energy drinks to wake them up and get them going for the day, as well as reaching for more throughout the day to keep them going longer. This is pretty much like giving yourself a drug all the time to provide you with quick, but 'bad' energy. It's *false* energy, causes harm, and puts a lot of stress on your body if it's happening on a regular basis.

In the case of coffee, I am not totally against it; it's certainly not unhealthy to have a coffee once in a while, and some say it's completely fine to have one or two each day and that in fact it can have very positive health benefits. But to rely on *many* cups to keep you going throughout the entire day is not exactly a good thing. A healthy body will already have the energy it needs to keep you going throughout the day without the need for regular stimulants. When coffee is consumed too much (more than 2 a day), the effect can be quite worrying. And for some even one cup a day may cause:

- Nervousness
- Irritability
- Fast heartbeat
- Muscle tremors
- Restlessness
- Stomach upset
- Bowel problems
- Rapid rise in stomach temperature by 10–15 degrees
- 400% increase in the secretion of hydrochloric acid (this is linked to causing Alzheimer's)
- 100% increase in urination – causing stress on the kidneys

- Increase in the cadmium levels in body due to coffee being the major dietary source of this toxic metal
- Stress to the lungs
- Narrowing of blood vessels in the brain, and in and around the heart
- Greater tendency for cells to mutate into cancer cells
- Enhanced predisposition to Alzheimer's
- Addiction

Alcoholics Anonymous counselors have noted that many of its members who are trying to kick alcohol tend to replace their drinking with cups of coffee; the average found was approximately 20 cups a day. The list above goes to show that drinking large amounts of coffee can lead a person to have health problems just as serious as what alcohol could do. So it makes sense to keep both at a minimum.

The rarely talked-about connection between coffee and Alzheimer's is also extremely concerning.[66] The rapid production of hydrochloric acid in the stomach after drinking coffee leads to the increased absorption of aluminum into the bloodstream. Aluminum and its derivatives are found in many common foods such as baking ingredients, in cooking utensils, prescription drugs (such as aspirin), deodorants, tea, water, and from air pollution. I think this fact alone is reason enough to keep your cups of coffee to a minimum. Alzheimer's is a cruel and degenerative disease that I wouldn't wish upon my worst enemy.

People who suffer with chronic fatigue or adrenal fatigue should also stay *right away* from coffee all the time (and chocolate too), but usually, they are the ones that drink it too much due to having a body that is unable to produce its own energy efficiently. Coffee gives them a sudden boost of short-lived energy, but then there is generally a big crash afterwards, making a person reach for more. It's truly a vicious cycle.

Coffee is certainly very powerful. I had quite a few cups myself during the writing of this book. I wanted to be able to concentrate and to get a lot done in one sitting and, wow, did it really give me a kick! Because I didn't have it very often, I was amazed at how it affected me, literally within minutes. Not only did it give me a lot of energy, but it also made me feel very happy for the first few hours. Both of these attributes are exactly how drugs initially make people feel, so it's easy to see how addictive it is.

Another concerning factor is that coffee is also sprayed very *heavily* with pesticides throughout the growing process. The coffee that ends up in your cup, and therefore in your body, is laced with pesticides too. And if you are having a lot per day, then it's definitely going to add quite a bit more to your toxicity levels.

When drinking coffee, always try and get organic and fair trade coffee. It tastes so much better too, and this way you will actually receive the health benefits that coffee does have in small doses.

Something else to consider is that the coffee trade is one of the *worst* for supporting slave labor as well. The ridiculous ongoing demand for cheap coffee in the Western world has created way too much competition, which means that the suppliers will sell their coffee for as little as possible to score the big contracts, and this means the workers – men, women *and* children – are treated absolutely appallingly. Therefore, buying organic fair trade coffee is one of the most ethical purchases you can make.

Stimulants are also now in lots of our food, which I have mentioned previously. They can give us a temporary high, only to make us need to eat more later on. And of course, alcohol, cigarettes and drugs are commonly used to relax us, make us 'happy', and to have 'fun'. But the downside is that the next day and over the long term it causes much stress to our body and brain. And, for many people these days, it's normal to drink every night of every single day and at lunches and quite heavily on the weekends. If you count up the drinks, it's certainly a lot.

If that is you, ask yourself *why* you do this. Chances are it's because you are not a truly happy person deep down, and the alcohol is trying to fill that hole we mentioned in Chapter 8, 'Removing Clutter'. Please don't think I am a saint; I used to drink a lot of alcohol, with huge amounts of dangerous binge-drinking on my weekends. I also know from experience that I was *very* unhappy, painfully shy and had very low self-esteem. The alcohol brought me out of my 'shell' and temporarily numbed my pain. I became a different person, the life of the party, but buried my problems deeper and ended up really making myself very sick later in life.

The amount of recreational drugs I did caused me a great deal of harm. My liver was in a *very* bad state. These days, I stay right away from drugs, alcohol and cigarettes. And I do not miss them *one* bit.

If you have a 'vice' and if it's that difficult to quit, there is perhaps something much deeper within you that is the real cause of this addiction.

Wine

It's true, a glass of red wine really does have some healthful benefits. So if you do enjoy a bit of a tipple, then one a day is OK. It's when that *one* leads to three or four that it's not good for you. Binge drinking is on the rise, and not just with teenagers and young adults fresh out of collage or school. More than ever before in the average household its typical for most working couples to drink every night to 'relax' after a stressful and busy day. It might be more 'normal' these days, that this is how most people are, but its certainly not OK for our long-term health. Liver damage can take quite a long time to show up on mainstream medical testing methods but damage can occur much earlier on, not to mention what regular consumption of alcohol can mean for your brain's health.

People also don't really make the connection, but with each glass of wine, you are actually swallowing a whole lot of pesticides and fungicides. If you check the list of non-safe non-organic fruits and veggies, grapes are really high up on the list. Grapes are commonly sprayed with so many chemicals – at least 22 different types of pesticides, fungicides and insecticides. A study carried out by the

European Pesticide Action Network found that '100% of conventionally grown wines contained pesticides, with one bottle containing ten types'.[67] So that's what *you're* drinking too. Yes, grapes and wine have many healthy qualities such as a high amount of antioxidants. But unfortunately wine causes a toxic reaction in the body because of the high chemical content, and the good effects go to waste. Also, the high pesticide levels and preservatives are a reason why, when you drink too much wine, you get a *killer* hangover the next day.

Here is something for you to try: next time you grab a bottle of wine, choose an organic sulfite-free wine and see how you feel the next day. I can guarantee you will feel a *lot* better. But that doesn't mean, go out and drink three bottles – you still need to be sensible. Try to limit yourself to not drinking every night in a row but to have a few evenings off; this will give the liver a chance to do its job.

Obviously it's not just wine; *all* alcohol is not safe to be included in a diet too regularly. Far too many people use alcohol to make them cope more with life, to feel happier in a not-so-great relationship, or to deal with depressive-type feelings and over a long period of time it *will* seriously affect your mental and physical state. That's a given. So if the future concerns you (as it should) and if you feel panic at the athought of giving up or cutting down drastically on on your drinking, then you may have in fact an *addiction* of some sort and perhaps need counselling for it.

To be truly healthy, we must let our liver deal with the least amounts of toxins as possible. Give it a helping hand rather than overloading it unnecessarily.

Cigarettes

I know, this should be a no-brainer. We all *know* that smoking is bad for our health. Yet look around: so many people *do* still smoke. You would think that if you worked in a hospital and saw people dying of emphysema, you would never smoke, but I have seen so many nurses and doctors smoke that it's really worrying. They, above all people, should be running scared from smoking. It's just that it's so addictive, and some say as hard to give up as heroin, so smoking is huge problem in our society.

Perhaps even you are a smoker yourself right now? Well, what I am going to do is just share with you what is in the cigarettes, and why it makes them so dangerous, and hope that this may help you to finally want to give them up. You see, it is *not* actually the tobacco that's harmful; it's the other toxins added to them that give people lung cancer. There are *4000* different chemicals in cigarettes and approximately 51 of them are proven to be carcinogenic.[68]

Inside the average cigarette and found in its smoke are the following chemicals:

- Benzene – a known carcinogen and associated with leukemia – also used as a solvent in fuel and chemical manufacture
- Formaldehyde – used as an embalming fluid, known to cause cancer, respiratory, skin and stomach problems – found in smoke
- Ammonia – commonly used as a toilet cleaner, often found in dry cleaning fluids, used as flavoring, stops nicotine from turning into a gas
- Acetone – also known as nail polish remover – highly flammable and is found in cigarette smoke
- Tar – once inhaled this condenses in the lungs and 70% of this is deposited in the lungs
- Nicotine – one of the most addictive substances known to humans – a fast-acting medical and non-medical poison – this is what causes the addiction
- Carbon monoxide – aka car exhaust fumes – tasteless and odorless, poisonous and fatal in large amounts – it's also the main gas which comes from a lit cigarette
- Others – arsenic (aka rat poison), hydrogen cyanide (used in World War 2 in the gas chambers)

Other chemicals found in cigarettes are: DDT (banned insecticide), butane (lighter fluid), sulfuric acid (used in car batteries), cadmium (used to charge batteries), maltitol (a sweetener not allowed in foods in the USA).

When we look back through history, remember that cigarettes were marketed as healthy (even by doctors!) and it took many, many years and huge lawsuits to prove that they were indeed the total *opposite*, that they caused many health problems and also contributed to millions of deaths.

If you find that you still cannot quit smoking, then please look for tobacco as pure as can be that comes loose, without all the chemicals, so you can roll your own. And you can also try and source a dioxin-free rolling paper. You can also purchase hemp and unbleached hemp papers. The websites listed below offer organic tobacco and unbleached papers for smoking.

- ✓ rollingsupreme.com
- ✓ organic-smoke.com
- ✓ motherearthtobacco.com

Energy drinks

These little cute-looking cans contain dreadful chemicals that do give you a boost but only temporarily and, also, with 'drug-like' effects. They are often touted as 'health drinks', yet are not the *least* bit healthy. Sure, they can have vitamins added to them and things like ginseng, but the main ingredients, such as a super-high dose of caffeine (often up to 7 *times* that of a normal coffee!) are just *not* good for your body to have to process. And these drinks are meant to stimulate the brain as well! They also harm the teeth much worse than regular soft drinks / sodas do. So acidic are these drinks that they can make the teeth enamel very thin – the same effect that battery acid would have on them!

Lots of people have these drinks instead of coffee, thinking that they are healthier (because of the misleading advertising), yet they are definitely not healthy at all. It's also quite alarming to see young teenagers drink them regularly. Having these before or during the school day will not be a good way to keep them listening and concentrating; it is more likely to cause them to have a nap at their desk during lessons!

Manufacturers make synthetic caffeine which goes in many of these energy drinks and is derived from pretty scary sources:[69]

- Trichloroethylene (TCE) – a chlorinated hydrocarbon commonly used as an industrial solvent. It's so powerful, the Air Force uses it to clean jet engines. Banned in Europe as a known cancer-causing chemical, it is perfectly legal to use in the United States.
- Sodium cyanide – a highly toxic, colorless salt used in gold mining to strip gold from rock.
- Sulfuric acid – a strong mineral acid used in car batteries, ore processing, fertilizer manufacturing and oil refining.
- Benzene – a known cancer-causing chemical used as an industrial solvent and in the production of drugs, plastics, synthetic rubber and dyes.

Many years ago, I remember going to a music festival with a friend who did not want to drink or take recreational drugs like most of the others who were there. Instead, she bought about 6 cans of a popular guarana-based energy drink and drank them all throughout the day.

A few short hours later, she ended up having to go to the emergency section at the festival to get help from the ambulance crew. She was having *severe* anxiety and panic attacks as her heart was racing way too fast from the huge doses of stimulants. Her body literally thought she had drunk about 50 cups of coffee.

The ambulance people advised her that what she had done was just as *dangerous* as drinking way too much alcohol and mixing it with drugs. It was a very, very scary experience for her (and me too after seeing her like that!) and one she learnt from. Worryingly, many clubgoers now have spirits such as vodka mixed in with their energy drinks, and I have tried them myself years ago when I used to go out clubbing.

Back then I was also on antidepressants so this made it even worse for my poor brain; all that chemical stimulation was just not what I needed! Even having just *one drink* mixed in with alcohol made me stay up until 6am, even though I had left at midnight to go home to try and sleep. The body just sees these types of mixtures as way too stimulating and often can make you feel quite ill the next day.

Red Bull, one of the most famous of all the energy drinks, has been banned in France after a basketball player died due to having 4 cans of the drink before the high-energy game. Even many doctors in the UK are trying to get the law changed so that there should be warnings on the cans to make people aware of the possible side effects.

There is even a drink labeled 'cocaine', which is just disgusting and it shocks me that it is even allowed to be sold!

There are ways of making your own drinks that can give you an energy boost with no harmful effects. In the recipe section there is a yummy chocolate drink you can make to help you feel more energetic. And in Chapter 28 there is some helpful information regarding natural energy boosters.

I also highly recommend a daily dose of Green Energy capsules by Touchstone Essentials. These contain a blend of organic decaffeinated green tea, enzymes and botanicals which is wonderful for helping you feel good all day. They also help with improving poor digestion due to too much protein consumed in the average diet which affects and decreases the way our oxygen is delivered to the cells. The less oxygen your cells receive, the more tiredness you will feel. 'Leaky gut syndrome' can be caused by too much undigested protein which causes the red blood cells to clump and 'stick' together. Leaky gut syndrome affects so many people these days, which I discuss in greater detail in Chapter 18. After using Touchstone Essentials Green Energy for a month, I noticed that I had less extreme sugar highs and lows so I wasn't having any sudden crashes in energy. Unlike with coffee, I was not having any racing heart symptoms and did not feel 'on edge' like coffee tends to make me (and most of us) feel. I also think it helped me breathe better too; each time I inhaled oxygen, it seemed to fill up my lungs better. A truly wonderful product.

Chapter 13

The Vital Importance of Detoxing

I have seen patients who had been diagnosed with illnesses including MS, Crohn's disease, liver cancer, autism, hay fever, arthritis, gout, rheumatism, type 2 diabetes, Desert Storm syndrome, migraines, chronic candidiasis and parasite infections, psychotic 'horrors' and a multitude of others end up hearing their doctors say, 'It was a misdiagnosis,' after completing HM&C (Heavy Metal & Chemical) Detox successfully. Heavy metals and chemicals interfere with cellular, enzyme, endocrine and neurological function. I never 'cured' any of those diseases, as the patients never had them to begin with. The HM&C toxicity manifested as those disease syndromes.[70]

Dr. Timothy Ray

I guess common sense tells you that if you have been living on this earth with no clue to all of these dangers until now, then you must be full of toxins already? I hate to scare you but, yes, that's the truth! Healthy people tend to have a body that can deal with things, but chances are because of the assault from *so* many toxins that are in our water, air, food, houses etc. you do have a lot of nasty things floating around in your body, possibly lying dormant, so you don't even feel like anything is wrong. You can literally go from being healthy and fairly low in toxins one year, to quite ill the next year, especially if you have gone through a lot of stress. The stress will cause the body to become sluggish to the point where the liver won't be able to do its job properly.

Someone that is very sensitive to chemicals may have any or more of the following symptoms

- runny nose all the time (rhinitis)
- nausea

- muscle and joint pains
- dizziness
- skin rashes and itching skin
- sore throat, cough
- headaches
- poor memory
- poor concentration
- light and noise sensitivity
- digestive problems
- stinging eyes
- sleep disturbance
- regular colds
- regular flus
- tiredness
- being prone to anger
- emotional outbursts
- depression

Not a nice list, is it?!

Chronic toxicity and the systems it affects

- Central, nervous and autonomic systems
- Hematological and immune system
- Heart and cardiovascular system
- Endocrine system
- Eyes, ears, nose and throat
- Respiratory system
- Skin
- Gastrointestinal system
- Liver
- Urinary system
- Musculo-skeletal system
- Reproductive system

So basically, every single part of the body will be affected by toxicity.

Now can you see why I believe that most diseases are directly related to chemicals that we are absorbing?

Colonic hydrotherapy – a fantastic way to detox

If you have heard of this treatment before, you may be automatically thinking, 'No way, yuck!', but please hear me out. Yes, having a colonic does mean sticking a tube up your backside and using water to clean your colon out – but, despite how scary it sounds, it does *not* hurt, can actually be very relaxing, and is *one of the most powerful things* you can do for your health. Far too many people are being diagnosed with colon cancer which is linked to eating a diet high in animal protein (particularly hormonally treated non-organic red meat) and low in fiber.

I only had my first colonic in 2010 and, oh my, did I regret not having them *years* sooner. What I am about to tell you, which is quite personal, is just to show you how many years 'stuff' can be left to rot in your colon. When I was having my first treatment my therapist was concerned as to why I had pitch-black dried-up bits of poop coming out. She questioned why that could be.

I immediately remembered back to my early 20s. I was, back then, severely depressed and attempted suicide with pharmaceutical pills on two separate occasions, which landed me in hospital. I was made to drink cups of charcoal which looked and tasted like black sand. Not only was it awful to drink (and yes, it probably saved my life), the charcoal was still *right* there in my colon, *10 long years later*! My colon could not process it well and had to store it there for a very long time.

My therapist said I also probably had remnants from burgers and fast food and other processed foods in there as well. So highly trained was she that she could tell what my little lumps were! When you eat things like McDonald's or KFC, these chemically based foods do not get digested well (or sometimes never at all), and in my case (having not eaten any foods like this for at least 10 years) parts were still there, perhaps from even *20 years earlier*!

Having a clogged colon puts a *massive* strain on your body. It has to try and deal with the blockage, and many times, parasites and other horrible things grow in the intestines and feed off all the waste that is trapped there, and then they *dump their waste in your body*. Yuck! That means that parasites poop in your body! Gross!

Some of the reported benefits of colonics are quite impressive. If you have a bad back, for instance, you may find that having a treatment could really reduce your pain. A clogged colon can put pressure on sciatic and lumbar nerves. Having parasites and internal worms can also make back pain worse. And people with drug and alcohol addictions have also reported they were able to finally stop being addicted once they had cleansed their colons.

Cleaning the colon will also help to remove heavy metals and other carcinogens and will help the body with its own vitamin production. For example, the colon helps produce B vitamins, folic acid, niacin, riboflavin, and pantothenic acid. It also aids in the pre-digestion of proteins and lactose, and in the important formation of amino acids.

If you suffer with constipation, nothing is better for it than a colonic! Constipation is not good to have regularly because it puts strain on the gallbladder, liver and bile duct. A clean colon also has a dramatic and positive effect on the immune system.

I guess we should look at the colon like we do a car's engine – that the car needs to have an engine running properly for the car to function without problems.

So, if this hasn't moved you to get a colonic, I don't know what else will. OK, maybe this statement, from Dr. Bernard Jensen in 1974, will help:

The colon is a sewage system, but by neglect and abuse it becomes a cesspool. When it is clean and normal, we are well and happy. Let it stagnate and it will distill the poisons of decay, fermentation, and putrefaction into the blood, poisoning the brain and nervous system so that we become mentally depressed and irritable; it will poison the heart so that we are weak and listless; poison the lungs so that the breath is foul; poison the digestive organs so we are distressed and bloated; and poison the blood so the skin is sallow and unhealthy. In short, every organ of the body is poisoned, and we age prematurely; look and feel old, the joints are stiff and painful, neuritis, full eyes, and a sluggish brain overtake us, and the pleasure of living is gone. Death begins in the colon.

Let this be a friendly yet very serious warning to you that your colon's health is very, *very* important to your whole life. And it's not just something you should do once in your life; keeping up to date with having a healthy colon is very important. The massive rise in bowel cancers is proof of this. And if you want to feel pretty much instantly better, a good colonic can really do this.

A great website which explains why cleaning the colon is so important is below:

✓ naturalflowtohealth.ca

Enemas

If the thought of visiting someone to have them administer a colonic gives you the heebie-jeebies, or is too expensive, there is another option, and that is to do an 'at home' enema. This involves using a bag (you can purchase this as a kit with the other items needed) which you hang up somewhere. Then you fill the bag with pure water (or you can mix it with things like organic coffee) and place a tube inside your bottom so that the water will flow inside. You keep the fluid in as long as you can, and release it into the toilet after a certain time. This gives the colon a pretty good cleanse (not as intensive as a proper colonic, though, but it still can give amazing results) and also exercises the intestines/colon. There are plenty of YouTube videos with helpful instructions. A very inexpensive way to give yourself a colon cleanse. And the private setting of your home makes it even more appealing. Some people find enemas so good that they actually become addicted to them, so of course, make sure you do them carefully, correctly and never too often.

Kits are available in the UK from:

✓ rawliving.eu

✓ detoxyourworld.com

If you are outside the UK just google 'enema kits' and purchase one that comes with instructions.

Foods that detox

Although I do think that zeolites (you will find detailed info on these at the end of this chapter) are the fastest (and easiest) way to detox, there are certain foods, supplements and herbs which you can incorporate into your diet that have a detoxing effect on the body. But if you have a serious amount of toxins in your body, you do need high doses of the right things, and for certain amounts of time, to get them out. And I would strongly suggest seeing a natural health specialist who can advise you exactly what to do.

To keep your body healthy, or at least put it on the right path, I can suggest the following foods you can include daily to help with the process: lemons, broccoli, cilantro (also known as coriander), artichokes, prunes, garlic and onions, green and white teas, chaga (a powerful mushroom extract), seeds such as almonds, walnuts, sesame seeds, chia seeds, pumpkin, sunflower and flaxseeds – all have detoxing abilities.

Start each day with a glass of warm water and lemon; this helps the metabolism and the detoxification process to get going.

Juicing

Another way to cleanse the body, and also very easy to do, is to juice for a period of anywhere from a few days to a week (some people do this for longer than a week but I personally feel that is too long), drinking nothing but organic fresh vegetable juices with minimal fruits. These detoxes can be performed a few times a year – but here is some advice: don't go overboard with them or get obsessed. More juice fasts does not mean better health for you. It does give the body and its organs and digestive system a chance to relax and can also pull out heavy metals (depending on the ingredients used) and other toxic build-up if you include coriander in the juices. If you don't want to give up eating on this juice fast, then I think it's definitely OK to eat light and simple whole foods as well. If you have gone from eating a standard unhealthy diet, then to start eating like this can do you a whole lot of good without being a total shock to the system.

I know of many people who do juice regularly and they absolutely glow with health! I also know some people who keep doing far too many juice fasts and are clearly not well. What works for one person may not work for another, so it's always best to listen to your own body. I don't personally think that juicing for weeks on end, many times a year, is what the body needs, and from what I have seen, it perhaps can be quite addictive for some people. Everything, as usual, is best in moderation.

Many recipes for juices can be found on the internet if you would like to investigate further. My personal favorite juice recipe is with celery, cucumber and kale. It's very low in sugars and if you have it every day, it can make your skin so much clearer and vibrant. The key is not to drink gallons and gallons of juice; you don't want to bombard your body with too much iron or too many vitamins. It's all about balance.

I have some yummy juice recipes you can try in Chapter 19.

Another great recipe book is Jason Vale's *The Fresh Funky Juice Book*. You can find out more about him and his juicing regimes at:

✓ juicemaster.com

Herbal teas

The Chinese have known for thousands of years that herbs are so powerful for the body. Wise Chinese people drink these teas till the cows come home and for good reason too: it keeps them free from disease and illness. Some of the world's longest-living people drink copious amounts of certain types of tea. You can find herbs in most health food shops, although sadly, many are becoming illegal due to a new law being passed by an organization called 'The Codex Alimentarius Commission'. Codex Alimentarius is a food code which was established way back in 1962. What is very insidious about this organization is that they are trying to deem many healthy foods, herbs, minerals and vitamins as 'drugs and or medicines' and are trying to get certain things completely banned, or to reduce the levels of a certain vitamin/mineral.

> Codex began simply enough when the UN authorized the World Health Organization and the Food and Agriculture Organization to develop a universal food code. Their purpose was to 'harmonize' regulations for dietary supplements worldwide and set international safety standards for the purposes of increased trade. Pharmaceutical interests stepped in and began exerting their influence. Instead of focusing on food safety, Codex is using its power to promote worldwide restrictions on vitamins and food supplements, severely limiting their availability and dosages.[71]

Many things have already been banned which were highly beneficial for people's health, such as certain herbs. It is ridiculous as many natural ingredients are very healing to the body and someone's overall general health, which help people to avoid going to the doctor or needing to take other things. Whilst its true, herbs can be harmful if taken in large doses and if you are also using certain medications, it does seem ridiculous to class them as a drug because they are in a natural form – they haven't been synthesized into a drug by laboratoires. It seems crazy to put them in the same category as medications when they (pharmaceuticals) are the ones that have much more harmful effects on people. And this is proven by statistics and evidence! Who has overdosed on too much chamomile or too much lavender?

This vitally important topic could be a whole other book, so if interested please go to YouTube to see what this means for our health freedom. There is a movie there called *We Become Silent,* narrated by Dame Judy Dench, which explains it all. Be prepared to be very outraged.

If you do get hold of herbs, *they must be organic*! I can't stress this enough. Herbs grown in typical places like China and India (if not truly organic) are *covered in many heavy metals and pesticides*. When looking for herbs try and make sure you know they are organic and where they come from. I would even avoid buying anything from China if I were you, due to the fact that there's been many cases where the manufacturers have lied about the purity of their products. There are bio-dynamic farms (Demeter association) all over the world (particularly in Europe), so you can try and contact them and see what they sell and where they distribute.

Here is a short list of herbs to help the body become stronger and cleaner:

- Nettle
- Burdock Root
- Horsetail
- Licorice Root
- Witch Hazel (bark, twigs and leaves)
- Milk Thistle seed

Herbs should *always* be used very wisely as they can be super-powerful, so always get advice from someone trained in that area. And remember, if you are on any medications, then this could cause a bad reaction (as I experienced personally!), so please be careful.

Supplements

I used to take handfuls of vitamins a day, only to realize that not only was I literally pooping them out (due to not absorbing them at all), but they unknown to me, were also quite toxic. Many vitamins today contain fillers, GMOs and synthetic ingredients. If you take Vitamin B for example, you are more than likely swallowing lots more things – you just aren't aware! Many people are overdosing with too many substances, for instance, thinking they need a super amount of antioxidants but the truth is, too many of them is not a good thing for the body either. I have really cut down on what I take. I am shocked when I think about how many I used to take, how toxic they were and how much money I wasted! The only supplements I take and trust are the Touchstone Essentials brand and some specialized things I take which were created by a doctor from the Czech Republic, who also treats the Russian astronaut space team. I discuss more about Touchstone Essentials products later on, and in another book I will one day write, I will feature more of Dr. Kucera's supplements and his groundbreaking work.

Chlorella, chlorophyll and in particular spirulina are amazing at detoxing the body and can remove heavy metals.[72] I would include these in your diet regularly to keep the body working to remove unwanted toxins. The ironic problem with these is that they are also said to be toxic (if they are sourced from oceans where the waters contain heavy metals) so you need to be aware that not all brands are good. Some companies sell products that have been purified so try and look for those.

- ✓ Mike Adams from Natural News has investigated this issue in great detail. He has discovered one of the worlds most purest Chlorellas. You can purchase it from: store.naturalnews.com
- ✓ Mercola.com also has some fabulous information about chlorella, spirulina and chlorophyll where you can purchase high-quality types
- ✓ In the UK you can buy from rawliving.eu

'Whole Being' detox – body, life and mind

While certain detox techniques, such as the ones I have mentioned above, can be very powerful, some experts say that for tip-top health, an intensive program will really get the body running and healing, to function at its best. For this type of advice, I have called upon Savannah Alalia, whom I really respect, to educate us about what this means and what it involves for the body.

Detox is about organ cleansing

OK, what does that mean? Well, let's look at it this way: If you imagine your body is a house and each room in that house relates to an organ. For years you have had all sorts of foods, or let's call them 'house guests', walking through your house. Some of those 'guests' have been clean and wiped their feet and moved through easily, other 'guests' have had great big muddy boots on and have been cheeky and had their feet up all over your furniture and maybe even taken up residence in one of those rooms... but you have not really been giving any attention to what your 'guests' have been up to.

I like this saying... because I think it fits here – 'House guests are like fish – after 3 days they start to smell.' It is the same with the food 'guests' that you have traipsing through your 'house' or body; if they get stuck there it can get a little whiffy inside...

And no one likes to smell... OK, I think I've got your attention...

Now you're starting to take a look at the reality that your 'house' is pretty grubby and a few of your 'guests' who smiled sweetly on their way in have now taken up residence... they looked lovely and clean on the outside, they tasted great, but on entry to your house they have wreaked havoc.

Only you know who or what you have consumed or let in to your house... but what we both know is that some of those 'guests' need to be shown the door...

It's time for them to leave, but how do you get them out?

This is where organ cleansing or detox comes in. Organ cleansing or detoxing is Mother Nature's way of cleaning out unwanted house guests. Ever thrown a party as a teenager and had your 'guests' overstay their welcome and begin to trash the place? Who gets called in? Mum... and she will tell them exactly what she thinks and show them the door, because no one messes with Mum. Natural Organ Cleanses are your Mother (Nature's) way of getting any unwanted 'guests' out of your 'house' or body.

(For all Miss Eco Glam readers I will give a free copy of the main organ cleanses I use and recommend. If you go to www.SavannahAlalia.com/MissEcoGlamPromotion you can enter your details and you will be sent these natural organ cleanses and detoxes.)

So Mother Nature helps us out, and we get rid of our unwanted food 'guests', but what next?

Staying clean is something we need to keep on top of, just like you do your actual house cleaning. A deep clean every season will get you on track with clear organs giving you organized (sorry couldn't help the pun ;) and clean 'rooms'. If there has been years of neglect it can take a little while to get it all sorted but if you still have a house or a body then the sorting process is possible and even pretty amazing.

So that's the basics of detoxing covered. Now we move on to diet but just to be clear on why detox is not just diet.

To stop having 'messy house guests' for 1 week or 2 weeks or even a month of say juicing or healthy eating simply means you are no longer adding more dirt to your space rather than cleaning up the mess you already have in your 'house'.

Most people do what they think of as a 'cleanse or detox' which is really no more that a diet change and after they have finished they invite the messy guests back and wonder why it hasn't made any difference…

A cleanse or detox for each organ individually is your starting point, then you can create a routine for the upkeep of 'your house'. A natural cleansing/detox process should be pretty simple, manageable, enjoyable and even easy. If you are fighting your way through a 'detox or cleanse' you are missing something.

So how do you know which 'guests' to invite?

Diet is about minimizing the toxic load that is coming into the body. I know Anna has got you covered on much of this with her thorough research into the 'nasties' in our day-to-day living, but I am just going to add a few points to consider.

Hopefully you are beginning to see how this is about a lifestyle approach rather than just a fad.

Getting to know your house 'guests' better, as in knowing the food you are consuming, will allow you to be aware of or keep an eye on how your 'guests', or your food, will behave in 'your home', or your body.

You get to begin to have a choice of what or who you will happily continue to invite in.

You can begin to see if your 'guest' (or food) is nourishing you, taking care of you and leaving having improved things rather than left a mess to clear up… this aware approach is about a lifestyle that allows you to feel great, look amazing and have rockin' energy levels.

Believe me, it's worth taking the time to acquaint yourself with your 'guests' or food.

Here are a few of the basics:

Fresh water (spring water ideally)

Water is a best friend to consider spending as much time with as you possibly can. Water will keep you clean, keep everything moving (quite literally) and will help you see if some other food is trying to con you into being 'let in'. Often dehydration is the issue rather than hunger. Drinking enough will keep you clear in so many ways.

Organic is a must

Why?! Well, as I know Anna has shared, if you eat anything other than organic you are giving a free invitation to chemicals from pesticides and other nasties to enter in and make a mess in your 'house'. Plus the nourishment you will get from 1 organic piece of broccoli is about equal to 5 pieces of non-organic broccoli; that's a lot of extra chewing. Eating non-organic will have you feeling hungry and unsatisfied and invite a load of tag-alongs to your 'house'. So you tell me, is it worth it?

At least 50/50 raw to cooked food ratio

Keeping this ratio will surprise many of you. The raw 50% will actually assist in the digestion of the cooked 50% and so your 'house' will be on sort of an auto-clean. Again really worthwhile! Try it and see for yourself.

No processed foods – this includes SUGAR

This one sounds obvious but let me share a little deeper. Processed foods are fake 'house guests'. They will lie, lie, lie from the second they enter; they will look good, taste right, but they will be constantly making a mess and disrupting other passers through. And just to be clear: normal SUGAR is processed.

No chemicals – this includes SWEETENERS

There are no substitutes for respectful 'guests' and we humans are like children trying to play grown-up when it comes to these 'guests'. The chemicals we create with special technologies are missing so many key factors, which makes these 'guests' more like zombies that will come in and steal from you, act as a parasite and have no awareness of your space at all other than it's a great host... Mother Nature has your back on this with a queue of natural 'house guests'... Why play with the living dead?

Whole foods

Whole foods are going to be your lifelong buddies. They make great 'guests' – they are well-rounded, cheery and easy to have around. They will even help clean up your 'house'. They are keepers as far as 'guests' go and I would suggest making sure they have a very regular invitation.

Wild foods

Wild foods are the superstar 'guests' – they will have you feeling incredible. Wild foods are packed full of nourishment and so will have you feeling fulfilled and excited to have them over again and again and again. I suggest remembering to let them in – you'll be so happy you did as they will always be the best of all company.

The two final basics are good exercise; that means regularly, at least a few times a week. And a clear mental state, which can be achieved through slowing the usual mental chatter and getting clear on what you are doing and why. Both the exercise and the mind are equally important and neither should be overlooked as they will give you the foundations needed to keep your 'house' in order.

This all sounds great but how can you get there easily?

After over 15 years of hands-on research, both personally and with thousands of clients, I have found what I feel is the simplest path to enliven your senses and awaken your natural instincts so you know who or what to say yes or no to and how you can do it easily. I have called this process HumanFood101, and it's a 10-week online food revolution process, with a community of other like-minded individuals that teaches you to get to know your body (your house) and what foods will actually nourish you (which guests to invite in).

At the beginning of HumanFood101 I encourage people to look at how the simple basics around when you are eating, where you are eating and what you are eating can affect how your body will feel on the food you consume. When you begin to learn how to be aware of what is affecting your life and vitality levels, it gets very easy to make decisions to get the foundations of 'feel great' in place.

I believe what you eat can affect your mood, your weight and your energy levels. I also believe 'health' around food is a lifestyle rather than a 'diet fad'. Yo-yo dieting, however 'healthy', can actually be harmful. Learning a step-by-step approach to cleansing and detox and then nourishing your body are the keys to feeling great... the whole way through :)

An illusion is that 'healthy' food is boring or there are no treats and this is the best-kept secret out there. Healthy treats are more delicious than anything you think you want now... if you try this you will begin to see that up until now what you thought tasted good was actually pretty bland and dull.

(I only run HumanFood101 a couple of times a year so if you're interested you can get onto the waiting list here... www.SavannahAlalia.com/MEGHumanfood101)

Please note: Savannah Alalia retains the ownership and the rights to this extract and she is just giving her permission for me to use her materials as it is this one time, it cannot be copied from this book.

Pure Body Zeolites – the essential way to detox

The most successful way to remove toxins that I have *ever* tried is 'Pure Body' by Touchstone Essentials. This is a truly *brilliant* zeolite product which can often have miraculous results. It certainly changed my life in a huge way. And it requires little effort on your part to get rid of all of the chemicals that are in your body. You simply add it to water, drink (or spray into the mouth) several times a day, and it works its magic immediately; within 4–6 hours that dose will have left the body. It's completely non-toxic, 100% natural *and* safe.

I will tell you something quite embarrassing. Unbeknown to me, apparently I smelt very bad. My husband said that he always knew I was sick because I had a strange smell that was coming out of my skin. Not just normal body odor – it was a sickly smell (like 'off' milk) and something just didn't seem 'quite right' with me. I always knew that I indeed needed to wear deodorants, but I had no idea that my actual skin itself and not just my armpits was giving off a nasty smell. My husband told me this a few weeks after I had started taking the zeolites and commented to a friend (in front of me also) that they were amazing because, after taking them for just 2 weeks, I 'no longer smelt bad'. Well… Wasn't I shocked to know that for the past 7 *years* my husband thought I was a stinker?! It made us both realize that you can tell a *lot* about someone's health by their body odor; this is a vital clue. And his comment also proved to me just how quickly these zeolites can act.

What are zeolites?

Zeolites are a 100% natural mineral that comes from volcanic lava. They are formed where the lava meets the sea. The particles are millions of years old, super super tiny, but do something so amazing it's almost very hard to believe. Under a microscope the zeolite actually looks like a cage and when it's suspended in a liquid, and traveling inside the human body, it will attract to its *negatively* charged structure anything that has a *positive* charge. So it basically acts like a magnet. And guess what? Most of the toxins that do not belong in the body are *positively charged*. Pretty amazing, right?

In the medical environment, doctors carry out a treatment on people who have been poisoned with heavy metals or other chemicals, which has similar effects to zeolite. It is called 'chelation therapy' and is said to trap the particles and then move them out of the body through urination and sweat. The problem with chelation therapy is that it's typically very intense because it also removes other precious minerals from the body as well as vitamins. And it's very expensive, so for many people chelation therapy is just not an option. And it's safe to say that this form of detox is very, very harsh, and could do more harm than good as you don't want to negatively affect the mineral levels in the body.

Pure Body Zeolites are far less invasive, as they only draw out the unwanted toxins in the body. They tend to have a phenomenal effect on high levels of mercury, so for people who have amalgam fillings (silver-looking fillings), you definitely need to get yourself on these zeolites as the longer the fillings are in your mouth, the more mercury you will have in your bodies as the fillings wear down over time. Each time you chew, mercury vapor is released into the body. There are over 300 studies found on pubmed.gov on the beneficial and positive effects that clinotoptilite has on the body.[73]

How you take them is like this. Each day you can take an approximate dose (for an adult) of 4 drops 3 times a day. There is no need to take more, even for an intensive detox. You put them directly in a glass of water, or spray in the mouth if you are using Pure Body Extra Strength – and that's it! The only downside is you will need to drink plenty of water so that the zeolite passes through your body quicker. Some people report headaches or slight nausea, but that is a good sign, it means your body is throwing the toxins out!

I don't rave too much about many supplements, because over the years, I tried so many and none of them really worked. I wasted *so* much money and just felt very dismayed that everything seemed to be a waste of time. Far too many supplements are not absorbed by the body. However, after the *first* time I tried zeolites, within 2 weeks only, I noticed a *huge* improvement in how I felt. I used to have very 'heavy' feeling legs, so that when I walked up stairs it was truly difficult. I just had no energy in them at all. Everything was such an effort. I also used to have chronic brain fog where I always felt like my mind was fuzzy and 'stuck'. I couldn't concentrate and always felt I needed to sleep to get rid of it, yet sleep would never actually fix it. I was showing classic signs of toxicity. After only 2 weeks, this all went *completely* away! And, lucky for my husband, my stinky smell also disappeared very quickly. Thank goodness!

Pure Body Zeolites is truly an *amazing* and, for many, can be a *life-changing* product because it can help with pulling out mercury, lead, pesticides, residues from pharmaceutical medicines, plastic particles from water bottles, chemicals from your beauty products and all the other areas of life they have come from. They really are truly an absolute miracle, and now with what I know in relation to the bombardment of chemicals around us, I think *everyone* should be taking them regularly.

They are also clinically proven and FDA-approved and are said to be 100% safe for pregnant women, babies and children to use. The company is not allowed by law to recommend this as such (hardly any supplements are ever approved for use in pregnancy) but you just have to know the right dose, although it's very good to know they can't be overdosed on.

Just so you know, there are only two zeolite brands I have personally tried and support. Waiora make a good one called NCD, although it is nowhere near as strong as Pure Body (you can tell easily because NCD is very clear-looking like water and Pure Body looks a lot more like a thin mud which shows there is much more clinotoptilite) and it's also *much* more expensive. Even toxin aware doctors are preferring their patients take Touchstone Essentials Pure Body Zeolite.

Doctors know the cumulative effects of pollutants, toxins, heavy metals and other carcinogens can have a devastating effect on our bodies. As a practicing physician, I know that prevention is clearly the best form of health insurance you and your family can get. In an age of rising health costs, zeolite provides an affordable solution to many of the environmental risk factors we face today. While there are many zeolite products on the market today, one zeolite product in particular meets the rigorous standards

medical professionals seek – a product called Pure Body.
Alex Lee MD, Board Certified, Internal Medicine, Gastroenterology – Assistant Clinical Professor of Medicine at UCLA

When you are researching zeolite, be careful, as there are so many other zeolite brands on the market. And most will say that they are the best, yet they aren't backed up by science. The information I have seen is that unless a zeolite goes through an itense cleaning process like Touchstone has developed, they are not safe as they are still full of heavy metals, because they are from the earth's crust – which if you remember from Chapter 3 is completely full of heavy metals that you don't want in the body.

Below are some impressive testimonials about Pure Body.

Helen Hooper

I started taking Pure Body Zeolites about 8 weeks ago now and if I am honest I wasn't expecting too much. Having been on a raw-food diet for about 7 years and having done lots of cleanses, juice feasting and fasting, all without too much effect, I didn't think that anything would have a big impact on me. Wow, was I wrong!!!

Within the first few hours of taking Pure Body my head felt as if it was in a vice and what followed over the next few days was a huge purging that seemed centered around my head and neck. On day 3 I was practicing yoga and while performing a shoulder stand I felt a huge release in my shoulders. Within hours I had developed a rash all across my left shoulder and up into my neck. This lasted a few days before it cleared.

In the weeks that have followed I have had purges and then lulls and then purges again. I have released kidney stones, had areas of extremely dry skin – almost like eczema, headaches, and a clearing of rheumatoid arthritis.

Just when I think things are coming to an end something else pops up! Which makes me realize that this is going to be a long but beautiful process.

So, a big and delightful surprise to finally find something that actually shifts things in a rapid and powerful way. I would happily recommend Pure Body to everyone and will definitely be using it with my own clients in the future.

Paul Cashmore: Red Bull and headaches

Having been provided a bottle of Pure Body Zeolites, I was intrigued as to its effects. I have suffered with shoulder pain and headaches for some time and in my time I had eaten quite a lot of canned tuna and grains and worked in London, drank alcohol, so I guess I have been open to a massive amount of pollutants.

As a Red Bull addict I cut it out and began my Pure Body regime. It doesn't taste of anything so that was a great start; the last thing I want is to be chugging some nasty medicine-type liquid down my neck.

Well, my headaches have gone, my face tingled for a while and my back, but this is my body ridding itself of pollutants and toxins. I detoxed my body and thought I would test my new body and consume a Red Bull. It was like being hit in the head with a sledge-hammer. OK, so the Red Bull addiction has gone and the ultimate result is no withdrawal headaches.

I would recommend anyone taking zeolites to combine with a detox plan and, man, you will feel the benefits.

Bob Goetz: organic pesticides

On June 20th of this year (2012) I was exposed to an organic pesticide that started a chain of events that led to 8 weeks of pain and suffering. I was in my yard preparing to spray the perimeter for rabbits and deer. I was using a pump sprayer. After pumping to full force I started to spray when the sprayer tip exploded and covered me with contents. I immediately headed for the hose. I stripped my clothes and continued to flush my body. After a while I went in the house and took a shower. The poison control center confirmed it was organic and should have no lasting effects unless I was allergic to an ingredient. During this time we were experiencing over 90°F high heat levels and we had no air conditioning.

On the 24th we went to a farm breakfast out in the sun for hours. When I returned home I was exhausted and lay down. All of these conditions started a 3-day bout of high fever (103°F), sweating constantly and inability to eat or function. When the fever broke it took a couple of days to get my strength back. I could not eat and lived on double doses of Touchstone. As I began to function Donna noticed very small red patches on my skin and within 24 hours these had grown into large patches that began to be painful. At this time I went to the clinic for a diagnosis. They asked if I had ever been in Asia and I replied yes, I spent 3 years in Vietnam during the war. Had I ever suffered excessive heat exposure? I replied yes. They said my sweat glands had shut off and my body was overheating from the inside out. It would have to run its course and I should drink lots of liquid and put ice packs on the affected areas. The rash moved over my entire body. As it appeared it would go from light red to red and then to black and become very hot and painful. The next day the top layer of skin would peel like a sunburn and then it would appear somewhere else, from my face to my toes. I was unable to keep ahead of the dehydration and lost 28 lb in the course of the 8-week duration.

I basically lived on watermelon, water, electrolytes and our nutritional supplements. On August 10th I went in for testing at the VA. The results were, there are no organs affected. I attribute this to the high levels of Touchstone nutritional supplements (particularly Pure Body) I was taking, plus high vitamin C. Thank God for the right things at the right time. As of August 14th my only deficiency is vitamin D. Almost 8 weeks to the day I was unable to be in the sunlight because it would worsen the condition. What a wonderful summer.

Rosa Haines: *heavy metal toxicity, depression, chronic fatigue, joint pain*

After taking the Pure Body Zeolite product, I feel like I've finally got my life back! I want to thank Touchstone Essentials with all my heart, for this product has truly changed my life.

For years, I suffered from chronic fatigue syndrome, depression, joint pain and heavy metal toxicity. I had been taking a different (well-known) brand of zeolite for years and it helped a lot, improving my chronic fatigue. However, I still had low energy levels and severe depression. It seemed as though nothing would lift the clouds of despair I felt.

Then I learned about Pure Body Zeolite. With a small zeolite particle size, the available surface area of the zeolite is much bigger, and that could mean a greater ability to attract toxins, so I wanted to try it.

When I first started taking the Pure Body, my head felt like it was being drained of some sort of toxic build-up. It literally felt like this numb heaviness was draining out of my head. This lasted for about 5 days. After a week of taking it, I woke up feeling the happiest I'd felt in years!

Words cannot describe how incredible it is to feel happy after having felt sad for so long. It is as though someone lifted the clouds and let the sun into my life.

Since taking the Pure Body, my energy levels have increased beyond belief. My sleeping is back to normal. My concentration is much improved, and I'm able to enjoy reading books again, whereas before I couldn't concentrate for more than 2 minutes.

With the sadness gone, I have rediscovered the joy that comes from everyday activities! I feel like I have gotten my life back and I am looking forward to what's ahead. I'm truly grateful for this amazing product. It is going to help so many people. Thank you!

* * *

I also have a *very* impressive story about how Pure Body helped an autistic boy start to recover; it's too long to include here but it's well worth a read. Click on the Touchstone Essentials section on my website and scroll through the articles; it's called 'Can Pure Body Help an Autistic Child?'

Pure Body by Touchstone is the *only* brand that I trust and have had the best personal experience with. I take it every day, and Lola is taking them, as well as many of my friends and family. There are tens of thousands of chemicals all around us, and it's so important to try and protect yourself from as many as possible. It's the most important supplement any person can take because if you don't keep heavy metals and other chemicals to a minimum in your body, then it is going to struggle to be healthy long term.

I also think that for people who have a limited budget and can't do much with changing their diets, beauty products or their environment at home, then by using Pure Body in their day-to-day life, they will be able to at least keep the toxic burden to a minimum.

Touchstone Essentials recently released a new 'Extra Strength Pure Body' which is in a spray bottle and is a colloidal solution. Instead of adding to drinking water, you spray it directly in the mouth. The results that people are having with this are absolutely amazing. The colloidal suspension is allowing the zeolite to reach very deeply into the body and from personal experience it's absolutely incredible. It is *750 times* more powerful than regular strength. It also has an ability to travel to different areas of the body, so using both regular strength and extra strength can give you exceptional results.

I tried it myself as I was sending my book to the publishers, and it was more powerful than I gave it credit for. The detox was very intense and I had to drink lots more water, and take it easy, but how I felt afterwards was absolutely incredible. If anyone thinks that zeolites are rubbish, they only have to take the Extra Strength and see what it does. It actually affected me within minutes of having a few sprays. I think this particular product is going to be huge in the health world because it really does work very powerfully and is 100% safe.

✓ The company's website is touchstoneessentials.com and you can also find more information about them on my website missecoglam.com

No one is in control of your happiness but you; therefore, you have the power to change anything about yourself or your life that you want to change.
~ Barbara DeAngelis

PART 2

THE PATH TO HEALTH AND HAPPINESS
– WHY IT MAY BE MUCH EASIER THAN
YOU THINK

Chapter 14

Why *Do* So Many People Struggle with Happiness?

There are many reasons why people struggle with happiness, but as you already know by now, I feel *very strongly* that it comes down to toxic overload in the body and, more detrimentally, the brain. Mercury, and other toxins such as lead, *directly* affect the way it functions, and it's never in a positive way either – it's *always* damaging. As we covered in Chapters 1 and 3, lead is a neurotoxin and is found in huge amounts in the environment. Mercury is in all of us too, as well as arsenic, cadmium and aluminum – to name but a few toxins. *All* of these metals have a harmful effect on brain function.

I have heard many stories about how, once people remove these and other toxins, they completely change, for the better, in person-ality and brain function. I know this from my own personal experience: having once being labeled a 'crazy' person (by myself and many others), I am now much calmer and find myself being very happy most of the time, whereas it used to be the exact opposite. I was always *very* unstable and rarely happy. To see this big switch in myself, after I had removed most of the heavy metals from my system, shows me a lot of proof that people who struggle with happiness, and have abnormal mood swings and anger problems, are more than likely being affected by these and many other types of toxins.

I also believe that unhappiness comes from being deficient in certain nutrients and deficient in healthy exposure to the sun.

Also, we now have a society which has conditioned us to compare ourselves with the 'rich and famous' who *seem* to have it all. We watch all the glamorous shows on TV and read about the stars in magazines – where people are now famous just because they are attractive and wealthy. Yet it's very rare that they report that they too can struggle with unhappiness at times and that money truly can't buy love. But if people look deeper into the lives of many of those in Hollywood, there are many stories of drug addictions and eventual suicides. Not to mention the huge rate of divorce that affects 'beautiful people'.

I also believe – and will be discussing this in much greater detail later on in Part 3, 'Rethinking the Way We Parent' – that we are creating desperately unhappy adults, mainly because of the way they were brought up. We need to completely take a look at the messages we give our children, and to make more of an effort to really bond with them from birth and to continue that bond well into later life. If as a society we were bringing up children in the way that we are meant to, then the rates of depression would not be as high. Something is missing in many adults today: they see themselves in such a poor light and view their place in the world as unimportant or worthless, only to go on living a life of deep unhappiness.

I think people have also lost the ability to connect with themselves, and are constantly unsure of why they are here and what they are meant to do with their lives. A lack of not knowing their own talents (of which we all have at least one, by the way) makes people lack true happiness. Over this next section of the book I will give you some tips to help you find your path to happiness.

Chapter 15

Happiness *Doesn't* Come in a Pill – The Real Dangers of Psychiatric Drugs

When you start looking at the brain, your treatment protocols radically change. We were taught to use certain anti-anxiety medications like Valium and Xanax, but as soon as I started scanning people, I stopped using them because I saw that Valium and Xanax and medications like that, pretty much work like alcohol in the brain, and over time they cause suppression of brain activity and I would go 'I am making people worse!'. If you don't look at the brain – you have no accountability for making your patients worse. Psychiatry is broken. Psychiatrists make more money if they see 4 people in an hour, so it's become 4, 6 people in an hour, here is the medicine, what are your side effects, does it work, let's try this, OK, I will see you back for $175 for 15 minutes, in a month. It's crazy, it's just a total, crazy mess. In order to really make a proper diagnosis, you need to understand their biology and their psychology, how they get along with other people, what's the social situation, what are their spiritual beliefs, not necessarily religious, but why do they care, what does their life mean, and when you treat them again, do it in a biological, psychological, social, spiritual way. 85% of psychiatric medications are prescribed by non-psychiatric physicians, your family doctor or your OBGYN or your internees, and I actually think they don't do a very good job. And the problem with medicine is we make symptoms, e.g. depression, as a diagnosis... and when you do that with depression, you dishonor it because depression is a symptom. It's got many causes and you end up giving a 'one treatment fits everybody' approach and it's really no better than a placebo. That's what we do in psychiatry and it hurts people.[74]

Dr. Daniel Amen, author, speaker and founder of the Amen Clinics

This is a very serious chapter so it's going to be a fairly long one as it's quite close to my heart. I feel an urgency to tell as many people as I can about this subject as far too many people are affected by the very real dangers of psychiatric drugs. For about 10 years, I took many different types of antidepressants and also other types of prescribed pharmaceutical drugs. After this fairly long experience, I now have no doubt that they only made my problems worse, and not any better at all, and I fear (as well as have some proof) that it is the same for literally millions of people all over the world.

I remember when I was first diagnosed with a 'mental condition', and that it gave me a big sense of *relief*. Finally someone could help me! Now that I had a real 'problem' which was described in one of the big medical books, surely I was going to get better and start to feel great? All of my worries and anxiety would now disappear?

Back then, I had *no* idea what I was *really* getting myself into, that I would begin a journey of taking many different types of powerful drugs, risking my life (from a possible suicide that could finally happen) and that the day I actually wanted to get off them would begin *another* nightmare because I would be so physically addicted to them that the withdrawals and sickness would be ten times worse than the condition they were prescribed for in the first place.

It's hard for me to remember those times now, as I have healed myself of that depression, but I was actually one of those people who had many deep problems and everyone close to me knew it. I was always crying, always angry (sometimes even becoming quite psychotic) and had many arguments with pretty much everyone I knew. I just had a life of pure chaos. And the most disturbing thing was, I had a deep hatred for myself that caused me to do many erratic things. I had a habit of self-harming when I got upset, and still bear some scars on my legs today that are a reminder of how low I used to get. I was a pretty bad case of being mentally unstable – someone that the mainstream suggested would never get better and would always need prescribed antidepressants and other medications. I believed that 'life sentence' for a long time too.

What I remember the most, and is the main reason why this chapter is so important for me to have in this book, is how *easy* it was to get a diagnosis and how *easy* it was to walk away with a prescription for a very powerful psychiatric drug. And what was even more shocking was that the doctors whom I would see would never ever tell me about the extremely difficult reactions I would have once I decided to try and get off these drugs. No one told me that *50% of all suicides* actually occurred in people who were on antidepressant medications at the time when they killed themselves.

What I have come to learn only recently is that most mass murderers were on psychotropic drugs when they committed their terrible crimes. Jeffrey Dalmer, infamous for killing 17 people, was said to be on tranquilizers and antidepressants, John Hinkley who tried to assassinate then President Ronald Reagan was on Valium, and in 2001 Andrea Yates was found guilty of drowning her five children while being on Effexor *and* Remeron. Every day, there are cases of seemingly *normal* people doing horrific things which most of the time will involve their wife, or husband, themselves and their children. Total lapses of sanity can turn into the most violent outbursts ending in tragedy. Many doctor's and educated professionals are now questioning whether these medications do more harm than good.

> I have to say, whenever I read in the newspaper of some violent act, one of the first questions I ask is 'Was the person on medications?'
> John Sommers-Flanagan, Professor of Counselor Ed., University of Montana

In the last 15 years, there has been an increase in children and teenagers committing acts of terror, usually at their school, as in the case of the Columbine High School massacre. One day in late April 1999, two students, Eric Harris and Dylan Klebold, shot 12 students dead and also killed one teacher. At the time of these murders, Eric had been seeing a psychiatrist and had complained of anger and depression, and was having suicidal thoughts. He was prescribed Zoloft (a very popular drug and one that is also linked to many other murders/suicides) but came off it as he stated that he felt unable to sleep and could not concentrate at school. Eric was then given the drug Luvox at the beginning of April.[75] Side effects of this particular drug included: loss of remorse, depersonalization, and increased aggression; it has also been found to make the patient 8.4 *times* more likely to commit violent acts than other types of medications.

And just recently Adam Lanza, who killed 26 people including 20 children in the town of Newport, USA, was allegedly on Fanapt, which is an anti-psychotic drug. Fanapt has a very shaky history of its own. It was originally given a 'non-approval' stamp for failing to be deemed as safe. It was found to cause severe heart problems in enough patients for it to not be passed by the FDA. And knowing what I know about how easy it normally is to get drugs approved these days, it sounds like Fanapt should *never* ever have been allowed on the market. Have a read below about what the side effects are:

Psychiatric side effects including restlessness, aggression, and delusion have been reported frequently. Hostility, decreased libido, paranoia, anorgasmia, confusional state, mania, catatonia, mood swings, panic attack, obsessive-compulsive disorder, bulimia nervosa, delirium, polydipsia psychogenic, impulse-control disorder, and major depression have been reported infrequently.
(Source: Drugs.com – side effects of the drug Fanapt)

For someone that just went to their school and opened fire on classmates, small children and teachers, with the premeditated intent to kill, don't the above side effects of 'loss of remorse, increased aggression and depersonalization' describe *exactly* what would be behind most people's behavior when carrying out these horrific acts?

What is really worrying is that among the side effects of these medications, this risk is actually there for all to see, if they only ever bothered to *look*, or their doctors were *made* (by law!) to warn you about them. Ironic, isn't it, or really *sick*, isn't it? If you were suffering from depression, and went to see the doctor *because* you were feeling suicidal, you would want to take something that would *stop* you from feeling worse so that you would *not* commit suicide, right? Well, sadly, these drugs have been known to 'increase the risk of death' or to 'increase the risk of violence', so much so, that these warnings are listed on the product inserts.

And what people do not realize is that when they are on these medications and decide to come off them, it may be the most *difficult and dangerous* thing they will ever have to go through. If you do it 'cold turkey', it could actually lead to your suicide or to acts of murder.

In May 2012, Felicia Boots killed her two children, Mason (9 weeks old) and Lily Skye, 14 weeks after stopping her antidepressant medication that she was taking for post-natal depression.[76] She wanted to breastfeed Mason but was concerned about what the drug would do to him, so she went off the medication 'cold turkey', and suffered increasing levels of paranoia which led to her strangling her children. She then tried to take her own life and left disturbing notes by her children's bodies. Now she says she does not know why she did it and has been in a psychiatric hospital ever since. A truly sad story and one that, unfortunately, is not rare.

Looking back, I would say that 90% of my lowest times, when I was self-harming, wanting to commit suicide and was at my most unstable, I too was on antidepressants. So YES, they certainly do increase the risk of suicide – take it from me, I know! And there's overwhelming evidence that proves taking them *does* increase the risk of suicide, ending in tragedy for many a family. Barry Grove author of *Trick And Treat* writes:

Dr Andrew Mosholder, an expert with America's Food and Drug Administration, reviewed 24 studies involving 4,582 patients taking one of 9 different antidepressants. They showed the drugs nearly doubled the risk of suicide among children and young adults. The FDA barred him from publishing his findings, but they were leaked to the press in 2004. In 2006, Mosholder's study was published. It makes for extremely worrying reading. More worrying, perhaps is that the FDA's principal role is guardian of public safety, yet it suppressed evidence for two years. How many children in that time took their own lives?

I also contemplated recently, that over the 10 years of taking both recreational drugs *and* pharmaceutical ones, the only drugs that I ever became addicted to were the *pharmaceutical* ones. After developing insomnia, I became addicted to sleeping pills and was also very much addicted to my antidepressants; I could not come off them very easily at all. In fact, it took me several attempts over 4 years, and I needed an entire 6-month period of not working, to finally be free of them. I even had a few side effects that lasted for a whole year after I stopped taking the last pill. I had to become unemployed on purpose, and literally needed to sleep the effects off, because getting out and about in public was so horrible – I felt confused, had weird tingly skin sensations, and was even more teary, angry and sad.

Due to this experience, which I call 'my own private hell', I have no qualms in understanding how some people who were either starting new medications, trying to get off old ones or were regularly on a combination of medications, ended up committing these horrible crimes. These drugs simply can overtake your mind and make you do things that are seemingly out of your control. And when I dug deeper into this subject, I found there were also countless cases of seemingly normal people who were going through a bit of a dark period in their life, who went on these types of drugs and had such a bad reaction that they would end up either killing their entire family and/or themselves.

Now, surely, with this knowledge, with this proof, alarm bells should be ringing in all of our ears? Sadly, hardly anyone is hearing them. In the USA today, a whopping number of people – over 100,000,000 people a day – are on psychotropic medications, with that number growing stronger at a super-fast rate. This statistic shows that in the US, for every three people, *one* of those is on these types of drugs. Back in 2009, the top 25 psychiatric drugs were prescribed through 300 million prescriptions just for that year alone.[77]

Now, I can't and won't say that no one has ever received some benefit from taking antidepressants or other psychiatric drugs. Many people swear that they did save their lives. I have a friend who said that they helped her immensely when her life was going through tough times, and for a short period while she was on them she was able to get her life back together. But could it be simply down to the placebo effect? In Februrary 2012, CBS's 60 Minutes aired a show on antidepressants being no better than a placebo. Irving Kirsch who is an author and Harvard Researcher said that these medications do not work because of the ingredients, nor do they have any effect on serotonin but because those that take them, *believe* they will get better if they take them.

Serotonin is said to be found in low levels in a depressed brain, hence why drugs called SSRI's (Selective Serotonin Reuptake Inhibitors) are prescribed. But is this theory even proven? In the groundbreaking book, *Anatomy of An Epidemic - Magic Bullets, Psychiatric Drugs, and the Astonishing Rise of Mental Illness in America*, author Robert Whitaker wrote about the commercial success of Prozac which was not backed up by any solid evidence that it actually worked.

Stanford University Psychiatrist, Dr David Burns, said in 2003:

I spent the first several years of my career doing full-time research on brain serotonin metabolism but I never saw any convincing evidence that any psychiatric disorder, including depression, results from a deficiency of brain serotonin.

And he isn't alone in this way of thinking. Colin Ross, an associate professor of psychiatry at Southwest Medical Centre in Dallas wrote in his book, *Pseudoscience in Biological Psychiatry:*

There is no scientific evidence whatsoever that clinical depression is due to any kind of biological deficit state."

So if this is true and serotonin *doesn't* play a role in causing depression or help in treating it, then *what* are those 'seratonin increasing' drugs *really* doing to our brains?

In the cases of severe bipolar disorder and schizophrenia, some people may need certain medications, as they could end up hurting themselves or others.

But, what is unknown, is what happens to these patients if they were to try detoxing, better diet, or other types of supplements first, which are known for helping brain health? I wonder if they would have had an even speedier recovery trying other things first. Dr. Daniel Amen of the Amen Clinics is a world-renowned psychiatrist and leading the way in incorporating a holistic approach to treating brain disorders, with great success.

✓ amenclinics.com

And, it's also not widely known but sexual and physical abuse has been noted in large numbers of people diagnosed with schizophrenia, which should shatter the myth that severe mental disorderes such as these, are 'in the genes'. Oliver James, author of *They F**K You Up* writes that it may even be down to parenting in most cases:

A remarkable amount of new scientific evidence that strongly bears out the argument of this book has been published in the five years since the first edition in 2002, requiring a second one. In just that short period, the main proponents of 'genes for' mental illnesses like schizophrenia or depression have wholly recanted their former position. Having pored through the genes identified by the Human Genome Project they have been forced to admit that it is extremely unlikely that there are any single genes for any mental illnesses. The new position is that it must be a question of clusters of genes. We shall see, but thus far there is little evidence for this theory. Meanwhile, the overarching importance of parental care continues to find confirmation. One of the most convincing demonstrations is studies of its effect on patterns of brain electricity and chemistry, and even, on the very size of the different bits of brain. For instance, it is becoming increasingly clear that subsequent good experiences, like therapy, can reset the levels to healthier ones and that bad ones do the opposite. One of the most significant scientific events of the century so far occurred this year when a whole volume of a highly respected psychiatric journal was devoted to the overwhelming evidence that schizophrenia is often caused by sexual and physical abuse. At least half of the people given that diagnosis suffered from this experience.

Pretty shocking, right? I certainly thought that this type of severe mental illness was something people were 'just born with', but now after looking into the effects toxins have on the brain and also the effects traumatic or unhappy childhoods can have on the brain, leads me to a new conclusion and that is: there is *lots* that can be done to help people with mental illness, and it might not come in a prescribed pill.

How do people get tested for diagnosis?

Before the introduction of Prozac in Dec. 1987, less than one percent of the population in the U.S. was diagnosed with bipolar disorder – also known as manic depression. Now, with the widespread prescribing of antidepressants, the percent of the population in the United States that is diagnosed with bipolar disorder (a swing from depression to mania or vice versa) has risen to 4.4%. This is almost one out of every 23 people in the U.S.[78]

When we speak of someone being depressed, we tend to hear people, as well as the doctors, say, 'Oh, they have a chemical imbalance.' Yet would you be shocked to know that there is no *blood test* or any other form of physical test that can find out if there truly is a chemical imbalance, and that it's *impossible* to actually test what is a 'normal' chemical balance in a happy and healthy person?

How people get diagnosed and then prescribed these at times, *very* strong drugs is purely from questions and surveys. Then, after the questions have been answered, the doctors tally up the scores and consult their 'psychiatric bible', the Diagnostic and Statistical Manual of Mental Disorders, otherwise known as the DSM, which is where the diagnoses come from, and how a billing code is created for the doctors to receive their payments. I know this because I have gone through the standard practice myself a few times and it's exactly how these diagnoses are carried out in every doctor's, psychologist's and psychiatrist's office today.

The DSM used to be a very small booklet; now it's a *massive* book, so heavy in fact that its difficult to carry and has a staggering 886 pages (being added to every year by the way) which lists at the time of writing, approximately 374 disorders, some of which sound absolutely ridiculous, I must add. Did you know that if you 'suffer' from shyness, you can be labeled with the diagnosis of 'social anxiety disorder' (SAD)? The questions to find out if you are suffering from SAD go like this: 'Do you feel nervous going to speak to your boss?' 'Do you feel nervous speaking in front of a crowd?' 'Um… yes to both' – that's what I would answer, as would millions of others, but does that warrant us being given a mental diagnosis for it or to be prescribed psychotropic drugs? NO!

Luckily, some of these psychiatrists have come forward, expressing their own concern at what is being added to this already enormous medical book. According to Natural News.com:

> Allen Frances chaired the DSM-IV that was released in 1994. He now admits it was a huge mistake that has resulted in the mass over diagnosis of people who are actually quite normal. The DSM-IV 'inadvertently contributed to three false epidemics – attention deficit disorder, autism and childhood bipolar disorder,' writes Allen in an LA Times Opinion Piece.[79]

So there we have it: someone who used to be responsible for what gets added to these psychiatric bibles, admitting that what they did, by adding new mental disorders, was in fact very wrong.

What could long term use of antidepressants do to your health?

If it wasn't scary enough knowing that antidepressants can increase the risk of suicides and provoke violent behavior, its even more alarming to know what the *long term* use of them can do to other areas of your health. According to Joseph Mercola from mercola.com the following effects and outcomes has been found:

- Diabetes: Your risk for type 2 diabetes is two to three times higher if you take antidepressants, according to one study.
- Problems with your immune system: SSRIs cause serotonin to remain in your nerve junctions longer, interfering with immune cell signaling and T-cell growth
- Stillbirths: A Canadian study of almost 5,000 mothers found that women on SSRIs were twice as likely to have a stillbirth, and almost twice as likely to have a premature or low birth weight baby; another study showed a 40 percent increased risk for birth defects, such as cleft palate.

- Brittle bones: One study showed women on antidepressants have a 30 percent higher risk of spinal fracture and a 20 percent higher risk for all other fractures.
- Stroke: Your risk for stroke may be 45 percent higher if you are on antidepressants, possibly related to how the drugs affect blood clotting.
- Death: Overall death rates have been found to be 32 percent higher in women on antidepressants.

Many of the drugs prescribed for psychiatric conditions can give the patient a variety of intensive side effects. A drug by the name of Abilify, which is used for the treatment of schizophrenia, bipolar disorder, autism and serious depression, has been found to have a whopping, 75 *different side effects,* including coma *and* death. With so many side effects linked to this drug, if you were to take it, you are pretty much *guaranteed* to have quite a few of them. Pretty frightening indeed.

The multibillion-dollar industry making money out of madness

When you look at the amounts of money these drug manufacturers are making, it's easy to see that they literally are making *huge* amounts of cash out of people feeling unbalanced and unhappy. And when you realise that drug companies are listed on the stock exchange, then they *have* to improve their profits, year after year - they 'owe' that to their shareholders. With this in mind, do you think that certain people and corporations, would actually *want* to end mental illness for good? And what I want to drive home here is, if there is *no effective testing* for a chemical imbalance, then *why* the hell are we thinking it's OK taking drugs that are powerfully and, more often than not, negatively affecting the chemicals in our brains? It really does *not* make sense, not one bit, to be trusting these types of medications after a diagnosis based quite often on silly questions!

What really makes my skin crawl with worry is what is happening to children in regards to psychiatric drugs. Are they being diagnosed too fast? Yes, it seems that way.[80] In America, *1 in 10 children* are diagnosed with ADHD (attention deficit hyperactivity disorder), ADD (attention deficit disorder), depression or anxiety. Children are becoming psychiatric patients at ages as young as 4. It is said that up to *8 million children* are taking medications for these disorders.

What is very *worrying* is the side effects of these drugs, which often affect anyone that takes them, are even more concerning in regards to children. Now can we see why shootings are becoming more common with younger people involved?

How long are these drugs tested on – for years, surely?

The answer to this is going to alarm you. The period of clinical tests which are carried out on these types of medications ranges from 4 to 8 weeks. *That is all.* The pharmaceutical companies then pay loads of money to 'fast track' them to be approved. And coming from me, who has been on many types of antidepressants, this time period is *horrifically* too short to test the drug for its safety and efficiency. It's actually quite disgraceful.

When a drug is fast-tracked, it opens the situation into a much bigger problem. If these new drugs haven't had enough scrutiny over the way they were studied in the first place (not forgetting how much corruption there is in the pharmaceutical world and that the FDA are not in control of Big Pharma as we think – it's more the other way around), then harmful drugs will be on the market and people will actually lose their lives. It is said that more than 40 people a day, across the USA, die from prescription pain medication overdoses, while more and more doctors are getting huge payouts from the drug companies to promote these medications. In the past 10 years alone, USA spending on prescription drugs rose *475%*.[81]

According to Business Highbeam.com:

> Healthcare professionals freely admit that medication trials have narrow inclusion and exclusion criteria, resulting in a greater likelihood of product success and thereby limiting the relevance of such trials. When it comes to psychotropic medication, a new study confirms that antidepressants are tested on only a narrow band of depressed patients but prescribed to a wide range of people.[82]

Why are we letting ourselves take these kinds of hardcore drugs that have only been tested for, at the very best, 2 months? Surely they should be tested over years and years so that we can be certain they really are safe? The problem is, the majority of people are just not aware. I recently asked some people how long they think testing should be carried out for if they were to take any type of drug. They all answered, 'Years'. When I told them it was just weeks, they looked horrified.

You would also think that the studies should continue afterwards for a long time to really see if people's lives actually dramatically improved, wouldn't you? The answer is sadly no again. When you look at how much money a drug company makes when it has a new drug on the market, it's in their interest to get it out there as soon as possible, and what is happening in the industry is that new drugs are being released onto the market which are actually no better than other drugs already prescribed yet are often touted as more effective. When you research into how drugs get passed so easily, how the studies get funded, it is very hard to trust any type of drug, especially the ones produced in the last 10 years.

We have the FDA in place to help us, but do they really? Are they *really* protecting us from dangerous foods and dangerous medications? It seems no and it may have been like this for decades:

The thing that bugs me is that people think the Food & Drug Administration is protecting them - it isn't. What the FDA is doing and what the pubic thinks it's doing are as different as night and day

Dr Herbert L. Ley Former FDA Commissioner 1969

Pharmaceutical ethics (the rampant lack of them) is a *huge* subject and of course, I can't cover as much as I'd like to. If you are interested in learning more about these types of practices that are happening at an alarming rate in the pharmaceutical world, I urge you to read the book *Bad Pharma: How Drug Companies Mislead Doctors and Harm Patients* by Ben Goldacre. One of the most shocking books I have read about the pharmaceutical industry. Ben is a doctor and science journalist and has a very popular column in the *Guardian* newspaper. I don't usually agree with all of his work but this book, in most regards certainly, is outstanding. Every single doctor, healthcare worker and scientist should read his book.

Another eye opening book is by Marcia Angell, MD, author of the New York Times Business Bestseller novel, '*The Truth About The Drug Companies - How They Deceive Us And What To Do About It*'. Marcia was employed for over 20 years at the New England Journal of Medicine where she saw firsthand, blatant corruption of the medical industry. With all of the court cases against many of our most famous drug companies, and the huge payouts they are ordered to make, it seems that it's actually happening throughout the industry and is a lot more than just a 'once off.' Because of this, I don't automatically trust many drug makers anymore, and you probably shouldn't either.

It's completely normal to feel ups and downs!

What is also highly worrying is the *types* of questions on these surveys (if you like, take one of them online so you can see what I mean – just google 'mental illness test'). Seemingly harmless enough, most of these questions describe normal life, which has ups and downs and highs and lows. It's normal to feel sad sometimes, and it's normal to get bursts of energy and feel very happy. Yes, there is a problem when it's so extreme it's causing your life to be an absolute misery (remember, this could be related to toxicity in the brain) but for most people who are going through a 'rough patch', they don't need to be given a label and a box of pills that are more than likely going to a) not solve the problem – the root cause, b) cause them to feel worse, c) possibly make them become addicted to the pills, and d) increase their risk of becoming violent or harming themselves.

I did a test for this book, from this website:

✓ gotoquiz.com/results/what_mental_disorder_do_you_have

And it's so true! These tests are just rubbish – the questions are so sneaky! Basically this test will give *anyone* a diagnosis because none of the answers were able to make you seem 'normal'. Even ticking 'False' as an answer was not a positive in the test's eyes (e.g. it asks you if you don't fear things and when you say no, not being fearful is *not* seen as a good thing). This test diagnosed me as having ALL of these conditions: OCD, manic depression, generalized anxiety disorder and paranoia! And the questions I answered were just normal everyday things, which I didn't find affected me, so I answered 'False' as in 'Nope, that does not apply to me'. I played around with answering different questions, and they all gave me a diagnosis. If you can, go over to the website and have a play around yourself and see what diagnoses they give you. Just don't take them too seriously.

Now, I *was* very mentally unwell years ago, and for a very long time so I do know what it's like to think certain ways and to show behavior that is not particularly 'normal'. But now? Do I really feel that I fit any of those diagnoses and need regular doses of medication? Definitely not! I am able to function very well every day, do not have extreme highs and lows anymore, and I have not had any sort of breakdown for years and years. This test would be almost laughable if it wasn't so serious. Can you imagine how many people do these sorts of tests, answer the questions as truthfully as they can, and end up getting all of these sorts of diagnoses? Then, because they are so scared, they will take themselves to a doctor and say, 'I did a test and it says I am this or that.' Then the doctor asks them the same sorts of standard questions again, and then they are told 'Yes, it's true! You do have this disorder or that disorder and need this medication.' A simple online test has now made you a potential lifelong customer of Big Pharma. And in the USA, these tests are being given to high-school students who may not even feel depressed. Yet after they take one these tests, which are very sneaky, using the same 'no answer is the right answer' questions, every single teenager will more than likely walk away with a new diagnosis.

To improve mental health, what people generally need to do is to *remove* heavy metals, as these 100% certainly affect the way the brain behaves and therefore how someone acts. People also need to start to eat better, cut back on sugar and chemical-based foods, stop drinking alcohol, incorporate more exercise, get more sun, check your hormone levels and get some counseling to learn to *deal* with the problems that they may have had stemming from childhood or due to something happening recently to them.

Lots of people have developed a brain/stress-related mental condition due to being extremely unhappy in their childhoods. This is something I will be writing about in another book one day, because it too is also an epidemic in our society. Many people with chronic fatigue report similar stressful childhoods where they were constantly upset, crying and just felt very lonely. The intense and ongoing stress from feeling sad, unloved, lonely, being angry and upset, affected them not only mentally, but physically too.

However, it has to be said, that there *are* some very *extreme* mental conditions out there and I am certainly not qualified to give you advice here about how to treat those, but I would definitely love for there to be a study undertaken with the types of patients who use chelation therapy or something such as zeolites first, to see if they have high levels of heavy metals such as lead or mercury in their brains, and what happens to their behavior after these types of treatments are carried out. I believe there also is a lot left to be discovered about the effects on the brain from what happens in utero to an undeveloped fetus from toxic exposure.

Before I detoxed my toxins out of my system, I was *extremely* paranoid, someone who worried about anything and everything 24/7, and at times had some mild to more extreme psychotic episodes. If I got into an argument with someone, it would quite often get out of control where I would physically lash out and say some absolutely horrible things, and it would be like someone else was actually in my body making me do these things. Then when it was over, I would forget what I had actually said and done to the person involved. This sort of behavior made me feel very unstable, and fearful of who I was and what I was capable of doing. I welcomed the 'help' from the doctors and was relieved to be taking medication for it. What scared me, though, was that I was always told, 'You will never recover from this. You will just have to learn to deal with it because there is no cure for your type of depression' and 'You will have to take this medication for life.'

Well, let me tell you this: that is absolute *rubbish*. I am here, today, to prove that is *not* true – you *can* recover, and without toxic medication, even from extreme suicidal depression. I have a very healthy and happy baby girl and a life that mirrors my now much more positive and happier demeanor. I am often told by many people how calming I am to be around and that they cannot imagine me as someone who was once called 'crazy'.

Now, that's not to say that I don't have periods of being in a bit of a bad mood or feeling a little down. But they last for only a day at most, or hours, instead of for 29 whole days out of each month. And I know now that to have these ups and downs is *completely normal* and I think that our obsession with having to be blissfully happy each day is another sign of how unhealthy our society has become. We have been led to believe that unless we are ecstatically happy all the time (although ironically even if we *were* happy all the time there is a psychiatric diagnosis for that too!) then there is something wrong with us and we will need to see a doctor to find out what we have and we will also need to take some sort of medication for it. I can now also see if something I ate, for example, something really sugary or high in chocolate, was what made me have a down day the next day.

Years ago, I always thought that the tiny little pill that I was given was going to sort my problems out, and I made no effort to look at my lifestyle, how I was eating, or to understand toxic exposure, to realize that I was actually only *adding* to the many health problems I had. I had no idea that it would be impossible for me to be on prescription medication and to suddenly become healthy, fit and happy. After being on many different types of psychiatric drugs over a 10-year period, I eventually realized that they weren't helping at all – I was still in just the same mess – and that I wanted to get off them and find another way.

Depression and Diet

I recently asked a family friend who is a psychiatrist, if she was able to advise her patients on the type of diet they ate. I was shocked at her answer. It was no! Some psychiatrists, depending on where they work are sometimes *not* allowed by the medical authorities to discuss diet and lifestyle with their patients. Nor do they get much training at medical school about the effects diet has on mental states. It's absolutely shocking and so very wrong, that doctors who are in charge of people's brain health, are not allowed to tell their patients what better ways they could eat for the sake of their moods. According to Barry Grove, author of *Trick And Treat*, sugar and certain carbohydrates are the *worst* things for depressed people to eat:

Are you feeling tired or depressed? You've all seen the adverts on TV for pick-me-ups, perhaps in the late afternoon: eat a biscuit, chocolate bar or other source of sugar. These advertisements rely on people's belief that a resulting rush of sugar into the bloodstream will give them a mental boost, that it will make them feel good and more alert. There have been many studies of the effects of these different meal patterns and different foods. Some tested and measured subjective things such as fatigue, vigour, anger, hostility, confusions, anxiety, and depression. In all of these tests, those who ate carbohydrate-based meals reported worse scores in all classes except anxiety, where there was no difference. In other, objective tests of alertness, auditory and visual reaction times, and vigilance, carbohydrate eaters again came off worse.

There is certainly evidence that eating sugar or other carbohydrate foods has the ability to improve your mood. The role that glucose is known to play in supplying the cells of the body with energy has led to the assumption that an enhanced source of metabolic energy is associated with feeling subjectively more alert and energetic. But in fact, much of the evidence is that consuming carbohydrate has a hypnotic effect. In other words, it makes you feel good by making you more relaxed and sleepy, rather than more alert. This is the reason why many dieticians recommend a carbohydrate meal in the evening – it helps you to sleep. But with depression, if you are tired, you really don't feel like dong anything it's an effort to get up, work, play, interact with people, get meals, and so on. And under these conditions, carbohydrates meals have exactly the opposite effect from what you might expect. They make you relaxed and slow your reaction times; protein/fat meals make you feel awake, bright, alert and quick–thinking and crucially, lift depression.

Coconut oil can be exceptionally good at helping those with depression. Whilst we've been told for years that too much fat is bad for you, the *right* kinds of fats do so much good for the body and brain that they are vital to health and wellbeing.

Authors Dr Mary Enig and Sally Fallon wrote about this in their book *Eat Fat, Lose Fat:*

> We know, you've heard that saturated fats are unhealthy. Who hasn't? Read on and you'll be surprised to learn about research published during the last 20 years in respected scientific and medical journals, like The Journal of Lipid Research, Reviews in Pure and Applied Pharmacological Science, and The American Journal of Clinical Nutrition, that shows that just the opposite is true. Your body needs not only fats, but saturated fats, to nourish your brain, heart, nerves, hormones and every single cell. Saturated fats form a key part of the cell membranes throughout your body. When you eat too many unsaturated fats, the kind found in polyunsaturated vegetable oils, these fats adversely affect the chemistry of those membranes.

So if you are someone that has been following a 'low fat' diet because you have been told this is healthy then it may have been doing you more harm than good. If you are feeling depressed, you may actually have a poor functioning thyroid (triggered by stress, drinking fluro-dated water, certain toxins, medications or poor diet) which could be over looked by most doctors.

Anji Sandage who wrote the *Everything Coconut Diet Cook Book* explains:

> 10 percent of Americans most likely have an undiagnosed thyroid disorder. If you are experiencing unexplained weight gain, fatigue, hair loss, insominia, depression and anxiety, you could have an undiagnosed thyroid disorder. Thyroid disorders can lead to serious problems, but very often the doctor will tell you to get more sleep and put you on antidepressants because your

basic thyroid hormone levels came back within the normal range. Often thyroid disorders get overlooked because without the proper testing, they can be hard to detect. If you suspect that you have a thyroid disorder, and you don't get a diagnosis because your doctor didn't order a full thyroid panel, you should get a second opinion. Adding coconut oil to your daily routine can also have a positive effect on the thyroid and can even reduce, or eliminate hypothyroidism.

Thyroid problems are at epidemic proportions, and the medications typically prescribed for it aren't exactly nice on your body. Side effects include heart palpiations, nervousness, insomnia, shaking, frequent bowel movements, too much weight loss, discomfort in warm weather, bone thinning and you may even increase your risk of a heart attack. And you may also need to be on this medication for life, increasing your dose as you age. I would suggest to everyone, to take coconut oil regularly, unless you are one of the very small few who are allergic to it, but generally it seems to suit everyone. I take 6 virgin coconut oil tablets each day and have noticed an increase in my energy, my mood and general wellbeing. It is amazing stuff.

If you have mood swings, it is recommended you take a very close look at the foods you are eating and try and take notice as to how you feel after eating them. Maybe even write a diary of what you have been eating, how they make you feel etc. Then once you have figured out what triggers bad or low moods, try and introduce foods that don't cause such dramatic fluctuations in your mood. Best to stay right away from sugary things and from Hi Glycemic Index foods that can increase your blood sugar levels too quickly.

Some books you might like to read to help you with diet in relation to treating depression, anxiety and other mental disorders diet are: *Potatoes Not Prozac: How to Control Depression, Food Cravings and Weight Gain*

Kathleen Desmaisons
What Your Psychologist Hasn't Told You About Anxiety & Depression
Cynthia Perkins, M. Ed.
*Gut and Psychology Syndrome: Natural Treatment for Autism,
ADD/ADHD, Dyslexia, Dyspraxia, Depression, Schizophrenia*
Dr Natasha Campbell-McBride

If you are struggling with depression then there are many things you can do to help yourself recover without resorting to pharmaceuticals. But if things get so bad that none of this stuff helps, then of course, see your doctor, and try and choose one that looks at your entire lifestyle.

Dr. Daniel Amen, whom I mentioned before, is a wonderful psychiatrist who has written many insightful and groundbreaking books on brain health. Seek out some of them and try and find a doctor who has had training with him or follows his protocol. If you live in America and can go and visit one of his clinics, I can assure you it will be well worth the effort. No one understands brain health like Dr Amen.

✓ amenclinics.com

To read more stories on how SSRI drugs have affected people's lives – cases which ended up in either newspapers or medical journals – please visit this website: ssristories.com where there are over *4800* stories which have been in the mainstream media linking suicides and murders to certain psychiatric drugs.

If you have had an adverse reaction yourself to a certain drug, you can visit this following website and report it. You can also do some research into prescription drugs you are curious about or have been suggested to try at:

✓ rxisk.org

Chapter 16

Why Sun Exposure is Essential for Happiness

It's a well-documented fact that sunlight is necessary for human survival, but we've been brainwashed into thinking that any exposure to sunlight is bad. This is both unfortunate and untrue. There really is no substantiated and scientific evidence to suggest that moderate sun exposure significantly increases risks of benign cancers or, more importantly, the most deadly form of skin cancers, melanoma.

Dr. Andrew Weil, Foreword written for Dr. M. Holick's book *The Vitamin D Solution*[83]

Now I want to share with you what can be done to restore the body's ability to heal and to help you feel naturally good and truly balanced. The powerful healing effects from the sun is where I want to start.

Have we been lied to about the sun? Yes, it appears that way – although severely *misinformed* is a better way of terming it. The sun is what gives our entire planet life. It is also what gives us life. Without it, we would wither and die, just like plants do. Because we are truly connected to Nature, we must see that means we are connected also to the sun. If a plant has too much sun, it may burn, but if it has the right amount, it thrives.

Just like we do.

Yet we now tend to really fear the sun, and have been led to believe that we must not expose ourselves to it at all, that we should cover up at all times because it gives us cancer and can kill us. But more and more information is coming out that we now need the sun to be vitally healthy. And not something coming just from a vitamin D pill, but from the real source.

The energy from the sun is actually a form of *medicine*. What we haven't been told is the right amount of sun we need, nor how to look out for the signs our bodies give us to tell us when enough is enough. So we have avoided the sun at all costs, and now some of us are paying the price with ill health, which also directly affects our mood.

I grew up fearing the sun, in a big way. Why? Well, I came from Queensland, a super-hot place in Australia which has a very high rate of skin cancer. One of the worst in the entire world. Apparently our ozone layer is very thin so the UV rays there are super-strong. Many people have died from skin cancer in Australia, and tragically, this includes the very young. My childhood was spent trying to avoid being in the sun at all costs, and when I was in the sun, I would wear thick stinky sunblocks to cover my skin to avoid being burnt.

Well, it appears now that most people who have followed this belief are now extremely vitamin D deficient and that the skin cancer rate is actually increasing. Isn't that strangely ironic? People are avoiding the sun yet there are more skin cancers than ever before?

Now, I want to get this straight: it's *never* a good thing to get burnt. This chapter is not saying, 'Go out and bake in the sun all day – it's fine to be in the sun all day no matter what.' Definitely *not*! Burning of the skin is never a good thing (neither is looking like a leather bag), but I think we all need to rethink our fears towards the sun and see that it's meant to give us life and vitality, but only in the right and sensible amounts.

The proven health effects of the sun

If I had to give you a single secret ingredient that could apply to the prevention – and treatment, in many cases – of heart diseases, common cancers, stroke, infectious disease from influenza to tuberculosis, type 1 and 2 diabetes, dementia, depression, insomnia, muscle weakness, joint pain, fibromyalgia, osteoarthritis, rheumatoid arthritis, osteoporosis, psoriasis's, multiple sclerosis, and hypertension, it would be this: Vitamin D.[84]

Dr. Michael F. Hollick

We all know the sun makes us feel good. Anyone that hasn't had it regularly and goes out into the warm sun immediately feels happier. It's an instant mood booster. Even animals show us how much they love it as well. Dogs and cats will lie in patches of sun and even crocodiles will come up out of the water to get warm. Reptiles which are kept as pets have been known to develop bone problems due to the lack of sunlight in captivity. But what can the sun do for *our* actual health?

Well, many, many wonderful things – and what is interesting to note is that doctors many years ago (going back more than 50 years) knew this and would actually advise people to go out in the sun to heal their ailments. Clinics were set up all over the world, some in high-altitude places where people could be as close to the sun as possible.[85] They would go for a month or so and their health problems would be pretty much gone after their time spent there. They would not sit out all day, yet would figure out what the best time was for them (approximately 20 minutes) and then cover up or go back inside.

The following diseases have been shown to dramatically improve with vitamin D therapy:[86]

- Heart disease
- Cancer
- Diabetes
- Inflammatory bowel disease
- Rheumatoid arthritis
- Multiple sclerosis
- Osteoporosis

And in relation to cancer this is how vitamin D can help. Vitamin D has a protective effect against cancer in several ways, including:

- Increasing the self-destruction of mutated cells (which, if allowed to replicate, could lead to cancer)
- Reducing the spread and reproduction of cancer cells
- Causing cells to become differentiated (cancer cells often lack differentiation)
- Reducing the growth of new blood vessels from pre-existing ones, which is a step in the transition of dormant tumors turning cancerous

Many of my super-healthy friends, who are into eating lots of fresh raw foods and regularly detox their bodies, often report to me that they don't burn as much now in the sun like they used to. And these are really fair-skinned people too. I think there is something, perhaps yet unproven, about being really healthy that means you have skin with a higher natural protection that won't be so suscep-tible to burning.

Unhealthy bones: an epidemic that is affecting so many of us

Girls today break their arms 56% more often than their peers did forty years ago. Boys break their arms 32% percent more often.[87]
Dr. Michael Hollick, author and discoverer of the activated form of vitamin D

It's common knowledge that lack of vitamin D causes bone problems, making them become very brittle. We have all heard of 'rickets' which used to seem to only affect people in Third World countries. But due to the overuse of sunblocks (which block out all of the healing rays) and the fact that kids now play inside rather than outside, most of them (and us) are vitamin D deficient and that means our bones are suffering too.

As I mentioned, growing up I lived in a hot country but I always wore thick sunblock and protective clothes – and guess what? By the time I was 15 I had broken *four* bones. And I broke *another* one when I was 25. My exposure to lead wasn't exactly beneficial for my bones, but I also think that lack of sun exposure was perhaps another cause to these broken bones. I always wore suncreams or stayed inside. I just wasn't exposing my skin to the sun in a healthy way at all.

Many people think that when their food is fortified with vitamin D, and they also take a multivitamin, that means they are getting the daily requirement. But the real truth is, we need *much more* than that and we need to get it from the *real* source. Also, if nursing mothers aren't getting enough sun, it means that their breast milk is more likely to be deficient as well, which is not a good start to life for the child. Osteoporosis is absolutely rife these days and it's always found in the countries where dairy is highly consumed and where people are warned about being out in the sun and urged to wear lots of high-SPF sunblocks. Maybe we should take more notice of this and ask why we are having so much trouble with our bone density?

What *should* we fear? The sun or sunblocks?!

One of the biggest concerns in regards to the sun should be our view and use towards sunblocks. Not only are they blocking out the beneficial healing rays which we all desperately need, but they also contain *highly* toxic chemicals.[88] These days we can buy products that have up to SPF 50 which makes people assume that they can stay out all day in the sun and not cover up. While you might not get burnt, what is happening deep beneath your skin is far worse than burning.

The chemicals in the sunblocks are seeping into your bloodstream via your skin and are seen as an invader, causing your system (and skin) to become stressed. You might not feel it, but your insides certainly will be reacting, as anything that is put on the skin has an effect. And if you eat a diet high in acidic and processed foods, your risks of having skin reactions is much higher. Also, if you are on lots of pharmaceutical medications, then these too will also affect how your skin reacts to the sun.

People often think that using these sunblocks is a way to make time spent under the sun safe, yet sunblocks are some of the *most toxic* products for your health you could ever buy. And because they usually cover your entire body, it's also one of the quickest ways to overload your toxin levels.

I know that so many people really feel very strongly about the use of sunblocks and are going to be alarmed at reading that they are dangerous. This is why I have included the following information in great detail.

Here is a list of the main chemical ingredients found in most sunblocks:[89]

Octinoxate (Octyl methoxycinnamate)
The most widely used sunscreen ingredient, known for its low potential to sensitize skin or act as a photo allergen. Estrogenic effects are noted in laboratory animals as well as disruption of thyroid hormone and brain signaling. Has been found to kill mouse cells even at low doses when exposed to sunlight.

Oxybenzone (Benzophenone-3)
Associated with photo-allergic reactions. This chemical absorbs through your skin in significant amounts. It contaminates the bodies of 97% of Americans according to Centers for Disease Control research. Health concerns include hormone disruption and cancer.

Octisalate
Octisalate is a weak UVB absorber with a generally good safety profile among sunscreen ingredients. It is a penetration enhancer, which may increase the amount of other ingredients passing through skin.

Avobenzone (Parsol 1789)
Primarily a UVA-absorbing agent, sunlight causes this unstable ingredient to break down into unknown chemicals, especially in the presence of another, active, octinoxate.

Octocrylene
Produces oxygen radicals when exposed to UV light.

Homosalate
Research indicates it is a weak hormone disruptor, forms toxic metabolites, and can enhance the penetration of a toxic herbicide.

Micronized titanium dioxide
Sunscreens with micronized titanium dioxide may contain nano particles. Micronized TiO_2 offers greater sun protection than conventional (larger) particles. These small particles do not penetrate skin but may be more toxic to living cells and the environment. Inhalation of powders and sprays is a concern.

Micronized zinc oxide
Same as micronized titanium dioxide, above.

Titanium dioxide
Appears safe for use on skin, due to low penetration, but inhalation is a concern.

Ensulizole (Phenylbenzimidazole sulfonic acid)
Known to produce free radicals when exposed to sunlight, leading to damage of DNA, this UVB protector may have the potential to cause cancer.

Nano zinc oxide
Nano zinc oxide offers greater sun protection than larger zinc particles. Comparatively little is known regarding potential health

effects of nano particles. They do not penetrate healthy skin, and thus appear to pose a low health risk in lotions. Inhalation of powders and sprays is a concern.

Nano titanium dioxide
Same as nano zinc oxide, above.

Zinc oxide
Zinc has a long history of use in sunscreen and other skincare products; little absorption and no adverse health effects are reported.

Padimate O (Octyl dimethyl PABA / PABA ester)
A derivative of the once-popular PABA sunscreen ingredient, research shows this chemical releases free radicals, damages DNA, has estrogenic activity, and causes allergic reactions in some people.

Menthyl anthranilate
One study found that it produces damaging reactive oxygen species when exposed to sunlight.

Mexoryl SX
Two hours of sunlight can degrade as much as 40% of this active ingredient. Low skin penetration.

Methylene bis-benzotriazolyl tetramethylbutylphenol
Not an approved active ingredient in the USA. Few studies exist on this chemical. It is photo stable and does not absorb through your skin.

Sulisobenzone (Benzophenone-4)
Can cause skin and eye irritation. Does not penetrate your skin to a large degree, but enhances the ability of other chemicals to penetrate.

Benzophenone-2
Not approved for use in United States sunscreens. Concerns about hormone disruption.

Make the connection

Despite sunscreen use being higher than ever, skin cancer is still on the rise. The most common cancer in the United States, skin cancer accounts for nearly 50% of all cancer cases.[90]

Can you now see how there *must* be a very strong connection between skin cancers being caused, not due to the sun, but from all of these chemicals found in sunblocks? Does it not make sense that something so irritating must be quite harmful and causes a reaction whereby the skin will not be able to function normally?

We see these products as a form of protection, but they are in fact dangerous and harmful. When the sun's rays hit the chemicals in these products, it causes a toxic reaction which affects what is happening on the inside of your body.

And if you are already toxic, the sun will do its best to draw those toxins out of you, as the sun's purpose is to detoxify and heal us! It acts like a magnet trying to make you well. But the message the skin is getting is one of utter confusion. We put on sunblocks to block the sun, yet the sun tries to pull out the other toxins from within your body. When they are brought to the surface, this chemical reaction can cause the skin to break down and become extremely sensitive and reactive, and the worst case scenario is that skin cancers *will* form.

And it is even more worrying that we are covering up our children with these types of products as well. Some companies say that their product is 'kid friendly', but the real truth is, they still contain many of the deadly ingredients! Children need sun regularly too, but again, only in the safe amounts. And if we want them to grow up happy as well, then they need to get the magical effects from the sun. If we are blocking them by using toxic sunblocks, then what is that doing long term to their body's own production of happy hormones?

The point of sunblocks is to block out the sun, which means blocking out all of the rays. UV light is made up of UVA, UVB, and UVC – all of which have their own purpose. All combined are healing, in the right amounts. It's when you stay out for far too long that you burn, which damages the skin. The key is never to burn! Get out of the sun before your skin has been burnt. Cover up with thick clothing and a wide-brimmed hat. Don't slather yourself with poisonous creams.

Many scientists now believe that skin cancers are being caused by the sunblocks themselves. Dr. Ackerman released his own study through the *British Medical Journal* back in 1996 to show that the regular use of sunblocks meant an *increased* chance of skin cancer due to the fact that people were not aware when they had enough sun, because there were no signs of redness, which is Nature's way of saying, 'Right, that's it – get out of the sun and cover up.' They simply had too much sun, which caused damage to the skin. Other scientists such as Rachel Haywood, who wrote a letter to the editor of the *British Medical Journal* in 2003, are expressing their concern at what they have found through their own studies:

We concluded that: since ultraviolet-A (UVA) forms at least 90% of solar UV which penetrates the earth's atmosphere, since protection against UVA by sunscreens is disproportionate, and less by a factor of 10, to that of ultraviolet-B (UVB); and since sunscreens by protecting against UVB-induced erythema encourage the user to stay more in the sun, they increase exposure to UVA and its damaging effects. Thus use of sunscreens may explain the increase in incidence of melanoma.[91]

We previously learnt that regular beauty products contain many unsafe chemicals, but the truth is, the chemicals in sunblocks make them look like a picnic. Sunblocks are typically very thick in consistency and are applied all over our faces and our entire body, usually leaving only the scalp without sunblock on it. Again, many of these ingredients have never been tested for safety. And as we will see, they are actually capable of catching on fire:

In 2012, CBS News reported on a story involving a man using his barbecue on a hot summer's day. The man caught fire, not because of an accident from how he was cooking the meat, but because he was wearing a spray-on sunblock.

> I sprayed on the spray-on sunscreen, and then rubbed it on for a few seconds. I walked over to my grill, took one of the holders to move some of the charcoal briquettes around and all of a sudden it just went up my arm,' Brett Sigworth of Stow, Mass., told CBS Boston.[92]

You can see the photos of Brett's injuries, on the CBS.com website, and they're pretty shocking. He was injured all up his chest, ear and back and arms. The fire went *exactly* where the sunscreen spray was on his body.

I think this story is a perfect example to encourage people to see that these sunblocks are perhaps causing more skin cancers than preventing them. I want to stress again, however, that I am not suggesting anyone goes into the sun for long periods of time without any sort of protection. I mainly want people to understand that regular sun exposure is healthy and can be safe, but using toxic sunscreens is not. The FDA have even *admitted* that they do not have any proof that the sunblocks actually help to prevent skin cancers. And, according to a report by the National Toxicity Program, the FDA also have admitted that one ingredient in particular, that of retinyl palmitate, is very dangerous and linked to causing cancers:

> 'Retinyl palmitate was selected by (the FDA's) Center for Food Safety and Applied Nutrition for photo-toxicity and photocar-

cinogenicity testing based on the increasingly widespread use of this compound in cosmetic retail products for use on sun-exposed skin,' said an October 2000 report by the National Toxicology Program.[93]

The sunblock industry alone is worth *$5 billion* per year – which is worth noting. What would happen if suddenly everyone knew these products were dangerous and were causing cancers and killing people? Many companies would go bust and quite possibly have huge lawsuits filed their way. And people would be absolutely furious with the FDA for allowing these to be seemed as a necessary health product.

Is there even any proof that the sun actually causes skin cancer?

I bet you think, 'Yes, of course there is!', like I used to also think, but shockingly, no studies have ever been proven to show that sun exposure *alone* causes skin cancer.

Many people of darker races, such as Africans and Aborigines, are getting melanomas on their torso and underneath their feet. Isn't this a bit odd? They are getting cancers on the unexposed body parts the sun never or rarely sees! And dark skin has such a huge melanin content which offers them natural protection – that's *why* they are so dark, because they need the natural protection to live near the equator. So it's *very* puzzling and hard to understand why they get these cancers on such odd body parts and on skin types that have their own natural high protection.

In other studies, the type of people *most* likely to get skin cancers are those that work in an office and do *not* have regular exposure to the sun.[94] There was even a study done on US Navy personnel between the years 1974 and 1984 which showed that the sailors who worked on the deck, and therefore were in the sun most often, were actually the ones *least* likely to develop skin cancers. The sailors who worked *below* deck, however, were the ones who got the cancers.

Another study, by Dr. Helen Shaw from the London School of Hygiene and Tropical Medicine, was published back in 1982 in the *British Medical Journal, The Lancet*. This study showed that those that spent most of their time exposed to natural sunlight in moderate amounts were at the lowest risk of developing skin cancer.[95] She also discovered that people in Australia (and also Britain) who worked in offices were developing skin cancers.

Healthy sun exposure

With sun exposure, it's always best to start up gradually and to *always* avoid getting burnt. Twenty minutes on the front and back is usually the safest amount, depending on your skin type and current health condition (e.g. if you are super-toxic you may burn faster). I spent 5 weeks in hot Costa Rica in April of 2011 and never used sunblock, not even once. Costa Rica is very close to the equator and if you are not careful you can easily get burnt. I always made sure I was exposed for about 20 minutes and then would cover up with clothing and a hat and would sit in the shade. I also used coconut oil on my skin, which has a natural SPF of 8. I was amazed that I never got burnt.

How lack of sun makes us sick

Over the years of living in the UK, I had not really seen the sun since I left Australia. That was 7 years ago. About a year after I arrived in the UK is exactly when my chronic fatigue syndrome kicked in very badly. I now believe without a doubt that the even less sun exposure compared to what I had grown up with was one of the main culprits for causing this, and the list below shows that lack of sun exposure is a direct cause of 'adrenal insufficiency' which all chronic fatigue sufferers seem to have.

If the sun can heal, and you are sick, you won't heal as fast without regular, safe sun exposure. You only have to lie in the sun for a short while to know that it's essential for us because it also feels so good!

A grumpy mood can turn into a bright and positive mood within no time. In the UK, when it is a sunny day, you should see how different the atmosphere is; people in shops greet you much more happily and they actually smile. When it's cold and grey, people reflect that too.

The following health problems have been attributed to vitamin D deficiency:[96]

- adrenal insufficiency
- Alzheimer's
- allergies
- autoimmune disorders including multiple sclerosis and rheumatoid arthritis
- cancers of the colon, breast, skin and prostate
- depression, seasonal affective disorder (SAD)
- diabetes, type 1 and 2
- gluten intolerance, lectin intolerance
- heart disease, hypertension, Syndrome X
- infertility, sexual dysfunction
- learning and behavior disorders
- misaligned teeth and cavities
- obesity
- osteopenia, osteoporosis, osteomalacia (adult rickets)
- Parkinson's
- PMS
- psoriasis

What can you do when sunlight is minimal?

What if you don't live in a warm country and receive only a little bit of sun each year? Well, apart from going on holidays somewhere hot as often as you can, it may be best to consider buying a sun lamp.

You can purchase these from Amazon or Ebay; they are called 'SAD' light boxes. SAD means 'seasonal affective disorder', a condition which even doctors recognize as a type of depression people suffer from during the winter months. If you have been used to sun all your life, like I have, you certainly will notice a big difference when you are without it. These little boxes can be put by your computer or anywhere near where you sit, and you switch them on for certain periods throughout the day. They provide you with the same health benefits as the sun but produce less UV light than normal sun does.

I really like the UK company Lumie, which sells all sorts of SAD lights for home and office use. Lumie light boxes are fitted with special filters so the amount of UV they emit is fractional. Not many brands have this feature, so it's always best to research as much as you can that the brand you have your eye on is actually one like this.

You can purchase the lamps from lumie.com in the UK. You can also get VAT-free lamps if you have SAD (a valid medical condition) so you can save yourself a bit of money.

I am not much of a fan of taking high doses of vitamin D in a pill. I keep hearing conflicting information about how much to take. Some say mega-high doses are needed, while others say that these high doses are quite toxic, so I feel it's best to try and get vitamin D from a natural light source. But if your healthcare provider seems to know a lot about vitamin D, then following their advice may really help you – I would just be wary of someone who wants you to take doses in the tens of thousands. Some supplements are good, which I will mention below.

You can, however, get vitamin D from certain foods – eggs, oily fish and mushrooms in particular. But diet alone won't be enough so, even if your diet is high in vitamin D, don't be fooled into thinking you are safe from being deficient. And because fish is so polluted these days, I don't tend to recommend people eat them, so I prefer to suggest mushrooms. You can't really eat mushrooms every day (well, you could but you might easily get very bored) so I do recommend taking the 'Super Greens + D' by Touchstone Essentials. These potent capsules not only provide an enormous array of phytonutrients and other minerals and vitamins from all of the green vegetables, but they also offer the body a good dose of vitamin D from the organic mushrooms. Taken 3 times a day, this can help your vitamin D levels. I also like using vitamin D3 sprays that can be used sublingually and are available in different types for adults, children and pregnant women. It's so vital that children get enough vitamin D3. You can purchase these sprays from rawliving.eu and mercola.com

For those that are really serious about their health, and if you have the money, you could perhaps consider investing in a sun bed. I never thought I would say this as I was led to believe that tanning beds were always dangerous, but they do have their benefits if used *wisely* and correctly.

A recent study found that bulbs with 6% UVB were twice as efficient at producing vitamin D (before erythema) compared to those with 2% UVB. For best results, some researchers recommend a minimum of 1.5% UVB. Does indoor tanning work? One study found that twice-weekly tanning raised vitamin D levels to a healthy 46 ng/mL compared to the average (and insufficient) 24 ng/mL seen in comparable non-tanners.[97]

On the market there are now tanning beds specially designed to boost your vitamin D, but they have had the more dangerous elements removed. They are either a sun bed or an upright tanning panel, which can be installed into your home where you and your family can use them. Mercola.com have designed their own beds and panels which are extremely well made and of the highest standard. They certainly aren't cheap, but if you can afford it, the difference to your health and wellbeing will be huge. You can use them for *short* periods only twice a week.

If you can't purchase one, then perhaps consider a visit to a salon to use their tanning bed perhaps once a week for 10 minutes only (this time frame is for the beds that people can stay in for up to 40 minutes, not the stand-up ones which are super-strong where only minutes are needed). The best type of tanning beds have high UVB ratio so when enquiring about booking in, make sure you get the salon to tell you if their beds offer this. And please remember to not use them too much. They really can be very dangerous, so *moderation* is the key here.

Safe sunblocks: is there such a thing?

Thankfully, yes! There are some that are far safer than the regular brands, which still offer you protection if you are going to be in the sun for a long time. I highly recommend Lavera and Green People products, both of which offer high organic content and have various SPFs from titanium dioxide, which is a fine white powder that comes from plants. There are also gentle formulas for little ones.

Remember that the sun will try and pull out toxins from inside your body and this will mix with whatever you have put on your skin, so it's always best to try and make the inside of your body healthy too. Personally, I only use organic and unrefined coconut oil to protect my skin if I need to be outside for longer than 20 minutes. It's absolutely brilliant and surpasses any other sunblock I have used, because I know it is safe, and it also makes your skin smell and feel great!

Remember these important tips:

- Avoid the sun and you are missing out on many precious health benefits and may end up causing serious deficiencies.
- Abuse the sun and you risk damaging your skin.
- By using the sun in the right way, you will help to super-charge your health.

If you want to know more about vitamin D and sunlight, and their effects on health, read *The Vitamin D Solution* by Michael F. Holick, who is a world-renowned expert on the subject. He was also the discoverer of the active form of vitamin D. In this insightful book, he gives detailed advice about how much time you should spend in the sun without sunblock in order to get your vitamin D needs covered, while minimizing your risk of burning and getting skin cancer. He covers this for people living in all continents on the planet.

For more information, articles and a buying guide for safe sunblocks, please visit the websites below:

✓ vitamind.mercola.com
✓ naturalnews.com/Vitamin_D.html
✓ breakingnews.ewg.org/2012sunscreens

Chapter 17

Nature and the Vital Connection We Have

Short of Aphrodite, there is nothing lovelier on this planet than a flower, nor more essential than a plant. The true matrix of human life is the green sward covering Mother Earth. Without green plants we would neither breathe nor eat. On the under-surface of every leaf a million moveable lips are engaged in devouring carbon dioxide and expelling oxygen. All together, twenty-five million square miles of leaf surface are daily engaged in this miracle of photosynthesis, producing oxygen and food for man and beast.[98]
Peter Tompkins and Christopher Bird, *The Secret Life of Plants*

To have an appreciation for Nature is the essence of feeling truly connected to *life*. Yet sadly, many people have become so disconnected from Mother Nature, and the wonders of the world, that they miss out on the incredible healing powers and comfort that Nature provides each of us. It's truly amazing when looking at flowers for example, how incredible Nature really is. To witness how things grow, and to think how they were created in the first place, and to see the vast array of colours, textures and shapes they turn into is for me, at times, purely *magical*. I quite often gasp at seeing all of the beautiful plants and flowers. It can bring moments of clarity and a meditative state, simply to just look at the wonders of nature.

How many of us live and work in high-rise buildings today? When was the last time *you* were out in Nature? For lots of people, it could be a very long time ago indeed. Maybe your feet literally haven't touched the bare earth in years? Or very rarely?

This is another important factor as to why our health is declining. More and more studies are being done on the healing abilities of plants and how they benefit us in many ways, emotional and physical.

We can improve our health simply by being near plants and trees!

In the book *Blinded by Science*, author Matthew Fox saw his son, who was struck down with chronic fatigue, fail with healing until he started to get closer to Nature. His son began to be drawn to hugging trees and, within a short amount of time, his health dramatically improved, as well as his state of mind.[99] Matthew went on to write his groundbreaking book, covering little-talked-about subjects such as the effect that the cycles of the moon have on us, how plants and trees heal and communicate, and how types of modern technology, such as mobile phone towers, are affecting bee colonies and also bird life in a very negative way.

It makes us question: just what is all this technology doing to us? The answer is quite alarming: it is affecting us in many ways and this is severely underreported in the media. Studies have shown that illness linked to electromagnetic radiation exposure include: many types of cancers, ADD, neurological conditions, sleep disorders, depression, cognitive problems, mineral disruption, cardiovascular irregularities, hormone disruption, autism, immune system disorders, metabolism changes, stress, fertility impairment, increased blood brain barrier permeability, DNA damage and much, much more.

Thankfully Nature provides us with many forms of healing and one that is very beneficial for countering the negative effects of EMF exposure: we receive health benefits by simply *standing barefoot* on the earth's bare ground. Yes, that's right, standing on the ground, with no shoes on, can make you *healthier*. Clint Ober writes in his groundbreaking book *'Earthing'*:

> Most people, even in this scientific age, are totally unaware of their bio-electrical nature. Practically no one has the slightest notion of an electrical connection between his or her body and the Earth. Nobody learns about it in school ... so nobody knows that

we have largely become disconnected and separated from the Earth. In developed societies, in particular, we have essentially lost our electrical roots. Our bare feet, with their rich network of nerve endings, rarely touch the ground. We wear insulating synthetic-soled shoes. We sleep on elevated beds made from insulating material. Most of us in the modern, industrialized world live disconnected from the Earth's surface. Although it is not something you probably have ever thought about, you may be suffering needlessly because of this disconnect. And you may be suffering severely, and in more ways that you could ever imagine.[100]

Human beings all have an electrical charge in their bodies. The earth, which is like one big magnet, has an ability to connect with that charge and will always 'ground' you, meaning that the current flowing through you gets pulled into the ground. This grounding means that no other electrical current can affect you, blocking out EMFs (electromagnetic frequencies) and other frequencies. The reason why this is important is because of the bombardment of modern technology. We are all surrounded by EMFs these days because of computers, mobile phones, radio towers, TVs etc. etc. These EMFs are a form of radiation. They are so powerful that they can travel through very thick concrete.

Because we have our own current, our bodies pick up other currents by our cells and this charge causes them a great deal of stress; they become confused and not able to function normally. Bee and bird colonies are also suffering and this is being linked directly to mobile phone towers and therefore EMFs as well.[101] People seem to be able to accept that this problem is real in regards to these animal problems but are more hesitant to believe it is affecting us. That seems a bit silly to me. We are not all superhuman on this earth; we suffer quite easily when our environment changes so much. And humans are animals too.

Walking on the bare earth, without shoes, as often as possible is one of the best ways to help get your body functioning in the way it's meant to. It's also a wonderful way to receive reflexology. When you walk barefoot on uneven ground, it presses on acupressure points of the feet, helping to get energy flowing into your entire body.

Think back to the first group of humans who were on earth. They were not living in houses made of unnatural materials. They did not walk around wearing shoes. They did not work in offices all day surrounded by computers and unnatural surroundings. They were out in Nature, walking barefoot *all* the time and sleeping on the ground as well! They were very active and surrounded by Nature. We think that shoes protect us – and yes, they might from the cold or from water when it rains, or keeps you from stubbing your toe – but they are actually blocking your natural connection to the earth.

The bottom of your feet is the only entry way into your body that the earth's negatively charged electrical particles have, and if you put shoes on, that entry way is shut off completely. And if it is shut off, your body has no other way of letting the 'earthing' effects in. So if you want to get healthy, then a cheap way of doing that is to get out into Nature and walk on bare earth as much as possible.

Remember when you last walked barefoot on the soft green grass. Didn't it feel amazing? Do you want to know why that is? Well, it's because as soon as you connect to the earth, you begin to heal due to the negatively charged electrons contained in the earth. We must use common sense to look at what has changed so much over the years and could be causing us problems. Put simply, it's technology! While we do need it to communicate with each other and I am sure none of us regret the Internet being born, we really have no super long-term proof of what EMFs are doing to us. Only time will tell.

Water is also very grounding as well, so swimming in the sea, springs, waterfalls, rivers or creeks is another way to connect you back to the earth. If you are somewhere near a lot of trees, then you will also be able to breathe in truly healthy air. I have on many occasions hugged trees and noticed straight away how peaceful and calm I felt. I know it sounds silly but give it a try and see how you feel! Or if you are a bit shy about doing that, at least try sitting against a tree trunk – this also is very calming.

If you find it very difficult to get out in Nature because of where you live, then you can perhaps consider buying an 'Earthing Sheet' or even an earthing computer pad. The Earthing Sheet is something you put on your bed (it's what you directly lie on) so that at night, when you are resting, the current from EMFs is stopped and won't affect your body. The bed sheet is made out of soft cotton and has silver thread running through it. You can plug it into a wall or it also comes with an earthing stick which can be literally stuck into the bare earth, if you don't want to use electricity.

I have had one for a year now and I must say that I haven't ever slept this well before it came along. I used to get odd feelings at night in my body as I was trying to sleep and I have a feeling it was from being too close to my computer and for far too long. The Earthing Bed Sheet allows me to have a peaceful and restful night's sleep.

There are also sleeping bags you can use, which means you can be almost completely insulated from electromagnetic energy. These bags are comfortable and also wonderful when you are traveling. My daughter's school recently had a lecture by a well-known neuro-scientist who is an expert in the field of WiFi. So concerned were the board members of the school that they have now introduced a ban of

WiFi in most areas of the school. Studies are pointing to it causing serious damage such as cancers and other types of health problems which are affecting our children. They are often at school for 8-hour days and if WiFi is also on at home, then they are simply never away from it. And if they are using iPads and computers to play on, then again, the EMFs are around them all the time. Most parents don't know this but there have been no studies done on WiFi to prove that it is safe for our children to be exposed to during the school day. I think once people look at the evidence, they will be very disturbed. If it concerns you, please contact your school and get them to watch the video found on YouTube titled *Dr Magda Havas – The Truth About Wired and Wireless Technologies*. Dr Havas is an associate professor of Environmental and Resource studies at Trent University.

When at home, please try and turn your WiFi off as much as possible, especially at night as you really don't need it to be on. And, if your kids do play with your phone, and iPads - turn them onto Airport mode.

For more information on EMFs and to purchase products please visit these helpful websites:

✓ blindedbyscience.co.uk

✓ rawliving.eu

✓ wirelesswatchblog.org/wi-fi-in-schools/

Air pollution

City air is full of harmful toxins such as petrol and cigarette smoke as well as a whole list of other things. Breathing the air in London (said to be one of the most toxic cities in all of Europe) or any other big cities, per day, can be the equivalent of smoking 200 cigarettes in terms of damage to your lungs. Other, even more heavily polluted cities such as Nanjing, China are double.[102] And because of millions of planes filling up our skies, the air quality in even far corners of the earth is becoming not so clean either. If we are not careful, one day quite soon we may have to purchase oxygen machines to have at home so that we can get pure oxygen to keep us well, or we will have to walk around with gas masks on.

Fresh mountain or forest air provides us with air the way as close to as it is supposed to be: clean(er) and healthy. You only have to go outside of a city to visit somewhere with lots of trees and you will immediately notice the difference in your breathing. Again it's more of a reason to stock your house with plenty of healthy-air plants and consider purchasing an air purifier.

Nature is good for your mind

Whenever we are stressed, instead of hitting the pub, or going to the fridge, we really should go outside and sit in a park, beach, garden or forest somewhere. If you suffer from stress, as we all do whether we feel it or not, then 'grounding', or 'earthing', such as walking barefoot, will almost immediately help to relax you. Think back to the last time you were in a park or forest somewhere. Did you feel much better, after breathing in such pure air, and were you able to think more clearly? Nature is immediately calming, soothing and relaxing, and can often lead you to great insight as to how to solve a particular problem. Being near Nature is a form of meditation. Your body and mind craves it! Try and go outside every day, if you can, to reconnect with this magical force.

Chapter 18

Why Your Stomach May Be Making You Unhappy

When you consider the fact that the gut-brain connection is recognized as a basic tenet of physiology and medicine, and that there's no shortage of evidence of gastrointestinal involvement in a variety of neurological diseases, it's easy to see how the balance of gut bacteria can play a significant role in your psychology and behavior as well. With this in mind, it should also be crystal clear that nourishing your gut flora is extremely important, from cradle to grave, because in a very real sense you have two brains, one inside your skull and one in your gut, and each needs its own vital nourishment. Interestingly, these two organs are actually created out of the same type of tissue. During fetal development, one part turns into your central nervous system while the other develops into your enteric nervous system. These two systems are connected via the vagus nerve, the tenth cranial nerve that runs from your brain stem down to your abdomen.[103]

Dr. Joseph Mercola

So many people today (adults *and* children) have a huge problem with their stomach's health and do not realize that this *directly* affects their moods and therefore their happiness. Their stomachs are just not digesting food well, have an imbalance of flora, and this can affect the way the brain functions, causing depression, anger, and in many cases can even contribute to extreme behavioral conditions in children such as autism and ADHD. More and more information is coming out about the 'gut–brain' connection. Because of this direct connection, whereby one cannot be healthy without the other being healthy, we are at times able to treat certain disorders through diet alone.

The gut relies on a certain balance of bacteria called 'gut flora', and with so much of an assault on people's health due to toxins and stress, this balance is becoming anything but balanced. In a healthy body, the good bacteria should be about 85% and the bad should ideally be about 15%. For most people it's more the other way: the bad is outweighing the good. These bacteria serve many purposes, and scientists are only just discovering some of them. These bacteria actually have been found to *communicate* to each other as a synchronized unit. When the levels are balanced, they can coordinate their defenses and attack incoming viruses.

And when gut flora are not in a harmonious state, it increases the likelihood of someone suffering from toxic-exposure health problems:

> The trouble is that in our modern society, we live in a world where a growing proportion of the population have damaged gut flora, because they have been exposed to repeated courses of antibiotics; women are taking contraceptive pills, which damage the gut flora quite profoundly, or any other prescriptive long-term medication. People are taking in toxic substances through their food and drink, and other ... environmental influences damage the composition of their gut flora. As a result, when they are exposed to mercury, lead, other toxic metals, or other toxic substances in the environment, their gut flora is unable to chelate it, and cannot remove it. It floods into their bloodstream, and settles in the body. Unfortunately, toxic metals have a particular affinity for fatty tissues in the body, so they get stored in the brain, spine, and in the rest of the nervous system. They also target your bone marrow and the rest of the high fat organs in the body ... Of course, when they're stored in there, they would cause leukemia, lymphoma, other immune abnormalities, and other problems.[104]

Audio interview with Caroline Barringer and Dr. Joseph Mercola

People don't seem to know this but 80% of the immune system is located in the gut, which actually functions as a 'second brain'. During the development of a fetus, one part of the gut turns into the central nervous system and the other turns into the enteric nervous system. Both of these are connected via what is called the 'vagus nerve' which is the tenth cranial nerve running from the brain stem down to the stomach.

Toxicity in the stomach can spread throughout the body and go into the brain where it may appear as autism, dyslexia, depression, schizophrenia and other mental disorders. Dr. Natasha Campbell-McBride, an expert in gut disorders, believes that children should be tested for 'GAPS' (Gut and Physiology Syndrome) before they are vaccinated. If they are showing signs of GAPS (which is already a sign of body toxicity) then vaccine-related injuries are far higher (due to the addition of more toxins to the body) than in children who do not appear to have GAPS. You can read more about this at her websites:

✓ GAPS.me and doctor-natasha.com

Stress can cause an intense growth of candida-type flora which can make people feel incredibly run down, unhappy and sick. If the stomach does not have a healthy environment, the immune system will not be able to protect the body like it should do and these bad bacteria will take over. Someone with this problem will be more prone to catching colds, and feeling nauseous constantly. They usually will feel constantly exhausted too.

To improve these problems, a healthy balance of flora must be achieved. It is also said that formula feeding directly contributes to this problem. Due to missing out on a variety of nutrients which are only created by breast milk, children who are formula-fed are much more likely to suffer with stomach issues when they are older, and some will show signs in their youth as they will be sick on a regular basis. It can often be highly beneficial to take a good-quality colostrum supplement.

Stomach health is a *huge* subject which I can't cover here in its entirety, but I will suggest some experts to go and look into further if something tells you your own stomach is not functioning quite right. Look into eating more fermeneted foods to help your improve gut health.

Candace Pert has written a wonderful book called *The Molecules of Emotion: The Science behind the Mind–Body Medicine.*

Also, Dr. Natasha Campbell-McBride has written the book *Gut and Psychology Syndrome.*

Just like the health of your colon, the health of your stomach is vitally crucial to a happy and healthy life. Please take an interest in the health of your stomach.

Chapter 19

Healthy, Easy and Tasty Recipes

Even when you realize the vital importance of a good diet, it can be very hard to know how to start incorporating new meal ideas. I have come across some wonderful yet very simple recipes, courtesy of some talented foodie friends I have met along the way. These recipes really can make you feel better in a short amount of time, because they do not contain any processed sugars or chemical-based foods and some are healthier substitutes for 'naughty' things like chips, chocolate and ice cream. I have chosen things that are very easy to make, don't require masses of ingredients and are very tasty. Who wants to feel overwhelmed when it comes to food? Not me! Try a few for yourself!

Breakfast smoothie recipes

- Protein Explosion

1 banana, a handful of parsley, half a lemon, 2 teaspoons of bee pollen, 1 teaspoon of spirulina, 2 cups of fresh water or almond milk. Add a healthy sweetener of your choice – or add an extra banana. Blend until smooth.

- Berry Bliss

1 banana, a handful of berries (fresh or frozen), 2 teaspoons of cacao powder, 1 tablespoon of coconut oil, 2 cups of fresh water or almond milk. Add a healthy sweetener of your choice. Blend until smooth.

- Orange Heaven

1 orange, 1 mango, 1 banana, 1 tablespoon of raw organic honey, 2 cups of fresh water or almonds milk. Blend until smooth.

Fruit Soups

This is one of my all time favorite ways to eat more fruit. Part fruit salad and part smoothie, a fruit soup is really just blended fruits made into a thin liquid, with chopped up pieces of fruit thrown in. There are many varieties you can make -

I often make the following fruit soup:

1 banana, 1/4 pineapple + 1 Mango, blended together. Pour the liquid into a bowl. Slice banana pieces as well as any other fruit like strawberries and kiwi fruit. Place the chopped pieces into the bowl. You can now eat as is with a spoon, and add some passionfruit (or any fruits) on top. Completely delicious and kids absolutely love eating their fruit like this – it's fun!

Juices

Juice does not contain any fiber, but it is the purest water with loads of vitamins and minerals extracted from the fruit or vegetable, which is so vital to the body. A juice quickly hydrates and allows you to take in the nutrients of the foods without having to go through the full process of digestion. Many people do prolonged juice fasts but you do not need to do this – an organic juice a day, taken on an empty stomach is just fine.

Green juice recipes
- 3 sticks of celery, half a cucumber, 1 apple, half a lemon
- 3 carrots, 1 apple, a handful of parsley, half a lemon
- 1 cucumber, 1 small head of broccoli, 1 apple

Juice in a cold-pressed juicer for best extraction method. Or if you have only a blender, you can blend and then press through a nut milk bag to extract the juice.

Super salads

A salad can be a complete meal when you use the right ingredients. You can include so many different vegetables and fruits that you can have a different and satisfying salad every single day. Making a salad is also a lot of fun; you can involve your family and children (at the appropriate age), chopping and cutting stuff and helping with the mixing of ingredients.

Salads can also look beautiful and colorful, which makes them much more appetizing to the eyes. Open the box of possibilities by using ingredients that you would not normally think could go into a salad, such as dates, apple, cinnamon, orange, walnuts, cashews etc.

See some delicious examples below.

Chop the following into very small pieces
- 1 big red pepper
- 2 small tomatoes
- 2 avocados
- A handful of spinach
- Half a red or white/brown onion
- A handful of parsley
- 5 dates
- 5 walnuts

Mix well and add olive oil, sea salad (sea weeds) and a dash of grapefruit juice.

Chop the following into very small pieces
- 1 head lettuce
- Half head of broccoli
- 1 apple
- 2 small tomatoes
- 1 avocado
- 2 garlic cloves

Mix well and add a handful of pine nuts, olive oil, sea salad and a dash of lemon juice.

Arrigazzi Soup

This wonderfully delicious soup is probably the healthiest and most re-mineralizing soup you could make. People with different ailments and conditions or simply people with the aim of keeping a healthy life have reported great benefits by having this soup regularly. It was used after the bombing of Hiroshima on certain patients who were exposed to the radiation.[105] Many who had this soup regularly survived and did not develop cancers.

The ingredients of this soup, combined as described below and adding the dressing as mentioned on the last step, creates the perfect formulation to help reactivate the immune system, balance alkalinity, detoxify heavy metals out of the body, providing at the same time an array of minerals and vitamins necessary for good health.

Add some fresh organic herbs and spices such as thyme, rosemary, pepper cayenne, basil, oregano.

You can prepare the soup in advance and keep it in the fridge for up to 3 days.

The ingredients for this soup
- Water
- 1 big white onion
- 2 carrots
- 2 leeks
- 2 stalks of celery
- 1 large slice of squash (pumpkin)
- 1 courgette
- 1 parsnip
- 2 large leafs of Swiss chard
- Seaweeds (find these ingredients in any health store)
  - Kombu
  - Wakame
  - Hijikie
  - Dulse
  - Daikon

Seaweeds should be soaked before cooking, when they will expand considerably. Save the soaking water for the soup.

Dressing ingredients (find the ingredients in any health store)

- Hatcho miso
- Ginger
- Lemon
- Flax oil
- Brown rice

How to prepare the soup

1. Put brown rice on to boil – this will take about 20 minutes. In another pot bring 1.5 liters of water to boil with 1 teaspoon of sea salt and 1 piece of Kombu, 1 piece of Wakame, the equivalent to 1 tablespoon of Hijiki, 1 piece of Dulse and 1 piece of Daikon.*
2. Chop all vegetables into very small pieces.
3. Place vegetables into boiling water and boil for 10 minutes.
4. Turn off soup mix and let stand for 30 minutes.
5. Take 1 tablespoon of broth from the soup and place in bowl.
6. Mix 1 teaspoon of miso and dissolve it into the broth.
7. Grate some ginger into the broth mixture.
8. Squeeze in 1 tablespoon of lemon juice and chopped parsley into the broth mixture.
9. Add 1 tablespoon of flax oil
10. Mix in 2 ladles of hot soup, with 3 tablespoons of rice.

Serve and enjoy!

Try and eat this soup every few days for best results or at least 3–4 days a week. Only add a small amount of miso if you do eat regularly.

*Due to the recent catastrophe that took place in Japan we suggest you avoid seaweeds coming from that region.

(Smoothie, juices, salads and soup recipe all courtesy of Frank Arrigazzi, CEO and creator of Purple Balance Super Foods)

✓ purplebalancesuperfoods.com

Delicious desserts

Usually, most people's downfall (as is mine) when it comes to eating is - sweets! Sugar is so addictive and very hard to cut out of a diet. But there are ways of satisfying your sweet tooth without using processed sugar. One of the most delicious and ridiculously simple desserts is ice cream. Instead of making or buying ice creams that are made from dairy and sugar, you can make a fruit-based ice cream which will knock your socks off. Using frozen peeled bananas in a high-speed blender is so simple yet tastes absolutely amazing. I have made this easy dessert for many friends and family, and when they eat it, they cannot believe it's made from bananas.

You can take frozen bananas and either blend them up on their own or add things to them such as vanilla powder, cacao (chocolate) powder, other fruits such as berries – or what I do is add some organic peanut or almond butter to the frozen bananas to make a peanut butter type ice cream. Truly scrumptious and as healthy as ice cream can get! It's what I will be feeding Lola when she is old enough to have 'treats'.

Simple and quick ice cream recipes

• Vanilla

2 frozen bananas (per person), 1 tsp vanilla powder (or to taste). Blend until it becomes smooth and whipped. You can serve with some chopped nuts, sultanas or berries.

• Chocolate

2 frozen bananas (per person), 1 tablespoon of cacao powder. Blend until it becomes smooth. Top with some cacao nibs if you want a choc-chip ice cream! You can also add some fresh mint to the blender to make it mint choc chip.

• Peanut/Almond/Hazelnut Butter

2 frozen bananas (per person), 1 large spoon of nut butter of choice. Blend until smooth.

• Berry

2 frozen bananas (per person), 1 cup of berries of choice mixed or

one type (per person). Blend until smooth.

• Tropical Delight

2 frozen bananas (per person), 1 mango (per person), ½ cup of papaya. Blend until smooth.

Young Living Essential Oils are so pure you can even use them in your food and drinks too. Lemon, lavender, peppermint, orange, mandarin and even basil can make some incredible-tasting ice creams. Ben and Jerry's, eat your (unhealthy!) heart out!

You can use many better and healthy toppings such as coconut flakes or desiccated, dried fruits (go easy on them though as they are quite high in natural sugars), nuts, cacao nibs, lemon and orange peels, cinnamon, nutmeg – the list is endless really! Remember: moderation is the key here; you can have too many natural sugars too.

Minty lemon & banana hot cakes

This recipe makes 2 small hot cakes.

1 organic egg

A few mint leaves –approx 8.

3 dessert spoons almond meal

1 dessert spoon desiccated coconut (1/2 – 1 teaspoon grated lemon rind (depending on your love of lemon)

1/3 of a large banana or 1/2 a small

1 heaped teaspoon coconut oil for pan

Organic Yoghurt of choice to adorn the top

Place a small pan on the stove on medium heat. Throw all of the above ingredients (bar yoghurt and coconut oil) in a blender (stick will do) and blend until well combined and smooth. Add the coconut oil to the pan when hot. Once melted plop 2 pikelet sized spoon fulls of the mixture into your pan and let them sit for about 2 minutes. Using an egg slicer gently check the underside, you want them to be golden before you turn them. When ready, flick them over and leave for a further 2 or so minutes. Pop them on a plate and dollop some yoghurt of choice on top.

Raw broccoli & spinach bites

2 cups broccoli

2 cups English spinach

1 1/2 cups sunflower seeds

1/2 cup pine nuts

1/2 chopped onion

4 tablespoons extra virgin olive oil

2 tablespoons chopped parsley

1 large garlic clove

1/2 - 1 teaspoon Himalayan or Celtic sea salt, to taste

1/2 teaspoon pepper

1/2 teaspoon nutmeg

Process the sunflower seeds until fine.

Add all remaining ingredients and blend well into a thick paste.

Place teaspoon or dessertspoon sized bites onto a teflex sheet or baking paper for your oven.

Dehydrate for 8-15 hours on your pilot light in the oven (approximately 50°C) or 40°C in your dehydrator. Turn the bites over after approximately 5 hours.

These will keep in the fridge for up to a week or freeze and use as required. Serve with pesto, salsa, hummous.

Amy Crawford from theholisticigredient.com kindly donated her Minty Lemon & Banana Hotcakes and Raw Spinach bites recipes for this section. Amy used to suffer from Chronic Fatigue Syndrome and got better by eating organic whole foods.

You can find more amazing recipes in her beautiful ebook 'A Nourishing Kitchen' which is available for purchase through my website.

Kale chips

If you are a chip addict you will love these and they may just convert you away from potatoes deep fried in trans fats when an attack of 'the munchies' strikes. After all, why do that when you could be satisfying your urges with vital, beautiful, natural, nutrient-rich whole foods?

Needless to say, there is no deep frying involved here. You simply make a 'sauce' to massage into the kale; then you put the mixture into the dehydrator and prepare to be amazed at how crunchy it goes. That's thanks to the nut-based coating which takes on that texture when dried. You'll also be amazed at how cheeeeesy they taste. It's the nutritional yeast that achieves this flavor. The only downside to this recipe: it is as messy to make as it is challenging not to eat the whole batch straight out of the dehydrator!

Ingredients:

- 200g curly leaf kale (if not ready chopped, you'll need to slice it into vaguely crisp-sized pieces, removing the stalks)
- 100g raw cashews
- 1 large red bell pepper
- Juice of one lemon
- 25–50g nutritional yeast
- 1 cm piece of red chili
- Himalayan crystal salt or Celtic sea salt to taste

1. Chop the red pepper into small pieces and add to a blender with the lemon juice. Blend until smooth.
2. Add the cashews, red chili and ½ teaspoon salt and again blend until smooth.
3. Add the nutritional yeast and blend again. Doing it in stages like this helps you to get the smooth consistency you need without overheating it.
4. Put the kale in a large bowl, then pour the blended mixture over it and massage it in until all the leaves are coated.

5. Place it on dehydrator trays with Paraflexx sheets and dehydrate at 110 degrees. After two hours peel off the Paraflexx sheets and place the chips-in-progress on mesh sheets. You can also use a regular oven too; turn on lowest setting and leave the door open and bake for 6–8 hours, checking often.

6. By the time they have been in for 8 hours they should be seriously crunchy. If they aren't, just leave them in until they are! Taste, and if they're not salty enough, sprinkle some over and then enjoy!

Try these and you'll swear that kale was put on the planet all those eons ago so that in the 21st century creative raw-chef genius types could identify its true destiny as a crunchy savory snack.

(Recipe courtesy of sarahbesthealth.com)

Chocolate Mousse

This is one of the nicest desserts you can make – so quick and easy too!

- ½ cup medjool dates, soaked
- ½ cup maple syrup
- 1½ cups mashed avocados, ripe
- ½ – ¾ cup raw cacao/cocoa powder
- ½ cup water/rice/almond milk
- 1 tsp vanilla extract/powder

Blend until smooth – makes 2 cups

(Recipe inspired from the nouveauraw.com website)

Chocolate Fudge

- Generous ½ cup almond butter
- 3 tablespoons agave
- 5 drops vanilla stevia
- ½ teaspoon pure vanilla extract

- ¼ cup cacao powder
- 1 tablespoon lucuma powder
1. Add the almond butter, agave (or other liquid sweetener), stevia, vanilla and a pinch of Himalayan salt to a bowl.
2. Stir it all together.
3. Add in the powders and stir again. Sift if your powders are lumpy OR throw all the ingredients into a food processor.
4. Press into a small container lined with plastic wrap. Press chopped nuts into the top (optional).
5. Chill and slice!

Chocolate Fudge recipe courtesy from the fantastic sweetlyraw.com website created by Heather Pace. Heather makes all sorts of incredible desserts, meals, ice creams, drinks and so much more. Look out for the eBooks that Heather has written.

Happy Chocolate

Cacao itself is a natural mood booster. It contains naturally occurring chemicals such as anandamide and serotonin, which shift our consciousness and elevate our spirits. It does this by strengthening the neural pathways and encouraging the brain to create more of these chemicals itself, in contrast to pharmaceutical antidepressants which block the natural uptake of neurotransmitters and so create dependency on the medication.

Two things to remember: First, I have included four of the most powerful uplifting plant herbs I know of; you don't have to use them all, but if you do, you'll be having a real party! The second thing is, because of the way pharmaceutical medication works, it is not a good idea to use these herbs, particularly mucuna, at the same time as antidepressants. If you, or someone you are close to, is on medication, it's best to see a trained naturopath who can support you or them in coming off medication first.

Ingredients:

- 75g (¾ cup) cacao powder
- 100g (1 cup) cacao butter
- 100g (1 cup) mesquite or carob powder
- 60 ml (¼ cup) agave
- 1 tsp mucuna powder
- 1 tsp he shou wu powder
- ½ tsp blue manna or e3 AFA mend
- ½ tsp Etherium Gold

Melt the cacao butter on a low heat. This is best done by chopping it finely first, then standing it in a heat-proof bowl in a pan of gently simmering water. Once it's melted, stir in all the other ingredients together. Pour into a tray lined with greaseproof paper or aluminum foil. If you have silicon molds, that's even better, because they give a nice shiny professional finish to your chocolate. Put in the fridge to set – should take up to 2 hours. Once it's done, store in an airtight container in the fridge. it should keep up to 8 weeks.

Macappucino Coffee Substitute

This is one of my favorite drinks! Really hits the spot; it's warm, comforting, calming and energizing and the perfect pick-me-up on a cold grey day. All these ingredients are strengthening and fortifying and provide energy without depleting the body's reserves or stressing the adrenals (unlike coffee). The grain coffee substitute is just there for flavor, if you like a deeper coffee taste; personally I usually omit it.

Ingredients:

- 1 tsp maca powder
- 1 tsp coconut oil
- ¼ tsp Reishi extract
- 1 tsp raw honey or agave
- 1 tsp coffee substitute e.g. Barleycup or Bambu (optional)
- 300 ml heated water

Boil the water as if you were making a cup of tea. Put all the ingredients, including the water, into the blender together and whiz for a minute. Pour this frothy, creamy drink into your favorite mug and enjoy.

Happy Chocolate and Macappucino recipes courtesy of Kate Magic, speaker, educator and author of several popular raw food books:

✓ rawliving.eu

Chapter 20

Why Exercise Is Vital: You Simply *Can't* Be Truly Healthy or Happy Without It

We all know we should do it, yet many of us don't. I was too sick for 20 years to do any regular form of exercise. I always knew that I was in a vicious cycle. I needed to exercise to get more energy but I always felt too tired to start. Being tired and unmotivated to exercise is a sign that you are lacking energy and something needs to change.

Movement is the key to vitality and it doesn't really matter what form it is in; we just have to do something, and every day too. It is important for us to move regularly because we need to get the blood and oxygen flowing around our body. We are not designed to sit around a lot and do nothing. There are many different types of exercise but I have listed the things that even Miss Lazy Bones (me) found to be really good.

Jump for fun

For people who find it difficult to motivate themselves, I would recommend getting a good-quality rebounder, which is also called a mini trampoline. These are not only so much fun; they are also incredibly good for you.

A NASA report published in the Journal of Physiology (posted on the website Rebound UK) cites that benefits are 'greater with jumping on a trampoline than with running'. Cellular exercise strengthens the cells of the body for more efficient oxygenation, and rebounding is one of the best ways to do just that.[106]

Rebounders also help to release endorphins which is what makes you feel happy. Anyone suffering from depression should jump as regularly as they can. The first time I did it, I loved it so much that I turned on some upbeat music and jumped all day – well, literally for 4 hours. The mental and physical high I experienced (which I hadn't had in years) was incredible. But please *don't* do it for as long as I did, because it could really hurt your back and legs – as it did mine for the next four days. Moderation is the key here. Bouncing for only 15 minutes a day (some say even 5 minutes is incredible beneficial) really helps strengthen the lymphatic system and can tone and tighten your muscles. It is also wonderful for strengthening bone density. And the best thing is, it's also very, very good for cellulite so, ladies, if that bothers you, get one of these little tramps and start bouncing.

A handy tip is to have it in the house where you can use it easily (not put somewhere like the garage where it's out of the way). I have mine in my lounge room and make sure I try and bounce for a good 15 minutes each day. Try to invest in a good one too because the cheaper they are, the more harsh the bounce can be on your joints and back. And wear a good supportive sports bra too, ladies, otherwise it will bounce and stretch your boobs till one day they hit the ground and may stay there.

Jason Vale, who is also known as the 'Juice Master', is a big advocate of rebounding for exercise. He has his own range of great-quality rebounders which he sells through his site. You want to find a rebounder that has a soft bounce so good quality is a must here. You can also purchase DVDs to help you do set routines while bouncing.

✓ juicemaster.com

Kettle bells

For weight training, I love using Russian 'kettle bells'. These funny little odd-shaped balls with handles are one of the best and quickest ways to tone your muscles, and are said to be much more effective than using regular dumbbells, and may mean that you can exercise for shorter periods to get a better result.[107] You only need to do a few sets every couple of days to notice impressive results. Kettle bells help to create tight abdominals, thereby helping to strengthen your very important core area. It's also been discovered that with regular use, kettle bell training can help improve oxygen consumption levels, which is very important for a healthy body.[108]

You can use them in a short workouts and still effectively train your body to become fit and strong. They can be purchased on Ebay/Amazon or from sports stores. And there are YouTube videos which will help you learn how to use them. A really great piece of exercise equipment – those Russians sure are smart! And another great reason to use them is that they burn fat really quickly too.

Lots of cardio for weight loss may be a big fat myth!

We have been led to believe that the more cardio we do, the more fat we burn and the healthier we will be. But is this really true? Evidence is suggesting the opposite. And I think it makes sense. Take a look around. When you go to a gym, what is really common to see? Many overweight people walking and running on a treadmill for long periods. And when you see the same people in the gym, day in and day out, quite often doing this, what does it make you think? Maybe what they are doing is not working perhaps? Information is coming out that too much cardio puts your body into a non fat-burning mode and leaves the exerciser with very poor results. It can work well for some people but I definitely don't think it's right for everybody and for each hormonal type of person. If it did, the overweight people in the gym slogging away for an hour would lose weight quickly.

While lots of cardio was once touted as the way to protect yourself from having a heart attack, it's now thought that too much cardio puts an enormous amount of stress on your heart. With the amount of men that suddenly drop dead while jogging (and in 2012 a female marathon runner also died during her race), I think we can all see that this has more than some truth to it. Also, long-distance running can cause your tissues to break down when the body is pushed into a catabolic state. Too much cortisol is then released (a dangerous stress hormone) which also causes catabolism but can then go on to create chronic disease. Too much cardio can put an enormous amount of strain on the immune system, causing it to weaken so that you get sick more often. And it can even cause insomnia if you choose to exercise in the afternoon or evening. If you are into doing marathons, watch out, because you are at greater risk of harming yourself through such vigorous and long stints of exercise. A study in Montreal, Canada, discovered that marathon runners were at a sevenfold risk of raising the likelihood of triggering cardiac problems.[109]

Now, I am not saying that any cardio is a waste of time, because some is needed to be healthy. The key is to do the correct amounts. What is becoming very popular because of very fast results is 'interval training' such as the so-called 'Peak 8'. It is so successful at showing quick results because these short bursts of high intensity cause your body to produce high doses of Human Growth Hormone (HGH), something that declines a lot as we age. We have a lot of HGH when we are young and it keeps us looking exactly that, but like all things, as we get older it unfortunately decreases, and quite quickly too.

This form of 'Peak 8' training has been shown to dramatically cause the body to produce high levels of the 'fountain of youth' hormone. This fountain of youth hormone makes you strip fat fast, as well as replace it with muscle very quickly.

For an idea of what Peak 8 is: I started doing 8 sets of 30-second sprints with a break of 90 seconds in between. I did this 3 times a week (no more is needed) and lost weight and saw muscle tone like never before! I had to stop when I found out I was pregnant but knew that this was what I would get back into as soon as I could return to exercise normally again. I also love the fact that I can squeeze a session in wherever I want. It also only takes 20 minutes to do in total (with the high-intensity part only taking 4 minutes) so there is no excuse not to fit it in three times a week! It's hard work, but also over before you know it.

I know it works because it is the only method I have personally used that has ever given me results with weight loss that happened very quickly. I was one of those people that thought long sessions of cardio was the way to get fit and healthy. It actually didn't do me any good and I didn't lose a scrap of weight. Other people who I know use this method (even those over 60) look absolutely incredible. Longer sessions of cardio may work for you, but if it doesn't then consider looking into Peak 8. Like most things in life, what may work for one person may not work for another.

You can find out more about Peak 8 fitness on mercola.com

Yoga

Yoga is one of the most popular forms of exercise these days. No longer is it just for the enlightened Indians to do; it's become so well known that you can pretty much find classes anywhere. And it's a very easy form of exercise to do from home in front of the TV with a great instructional DVD.

Yoga is so good for the human form because it puts the body in untypical positions, and therefore uses many different muscles that are usually never used. This helps the body to become toned and supple, and it also has an anti-aging effect. Look at any serious yoga person: they tend to never look their age and their skin tone is very healthy and vibrant. Certain positions in yoga can actually help to detoxify the body as well. There are twists and other poses that you can do which squeeze and put gentle pressure on the kidneys, liver and other organs to encourage them to function more efficiently.

If you are pregnant then doing yoga throughout your pregnancy is one of the best things you can do for a successful labour. The stronger your core is, the easier it will be to help get the baby out and also for your body to bounce back into shape. Always consult an expert though if pregnant to help with choosing the right kind of poses.

Yoga is also incredible for the mind and is a form of meditation. And for the guys reading this out there, do not think that yoga is for girls! There are many forms of yoga, such as *ashtanga*, which is very heavy going and takes a lot of strength and co-ordination. I always suggest to people who are new to yoga to try the *hatha yoga* style. It is very easy to follow, not too strenuous and very fun to do. Yoga not only helps you to become fit and supple; it also may help you to overcome anxiety and depression and just change your life for the best overall!

I have included a few personal stories below from people who found that yoga not only made them much fitter, but also completely enhanced their lives.

How yoga changed my life
by Helena

I was badly injured from teaching too much aerobics, aged 26, and also into the cocaine lifestyle with weekends of champagne and sleepless nights, when I peered through a gym studio windowed door and saw what was called an iyengar yoga class going on!

Being arrogant and very fit, I imagined that this non-aerobic class was not for me; how wrong was I!

My shoulder was recovering from tendinitis and my ripped calf muscle was sore, but I decided to take the plunge and took a class the next week. The teacher was very iyengar, bossy and strict, and I wasn't that impressed, but the next day I could not believe the effect it had on my body. I was in agony... and as I was into 'no pain – no gain' at that point of my life, I loved it!

I started attending twice a week. My body became stronger and stronger. I couldn't meditate (that took years) – the very thought of that side of yoga bored the pants off me – but I knew something was going on. I began to enjoy the relaxation and that was massive for me!

From there it just grew. I stopped taking drugs a few years after and I added body balance to my CV and taught that successfully in and around London. I stopped teaching aerobics altogether then and assisted a friend of mine on a yoga retreat in Lanzarote for 9 months

– this is where the real yoga began. This is where I had an awakening: the total peace of existence flooded my body and I felt total peace after a pranayama session for the first time EVER!

I was also studying with Barbara Wren at the College of Natural Nutrition at this time. The new peace I found encouraged me to take responsibility for my own life and health and I healed myself naturally from an underactive thyroid, amenorrhea and eating disorders.

I completed my yoga teacher training and got a distinction; taught in retreats all over Europe; deeply detoxed and cleansed my colon and mind (which are very closely linked); and continued to learn with amazing yogis and friends all over the world.

It just doesn't stop! Yoga isn't about doing a headstand or sitting for 20 minutes each day; yoga is LOVE so it resonates in all that we do and allows us to be our own truth without judgement or criticism.

They call yoga asana 'your practice', as it takes years of practice to really feel and understand what's going on with it all… and then you just keep learning and feeling and opening.

Keep going… it's so worth it in the end.

How yoga transformed my life
by Dr. Claire Maguire

My idea of yoga was old ladies stretching. I'm not sure where this idea came from, perhaps from the image, which had lodged in my brain at the tender of age of 10, of my friend's mum doing yoga. Thinking about it now, that friend's mum was probably only in her mid-30s and yet I had made a mental association of her being old! And here I was now in my mid-30s, not feeling old at all, contemplating yoga. For I had tuned in a bit and begun to realize that yoga was getting popular as a way to keep fit. Just what I needed, and hey, I was pretty flexible. So I thought, with my ego, that I could go along and show the old ladies a thing or two!

In I stumbled to my local village hall with a small group of people around my age, all dressed in white. Strange. We started off with a chant. Even stranger. We breathed, did movements. This was fine. Then we started to chant while bent over, moving our heads from side to side, opening up our throat chakra, I was told. Whoa… this took me completely out of my comfort zone. What the hell was that all about? Chanting strange words! That's not for me, I thought.

But as one to give something another chance, I strolled up to the yoga class the following week. It was the same as the week before: opening chant, breathing, moving and then that chant again with the head movement. I was prepared this time and embraced the strangeness of it (relished the idea of my throat chakra opening).

We finished with a group meditation, which the week before I had dismissed as strange, odd, not what I do, yet this time… something within me stirred. I felt tears spontaneously fall down my face. This was not normal, surely. I mean yoga was to get fit, right?! However, those tears that fell felt so right, for I knew within me the search I had been on, a search to feel a path to my heart and desires, had been found. The tears that fell had dislodged something profound inside me. I didn't know what. I just felt. And I was hooked.

For my life was in turmoil. Wracked with self-doubt, low expectations, unsure of who I was. Confused by the yearning of ambition to create a difference and unable to express what I could offer the world. Trapped in mayhem. Surrounded by chaos. Living in a mutually self-destructive relationship.

Therefore, for me, *kundalini yoga* became something more than a mere way to get fit. It enveloped me in the exquisiteness of the wholeness of the person. I went week after week, and it opened up greater parts of me. I felt sensations that wracked my body with joy. I felt energy buzz around me in a heightened way. Nothing had touched me like this before.

I explored deeper, wanting to know more and more about this form of exercise. As I did, my body and mind subtly shifted. I felt better within me. I stumbled from yoga into raw foods and, as I did, so a greater transformation occurred.

I took a hard look at my then current life and made the decision that I didn't want the destructive relationship I was in. I left my husband, the father of my children, after a relationship of 11 years, to set myself upon a new path of freedom. It was scary and liberating. Kundalini was beside me throughout.

I committed to a 40-day *kriya*, as I had heard that the way to get the most benefit and transformative power out of a particular kriya was to practice the same one for 40 days. It was profound. I felt truly renewed by the end. I felt a new woman. It was unbelievably amazing, uplifting, inspiring. I was unrecognizable and my mind was clear and free.

I love the fact that kundalini yoga goes much deeper than the mere physical body, that it takes you to a full expressive connection within your mind and soul. It creates a sense of harmony of emotions and a compassion for yourself.

I am thankful that kundalini yoga has now become a part of my life, as it forms the backbone of the wellbeing retreats I have the privilege of running. The pleasure of introducing other women to feel the power of the kundalini and to see something stir within them fills my heart every time.

Dr. Maguire runs retreats in Yorkshire which have an emphasis on raw food, personal transformation and empowerment. She also teaches yoga throughout the retreats.

✓ splitfarthinghall.co.uk

Hot yoga

Another method of yoga which you may love is 'hot yoga'. Hot yoga, also known as *bikram yoga*, was named after its creator, Bikram Choudhury, who took yoga to a new level. Incorporating hatha yoga poses, hot yoga is different because classes are taught in very hot rooms, allowing the attendees to work up a real sweat. With temperatures up to 40 degrees Celsius, it's not for the faint-hearted, and if you have a heart condition this type of yoga is not for you.

Personally, I have not yet tried it as I am not too good in really hot environments but I have several friends who swear by it. The intense sweating would help you detox through your skin but I imagine the rooms would also be full of some not-so-nice smells.

Hike, run, walk, dance, swim or just do something!

The key to any regular program of exercise is to find something that you love, which makes you feel good and increases the chances of you doing it more often. If you push yourself through difficult routines that you really don't like, then it usually means, over the long term, you won't continue doing it, and before you know it, it will be 6 months before you have done any form of exercise. Gosh, don't I know that from personal experience!

Always try and walk as much as possible; avoid elevators and walk upstairs if possible. If you work in an office, whenever you go to the bathroom, do some squats near the toilet, so that you are stretching the muscles in your legs and butt. Walk down the stairs to lunch; even if you catch the elevator to the lower levels, get out and walk the last few flights down. These small things make a big difference as exercise is accumulative too.

One of the reasons elderly people have so much trouble with their joints later in life is simply due to lack of movement when they were younger. So if you want to avoid having aches and pains when you're older, get up and move about starting today.

Some surprising benefits of regular exercise[110]

Most of us know why we should exercise – to keep our weight down, to keep our hearts healthy and to live a longer life – but there are quite a few more reasons which aren't really well known. Here are some fascinating and appealing effects that regular exercise may give you and may provide better reasons for you to do some.

Spice up your sex life

Benefits from increased blood flow, improved stamina and better body image may help improve your sex life. Exercise has been shown to increase arousal in women and reduce the risk of impotence for men.

Increase your immunity

Despite people thinking that when they come down with a cold, they should stay in bed, moderate exercise is actually one of the best medicines for cold and flu prevention. Studies show that people who exercise regularly get fewer colds and need fewer sick days than those who are more sedentary. Exercise boosts our immune system in quite a few ways: It gets rid of bacteria from the lungs, so reduces your risk of catching a cold or other illness. It speeds up the delivery of disease-fighting antibodies throughout the body and temporarily increases body temperature. This helps to prevent bacterial growth and allows the body to fight infection much more quickly and slows the release of stress hormones, which increase the risk of illnesses. Please note: Very intense exercise might have the opposite effect on the immune system – so don't overdo it!

Boost your brain

Exercise increases your ability to learn and also helps you to be a much better multi-tasker. It can also protect brain health and general brain function.

Get better sleep

With so many of us suffering from poor sleep, if you aim to get 150 minutes of activity per week it can help improve sleep quality by 65 percent, according to a study in the journal Mental Health and Physical Activity. The timing of your workouts is also important, as exercising too close to bedtime can actually interfere with sleep. It's best to avoid exercise at least 3 hours before bedtime.

Increase your pain tolerance

German researchers found that athletes often have higher pain tolerance compared to that of non-athletic yet still-active people. The two groups began to feel pain at similar times, but the athletes were better able to handle it. There is evidence showing that regular exercise makes your mental strength better too.

You can eat all the best food in the world, but if you don't do regular exercise it's not going to help you that much to lead a long and healthy life. So let's (me included!) do something energetic today.

Chapter 21

Finding Your Spirit to Discover the True You

Spirituality is not a religion. It is a journey and an inner connection. For some of us, it is a natural part of our way of being and living, but for others, it sometimes takes a crisis to bring changes of outlook and lifestyle. Illness, for example, can be viewed as a positive experience, an open door that invites us to change. We can take the opportunity to leave behind our old patterns, and embrace new ways to live and relate. But why wait for a crisis? By becoming more committed to our spiritual journey, a whole new world opens for us.[111]
Glennie Kindred, author of *Earth Wisdom*

The Story Of Paul

I spent some time with a family friend who really brought it home to me that working on our inner sense of happiness is much more important than I ever originally thought. I will give you a little background history so that you can see how an unhappy life begins and how it can end up if you don't do something about dealing with your inner pain and find out who you really are underneath it all.

My friend Paul, had been brought up in a house with a very emotionally abusive mother. She pretty much displayed psychotic tendencies at times, which meant that Paul always feared what mood she would be in. Would she be nice today and make him feel loved and would they have fun, or would she fly into a spiteful and cruel rage today and say the most horrible things to him, confusing the memories of a past good day.

This emotionally abusive roller coaster and ill treatment from bad parenting, of course, created a deeply unhappy childhood for Paul, with the harmful effects still being there even though he was now well into his 60 s. In fact, the effects, for him, were worse than ever. Paul had never known how to sort out his emotional baggage and as the years passed, he was never really able to experience true joy. He was so disconnected from his feelings that even though Paul wasn't happy, it never occurred to him to ask himself why and what he could try and do about it. Paul just thought that was how his life was going to be.

Despite saying to himself he would never turn out like his mother, he actually *was* almost turning into her. His mother had always been terribly negative to be around, treated people badly, never gave anyone respect so many family members had simply stopped having anything to do with her.

Paul had kids of his own, all successful in their own way, but never tried to get to know any of them genuinely and found it much easier to put them down or instead, to be negative about their choices in life. Paul could not listen to their point of view, instead he always was the 'right' one and the kids never were in his eyes. Instead of being his own kid's biggest fan, he was their *biggest* critic. *Just like his mother was to him.*

Paul always had to be centre of attention and would get upset if he felt ignored, yet he would never make effort with anyone else. He never asked how someone was, or what they had been doing or what hobbies they had. He had been treating his kids like this ever since they could all remember. The time they spent around him now pushed a lot of buttons and it left them all feeling very upset and angry.

After working very hard for many years, Paul was just about to retire. One would think he would be so happy about this exciting new chapter in life, but it looked like he almost couldn't handle this newly found free time, away from the job where he got so much praise and attention. Every day, so many things were constantly being complained about, and from what an outsider could see, most were actually absolutely silly things. Car spaces were too small, everything was too expensive, people were all bad drivers, newspapers were the wrong size, meals didn't taste good and the service was too slow. It was just endless amounts of complaining. What came out of Paul's mouth was mostly always negative, and it was clear to see, nothing made him feel truly happy for long. It was hard to be around him because the negativity just alienated people. Even his kids were saying that they didn't really want to be around their own dad anymore. He was just too negative and didn't talk about anything interesting except to him.

Spending a few weeks witnessing this constant unhappy behaviour, made *me* realise just how many people spend their *entire* life, feeling like this. And I realized that unless one does something about it, those feelings will only get much worse. It *won't* just go away. That unhappiness and discontentment you have with your life now, won't disappear without *work*. And don't be fooled into thinking that 'doing things' will always make you happy.

Despite the good money Paul earned, or the wonderful places he traveled to or the lovely grandkids he saw grow up, there was always this melancholy and depression that was hanging around him. He was so engrossed in his negative way of thinking, that he couldn't even see that he was causing all of this unhappiness - no one else, just him. He had spent all these years working so hard but now that he had all this new free time, all the problems he developed from his unhappy childhood, were now rearing their ugly head in a big way, because he just didn't like dealing with his own thoughts. His unhappy times, were really only just beginning because now, more than ever, he had lots of time to think about all the things that made him miserable but made no recognition of needing to do something about them.

I would hope that by the age of 60, most of us will have found inner peace and happiness, but truthfully, unless you are born with a naturally happy personality (which some lucky people are) then you may have to really really work at it. Happiness takes effort. It's not something you just become, you have to create it. We are living in what could be called the most stressful times in history. We may have 'more' than ever before, but it's not made us any happier, only worse. We have to deal with seeing others have more than us, even if we have a lot more than other people, and society has made us not be grateful for it and the media constantly downloads more desires that we feel we must achieve.

And, if we *do* live a long life, we may end up living completely on our own in our final stages of life on earth. We also may end up as widows. And, if you aren't a nice person to be around, then your friends will be minimal and your family probably won't want to visit you and the visits that you look forward to because you are so lonely, may become less and less regular.

Any discontentment with your life, how wisely you spent it will be much more obvious in your elderly years.

I personally think a life well spent means that we have prepared ourselves for the future and for the day where long periods of time may be spent completely on our own. This is not me being negative, it's being realistic, as not many have the luck of living with family until their time is up. And this means, we must be able to be there with ourselves, to sit with our own thoughts and memories and to be able to look back on our life and think, 'It's been a good life, I laughed a lot, I loved my friends and kids, I experienced so much, I was lucky. I can sit here with my thoughts and I like who I am, who I was to people and what I did for society. I spent my time here wisely.'

This story is why I feel *very* strongly about working on improving our mental health, sorting out our problems carried on from our childhood and, on finding our spirit - our real purpose in life. And to know that this is *why* we are here. Despite us all probably knowing someone like Paul, his story is *not* one that you want to have in common with.

What IS Your Purpose?

I'm sure you have already asked yourself, 'What is the meaning of life?' or '*Why* am I here?' I know I *certainly* asked myself these questions time and time again for many years, and, as I was never able to answer them properly, I was left feeling very confused and deeply unhappy. I just didn't understand what my life was supposed to be about. It was depressing to feel useless and not able to do anything of benefit.

Finding your spirit also means connecting with what is called your 'intuition' – you know, when you have to make a decision and you can sense the right answer? But for many, they get the wrong answer because they haven't learnt to really listen to their inner selves. Finding your spirit also means getting in touch with your soul.

One way of connecting to your spirit is through meditation. Meditation has become a very accepted form of stress relief these days with many doctors now recommending it. Through the act of sitting, being still and deep breathing, within seconds the body and mind is able to achieve a very relaxed state. Hypnotherapists also use this technique to get into our subconscious minds where they can help us to overcome fears and anxieties, unlock past memories, and actually 'reprogram' the mind. It's interesting to know that the word 'inspiration' is not only used to define breathing, but that we use it to describe what drives and motivates us.

So to become *inspired*, we must perform *inspiration* through deep breathing. Yoga and getting close to Nature, are forms of meditation too. Try to sit still for at least 10 minutes every day; don't try and shut your thoughts off, but instead pay attention to them and see what keeps coming up. The more you do this, the more you will find yourself less stressed and will often also be able to deal with tough situations much better. Meditation allows you to be still with your inner thoughts and can bring a profound sense of peace. By practicing meditation, you can really get to know yourself, through seeing how you 'talk' to yourself, what memories come up and what you feel you need to improve.

If you have trouble meditating, like so many do, myself included, the following tips, inspired by the book *Falling into Easy* by Dee Willock[112] may help.

Sitting in the right position

This is usually cross-legged or sitting on a chair. Lying down may mean that you fall asleep, so sometimes being a bit uncomfortable will help you to meditate. When I try, I find myself getting super–itchy and cannot sit still! This is common too and only goes away the more you practice.

Making a space just for meditating

If you want to get serious about your practice, then it may be a good idea to create a little area just for this. You can get comfy cushions, or a nice chair, and surround it with incense (the non-toxic kind of course!), aromatherapy, music, candles and crystals. Buddhists will have status of Buddha to look at and may also use beads to hold. You can make it whatever way you like, but just be sure that it's an area that relaxes you.

Finding the time

Like most things, the more regular we are, the better and easier it becomes. Meditating is exactly the type of thing that responds to regular sessions. Some say it's best first thing in the morning and those that are serious may get up before the crack of dawn to meditate as the sun goes up. If you can't manage sessions every day, try to do it a few times a week, even if it's just for 10 minutes.

Breathing correctly

Breathing is so powerful. It can relieve us of tension and pain and get us quickly relaxed in no time at all. Women who do hypnobirthing say that they had a pain-free birth purely down to the way that they breathed, as well as visualizing and practicing the technique. I didn't exactly have a pain-free birth but I did manage to have it without drugs and I do credit the deep breathing with this. When meditating, breathing deeply is very important. There are many types of ways to breathe during meditation; some prefer breathing slowly, while others will do more vigorous types of breath work such as pranayama. If you want to find an example, YouTube have plenty of videos on this subject.

Letting your thoughts think

It used to be that we were told we must 'empty our minds' to meditate properly, but now so many are saying: No, that's not always right. You can let your thoughts enter you mind; take notice of them and then let them go. You can learn a lot about yourself when certain words or memories pop up in your mind; some will be a bit silly or odd and others may be quite profound.

* * *

If you find these tips still don't really help, you might like to read the book, *Falling Into Easy: Help For Those That Can't Meditate* by Dee Willock.

There are many ways to get to know your inner self better. Lots of groups and organizations are out there which you can join to meet like-minded people and to also learn other ways to view the world. You might find lots of inspiration from Buddhism, or from other faiths, but you also don't necessarily need to join any. I think that when you sit by yourself and really go within, you can learn so much about life and what you want out of it. We just need to give lots of time and dedication to that part of ourselves which often gets ignored.

I will admit, I haven't done too much work on myself in regards to meditating. I don't do it very often (although I did do lots of hypnosis throughout my pregnancy) and it's always something I intend on doing soon. I have, however, found a big part of my spirit through writing and reading. I feel I have found my purpose and this makes my soul happy. I also listen to myself lots more now and trust my instincts.

If you are interested in finding out more about spiritual methods, a really great and fun book is *The High-Heeled Guide to Spirituality* by

Alice Grist. Alice spent a few years testing out many different spiritual subjects and shares her views on how effective they were for her. Heart-warming and very funny, this book really opens you up to the world of spirituality but in a way that is perfect for our modern times. It will give you some great ideas about things you could try and some that are completely fascinating to read about but not necessarily the right ones for you. A very enjoyable book.

Chapter 22

Kindness to Others Is the Key to Loving Yourself More

One of the best ways to love life more, and therefore yourself, is through acts of kindness to others. This may be the real key to a happy life. Look back to a time when someone did something very kind for you that really took you by surprise. And remember back to a time when you did something kind to someone else.

If you have no or few memories of these, do not worry – you can change that today. I believe that one of the greatest ways to experience love and joy is through acts of kindness.

I would like to say that I have spent my whole life doing kind things, but the truth is, I was often so miserable and self-absorbed that I rarely was able to see outside myself to help others that were in need. It was always about 'me', and at times it still is, so I have to remind myself to be more thoughtful. The older I have become, the more I have realized that I prefer to *give* things, rather than to receive. For example, I used to love receiving gifts, yet now I prefer to give gifts to people. I love the look on people's faces when I surprise them with something. Giving to them gives something even *better* back to me! It's such a beautiful exchange of energy, which really can make someone's day memorable. And kindness is infectious! When you do something kind for others, they may pass that desire to be kind to someone else. And studies have discovered that when you are kind to others, it gives you the same physical reactions that happen when someone is kind to you.

I feel that being kind, and giving something to others, is the quickest way to feel happy and to feel joy. So the more you do it, the happier you may be and the more joy you will experience. You don't have to always spend money on people to be kind; you can do random things that don't cost anything.

I did something last year that really shocked the person I did it for. It wasn't even a big deal but I could tell it made her feel really good. I was waiting at the bus stop near my house in the rain where I was standing underneath my huge umbrella. I saw a lady near me that was without one and was getting very wet. Without hesitation, I said to her, 'Can I share my umbrella with you?' At first, I could tell she was a bit shocked but after she said yes, she gave me a huge smile and she began to talk about her day ahead. I saw a whole bunch of people in front of us that also had big umbrellas but they didn't even think of offering it to her. What I did is not really that much, but I could tell that it put her in a good mood and I felt great too. So simple, yet a kind gesture that made a stranger's day just a tiny bit better.

It's very sad that we often ignore people suffering in front of us. The truth is, this happens every day in all corners of the earth. Many horrific crimes are carried out right in front of people where no one stepped in to help. Sometimes it may be dangerous to help, but more often than not, there is something that can be done, especially if a group of people band together and try to help the victim.

I remember being on a train once and noticed a lady sobbing. People were staring at her, yet not offering to help. I too was very shy about saying something then and there, but when the train stopped at where I was getting off, I gave her a tissue and said, 'I hope you are OK.' I never saw her again of course, but hoped that just that little bit of reaching out made her feel a tiny bit better, that someone who didn't know her saw that she was in pain, and that it concerned them. Everyone needs to know that they are worthy of concern.

I also remember being at a nightclub and seeing an underage girl who was obviously having a very bad reaction to some kind of drug. Her eyes were rolling around and she could not stand on her own. Her equally young friends sat around and weren't doing anything to help her. Knowing how young they were, it made me realize they were out on a night when they should have been at home, and their parents most likely had no clue they were among adults in the pretty seedy nightclubbing world. I went straight over to the bouncer and said, 'Look, that girl over there is on drugs and she doesn't look to be doing too well on them. I think she needs medical attention.' To the horror of her friends, the bouncer went over and started talking to them and later I saw the girl get carried out to an ambulance. I don't know to this day if that girl ended up being all right, but I am glad I did do something. Imagine if I didn't and she had died?

I always try and help in situations like that, even if it doesn't seem quite like my business to. To just do something is always worthwhile doing, rather than ignoring a situation. Too many people think, 'Oh, it's got nothing to do with me – I'm not going to get involved', yet this is quite selfish and often has dire consequences. A friend of my family died from a drugs overdose of Ecstasy, in Sydney back in the late 1990s, and it was all over the Australian media. Anna Wood, a beautiful girl with a bright future, on a Friday night took some Ecstasy with her friends and went out nightclubbing. After becoming violently ill, and subsequently drinking far too much water, her friends took Anna back home, thinking she would 'just sleep it off'. Due to being so young at the age of 15, they were scared to tell anyone, until of course, it was too late. After they ended up telling Anna's parents almost 12 hours after she started having a reaction, Anna was taken to hospital by ambulance and died a few days later after falling into a coma.

Now, imagine if *you* had seen this girl at the nightclub being very sick. It was later reported she was unable to stand and was seen vomiting a lot outside. If only someone had notified the bouncer that a young girl seemed to be very ill and needed emergency help! Anna would have received the urgent medical care she desperately needed and would probably still be alive today. That night, many people would have seen Anna – she was in a crowded nightclub surrounded by hundreds of people. But that night, too many people thought, 'It's not my business.'

I once lived next door to a woman who used to get beaten up by her partner. It was awful, hearing him yell at her and hearing her cries. It was obvious it was more than just a screaming match and it seemed he was definitely laying his hands on her. Because I had an abusive boyfriend years ago, I knew exactly what it was like to have your cries for help go unheard. It makes the abuse just so much worse because you know that the person who is being abusive to you doesn't really care, and the people around you who are hearing him do this to you obviously don't care either, as they aren't getting you help. That night in Sydney, I rang the police who then came over and took the man away. I don't know what happened after that, I don't know if that was the end of their relationship, but I don't like thinking about what *could* have happened if I hadn't helped.

The most disturbing case of abuse I witnessed was a small child, aged about 5, being yelled at and hit by her own mother, a neighbour of mine. I used to hear the child scream and would often go and peek out through the back window to see what was happening. I needed to see if it was as bad as what it sounded. The mother was very scary indeed and there was no father around to be seen. This poor child was still in nappies at age 5 and would quite often come down to the end of the garden where our fence was. I saw her try and climb over towards me, countless times, as if to try and get away. My other neighbor witnessed this abuse as well, yet instead of showing concern she said some awful, racist and careless things about the mother and child. She didn't seem to care that not only was this abuse against the law, but that the child's *human rights* were being violated by her own *mother.* After seeing enough of this behavior from the mother towards her little girl, I rang Child Protective Services and told them exactly what I had seen on way too many occasions.

It was a tough decision to make, as I knew that getting protective services involved sometimes may not be the best thing as they can literally take the child away from the parents and put him or her into foster care, which may not be the best care for the child. But, due to the repeated horror of what I saw, I knew that leaving this situation alone was far worse. That child should not have been living with her mother. It was much too abusive.

A few days after I told Child Protective Services what was going on, I had a knock on the front door. The father of the child knew I lived next door because of the report so that he came to speak to me. It seemed he had been trying to get his daughter away from his ex for years, because he knew that she was being abused by her. But he had no proof and was told that he couldn't do anything. After I signed the affidavit for him, he was able to go to court and fight for custody. He went to court and won sole custody of the little girl. I saw him with his daughter later in a shopping court and the child, to my relief, was happy and appeared to be very well taken care of. I was *very* glad I had stepped in on this occasion.

Daniel Morcombe, who went missing in 2003, dominated the Australian press for years. A huge PR campaign was launched to find out where Daniel had gone. After the Queensland police asked for witnesses to come forward, many people reported the same thing: they had driven past Daniel standing by the roadside and had seen two men speaking to him. They all felt that they knew something was 'not quite right' with this situation, but kept on driving and didn't give it another thought until they heard about the missing boy. If only they had stopped to ask him if he was alright! IF only they had listened closer to their intuition to stop and act upon it.

Please don't get me wrong here. I am not telling you these stories so you can think what a wonderful person I am; I'm not on an ego trip here, I haven't always done the right thing for others. I am no saint – I don't go around behaving like Mother Teresa every day – but I do try to do something when I can. Especially in cases where someone is having a hard time on drugs or alcohol or someone is being physically abused. I don't want to turn away from other people's suffering. We all should know that we are connected to each other and when someone else hurts and we ignore it, then it's not going to do us any good either. We need to show *far* more concern for those around us.

Over my deeply troubled years, I had many extremely kind people reach out to me during my tough times and I know, without a doubt, that their *actions* and kindness out of concern kept me alive. I was on the edge more times than I can remember, yet someone was always there to keep me from giving up. Even today, I will often have a friend do something for me that touches me in a way that brings tears to my eyes.

There are certainly much bigger examples of being kind out there, but even small actions, I believe, can be very powerful for others. Especially if they come from a stranger who does not *have* to help. We are all bound together by common things – that is, we are living, breathing, human beings and, if you go back in time, we are all related to each other, albeit very, very, very distantly. So we need to see strangers as *part* of us and that we all deserve the same things, such as kindness and empathy, and we do not deserve to be ignored and viewed as meaningless. Every human being wants to be loved, accepted and validated.

I always find it funny how lovely everyone is at Christmas time. You get wishes of 'Merry Christmas' and 'Happy New Year' from total strangers. It's so lovely, but shouldn't we be that kind and considerate *all* the time? Shouldn't we want to offer help to people around us all the time?

In the brilliant book, *Am I Being Kind?*, author Michael J. Chase explains the 10 ways we can be kind to people each and every day. Michael himself has a truly remarkable story: once very depressed and minutes away from committing suicide, he thought about the love and selflessness his cousin had always shown him throughout his life. Thinking of her, and how she was, stopped him from ending his life. She had constantly been very kind and generous to him and he knew that if he killed himself, it would kill a part of her too. He just couldn't do that to her. He vowed that day to be more like her and started to use kindness as his life's motto.

Michael has now founded The Kindness Centre, which teaches others that to achieve a spiritual connection with *all* things and to live a life of real joy, acts of kindness must be seen as vital. Michael shares his stories, such as visiting homeless shelters and taking flowers to give to people as well as listening to their stories, giving out free hugs and telling them that they do matter.

Michael also has devised the following 'Five Keys to Kindness':[113]

1. Being aware of one's own thoughts, words and actions
2. Always asking, before you do anything, 'Am I being kind?'
3. Adopting the 'Living Kindness Philosophy'
4. Applying the '9 Elements of a Kind Heart'
5. Regularly performing acts of kindness.

You can start implementing these keys in your life right now. In fact, a great way to start is to tell yourself that today you will do five kind things to strangers, neighbors, loved ones or friends. There are many ways of being kind, and it doesn't have to be big things. You can always offer any of these things to help others:

- Your time: Perhaps someone needs help with fixing things around the house, but they cannot afford to pay someone to do it. Your effort in helping them could be the best gift you could give to them, especially if they live on their own.
- Your money: Money directed at the right person or situation can often be a lifesaver.
- Your things: Do you have any items you don't need anymore which would benefit others?
- Your skills: If you have many skills, then sometimes these can be a big benefit to others.

You could always help people who are struggling with their shopping, or by baking something and giving it to your neighbor, taping enough money to a phone box along with a note saying, 'This next call is on me.' Sometimes, even being polite to someone in the street can be an act of kindness. Just lending a friendly ear to listen to someone's problem is a form of kindness.

As an experiment, Michael set goals over 24 hours to take groups of people out into the streets, handing out food, balloons, flowers, hugs and just spreading good cheer. It not only makes the receivers feel amazing, but the givers too report glowingly happy good feelings! Some people's *entire* outlook on life was changed from that experience.

✓ Visit the kindnesscentre.com

If you have young children, it's *very* important for them to see you behaving kindly to others. Because children often mirror our behavior and are influenced by us, it makes sense to let them see you care about others. There are many ways you can help to create a considerate nature in young children. Despite knowing that there are some very unfortunate people in the world who suffer greatly, we may at times want to shelter our children from knowing this. I believe this is a big mistake. If they understand at a young age that not everyone lives in the same way – some don't have enough to eat; some don't have a roof over their head – then it is more likely going to impact a child to want to help. Children are naturally compassionate when young, so at the right time, act on it. Doing some volunteer work and bringing your child along is a great way to do this.

If you educate your children that one person's behavior can really impact others, then they are more likely to want to try to be kind. Let them see articles in newspapers that show someone's bravery or kindness to others, so that they can see how it affected someone. And knowing that it ended up getting the kind person some media attention might make your impressionable child think, 'Cool, that could be me!' You can also choose children's reading books that have stories about a hero who did something kind or brave to help others.

Some inspirational books to read about how kindness affects people are *The Bond* by Lynne McTaggart and *Paradise Built in Hell* by Rebecca Solnit.

Chapter 23

Why Forgiveness Is the Best Gift to Give to Yourself

If there is one aspect to life that causes so much pain to people, it's the inability to forgive.

I spent my own life being so bitter towards others that I know it also made me very sick. I blamed *everyone* for my own problems and latched on to such dark feelings for years and years. I would think about what certain people had done to me each and every single day and would also repeat those stories of abuse, neglect and subsequent heartache to anyone that would listen as to how badly I had been treated. While some of the things that had happened to me weren't exactly nice, and it was normal to react that way to them, what I was doing to *myself*, due to continuously being so bitter, was even worse. I had no idea that constantly thinking someone 'owed me' was more punishment than what the original issue was even about. I was using all of my thought space thinking such negative things, to the point where I was not able to think positively at all, and therefore my life completely *mirrored* my negativity.

Some people have had the most horrific things happen to them: perhaps they were physically or sexually abused or even lost their loved ones in extreme cases such as murder or something else just as tragic. While it's *completely* understandable that they would go through a period of intense pain, anger and sadness, these feelings must be dealt with eventually if the person is to *move forward* with their own lives. If they are to continue to be unable to forgive the people that hurt them or their loved ones, they will never ever move on from that event and it can even make them sick – and desperately unhappy in the process.

In a way, the perpetrator 'wins' again because the sufferer continues to feel pain from what they have done. Some people, unfortunately, can be so displaced from their own soul that they take glee in someone else's suffering. They won't try and make up for what they have done; they will only feel good about hurting you. So it's always important to try and break free by letting go of the anger you feel due to how they treated you.

The inability to forgive also affects many different extremes. There are many ways of being hurt, some minor and some major.

It always causes me much dismay when I read news stories about people in jail who are on death row, about to be executed. People sometimes camp outside the prison with placards displaying horrible words, *wishing* the death of that person. It's understandable to be shocked and disgusted at how cruel someone was to another human being, but to be *so* angry and wish pain and even death to that other person is just not how we should be.

When a family is affected by crime, more often than not, they will spend every waking moment thinking about what that person did and wishing revenge on them. While it's true that some people should not be allowed to be a part of society (they may not be able to be rehabilitated no matter what), the victims left behind go on suffering again and again because of wanting 'justice' for the other person. Because of this, the victims rarely ever move on. So the pain and anger continue day in and day out, causing a life of deep unhappiness. It is rare that someone can forgive after such terrible atrocities, but it does happen.

Back in 2006, a man shot fire at 10 schoolgirls in a school in the Amish county of Southern Lancaster County, USA.[114] Five of the girls died, but the five who survived were in critical condition. To this peaceful community of Amish people, who were known to be very gentle and always kept to themselves, this senseless act of violence was beyond shocking. People were outraged that this man could be so awful, and wished revenge upon him. But to the Amish, who were the ones that truly had the 'right' to be angry, it seemed that all they could do was forgive him. The *entire* Amish community, parents of the deceased children included, all gathered around to say that they had forgiven him. They later learned that he had lost his own daughter years before, and had suffered such intense grief and was so distraught that he had temporarily lost his mind. The gunman also ended up taking his own life in the school yard that day.

The parents who lost their daughters, as well as the community, did not take weeks or months to say they had forgiven the man; in fact, it only took them 6 hours. And not only were they quick to forgive – they were also very upset for the gunman's *own* family. A big group of them visited his family to express their sorrow at what had happened and to see if they were alright. When Charles Roberts (the gunman) was laid to rest, over half of the mourners in attendance were the Amish. Some had even tragically buried their own daughters the day before. Astounding, right?

The world was absolutely stunned by this compassionate act of forgiveness. Some people simply could not understand. How could these people so quickly look at this terrible man with such caring eyes? How could they not hold any anger towards the gunman who took away their precious daughters?

The Amish said it was because they had always known that the way forward is never to be hateful or vengeful, and that being unable to forgive is so negative for their *own* lives and that it serves no useful purpose. In the Lord's Prayer (the Amish are devout Christians) it says the following: 'Forgive us our transgressions as we forgive those transgressions against us.' The Amish literally have taken this to heart and this is why they were able to forgive the gunman so easily.

When someone commits a terrible crime, rarely does the media (or people in general) bother to look into someone's past to see how they were brought up. Many times these dangerous criminals have had very troubled childhoods (some so horrific we can't even being to imagine) and, when given a little bit of insight into someone's own world, we may be able to understand why they lashed out like this.

Families with poor communication and weak family bonds have been shown to have a correlation with children's development of aggressive/criminal behavior (Garnefski & Okma, 1996). Therefore it seems obvious to conclude that those families who are less financially sound, perhaps have more children, and who are unable to consistently punish their children will have a greater likelihood of promoting an environment that will influence antisocial or delinquent behavior. Another indicator of future antisocial or criminal behavior is that of abuse or neglect in childhood. A statistic shows that children are at a 50% greater risk of engaging in criminal acts, if they were neglected or abused.[115]

Another rarely considered fact is that they may have huge doses of heavy metals in their brains. Many of these criminals often have behavioral problems such as ADD, ADHD and other personality disorders.[116] While it does not excuse their shocking acts, it still pays us to think about *what* may drive someone to do these things. Was it 100% their fault or were they victims of circumstances they could not control? I really believe that toxins in the brain are one of the missing links we need to look into much more in regards to criminal behavior. Imagine if we detoxed people and kept them out of jail! Much better for the taxpayer and far fewer crimes and murders would be committed! And of course we have mentioned previously, in reasonable detail, about what certain psychiatric medications are capable of doing to people's behavior too.

I once met a psychotherapist who worked in a jail in Australia. I was absolutely fascinated by her job and would often ask questions about the criminals: what were they like, were they scary, etc.? Although of course she would never name names, she would sometimes tell me about some of their pasts and childhoods, and I was regularly *shocked* and horrified at how these people had been brought up. Some had *never* known love or even received much attention, and some had suffered such horrible abuse by their parents that it made me think that if anger and violence was *all* that they had ever known, then no wonder they continued that cycle as adults. No one had been able to show them hope or show them what love really was, so therefore all that they could do was try and offload their pent-up anger by being cruel and dangerous to society. It was the *only* way they knew how to be. Absolutely tragic, isn't it? And it makes you see criminals in a whole new light. They are not just 'bad' people, but victims of awful childhoods that go completely against what Nature wanted for them.

Forgiveness towards someone else is the best thing you can do for *yourself*. Most of the time, the other person may not even know that you have forgiven them, but at least *you* will be free of the bitterness, pain and suffering that you have been dishing out to yourself. And forgiveness does not mean that you have to take have these people into your lives again; sometimes things are just irreparable, but at least if you can let go, then whatever happened won't play on your mind so much, impinge on your happiness or even contribute to high levels of stress which can lead to serious illness.

If you are holding grudges of any kind, I strongly recommend that you try and work through them, for your *own* sake. Letting things build up over time is so stressful to your health. There are many wonderful books on the subject, which can help you to try and overcome what happened, no matter how big or small the initial situation was. Forgiving someone may be one of the hardest things you ever do, and it may take years for you to get to that point, but let me assure you, from my own personal experience, it *sets you free when you let go.*

The ancient Hawaiian practice that is called *Ho-oponopono* may be well worth looking into if you want to work on forgiveness of others or even towards yourself. People that practice this modern-day interpretation of the original prayer say daily, 'I'm sorry. Please forgive me. I love you. Thank you.' It can have very powerful results.

Chapter 24

The Art of Being Content – Why Less Is More

So many of us are not happy with where our lives are, and this can often be because we have grand ideals (and sometimes quite far-fetched) of how we want ourselves to be and how we imagined our life would turn out. While I do believe that if you change the way you *use* your thoughts into a more positive and focused manner, you *can* create the life of your dreams, I also have realized that when you get more in touch with yourself, with your *soul*, quite often you end up changing the nature of your dreams to desiring something much more simple and less superficial.

Take mine for example. Years ago I lived in a very wealthy part of Sydney, Australia. It was pretty much Australia's version of Beverly Hills: multimillion-dollar homes lined up against each other with huge pools, harbor views, the best restaurants, and shopping areas with Chanel, Gucci and other top designers. I was working in a very famous hair and beauty salon and all our clients were either celebrities or the super rich. The houses in that area were all worth so much money – homes that 99% of us can only 'dream' about – and the lifestyles that most of these people had, to me, seemed so fabulous. They went on luxury holidays all the time, and enjoyed huge shopping sprees and regular dinners out in the best restaurants. They knew the very 'cool' people too.

I used to think that if I could have a house like them, have expensive jewelry and do all the things they did, then one day I would be blissfully happy too. I really used to envy them and wished that my life could just be like theirs. That desire created quite an uneasy feeling in my life back then, as I thought I could not be happy unless I had all of that.

Now, much later in my life, after much personal growth, all my priorities have changed. I have seen through the glitz and glamor and realized that it does not equal happiness. Yes, I still want a lovely home, but it doesn't have to be something that costs millions, nor does it have to be a huge mansion (too hard to keep clean, for one thing!) and I don't even want to go on spending sprees to designer shops (this is a pretty big deal for an ex-shopaholic). I don't have to be seen in the best restaurants or bars and now like nothing more than to share a healthy dinner with good friends or family. If I do buy things, I love to purchase second-hand or environmentally friendly goods or things that are of exceptional and long-lasting quality. Now *that* kind of shopping does give me a good feeling!

I realized that, back then, I was chasing a *fantasy* – a superficial dream of all these things that I *thought* would make me happy. But when I was able to step back and realize that all that I really want now is a simple, yet comfortable, *healthy* life, I could see that I was actually not too far from *that* very dream. It was much more attainable, satisfying and real.

I have realized that I don't like city life anymore – the hustle and bustle is just too much noise and pollution to me – and I now crave the countryside with fresh air and healthy food. I want to learn to garden and to learn more about Nature. I want this for my children too, rather than offering them a lifestyle that is 'glamorous', including elite private schools and giving them all the latest gadgets. I desire to spend lots of time with them, cook and play in Nature, and see them grow up to be healthy and happy. I want them to know, from a young age, that simple ways of living can be the most fun as well.

While I know that some privileged people can of course still bring up their children in a loving and secure way, for me, I felt that if I had all of those material things like they do, it might draw me away from what matters – a connection with the earth and an appreciation for being content. It's only the very strong who are not seduced by lots of money and, despite saying it won't change a person, most of the time it does.

What is quite interesting to see, particularly on the many reality shows that are on TV these days, where we are given an 'inside' look into people's lives, is that most very wealthy or famous people are quite often sheltered from the *real* world. Because they have their every whim catered to, things that to most of us are small and insignificant can become a real problem in their eyes. People being late to a party, a broken nail, not being able to get the right dress for an event, or having a 'bad hair day', or even one tiny pimple, can make them feel like they are having a terrible day! They have no clue as to what others go through in an average day because they are rarely around the majority of those types of normal people. They don't use public transport but are driven around in limousines and fly on private jets – five star all the way. They really do live in another world, one that only 'the 1%' ever experience.

When life is based around getting things handed on a plate, where money is no option, people may not be able to see what really is important in life. I have seen many wealthy people like this. *We* may assume that they have it all, and are therefore going to be the happiest types of people, yet the truth, most of the time, is that they are often very uneasy with their lives. They are surrounded by similar rich friends who don't really talk about anything real; they can't admit that they have problems, and their whole existence is about holidays, what they own and what parties they are going to. This is a broad stereotype, of course, as there are some lovely people who are privileged and who often use their money and contacts to help others, but the majority of people in those circles are still quite lost in their lives. And they may not ever really get to know what their purpose really is, nor connect with their own spirit and the meaning of real happiness. They need clothes and jewelry and 'things' to make them happy because that's all they are used to getting. Sometimes their own parents work so hard that they rarely see them and may even have to schedule 'meetings' with them for some time together. When you're a child, you don't really care about money; you just want regular loving attention from your family.

During my year working at that famous beauty salon in Australia, I personally saw many wealthy customers get so upset about the littlest thing, and they were also at times extremely rude and looked down on people, and at times down on me. I always used to think, 'Why are they like this? Don't they have everything – shouldn't they be blissfully happy?' I soon realized, through salon gossip, that many of the housewives of rich men were unhappy because their partners were always away on business and many of them were having affairs with much younger and prettier women. The wives were miserable but had no way out, because the husbands controlled the purse strings and if they got divorced the woman would be out on her own, away from her 'fabulous' life. It felt like a trap for many of them and that's why they ended up being so fussy and hard to please, yet just shopped and spent money. It was the only way they could vent their frustrations, or to achieve a short burst of happiness

Due to envying wealthy people (and not yet realizing that they weren't always happy), I spent far too many years not appreciating what I already had; I always compared myself to others and was never happy as my dream just seemed so far away. Now I look around myself and count my blessings and realize that I actually had a lot all along. And I bet you actually do too.

The happiest people in the world are generally not the ones you automatically think of. In a Gallup poll released in 2012,[117] the happiest people were said to be from developing countries. Those in Latin America, Asia and the Caribbean. Costa Rica, Panama, Paraguay, Trinidad and Tobago, Thailand and the Philippines all came very high up on this poll. And all of these places have a few things in common. They are surrounded by the most beautiful areas of Nature and the people come from backgrounds with very strong family values. It was very common that people shared their time with many others, even with distantly related family members. So this sense of belonging and being surrounded by stunning scenery can make people feel loved, content and happier overall.

When you appreciate and give thanks to the wonderful things in life, which sometimes can be the simplest of things (like having a warm bath on a cold night, touching soft grass with your bare feet, playing with your pet, receiving a hug from a friend or loved one), it also helps the Law of Attraction to work, helping you to perform much better as well. It's as if the Universe knows that you are grateful and loving, and will reward you with even more great things.

Chapter 25

Change Your Thoughts to Change Your Life – The Power We *All* Have to Create Our Ideal Life

Remember that the Universe listens to every thought and every word you say and will always make them come true. Make your thoughts only positive and your whole world will change positively.

Boy oh boy. Did it take me a very, *very* long time to figure this out! Because I was so unhappy growing up, I behaved like one of the most negative people there ever was. I was so miserable I was even angry that I had been born, as I hated my life and found it so very painful. I blamed everyone and everything around me, including myself. I had a terrible time wherever I went. I had dramas with friends, my family, and even ended up in very destructive romantic relationships. One was even physically abusive.

I felt that I deserved everything I got. Yet I always *wanted* to be happy; I just never knew how to achieve it. It seemed impossible to me. Because of my lack of being able to be positive, I developed a drug problem, a sleeping problem, eating problems, and also shopping and money problems – and all of them happened at once. Everything was out of control because I could not change my thoughts and therefore could not change my actions. I never realized until I was about 28 that my life was *exactly* the way it was because of my own destructive, negative mind. I had thought until that moment it was because of other things that I simply could not control, that it was not all my fault; it was mostly everyone else's and the entire world's fault.

My inability to change my thoughts was because I played a 'tape' in my head over and over again, each day with the same dark messages. My mind was flooded with doubts, anxieties, worries and fears. I told myself I was 'no good', 'unlovable', 'had no talents', was 'hideously ugly', that my life was 'terrible' and '*nothing* would ever change that'. Because I felt I was unlovable, that was exactly what I *got* in all of my relationships with males. I would attract guys that could not love me in the real sense of love. I told myself I didn't deserve happiness, so that's what I got.

I was never able to let myself be free of it and didn't even know that I had actually *brainwashed* myself into being so unhappy. Despite a few people being pretty mean to me growing up, and throughout my teens and 20s, 95% of the horrible words and abuse that I heard was what I *gave* to myself!

I survived a few more painful years of my life feeling like this until 2009, when I read the book *The Secret*. Then *everything* began to change. While reading, each and every word spoke to me in such a deeply profound way that I knew, right up until that very moment, everything in my life that had happened was because of me. Even all of the truly terrifying moments in my life. I knew that I could turn it all around, as I finally understood and knew what I had to do. I had the tools that were necessary to change everything. No longer would I think wistfully about people that I knew who were happy and successful, and no longer would I envy them and be disappointed with myself because I was not like them.

Now I knew what they did to become successful! It was completely down to how they used their own thoughts. You only have to look at most successful people – you know, the ones that have come from nothing and have created empires, invented something amazing or achieved seemingly impossible things. These people come from *all* corners of the earth, but they all have one thing in common. They have a mind that is *positive* and one that *never* gives up, no matter what they are faced with. It's this *determination* which sets successful people apart from those that 'wish' they were successful. A positive action creates a positive reaction.

So how do you become a positive person?

Well, first of all, it would be a good idea to really pay attention to the thought process in your mind. Pretend you're an outsider, looking in at your own mind. Is it always behaving completely negatively? Or do you have good ideas and thoughts, only to become scared after you start thinking that something might stop them from happening? Get used to listening to your mind, and try to understand where all of this negativity is coming from. Did you hear it from your parents, or kids at school? Have you just gotten used to hearing such bad things that now you say them to yourself? Most often than not, if you really, truly ask yourself if you think you're a bad person, the answer is 'No, you're not!' Your *soul* really knows you are not bad; it's either your ego that is in the way or it's down to emotional baggage from the past.

Think about what you want and go get it!

What I always suggest is to always focus on what you *do want* in your life. This is the key! Look back to your thoughts, and take note – I bet they are usually focused on what you *don't* actually want. For example: Do you tell yourself that you can't stand your job, your life, your weight, or yourself?

What about if you started to think about what you did want?

If you spent the same amount of time thinking positive thoughts, *instead* of negative thoughts, your whole life would change very quickly! I can guarantee this! When I started using the Law of Attraction, my own life changed in a big way that quite often would completely surprise me. I have been able to create many things in my life that I now look back on and think, 'If someone told me years ago I was going to do this or that, I would have laughed in their face and said "I wish!"'

A good example is this: When I started my Eco Travel Website, I was able to do little trips around the UK, visiting environmentally friendly holiday places. I thought to myself, and said out loud to a few friends and loved ones, that I would really like to 'start going on overseas trips for my job' and that my dream would be to go to tropical places like Tahiti, the Maldives, Costa Rica, and to visit eco resorts and hotels.

Not long after, I saw a press release come through for a week-long, all-expenses-paid yoga trip to Tuscany and that ten journalists were wanted. I immediately wrote an email to the PR lady telling her what I did and that I would absolutely love to go on the trip. She explained that she would have to get back to me as there was now a whole list of other journalists who wanted to go and that she had had a big response.

Some people might have been disheartened to hear this, and perhaps have already started thinking negatively: 'I probably won't get the gig', 'I can't compete with the big travel magazines', 'My website is too unknown'. These thoughts never entered my mind and actually did not worry me. I spent that week *imagining* myself going and even said to my friends, 'I'm going on a yoga trip to Tuscany in October.'

Sure enough, the lady contacted me a few days later and said that she would love for me to go with the group; something about my positivity, she said, made me her want to accept me. During my amazing trip away in Tuscany, I realized that this was just the start of my dream job, to travel around to amazing countries visiting eco resorts and going on yoga trips. I just hoped I could keep doing it.

Well, lo and behold, on the Tuscany trip was also the editor of a major health magazine. I took the liberty of mentioning that I was absolutely loving this experience, visiting other countries to review places, and that if there was any chance I could be given a shot, then I would love to write a piece for the magazine. I was told to send in some examples of my work so that the editor could decide if I was good enough to write an article for the publication.

Now, just so you know, I am not a trained journalist. I never went to university or studied travel writing; it's something that just happened out of dreaming. I had an idea of visiting Costa Rica, which is one of the most environmentally friendly and health-conscious countries in the world. There were many amazing places to visit there so I pitched an idea to the editor. While I was waiting to hear back, I imagined every day that I would get the gig and spent the next few weeks picturing myself in Costa Rica. I looked at lots of information on the internet to get myself familiar with the country and started to make a list of places I wanted to visit. I put up a map of Costa Rica next to my computer with these places marked so that I could see it every day.

A few weeks later, I finally heard back, and the answer was yes! I was over the moon. My dream of being a travel writer was really well and truly on its way to becoming true and more than a one-off.

In April of 2011, I spent 5 *incredible weeks* in Costa Rica, where I went on a trip of a lifetime. I visited 12 places – resorts, retreats and beautiful hotels. I met the most amazing people, experienced the beauty of Nature like never before, and finally felt that I could break free from the misery of my past. The trip probably would have cost around £14,000 (about $21,000) if I had paid for it, but was mostly free. It was, without a doubt, incredibly *life-changing* and would not have been impossible unless I knew how to use my thoughts to make this happen.

I *allowed* myself to attract these things by being positive and also by imagining that they were real. Many of my friends, who see what I have been able to do, ask me what my secret is. It is simply down to not only being positive, but knowing *exactly* what I want, then *picturing* myself in the future as having that thing or as actually doing it. And it's not because I am a lucky person either, because growing up, when I was caught up in being completely negative, I was definitely not lucky!

Another person whose story is very inspiring and impressive is Denise Duffield-Thomas, who actually is now a Law of Attraction coach and author of two wonderful books: *Lucky Bitch* and *Get Rich, Lucky Bitch*. Denise and her husband Mark entered a competition called 'The Honeymoon Testers' in 2010. They were literally up against thousands of other people (30,000 to be exact!) and had to complete many difficult challenges.

Denise and Mark *won* and spent 6 whole months traveling the world testing luxury honeymoons. Their trip was worth over a whopping half a million pounds! They were even given *30,000 Euros* to cover their rent and other bills while they were away... They basically were *paid* to take amazing holidays.

Denise told me she always knew they would win because she knew exactly how to use her thoughts in the right way, and focused only on the positive outcome of what she wanted to create. She also discovered other ways to show the Universe that what she wanted was already true.

And guess what? Denise's story inspired *me* to do travel writing! When I read what she had won, instead of me being jealous of her (which would have been an easy, but also very negative way of thinking for me), I thought, '*That could be me!* That is what I want to do too.' So then I set off on my own journey to create my dreams of this coming true for me.

Ever since I visited Costa Rica, I have also visited Greece and was offered the chance to visit Tahiti and Thailand as well. All in the space of one year, and only because I now see just how I can make things happen. I fell pregnant a few months before I was meant to visit Tahiti so I had to cancel the trip, but I was still able to manifest it to be a definite possibility to go. And I know that this is not the end of my travel writing trips; in fact I am heading to the Maldives in 2013 and have other story ideas for future trips to pitch to the editor.

I also manifested this very book which you are reading. If you asked me years ago if I was to one day become a published author, selling books internationally, I probably would have laughed at you and assumed you were on some kind of strange drugs, or getting me confused with another person. But in the space of 3 weeks, I was drawn to the John Hunt Publishing Company. I was asked to send in my draft, and heard back within 24 hours that they wanted to see more. And after I gave my final basic proposal, I was given the book contract in the space of a very short time (3 days!) and not just their lowest level contract either. I was given the highest level they offered their authors, the one with 'most promise to sell', and one that they help to promote as much as they can. Pretty amazing, right?

Again, this contract was another thing which happened to me out of the 'blue' and was seemingly so easy! After I sent in my draft, I just began to *believe* it would happen. And lo and behold, only one week later I had signed my contract and my book was *really* going to happen. Book deals are something most people say is very hard to get, as I thought too, but I now think if you really know how to use your mind, and take action too, write from the heart, it is more than likely going *to* happen, rather than not!

You can use the Law of Attraction for lots more than just bringing material goods into your life. You can even help heal physical ailments, repair relationships, attract that perfect job plus lots more, by focusing on what it is that you want. Some say that if we all tried to attract 'world peace' it would happen, and I actually believe that to be true. We just need more people to understand how the Law of Attraction works and to want the world to be a better place. Unfortunately, as we have discovered previously, there are corporations and governments that just don't want to help this world become better. Perhaps we can use the Law of Attraction to get them to change their ways.

It might be worthwhile sitting down and writing a list of all the things you wished you had so that it gives you something to work towards. Even write down things that seem a little bit far-fetched and not immediately possible. Positive thinking is something you have to *work* on every single day. Our negative mind or what we call 'the ego' is usually waiting and lurking in the back of our minds, wanting to cause a few unnecessary dramas. I am not always positive and sometimes have a few down-in-the-dumps days, only to snap myself out of it and get back on the positive wagon again where I turn things around really quickly.

The key is knowing what to do each day to help create a positive future.

Affirmations

Saying affirmations, also known as positive statements, really helps to make things happen, as this is reinforcing the good things you want in your life. It is best to say them in front of a mirror, directly to yourself. I know, it feels a bit silly at first, but once you start getting into a habit it will be very easy to do and you won't feel odd talking to yourself! In fact, just saying those words to yourself automatically puts you in a better mood. When you look at how thoughts work, if you grew up hearing negative things, that's why you believed them because it was said to you quite often, so, if you turn those words around into positive, you *will* start to believe those also.

Affirmations and positive thoughts have been proven to help people recover from illness as well. And even more incredibly, studies have been done on the effects of other people thinking good and healing thoughts about someone else, who may even live far away halfway around the world!

A really great book for discovering what affirmations will work is *You Can Heal Your Life* by Louise Hay.

Negative thoughts affect far more than just how you feel about your life and what's happening in it. They also can *dramatically* impact your health. In the book *All Is Well – Heal Your Body with Medicine, Affirmations and Intuition,* co-author Dr Mona Lisa Schulz writes:

The Human body is an amazing machine, and as a machine it requires regular maintenance and care to run as efficiently as possible. There are a variety of reasons your body can break down and get sick: genetics, the environment, diet and so on. As Louise found in her career – and published in *Heal Your Body* - every illness is affected by emotional factors in your life. And decades after Louise presented her conclusions, the scientific community has put forth studies that support them.

Research has shown that fear, anger, sadness, love and joy have specific effects on the body. We know that anger makes muscles clamp down and blood vessels constrict, leading to hypertension and resistance to blood flow. Cardiac medicine tells us that joy and love tend to have the opposite effect. If you look at Louise's little blue book, a heart attack and other heart problems are 'squeezing all the joy' out of the heart, a 'hardening of the heart' and a 'lack of joy'.

Dr Schulz also writes about how harmful chemicals are produced by our bodies due to our negative emotions:

Specific thought patterns affect our bodies in predictable ways, releasing certain chemicals in response to each emotion. When fear is your dominant mood over a long period of the time, the constant release of stress hormones, specifically cortisol, triggers a domino effect of chemicals that lead to heart disease, weight gain, and depression. As with fear, other emotions and thoughts follow a typical pattern as they are projected onto the body in the form of illness. In my work, I have also found that while emotions travel everywhere in the body, they affect organs differently depedning on what is happening in your life. This is where intuition comes in.

Dr Masaru Emoto became a pioneer on the subject of thoughts and how they affect frozen water particles, and gave us a completely new way of looking at consciousness. He carried out experiments with bottles of water that were set under a positive or negative influence. For example, he would put notes wrapped around a bottle that were positive or negative, with the words facing inwards. He wrote positive things like 'thank you', 'beautiful' and on other bottles, negative notes like 'you fool' 'ugly'.

He then looked under a microscope and what he saw startled him. The frozen ice crystals *always* mirrored the words or thoughts directed at the bottles. When a positive thought, or even beautiful classical music was played, the ice crystals were absolutely beautiful. And when looking at the frozen ice particles of the negative bottles the shapes were misshapen and malformed. Dr

Emoto photographed these images and spent years repeating these studies again and again.

The fact that we are at least 70% water is something to think about in relation to all the negative thoughts and words we aim towards ourselves and what they could be doing to our health. Our cells contain water, and if we are constantly saying to ourselves, ' I am stupid, unloveable, fat, no good' etc., then how can we possibly have health that thrives? Our cells will *not* be able to function at their best.

You can read more and the see the stunning photos, of the fascinating effects of thoughts on water at masaru-emoto.net/english

Or you can learn about it through his international bestselling book *'The Hidden Messages In Water'*.

Before you sleep

You can also help yourself by imagining what you want as you are going to sleep every night. When your head hits the pillow, start to breathe deeply and relax your whole body starting from your feet and working all the way up to your head. Now, imagine that all of the things that you want to be true are *actually* true. Picture yourself in this dream. If you imagine going away on a holiday somewhere, then imagine yourself being there. If you want a new job, imagine that too. If you want your relationship to be stronger, then imagine that too. If you want a new house that is up for rent or for sale, then imagine you are living in that house. Sure, thinking this way won't make these things automatically happen overnight, but by regularly focusing your intention on them, they are more likely to make other things come your way which will help these desires to come true e.g. you may meet someone who has a job opening for you.

If you want to have better self-esteem, say affirmations in your mind. Say that you are 'a positive, kind and loving human being' or that you are 'getting stronger each and every day', or you are 'a great and worthy person who feels good about themselves'. There are so many affirmations that you can choose; you just have to know how to word them properly. Being relaxed before sleep is a very powerful time to get things really locked into your subconscious. Again, focus on what you do want, not what you don't want.

Imagine things to be real and let your mind go wild with what you want to create!

Dream boards

Dream or 'vision boards' are a very helpful way as well to visualize what you want to happen. You basically make a big collage on a large piece of cardboard that has images and words of the things you want to have happen in your life.

Grab some magazines and cut out the words and pictures of things that you want to come true. Stick the words down onto your cardboard or cork board and place it somewhere you will see it every day. And look at it very often and think about those things coming true. These *thoughts*, and this constant attention, will make them turn into actual *things*. I used words like 'travel', 'healthy', 'happy', 'Costa Rica', and all of those things came true after a year (some even earlier!) of looking at my image. You must specify what you want though, as sometimes the wrong words can attract the wrong things. I made a collage years ago and forgot about what was on it. A close friend reminded me last year after I had Lola that she remembered seeing my pink collage with all of my cut-out pictures and words on it. I even had a little girl with sandy blonde hair on the collage. Most of the things that I had on that collage came true and I had my friend as a witness.

For help with this, please go to the following websites:

✓ deniseduffieldthomas.com
✓ theamericanmonk.com
✓ mindmovies.com
✓ tut.com

Denise has also written a brilliant book called *Lucky Bitch* filled with lots of inspiring information including her tips on how she makes things come true. She has also just brought out another one, as equally as inspiring called *Get Rich, Lucky Bitch*.

How you can tap away your problems and make way for positivity

Sometimes, if we are so bogged down with negativity, we may actually need to dig really deep into ourselves to sort them out. A technique which can work wonders for ridding yourself of emotional pain is EFT, otherwise known as the 'Emotional Freedom Technique'. It involves tapping certain parts of the face, body, head and arms, which is said to trigger a deep release from unresolved issues. It is so powerful that many people who have tried it reported that their long-term fear of flying, fear of snakes or other phobias completely disappeared within one session! It also can help with anger issues, relationships, self-esteem, addictions and just about anything that is weighing you down.

It is a wonderful therapy; I have tried it myself and found it to be very helpful. I knew it was immediately powerful because from only *one* session I went from being an absolute cry-baby (I would literally cry every few days about something and it could lead to complete breakdowns) to only crying at soppy movies. To see this big difference from just one session made me see the power that this technique can have.

I also love that you can *save* loads of money by doing this technique as you can quite often sort out your problems without needing to regularly pay a therapist. I had one paid session of EFT and found it so easy to do at home on my own that I didn't need to go back. Unlike regular counseling sessions which you may need once a week, and can cost up to £100 (about $150), this is a therapy that you can do anytime, anywhere (OK, maybe *not* in public unless you want to be stared at!), and it doesn't cost a cent!

I used it throughout my pregnancy so that I could unlock my big fears around childbirth. It was totally amazing. I did one session around having fears of the pain of childbirth and I programmed the words into my mind, whenever I thought about the labor: 'You can do it.' I actually heard those words whenever I thought about the birth.

If you are interested to learn this technique yourself, please visit eftuniverse.com.

If you still suffer with unhappiness that you can't seem to shift after trying these things (and removing toxins), it might be worthwhile investigating what is the root cause. A great book to read is Dr. Amen's *Change Your Brain, Change Your Life*.

Chapter 26

Happy Loving Relationships – How Important They Are and How to Create Them

Sadly, it's no longer shocking to us that the divorce rate is sky-high these days, as more and more people are unable to sustain long-term relationships, or if they do, they are often quite miserable. Unhappiness in romantic relationships these days is so common that it's rare you find a couple that seems blissfully happy. It's another tragedy of modern society – we simply find it so hard to communicate and to understand each other. We can quite often feel that we are not only from different planets, but from completely different universes.

You can try and get as fit as possible, eat the best foods, work on finding your spirit, detox your body etc. but if you are in a relationship that is stressful, or you're in one where you feel lonely most of the time, that is most certainly *not* going to help you have the best life possible. A happy relationship with someone you share your life with is *essential* for a healthy life too. And while I mainly will touch on romantic relationships here, I really mean for all of your close relationships too.

So many people feel instantly attracted to someone, fall in love, get married quickly, have children and then the cracks begin to quickly show. The initial feeling of love is like a powerful drug, intoxicating, can't-get-enough-of, and then it can all come crashing down, turning into a big mess because you start to see that the person you fell in love with is not perhaps what you thought.

And, to them, *neither* are you.

The most common cause of problems in relationships is when two people start a relationship yet still have issues from childhood that they carry with them into adulthood. For example: just say you grew up in a house where your father (or mother) was not able to show you love. You were perhaps put down regularly and were never listened to, causing a feeling of inadequacy and lots of sadness.

Growing up feeling like you did not matter to your father (or mother) may have left you with damaged self-esteem, and a hole in your heart that you desperately wanted someone *else* to fill.

You meet a man (or woman) that seems perfect for you, but after a few months of being together, you notice that the way he/she sometimes treats you reminds you exactly of how your father/mother made you feel. Your partner often does not listen to what you are saying, puts your ideas down, and you end up feeling like you are not respected or validated. And the reaction from you may be exactly the same way as how you reacted in childhood. You may answer back to your partner in an immature way, and perhaps even go off and sulk for a while. You may even be behaving like this while being 45 years old!

This is happening because you never knew how to deal with this sort of situation when you were young. Your emotional needs were not met by your parents. You were perhaps not shown how to express your anger or to voice your concerns. And now, as an adult, it's happening all over again. In your partner's eyes the story may be the same, but in reverse. Perhaps his mother was very emotional or opinionated, always talking about ideas and subjects that were not something he agreed with and the way she went about arguing her side always triggers off an angry reaction, causing him to retreat into a shell or say negative things. Maybe she was a very strong-minded woman who put him down. But maybe she was also very nurturing, kind and had quite a few good points. A real mix of good and not so good.

So he meets you, who, unbeknown to him, has very similar traits to his mother with a strong and opinionated mind who likes to discuss certain subjects that leave the both of you arguing. During increasing arguments, you storm off because he has pushed buttons like your father did during your childhood, by putting you down or not listening. He storms off too as you pushed his buttons the same way his mother did.

The fights never really get sorted and it's a vicious cycle, because you keep being transported back in time to your childhood. And as time goes by, your feelings get even more hurt, as do his, and you both become more resentful and feel very unhappy. And the future for the two of you doesn't look very good.

Sound familiar?

Well, this sort of dynamic in a relationship is *so* common. It happens with all sorts of relationships, gay relationships, with work colleagues, etc. And the extreme and tragic side to this is that people who grew up abused or neglected emotionally by a parent will quite often go on to attract abuse again with another partner or perhaps many.

Yet most people are not able to recognize why this is happening. They might feel like they 'do not know' the person after all. But in fact they know that person very well – that is the problem! But they haven't been able to *understand* or see that the pattern in their childhood has affected their choice of partner later in life.

By the way, if you are in a relationship like this now, it does not mean you are not right for each other – definitely not; it just means you have to find the right sort of guidance to work through these problems. However, it must be said that anyone who physically, sexually or emotionally abuses you is usually someone best to walk away from unless they really, really want to help themselves. And they must not just talk about it; they must show you through their effort and actions. People deserve chances but not at the cost of your happiness.

Whenever a relationship is in trouble, counseling and therapy is always recommended. But some forms of therapy for this type of problem do not have a high success rate. One way of really helping to break this cycle is through the highly effective 'Imago Therapy'.

Harville Hendrix, author of many brilliant books on this topic, is a brilliant psychotherapist who has developed a form of therapy, which he termed 'Imago', that couples do together, and often with truly incredible results. Many couples on the brink of divorce discover this therapy, do the practice, and often end up having a partnership so powerful that their current relationship and childhood issues will both be healed and become a thing of the past, allowing them to live together, having a healthy and fulfilled relationship.

The therapy involves a special 'dialogue' that Harville has created after spending many years evaluating his patients, noticing that they would always say, 'Oh, she reminds me of my mother!' or 'He puts me down *exactly* like my father did!' This dialogue helps you to speak and listen to each other properly by learning to repeat back to someone what they have said to you about their feelings. When you try it, it's amazing how you actually *do not* really hear what your partner is saying most of the time. Nor do they really hear you.

It is an absolutely amazing form of therapy and, if both of you want to commit to it, it can dramatically change your lives for the better. Not just healing the relationship, but healing your childhood too. Allowing you to be free of emotional blockages that kept you stuck back in the past.

The website below will steer you in the right direction. You can also search on the web for 'Imago Therapy' for a therapist who is trained in this type of counseling.

✓ www.harvillehendrix.com

What's your love language?

Another way to dramatically improve your relationships (where you may not even need therapy) is to learn about all of the ways we can give love to others and also to figure out the way you need love to be shown to you.

In the wonderful book *The Five Love Languages: The Secret to Love that Lasts*, Gary Chapman has figured out that we all have different needs in terms of how we want to be loved. And that we also may show love in the wrong way to someone, which causes upset and drama in a relationship.

Being truly loved can make us feel full. And feeling unloved can make us feel like an empty vessel. Gary calls it a 'Love Tank'. When you feel deeply loved, your love tank is full and when it is empty you do not feel loved, can be very sad, have low self-esteem and basically feel very unfulfilled.

After years of counseling countless families and couples, Gary has ingeniously worked out what the 'Five Love Languages' are:[118]

- Physical Touch – do you need affection?
- Words of Affirmation – do you need words of encouragement and validation?
- Quality Time – do you need someone to spend quality time with you?
- Gifts – do you need someone to show they care by giving you thoughtful gifts?
- Acts of Service – do you need someone to do things for you to show they care?

In my relationship, I needed words of affirmation from my partner. I grew up very self-conscious and unsure of myself and was used to hearing negative things from people around me and from myself. So I realized that what I needed from my husband was to hear him say positive things about me *to* me. He, on the other hand, needed physical touch. He grew up with a very affectionate mother and was always used to someone hugging him and showing they cared through touch. I, however, am not naturally affectionate, so because I did not display much affection, he felt he was really missing out on the love that he needed.

We began to notice big problems between us because we were not giving each other what we needed. When we rectified this, and learnt about Love Languages, we became much closer and were able to close the gaps of loneliness and unhappiness. If you can figure out what is the best way for you to receive love and also to discover your partner's best way, by changing your behavior towards each other it can bring about a huge change in the dynamic of your relationship in such a short space of time.

This technique may be the most brilliant way ever discovered to change a relationship between two people that have previously had so much trouble getting along.

For people with deep childhood issues *The Hoffman Process* is apparently particularly very good to do. This is an 8-day retreat where you do intensive therapy with instructors and involves psychodynamic, behavioural, cognitive, transpersonal & gestalt therapies which work on emotional, physical, intellect and spiritual levels and helps people to develop new approaches to dealing with life's problems. The courses always have 1 instructor to 8 students so much care is taken to help individuals. It's not inexpensive, at around £3000, but as past students have said, if you add up all the years of therapy lots of people have, which may be no where near as effective, it might pay to do it all in one go.

✓ hoffmaninstitute.co.uk
✓ hoffmaninstitute.org
✓ hoffman-international.com

Other Therapies for improving relationships and personl development are:
✓ Family Constellations - centreforsystemicconstellations.com
✓ BodyTalk System - bodytalksystem.com
✓ Non-Violent Communication - cnvc.org
✓ Woman Within - womanwithin.org
✓ Shadow work - shadowwork.com
✓ Mankind project - mankindproject.org
✓ Matrix Energetics - matrixenergetics.com

Chapter 27

Mirrors and Body Image

I sometimes wonder how different the world would be if there was no such thing as mirrors.

Wouldn't it be completely different?

We would not be comparing ourselves to others, thinking we are not as good and wishing we had what 'they' had; people would generally be more confident, probably kinder to each other, and there wouldn't be the millions of people there are today who have such destructively low self-esteem.

Because of the media portraying the idea that happy successful people are always beautiful, thin and rich, girls as young as 5 are now succumbing to serious eating disorders. They not only grow up with mothers who hate their own appearance and are always talking about this diet or that diet; they also see what is on the television and in movies. Teenage girls are becoming addicted to magazines, TV and makeup and are dressing in ways that are far too old for them. They have learnt at a young age that to go anywhere in life you have to be 'famous, sexy, pretty and rich' and they desire to be in the magazines or on television at whatever cost. They want at least their 15 minutes of fame. The messages that they are being bombarded with are simply too invasive for them to ignore. Even young boys/teenagers are becoming victims of low self-esteem and some end up with eating disorders too.

Children are like sponges and will pick up on absolutely everything that is said around them. If such low self-esteem starts in childhood, it can set the person off for a very troubled time growing up – they need positive reinforcement and if no one is giving it to them, they are more than likely not able to give it to themselves.

Dr William Sears, one of America's most famous pediatricians, wrote the following foreword for the groundbreaking book *'Hidden Messages - What Our Words Are Really Telling Our Children'* by Elizabeth Pantley:

A child's self-image is affected - for better or worse - by the messages he or she receives from parents and caregivers. As a paediatrician and father of eight, I have the privilege of knowing many families. Their approaches to child rearing as a different as the very children they raise, but the vast majority of parents have one thing in common: they want only the best for their kids. These parents try, on a daily basis, to do the right things and to make good parenting decisions. Many of these parents, however, actually make fault decisions based on, or in spite of, those good intentions. These mistakes are sometimes insignificant, but more often, they have enough impact to cause problems that can affect the futures of both the child and the entire family. So why do good, well-intentioned parents make bad choices? Sometimes it's a matter of bad advice; sometimes love for a child makes a parent vulnerable to unhelpful advice; sometimes it's a set of incorrect assumptions; sometimes it's a lack of knowledge. But the most tragically common reason is that they are simply not aware of the full impact their words and actions have. At best, the evolution of a good parent is marked by moments of revelation, in which the parent is shocked to see the potential long-term effects of a mistake - and is able to change course quickly. At worst, the discovery is made much too late, the wrong path already taken.

Celebrity Obsessions

Children of today, look up to celebrities as their role models more than ever, but most of the time these people are admired *only* because they are 'beautiful', (with their idea of 'beauty' being women who have had lots of plastic surgery, who often wear very revealing clothes and far too much toxic makeup) rich or famous, not because they have done something truly amazing, such as helping women or children in Africa or in their local community to help people who are suffering. Society totally values the *wrong* things today and it's why a lot of the world, and its people, are in complete disarray.

My own damaged self-belief in my youth, and therefore intense focus on my looks, became a terrible daily obsession. I constantly checked my appearance in mirrors, always compared myself to others, and thought that life would only be OK if I was accepted for the way I looked. I was not focusing on what was truly important: my purpose, kindness to others, and my inner health. I had no clue that *real* beauty came from within and that *anyone* can be beautiful if they are truly a healthy, kind, loving and happy person.

Glossy hair, healthy skin, clear eyes and a healthy weight are achievable for most and look good on anyone! But sadly today, beauty is more about what someone is wearing, what their makeup is like, and how pretty and how fashionable they appear to be. Beauty today is also very, very false; it's fake hair, fake tans, new teeth, bodies and faces that have been altered by methods of surgery and/or chemicals.

Because of this, many people aspire to be like this so that they can change the way they look and fit in with society. I too was like one of these women. I felt I could not be happy with the way I naturally was, and opted for plastic surgery. I was bullied through school and people made nasty comments about my nose. I thought if I changed the way I looked then would life would be perfect and everything else would be wonderful too. I didn't care about the risks; I just wanted people to think I was OK so that the teasing would stop.

When I had my operations I had no idea that I was walking around with a slight heart defect. From all of the years of stress I had been under, my heart was not 100% healthy. In fact, for years, I used to get heart palpitations for no reason and almost blacked out a few times. I had some typical medical testing but they could never tell that something was wrong. It was not until a few years later when I met the doctor who helped me get my health on track that I had some intensive testing done (tests the Russian astronaut team uses) and discovered I had about 13% damage to my heart – there were areas that were not functioning well – that's why I had those palpitations! When I told my doctor about my operations, he said that I could have died, that heart irregularities and weakness can cause heart attacks under the anesthetic. Yikes! I even remember that, while being in the hospital after my operation, it had been very difficult for me to wake up after the anesthetic and that I had very high blood pressure. This operation put a lot of stress on my heart and also had put my life at risk, just because I didn't like my looks. It seems pretty crazy now that I can look back.

Although the results did stop me focusing so much on the features that I had changed, my thoughts then focused on to other areas of my body and face that I did not like. My self-esteem was so damaged that I needed everything on the outside changed, not realizing that I actually needed to change from the inside, from within. I needed to love me and find myself as great, just the way I was.

So how do we learn to love ourselves?

I believe that working on your health and happiness is a guaranteed way to make you love yourself more. When you exercise and eat well, it makes you feel good and feel proud of yourself.

In my early 30s, I did a bit of modeling. When I was doing photo shoots a few years back, it was actually when I was my most ill. Without makeup, I looked pretty awful. My eyes always had a yellow tinge (indicating a toxic liver), my skin was blotchy, dry and uneven (from not being able to absorb nutrients), and my body shape was not toned or at all genuinely healthy-looking. I even was on the cover of a *health* magazine, yet when I look back to the pictures, I can see how unhappy and sick I was. I was certainly *not* someone who should have been promoting a health magazine.

For me to look 'good' in the photos, I had to have lots of heavy makeup applied and afterwards they were air-brushed intensely, to make it *look* like I was healthy. Because of this, I ended up feeling like a big hypocrite and would always be shy meeting people for the first time in real life in case they were expecting me to look the picture of health, because I certainly wasn't.

I also saw myself start to age quite quickly because my body was not absorbing any nutrients, no matter how much healthy food I ate. So damaged was my digestive system that nothing was able to feed my body, skin, hair and nails with what was needed. It wasn't until a few years ago that I started to heal and noticed things getting better with my appearance as well as my self-esteem. And when I started to heal (removing toxins was the first step!), my eyes became clearer and whiter, my hair began to grow very fast, my nails became strong, my skin started to look better and my weight started to sort itself out.

So this means that now I can see myself looking much healthier and that also means that I feel better about myself. Instead of seeing all my faults, how sick and unwell I looked, I am now marveling at the incredible power that the human body has to heal. When you feed it the right things, remove the toxins and start to exercise, your body will start to thrive and soon you will dislike yourself less and love yourself more.

Try to stop comparing yourself to others and see yourself as *who you really are*. We all have good points; we just have to open ourselves up to seeing what they are. Working on being kind to others (which we have covered in Chapter 21) will also help you to love yourself more.

A good affirmation to say to yourself is this:

Every day, in every way, I am starting to become healthier, happier and more beautiful.

Or:

The Universe loves me and it wants me to be happy.

Nature provides the most ancient wisdom of all about how to heal the human body, and we have barely begun to tap it's resources. Some revealing statistics about the rich diversity of its potential for health and healing can be found in a collection of essays on ecology, *Nature's Services*

In tropical forests an estimated 125,000 flowering plants exist, few of which have been studied by laboratories for their medicinal propercinal potential – fruit, flowers, leaves, stems, and roots – and up to 750,000 potential healing extracts might be found. Not only that, but our planet supports about 75,000 plants that are edible, yet only three thousand or so plant species have ever been utilized as food during human history. Of that number maybe 150 have been cultivated on a large scle. The unexplored wealth of food nutrients and healing compounds from botanicals – edible or not – is amazingly diverse and immense, a true Garden of Eden

Randall Fitzgerald Author of *The Hundred Year Lie*

Chapter 28

Natural Alternatives, Supplements and Helpful Healing Tips

Health is not something that can be bought with an insurance policy. If hospitals and drugs could give us better health, we'd already be better. That is why holistic medicine is growing so fast – it's a question of survival.[119]
Dr. Timothy O'Shea – The Doctor Within

Nature is truly amazing and has pretty much provided us with everything we need; if that weren't the case, none of us would be here today. Nature also has a treasure chest full of natural remedies that can help us to get well and stay well. Despite the medical world pretty much ignoring natural health, and going as far as saying it's 'witchcraft', 'rubbish' and even 'dangerous', when it comes to actual causation of death, the statistics proving the *opposite* are quite plain to see. As read in the book *Work With Your Doctor* by Ty Bollinger and Dr M.D Farley, taking herbs, and natural supplements, is by far *much* safer than using medications and having certain operations. According to acclaimed researcher and scientist, James Duke (who is a former head of the USDA Botanical Division) the chances of dying from things are as follows:

- Herbs: 1 in 1 million
- Supplements: 1 in 1 million
- Non-steroidal anti-inflammatories (ibuprofen, aceta-minophen, Aleve, etc.): 1 in 10,000
- Hospital surgery: 1 in 10,000
- Improper use of drugs: 1 in 2,000
- Angiogram: 1 in 1,000
- Alcohol: 1 in 500

- Cigarettes: 1 in 500
- Hospital caused infections: 1 in 80
- Bypass surgery: 1 in 20

With these *glaring* facts in mind, I know I would *much* rather take my chances with organic herbs and natural remedies first, before resorting to medications.

There are so many things you can use to help balance and regulate the body without having to resort to toxic medications that may actually be highly unnecessary for you in the first place. The key is to find out what works for you. Combined with a healthy diet, regular exercise and positive thinking, certain types of supplements can really help treat many health problems you may have. Now, I can't advise you on the dose to take, so please get some professional advice as to what dose and combination you may need. I have, however, included a little bit of information about why these supplements are said to be so good.

Energy boosters

Lack of energy is a *real* problem most of us suffer from. And it is a big reason why so many people turn to recreational drugs or, more commonly, reach for coffee, energy drinks, sugary foods and other stimulants. The following are some popular things people to take to boost their energy levels.

Yerba mate tea

Yerba mate originates from South America where the health benefits have been known for hundreds of years. Originally a small tree, the leaves are dried then placed in hot water and drunk as a beverage. The leaves contain three xanthines, which are stimulants: caffeine, theobromine and theophylline (interestingly, caffeine and theobromine are found in chocolate). Despite this sounding like it would be super-stimulating, it has been reported that it is very mild and does not give people the shakes like coffee can, nor does it cause withdrawals. It is said that it also strengthens the heart tissue and is helpful for weight loss and treating depression. To get the best benefits you need to drink it a few times a day.

Spirulina

This blue-green algae has become so popular over recent years. Spirulina is said to contain a whole chain of essential nutrients, proteins and vitamins. It is energy boosting due to its rich amount of B vitamins such as B12, which is often lacking in people who suffer with fatigue. Spirulina also contains beta-carotene and minerals including iron, magnesium, manganese, calcium, potassium, selenium, and zinc. Not only is it beneficial for general health and energy levels; it is also a brilliant detoxifier and many are now using it to ward off radiation effects from the Japan nuclear power disaster. It is a supplement you take daily either in powder form or in tablets. Because spirulina is grown in the oceans and on lakes, it is essential you get it from a mercury-free source.

Ginseng

The Chinese have known for thousands of years about the powerful properties of ginseng. There are a few types of ginseng but the most popular and effective is 'panax'. When used regularly, panax ginseng boosts energy, and improves mood and cognitive function. Males report that it is great for sexual function as well. Ginseng can be very stimulating and must not be used in conjunction with some medications. This is something that when used correctly can be incredible, but you must find out if anything you are currently on may give you side effects. Ginseng is commonly taken in tablet form, tinctures or in tea.

Maca

Maca comes from ancient Peru and is widely used today, especially among those in the 'raw food' world. This light-yellow powder is also called 'Peruvian ginseng' due to its energy-boosting effects. It does not actually belong to the Chinese family of ginseng though – it's just a nickname. As with many natural supplements, studies have rarely been done in a manner which achieves support from the medical world. But ask any Peruvian and they will claim that it not only helps with energy but with fertility and sexual dysfunction in both men and women. Some are calling it an 'adaptogen', which means that it can change its effect according to what your body needs. Many people who suffer with adrenal fatigue include it in their daily diet, to help strengthen these stress-balancing glands. You can use maca either in powder form or in tablet form. Many people love adding it to smoothies, desserts and chocolates. It has a caramel taste and this is one of the reasons why it's so popular.

A good night's sleep

This is really just common sense, because if you are not getting enough sleep then you won't be able to produce enough energy. There are some tips in this chapter about how to help your sleep become much easier and more regular.

Sun exposure

One of the best ways to boost your energy is to get out in the sun! If you cannot do this as often as you need, I highly recommend the regular use of a sunlamp or SAD box.

Breathing

A little-talked-about but so important subject is breathing! So many of us are not breathing properly (myself included!) and therefore do not have enough oxygen in the blood, and this leaves us regularly feeling tired. If you have been under a lot of stress over the years, you may find that you automatically breathe very shallowly. I have been doing this for years and I find that I really have to remind myself to take deeper breaths as I have just gotten so used to using such a small part of my lungs.

If you are not breathing well, it doesn't matter how many amazing supplements you are taking; they will only be really effective if you are breathing correctly. The body needs plenty of oxygen to function efficiently. A really great way to help yourself learn how to breathe is by doing 'pranayama', which is an ancient technique discovered by the Indians. *Pranayama* is a Sanskrit word meaning 'extension of the prana or breath'. It's a series of exercises which help to increase the lung capacity and general health. It is amazing what a ten-minute session can do. Your mind, body and even skin will respond so well to practicing this technique and it is suitable for everyone.

When you first start doing this, you realize how you are just not used to having plenty of oxygen as it can make you a little light-headed – but please, stick with it – it will soon show you the rewards. You can find helpful videos on YouTube and there are even phone apps you can download onto your phone. Try and do it every day or at least three to four times a week.

Happiness helpers

So many people feel that they could be do with being much happier in their lives! Happiness, and indeed unhappiness, is related to many things: diet, lifestyle, relationships, self-esteem, and too many toxins. If we report to our doctors that we are feeling down or sad, they may be inclined to prescribe antidepressants that may not actually help in the long run, not with the root cause anyway. It is always a good idea, if possible, to try something natural first, before you have to go down that route.

I think that happiness comes from sorting out lots of different aspects in your life, and unless you have a balance of all of them, it may be hard to achieve it from making just one change. Eating too much sugar, for instance, can really affect your mood, as can lack of exercise. However, many people report that they have noticed huge benefits from taking the following supplements.

St. John's Wort

Touted as 'Nature's antidepressant', this is said to be so effective that even some in the medical community sing its praises. St. John's Wort, otherwise known as Hypericum perforatum, comes from a very pretty yellow flower. Dr. Klaus Linde, from the Centre for Complementary Medicine in Munich, studied the effects and found it to be 'as effective as Prozac' for patients with mild to moderate depression. Those suffering with severe depression will more than likely have other problems contributing to them feeling like this (perhaps an over load of heavy metals) and will need more help than just taking St John's Wort. You must also not be taking any other antidepressants with this supplement. It's available from most health stores, but getting advice for the correct dosage and brand is highly recommended.

SAMe

SAMe (pronounced sammy) is a nutritional supplement which has proven mood-enhancing benefits. We have SAMe in our body (S-Adenosyl methionine). It's a molecule that all living cells, including our own, produce constantly. Some research, including multiple clinical trials, have indicated that taking SAMe on a regular basis may help fight depression ('Investigating SAM-e', Geriatric Times, 2001. Retrieved 2006-12-08). Other reports have said that SAMe can also help with arthritis and liver problems. SAM is produced and absorbed in the liver. Interestingly, many healers also say that if you are an angry person, it may mean that your liver is under strain and may be full of toxins. As with all mood enhancers, it's best to get advice from a professional about what dose would be best for you.

5HTP

5HTP is an amino acid in the body which comes from the naturally-occurring Tryptophan which is calming and it's why babies sleep after being fed. It is reported to be very effective for helping with depression and mood. 5HTP also helps the body to produce 'melatonin' which is what triggers the brain to sleep. Users have reported less anxiety, better mood and less of an appetite. It is suggested to take a few doses throughout the day so that the effect is balanced. High quality is essential here.

Immunity boosters

Immune problems are so common that most people think it is normal to be run down. It certainly isn't, but luckily we can do lots to help boost how our immunity functions. Of course, I recommend taking zeolites first to get all of the toxins out because these can inhibit how the immune system functions. The following are a few things that when taken regularly can really help to keep our immunity healthy and strong.

Milk Thistle

Milk Thistle, Carduus marianus or Silybum marianum, is sometimes also called St. Mary's Thistle. It has a long tradition of being highly effective in easing symptoms of liver disease, as well as other liver complaints such as jaundice, gallstone formation and gallbladder problems. Many people also use it for its liver-restorative powers and it is known as a brilliant hangover cure after consuming excess alcohol. It's great to use this every day to keep the liver functioning well.

The herb Milk Thistle can be used to treat:

- Hepatitis
- Exposure to pollutants and conventional drugs
- Gallbladder problems
- Liver damage or disease including abnormal function and fatty liver
- Gallstone formation

I like taking Milk Thistle in a tincture – this is very easy to add to juice and is absorbed very quickly. Try and look for an organic source.

Probiotics

I cannot stress the use of these enough; they are essential for *all* of us to take – to keep the flora in our stomachs at a healthy level. Stress from all corners – lifestyle, relationships, work, diet – affects our stomachs more than one would think. When you have been affected by too much stress, the flora in the gut is heavily compromised, leaving many with major health issues. If your stomach is not able to absorb nutrients from food and supplements, then over time, this is a recipe for disaster as your body will not be 'fed' and other problems from deficiencies will arise.

It is *vital* for our immunity that we have a healthy balance of gut flora. Due to the mass over-prescription of antibiotics, many people are walking around with stomachs that are in desperate need of support. Probiotics are known as 'Nature's antibiotics' – they really keep the bacteria balanced rather than kill the 'bad' ones off. They are something you need to take regularly to keep the stomach healthy. It is also vital that you choose the right brand as many are said to be ineffective. Some say that they must be refrigerated and others say as long as the right balance of all the different types of bacteria are in there, then refrigeration is not necessary. I have tried both kinds and found both to be effective. Advice from a trained professional is recommended, and one from a health food shop as opposed to a pharmacy – unless they also have a background in Natural Health. I also think that Dr. Mercola makes a very good probiotic. It is available at mercola.com

The Raw Living website stocks the brand 'Primal Defense Ultra' which contains 13 species of beneficial cultures. Some of the strains are also fermented which makes the friendly bacteria even more powerful. Primal Defense contains plant-based minerals, grass juices, and a whole list of amazing bacteria to help restore the gut function. Look out for Raw Living's Sunbiotics chocolate bars which have billions of probiotics in a yummy raw chocolate bar.

✓ rawliving.eu
✓ Sunbiotics is also another high quality probiotic supplement

you can take. This vanilla flavored powder contains 28 billion CFUs of 4 well researched probiotic strains. You can add it to water, juice, meals or your favorite smoothie.

✓ sunbiotics.com

Oregano oil

I have only recently discovered this incredible oil and urge everyone to consider having some at home, to be either taken regularly to strengthen your immune system or when you or someone in your family suffers from a health concern that would normally be treated with antibiotics. It is fantastic to take when suffering from a cold or a flu as it can clear congestion quite quickly. Oregano oil acts as an antiviral agent, is an anti-inflammatory, reduces negative effects of menopause, and is an anti-allergen (so essential for those suffering with allergic conditions such as hay fever). It is also a powerful antioxidant and pain reliever, and helps the digestive system work much better. One of the reasons oregano oil has gained such popularity is that it has very strong anti-fungal qualities, and is used when someone is suffering from parasites. You only have to taste a bit of it to know that there is something very medicinal about this oil. It has also been extensively studied and has been found to be as effective in killing germs as many of the top prescription antibiotics. There was a six-week study done on patients with parasites who were treated with 600 mg of oregano oil taken daily and every single patient was parasite free after the treatment. It also contains many vitamins and minerals. A must for everyone's natural-based medicine cabinet! As always, try and source an organic or wildcrafted oil.

Try the naturalnews.com store or iherb.com

Vitamin C

Most of us know that vitamin C is essential for good health, but many only take it when they are suffering from a cold. It really is best to take it regularly, as in each day, to keep those colds and flus at bay. And a high dose of at least 1000–2000 mcg is the suggested daily dose. When you do have a cold, you can take much more than this to help knock it out of your system. Side effects may be some runny bowels, but as vitamin C is a water-soluble vitamin, it is never stored in the body for too long and you will just excrete it. This is why it's best and recommended to have some every day. I prefer the abscorbic powdered form, and like to add it to my juice.

More studies are proving extra health benefits from regular use of vitamin C and they are very impressive. Some are claiming that cancers can be cured when using IV high-dose vitamin C. Vitamin C also has effective detoxification abilities and can help to remove heavy metals. It is an anti-aging vitamin as well, which is why it's in so many beauty creams (although usually not the right type of vitamin C). Vitamin C is actually not produced naturally by humans, but in animals it is and at very high doses. We need to either get it from our diets or from supplements. And please don't think that a glass of orange juice is enough to get your requirements from. Sadly it's a big myth; there are many other ways to get your vitamin C which have much larger doses than that of orange juice. Always choose a source that is GMO free as many come from genetically modified corn. You don't have to spend a lot of money on powdered Vitamin C, you can get a big tub for under $10.00. I cannot stress enough how beneficial taking this vitamin is, regularly, for health and wellbeing.

Echinacea

This pretty pink flower does more than look attractive; it also happens to be very powerful for building the immune system. Native American Indians have been using this for health for thousands of years. It is reported to help with toothache, and fights bacterial, fungal and viral infections. Most commonly used in conjunction with a cold, echinacea helps fight so many other problems. It comes in the form of lozenges, tinctures, tablets and capsules. Daily use of this is highly recommended. When used with a cold, it can really help to reduce the length and severity.

Sleep remedies

Sleep problems are absolutely rife these days, with 30% of the population suffering with regular sleepless nights. In fact, I don't know of many people who have a good night's sleep every night! I personally suffered with terrible insomnia for years and even became addicted to sleeping pills for a short time. It was horrible. It took me years to be able to sleep easier, and even now, if I use the computer too much I tend to have trouble falling asleep. But after sorting my health out, it's a huge relief to know that I can now sleep unaided. For many years I had to take something very powerful to trigger my brain that it was sleepy time.

Due to us leading such stressful lives, it's so common to have irregular sleeping patterns, and once you have developed one, it can be a tough habit to break out of. There are things you can do to help sleep happen easier: exercise regularly (but not in the afternoon or early evenings) and stay away from stimulants. That means chocolate too (especially raw as its caffeine content is even stronger than cooked chocolate). If you are to have some only have it before about 2 or 3pm so that the caffeine effects wear off. If you like carob, have that instead. However, there are a few natural things you can try and take which are said to be highly effective.

Melatonin

Melatonin is a naturally occurring hormone found in the brain. When we have the right amount, it triggers the brain into falling asleep. Due to being so busy with so much responsibility, many of us are now not producing enough melatonin, which leads to sleep deprivation. Bright lights can also really confuse the brain into thinking it's daylight so you may need to get into a routine of keeping lights low after a certain time. Taking melatonin can be a brilliant way to fall asleep. I have found it highly useful myself and, out of all the natural aids, this one, for me, was the best. You can take it in tablet form and it is also available in a spray. Best to take it about 30 minutes before bed and you may only need a small dose. Don't take it too late at night if you need to get up early in the morning; you may feel a bit groggy. Sleep problems can sometimes be connected to emotional problems as well, so you might need to really have a think about what is keeping you awake at night so often.

Mercola.com make a very good spray and I also have bought some other high-quality brands such as nowfoods from Iherb.com.

Meditation

Problems with sleep may simply be down to stress, and one of the best stress relievers is meditation. If you can get into a routine of having some quiet time, this form of relaxation may be just what you need to have a peaceful night's sleep. Meditation takes practice and commitment to get the best benefits. It may be hard at first, but if you stick with it, the results will be evident and soon you may be sleeping like a baby.

Chamomile

One of the most common sleep aides is a pretty little herb called chamomile. Used in teas at night, it has soothing and calming properties. It is also now being reported that it lowers blood sugar levels and can help to manage diabetes. I personally don't think it helps much in people who have a major sleep problems (it didn't work for me) but it can certainly help for those with mild and rare sleepless nights. If you make a routine to sleep (warm bath with lavender, low lights, no TV) and add this to your evening's activities, you may find that it really helps. Chamomile is readily available in tea form and you can also easily grow it yourself!

Herbal tinctures

A good homeopath or herbalist can mix you up a special concoction to help you sleep. Taken 30 minutes before bed, it can really help you to drift off to sleep peacefully. Common herbs used are lavender, valerian, skullcap and chamomile. I use one myself and it's been very effective, much more than I first gave it credit for. Remember to tell the person dispensing this to you, if you are on any medication.

Valerian

Valerian is another herb which has been used for thousands of years to help relax and trigger sleep. It is a small green plant and the leaves are dried and used in teas. Many users take valerian to help with nervous and anxiety problems as well due to its calming effects. Lots of users like it due to the fact that it does not leave you feeling tired the next day. Herbs are powerful, so again, use it in the right amounts, get some advice on how and when to take it, and make sure you are not on any other medications. Valerian is available in tablet form, tinctures and in its natural state.

Common items in your cupboard which may improve your health and wellbeing

Our kitchens are often home to many valuable items which can really help to boost our health. It is amazing what foods and spices can really help us with common ailments and below is a list of the most common ones that I am sure you have heard of.

Apple Cider Vinegar

Apple Cider Vinegar (ACV) really is truly astounding at what it can do for your health. And it can also be used literally in many ways around the house too. A recent study shows that regular intake of ACV may help to curb appetite and to help speed up the metabolism as well as playing a role in blood sugar control. To show you what apple cider can do for us, I would have to write a new book. In fact on my book shelf at home, I have a book called *101 uses for Apple Cider Vinegar*. This book is really just for things around the house (cleaning, laundry etc.) but you can find books on what it can do for your health and wellbeing. Because ACV is fermented, it contains so many important acids, vitamins, and mineral salts. There are promising studies showing positive benefits for the treatment of: diabetes, high cholesterol, heart health, cancer and weight loss. Many are saying that it helps with the immune system, increases energy levels, reduces sinus problems and sore throats (great to take when struck with a cold/flu). It improves skin conditions such as acne and helps to improve digestion and constipation.

You can take it internally with a dose of two teaspoons a day. Some people make a tasty ACV drink they consume daily with honey, lemon and ginger.

When making salad dressings look for recipes that include ACV. And when purchasing it, look for Organic, Raw Apple Cider Vinegar.

Garlic

Garlic is a super-powerful healer which has so many benefits. The ancient Egyptians used it often for health ailments. You can take it when you have a cold as it is said to be an antibiotic, and you can rest assured it won't kill any of your good bacteria either. It also can help with earaches and other infections. It's cheap too. You can use raw garlic cloves or can purchase garlic oil from health food shops. It's reported that you can also use garlic to help balance high blood pressure. If you are using pure garlic, make sure it's raw as it's in its strongest state. If you are worried about garlic breath, the capsules are often very good at giving you the health benefits but not the smelly breath.

Ginger

Ginger is another helpful item found in most people's cupboards. Not only does it smell and taste good, it is also very effective for helping with digestion and viral problems. If you are suffering from nausea, you may find that ginger tea can really make your stomach feel better. It can help asthmatics to breathe easier, minimizes mucus in a cold, and can be a great pain reliever. Some are saying that ginger has anti-cancer components and are adding it to their cancer therapies. You can buy ginger tablets but I love using the powdered form (make sure it's organic though) or making a tea from the real thing.

Lemon

Lemons are perhaps one of the most amazing fruits that Nature has provided us with. Many people who start their day with warm water and a squeeze of lemon juice say that it's something they can't live without. Lemon has brilliant detoxing properties and this is why it's recommended to have some every day. The liver functions very well when lemon is taken regularly. It also helps with bowel function, and reduces phlegm so is very beneficial to use when you have a cold. It is also very good at balancing the acid–alkaline levels in the body. Lemons are very high in potassium which tends to be quite deficient in people who suffer with depression, anxiety and memory problems.

Try and have lemon in water every day, and use it in salad dressings. You can even add fresh lemon to juices and smoothies.

Manuka honey

This honey from New Zealand is said to be one of the best in the world. It's also one of the most expensive forms due to its popularity and healing benefits. Manuka is a white flowering plant found in New Zealand which has been used by the native Maoris for hundreds of years. The bees produce honey which has many proven effects, and even has the support from many scientists. It is highly anti-bacterial and healing and even hospitals are recommending the use of it over burns and other skin problems which have become resistant to antibiotics. All honey (in its raw form) has healing benefits, but manuka is known as having the most powerful qualities. It is not cheap, but if using the right brand (high quality is a must) it may be worth the money! Manuka honey is given a UMF® ratings with 10 being the lowest – a higher rating means it's more powerful and more expensive. Raw organic honey is still quite effective too, so if you can't get hold of manuka, it's certainly worthwhile to stock this in your kitchen.

Organic raw honey in general is very helpful for many ailments, and super-good for the immune system – it's very beneficial to have a spoonful a day. Some people mix it with raw apple cider vinegar for a very powerful combination.

Cinnamon

This delicious spice was favored by the ancient Egyptians who knew about its health benefits. The Chinese have also known that it was very effective for healing certain ailments. And the Ayurvedic Indians have been regular users of this popular ingredient. Its reported benefits include helping with the severity of a cold, digestion, menstruation pains and diarrhea. Researchers have also reported that it is beneficial for diabetics as it helps to stabilize blood sugars. Cinnamon is said to have antioxidant qualities as well. You can drink cinnamon in teas, or sprinkle it over foods such as fruit and include it in smoothies. Baking with cinnamon is popular, but intense heat is definitely going to affect its potency. Always source organic forms as well and if you are pregnant steer clear of it as it can thin the blood. Honey and cinnamon used together are said to have anti-cancer benefits as well as helping to stabilize weight. It's best to have cinnamon in liquids, as opposed to eating, as the liquid apparently makes the cinnamon more active.

Turmeric

Another spice gaining popularity in the heath world is turmeric. This yellow spice, used in Indian food to give it an authentic color, also has many benefits for health and wellbeing. Turmeric displays anti-inflammatory properties and reduces oxidative stress. The yellow color comes from its curcuminoid polyphenol antioxidants. This antioxidant has been shown to stabilize blood sugars and improve the cardiovascular system, and has anti-aging effects. It's also said to be very effective in some cancer patients. In studies turmeric is the fourth highest antioxidant-rich herb with a super-impressive ORAC score of *159,277*. Use it every day in your diet if you can. Always buy it from an organic source. Turmeric root is found in the Touchstone Essentials Wellspring Daily Supplement.

* * *

There are many other powerful spices and foods in your cupboard but I feel these are the most common and easiest to get hold of. You can make a yummy drink out of warm water with honey, lemon, ginger and cinnamon, and it's so beneficial for a cold, or even having daily to keep colds and other viruses at bay. I sometimes throw in some garlic and turmeric as well to the mix, as I know it's so good for my body.

Coconut oil

For many years, coconut oil has been seen as a 'bad guy' and has been avoided by many people. Because it's a thick white fat, it must be bad for you, right? But the opposite is actually true. Coconut oil actually is shown to help your body balance the metabolism by burning fats faster. But it does so much more than that! When researching for this book, I wanted to give you the list of all of the benefits coconut oil has, but the list is so long I can't include them all here! However, here is a condensed short list:

- Promotes weight loss, when needed
- Supports your immune system health
- Supports a healthy metabolism
- Provides you with an immediate energy source
- Keeps your skin healthy and youthful looking
- Supports the proper functioning of your thyroid gland

It's ideal to have a tablespoon at least a day of raw organic virgin coconut oil. It's something you can eat on its own or mixed into smoothies/desserts/raw treats or on breads/crackers. And of course, it's great on your skin and used in your hair too. And you can give it to your dog too. Pets love it! I take coconut oil tablets to make sure that I always have it every day. I have noticed that I am able to maintain my weight and also easily lose a few kgs if I need to.

✓ For much more detailed information about coconut oil please check out coconutresearchcenter.org

* * *

It's impossible to list all of the things you can add to your diet to help you heal and stay that way. What has amazed me along this journey is understanding just how incredible the plant world is. Scientists are discovering new powerful qualities in certain plants and foods all the time.

For learning more, here are some wonderful books which can point you in the right direction:

Raw Magic by Kate Magic

Adaptogens by David Winston

Supplements and vitamins: the ugly truth

Mark Hyman, MD, founder and medical director of Ultra Wellness Center in Lenox, Mass. and author of The Ultra Simple Diet, writes: *'If people eat wild, fresh, organic, local, non-genetically modified food grown in virgin mineral-rich soils that has not been transported across vast distances and stored for months before being eaten … and work and live outside, breathe only fresh unpolluted air, drink only pure, clean water, sleep nine hours a night, move their bodies every day and are free from chronic stressors and exposure to environmental toxins, then perhaps, they might not need supplements.'*[120]

Sadly, this does not describe any single person on earth who lives like this anymore. Toxins and food lacking in minerals is how it is these days. So we are needing, more than ever, to really make our diets the best that they can be, and even then, the food is still lacking in the levels of nutrients that they once had before factory farming and Big Agriculture was invented (foods are said to be 55–85% less nutrient-dense than 60 years ago).

So to the question of 'Do we even need supplements?' the answer is usually a big yes! Pretty much every single one of us cannot remain truly healthy without taking some things these days. Yet, sadly, we have been led to believe that we can always trust where our little vitamin pills come from – they are all healthy, right?

Unfortunately, *no*. Buyers must be aware that, as with most things, where you source your vitamins and supplements from is *highly* important. Many vitamin companies are actually now owned by pharmaceutical companies (who see that the growing market is booming and want a piece of the pie) and they are also putting very toxic and cheap fillers into their products or making the supplements so low in strength that they really do absolutely nothing for us. Also, due to the epidemic of digestion problems, many supplements are not being absorbed into the body the way they should be.[121] It can be like literally throwing money down the drain or down your toilet. Many people who work at outdoor festivals and have the charming job of emptying the porta-loos report that they find hundreds of completely undigested vitamins in the bottoms of the toilets.

It was only recently brought to my attention that I too had naively been consuming vitamins that were all from synthetic and unsafe sources which were really not doing a lot of good. Years ago, when I first became interested in Natural Health, I literally took handfuls of tablets every day. At one stage it was about 30 or so every *day*. Now, with my knowledge about synthetic vitamins that have dangerous fillers added to them, I cringe thinking about the harm I was doing to my body from something that I was led to believe was supposedly healthy. It's got to be said that the natural health world also has a *lot* of misinformation sprinkled in among the genuinely good products and advice. There are many people involved in this industry too, who are not really ethical and only want to make money.

Synthetically produced vitamins are what most of our supplements are made from (it's said up to 99%) and they include many toxic sources. For example, if you were taking a vitamin K tablet it would be most likely made from a coal tar derivative with p-allelic-nickel. Coal tar is used to make roads, and is found in anti-dandruff shampoos, conditioners and synthetic paints, dyes and photographic materials. Why, then, should it be OK to be added to our vitamins?

For more examples of these scary ingredients used to make our seemingly trusted brands of supplements, please refer to the following chart found on the Touchstone Essentials website:

✓ touchstoneessentials.com/the-five-problems-with-vitamin-supplements

Isn't it scary where most of our 'vitamins' actually come from? I was gobsmacked when I really knew the truth. Because of the fact that our soils are lacking in vital nutrients from over-farming, and most of us are simply not eating enough healthy foods, I realized that many of us are quite malnourished, despite eating regular meals. And due to this alarming information about what our supplements are most of the time derived from, I needed to try and find some that were *genuinely* good for our health. I have to admit, due to the majority of companies producing utter rubbish it was very hard to come across many decent brands who were making high-quality real food supplements. I also needed to source *organic* whole-food supplements which had the vitamins and minerals intact, and were coming from *real food* sources. As I have discovered, things from Nature are always the best.

The best brand by far that I discovered in 2012 is Touchstone Essentials. This is a USA-owned company and one of only five brands in the *entire* country who make these sorts of food-grade organic wholefood supplements. Touchstone have managed to produce supplements that are as close to *real food* as you can get. The production method, which is unique to Touchstone, has enabled them to keep the ingredients as pure as possible because they have only used cold-pressed manufacturing methods, so in actual fact the ingredients are still 'raw', allowing you to get as much nutrition as possible from these supplements. And, yes, while it is best to eat your nutrients from real food, no one will be able to eat the equivalent, every day, of what is in these little capsules.

In the 'Essentials', which is Touchstone's multivitamin equivalent, check out what is inside their capsules:

Grape extract from grape skin, grape seed, and fruit; stabilized rice bran, green tea extract (decaffeinated), cinnamon extract, broccoli sprout concentrate, organic agaricus blasei mushroom, organic pomegranate juice, organic apple juice, quebracho extract, noni extract, acerola extract, acai extract, mangosteen extract, pomegranate extract, blueberry extract, blackberry extract, strawberry extract, cranberry extract, organic Jerusalem artichoke, Amylase, Amylase II, Protease I, Protease II, Peptidase, Lipase, Cellulase, Hemiseb™, Lactase, Maltase, Invertase, Bromelain, organic blackberry powder, organic blueberry powder, organic tart cherry powder, organic cranberry powder, organic lemon powder, organic mango powder, organic orange powder, organic raspberry powder and astaxanthin.

And this is what is in their 'SuperGreens + D' Formula, which provides 1000 IUs of vitamin D per serving:

Organic Barley Grass Juice, Organic Parsley Juice, Organic Spinach Juice, Broccoli Extract, Amylase, Amylase II, Protease I, Protease II, Peptidase, Lipase, Cellulase, Hemiseb™, Lactase, Maltase, Invertase, Bromelain, DDS-1 Lactobacillus acidophilus, Bifidobacterium bifidum, Lactobacillus bulgaricus, Lactobacillus plantarum, Lactobacillus salivarius, Streptococcus thermophilus, Bifidobacterium infantis, Lactobacillus longum and Lactobacillus rhamnosus.

With ingredients like those, you can probably see why I am such a big fan of this company. What I also love about their supplements is that they are not only completely safe, but highly recommended for children and pregnant women, due to the fact they are food-based supplements. And they are very good for people who are not able to eat much food, for example those who have just gone through treatment or are going through chemotherapy, which is often making them very nauseous.

I also love the company's genuinely good and compassionate ethics, and that they don't make any over-the-top claims. They are just offering people top-quality nutrition through the best farming methods, and the way they turn the food into the supplements is cutting edge. They also donate money out of their profits to their Touchstone Essentials Foundation, which goes to children in need. This is why I promote this brand, as I feel that there are too many great reasons why people need to know about them.

For every single person on the planet, we really only need to do a few things to be healthy: we need to *detox* the heavy metals and chemicals, and *nourish* our bodies with the right nutrition, from *food*, and not always from synthetic chemicals. Sometimes we may need to turn to synthetic vitamins if we have to take something like CoQ10 or Carnosine that is required in much higher doses as we age. But to take synthetic vitamins all the time, which have lots of added fillers is not the best for our health.

After trying Touchstone's supplements over just one month, I could see very quickly how incredible they were from my own improvements in skin quality, digestion, energy, nail strength and general health. I had never seen that from any other vitamin products before. I also love the fact that the supplements are all raw as they have been cold-processed and are so beneficial and safe that kids can take them. I discuss their Pure Body Zeolite for use with children in Part 3 of this guide.

You can find out more info about Touchstone Essentials on my website:

✓ missecoglam.com

Chapter 29

Four Weeks to Better Health – See How Quickly You Can Turn Your Health and Energy Around

Dr. Prasanna Kerur, Ayurvedic Consultant at the Ayush Wellness Spa, Jersey, advises the following tips to feel more energized and healthy:

- Start the day with 'honey water', using a teaspoonful of good-quality honey (like manuka) to half a pint of clean still water.
- Eat light with a combination of raw and freshly cooked, easily digestible food.
- Stick to regular eating patterns and avoid skipping meals.
- Sleep is vital to keep our biological rhythm in balance, so avoid too much or too little.
- Eat wholemeal grains and lentils and avoid processed, sugary foods
- Use healthy herbs and spices like fresh ginger, turmeric, garlic, cumin seeds and black pepper in routine cooking that have properties to reduce bad cholesterol, protect vital organs and trigger the body's metabolism.
- Exercise regularly.
- Fast for a day once a fortnight to allow the body's systems to have a rest, which will help to regularize the metabolism. Drink lots of lemon water during this time.
- Eliminate red meat, pork, shellfish, excess dairy products, excess wheat and alcohol.
- Drink fresh juices like wheat grass, spinach, ginger and carrot with a hint of honey.
- Eat plenty of fresh vegetables in your daily diet but reduce your intake of potatoes, mushrooms and aubergines.

- Take a teaspoonful of organic flax seed oil every other day.
- Body brush a couple of times a week to enhance circulation and stimulate weight loss.
- Avoid stress.
- Do regular exercise 5 times a week, walking for 30 minutes.

Chapter 30

Real-Life Inspiring Stories from People Who Turned Their Lives Around – Naturally!

Here is a small collection of stories from people who suffered from illness, depression and anxiety – people who became very sick from prescription medications or found that medical help wasn't able to do anything for them. Some of the lifestyle changes are simple and were just about diet, and some took a bit more effort. All are inspiring!

Frank Arrigazzi: my journey to health the ancient way

I didn't have any idea as a kid that the way I was been brought up would make such a difference to my life. I had been taught to always see my body as a 'perfect machine'. I heard many times my father saying, 'Your body is expressing itself with a non-verbal language; it speaks to you with "symptoms" and if you shut the symptoms off you will deplete the life-force potential of your body. But if you look and listen to your body symptoms, understand, and address their root cause, then you will always have a perfect body.'

These words have been with me all my life, and when I left home at the age of 18 I did not think that I would necessarily have to think about 'being healthy'; I just thought that being healthy was something natural, which should be the case when following a natural path. But living in a big city so disconnected from Nature, exposed to polluted environments, eating foods depleted of minerals which are loaded with pesticides – this is not what Nature intended for us.

Soon after leaving my family home, I found myself exposed to an unnatural and polluted world, not much easy access to natural foods, constantly eating sugary processed foods… To tell you the truth, I was quickly led to believe that if everyone else was following that way of life – eating fried foods, using microwaves, having processed chemical-based foods and they were still 'walking and living' – then maybe isn't wasn't too bad to live that way? That it was normal?

Reading my body

As a child I was encouraged to observe and use the subtle signs of my body as my main thermostat to understand my health: the color and wrinkles of the skin in my face, signs under my eyes, in the whites of the eyes. The levels of energy and vitality felt in the mornings, the quality of nails and hair. And interestingly, what I started noticing in myself after living in an unnatural manner for a few months was that the whites of my eyes were starting to look yellow, my skin was quickly showing more wrinkles, my hair was even falling out. I was waking up in the morning tired, drained. I felt depressed and was very uncertain about everything. I was only 18!

I began to feel that perhaps my destiny was to be unhealthy. I didn't remember with clarity anymore all the things learned as a child and what the word 'health' really meant. I observed my signs but didn't have the will to understand more. I was going out, smoking, drinking and letting that 'other' side take me over. I didn't think that living in this way could have more effect than just bringing a little bit of fun...

But nothing could be further from the truth. I was escaping from being fully in charge, and avoiding taking full responsibility for my fears and concerns. I was simply living the false belief that we are meant to 'have fun', and if that was the case, at what price?

Understanding the sacredness

It was after developing severe outbreaks of panic attacks and deep levels of anxiety that I started to reconsider where I was going and what was really important. It all reached a point where I couldn't walk comfortably in public spaces without feeling completely overwhelmed by the devastating feeling of losing control. I was totally overtaken by deep states of fear and stress every time I was exposed to an open public space, such as supermarkets, trains, restaurants. Now I was even replicating this state just by being in my house on my own. What was happening? I couldn't understand how this could happen to me... And then, after experiencing a very shocking outbreak one night, I suddenly remembered everything: 'Every symptom in your body has a code, a meaning. Your body is a perfect machine that expresses itself with a non-verbal language; it express itself with symptoms.' 'Whenever you become silent, present and listen to your body, you will understand its sacredness.'

Everything started to make sense – I was running from myself and didn't have any space for feeling where I was going. Instead I was just living on 'autopilot', and acting with no meaning or purpose whatsoever. And of course, my body was manifesting through each and every cell the deep discomfort caused by my actions. This was my understanding and I was determined to make a change.

Transforming the subtle energies

A decision was made and I started to take responsibility for every action in my life. I wanted to know what I was doing and how different things would affect me.

First thing I was committed to change was my daily routine, so I started to practice every morning a little bit of yoga. And, by adding a few simple exercises before my breakfast, I felt a huge difference in how I was feeling: much more energy, with a feeling of calmness, and I was more focused and present. I also researched how the electromagnetic fields in our environment coming from cell phones, computers, antennas were affecting the fractal energies and natural rhythms of the body, so I decided to reduce considerably the use of those in my life and started to go more often for walks in Nature.

I wanted to shine, to feel great, so the more I wanted that feeling, the more action I would take.

I also started doing colonic irrigations – a practice used from ancient times to clean our colon from toxins and impurities – and also added into my routine fresh juices, raw foods, whole foods, super-foods and herbs, and soon enough I started noticing a big difference in my skin, my hair stopped falling out, and it had just been a few weeks of discipline!

I continued challenging my old habits by adding new ones and naturally I stopped smoking and drinking. I noticed that I also attracted people into my life who inspired me to carry on throughout this journey and I reminded myself daily where I was going, by putting messages and pictures all over my room.

The yellowish color of my eyes started changing, and they became white again, my wrinkles started disappearing, and my hair stopped falling out completely. A few months later the panic attacks were completely gone and now it has been already been many years and I have never ever looked back.

Frank is the founder of purplebalancesuperfoods.com

Jesse Bogdanovich: my long road back to perfect health

I was born perfectly healthy, but an allergic reaction to a live polio vaccine at the age of 10 months almost killed me and left me with convulsions, seizures and paralysis. At that time doctors did not have to report such reactions, so they treated my condition as symptoms of flu and fever and dosed me up with antibiotics.

They also advised my mother not to breastfeed me any longer (thankfully she refused to listen to them) and recommended all sorts of wrong foods. My parents tell me that before I got the polio shot I was walking almost perfectly. But after it, it was a long time before I could walk again.

I remember as a small child having no strength in my legs or arms, and feeling very tired and needing lots of sleep. Doctors put me in braces and did all sorts of other things that didn't do me any good. They also recommended ligament surgery to loosen up the tightness in my limbs but fortunately my parents refused to do that.

I was so uninterested in food that I was very underweight; the doctors' solution was to force me to eat dairy, fats and junky, processed foods. Needless to say, this only made things worse and led, among other things, to juvenile diabetes and digestive problems.

It boggles my mind to think how hard my parents tried to feed me naturally and how opposed the doctors were to anything that deviated from the Standard American Diet. Not surprisingly, as time went by, my health deteriorated further. My parents took me to doctors of all kinds – from one opinion to the next, and from America to Europe. We went halfway around the world looking for a cure, not realizing the cure was in the proper nutrition found in our own garden and in the wild.

One day, when I was 12, my mom took me to a specialist who was supposed to be a world expert. He made me take off my clothes and had me try to stand up and walk across the floor, which was very cold. He then picked up a tape recorder and proceeded to talk into it about me. He painted such a grim picture, saying that I would never be able to walk, that my condition would only get worse and that I would die from the hormonal changes of puberty. I was crying and my mom almost passed out. Then she whispered to me, 'Do not believe a word he is saying. Let's go to the pet shop.'

The doctor was so engrossed in what he was doing that we snuck out and left. Sobbing, I told my mom I would prove the doctor wrong. On another occasion, my dad took me for a check-up for an ingrown toenail that was infected. My legs were turning purple and pus was coming out. The specialist wanted to operate and cut my toe off immediately. When my dad asked him to 'let us think it over', the doctor got mad and told us that I would lose my toes and my foot. Again we left, and I remember feeling devastated and really starting to think more about the why of things.

I had refused wheelchairs from the beginning. My dad carried me all over the place. When I was sitting down, I would sit so no one could see that I couldn't walk properly. I avoided walking as much as possible, since it was always difficult, what with swaying back and forth and sideways. But I couldn't avoid it at school, and it was very difficult to be around other kids because they made fun of me and wanted to fight and push me around. Those were dark days and I remember the pain of it being so great I wanted to die.

One day I broke down and told my parents I would rather do anything than go to school again. My parents heard my heart and from then on they home-schooled me. It was much easier on me and I got to see the world as I studied and traveled all over with my parents.

This approach caused me to want to learn, and I was allowed all the time I needed to explore the subjects that interested me. I did not have to study the unnecessary things that most kids have to learn in order to graduate, and one big advantage to home-schooling was that my studies would be done in a few hours rather than a whole day at school.

This education made me think and look at things in a more real and logical way and gave me an advantage over other kids my age. One day I told my parents that if someone dropped me off at the other side of the world I would know how to function and would make good of it. Even though I had health issues that other kids did not have, I felt very fortunate.

There came a time when we did not go to mainstream doctors anymore. My mom became a naturopathic doctor so she could learn what she needed to know to help me. By then we had discovered that doctors do not learn anything about nutrition during their studies, which is why they insist that nutrition has nothing to do with healing.

The first breakthrough in my health happened after my dad became interested in Paul and Patricia Bragg's fasting techniques. My parents took me to see Patricia and I fasted many times for 1–3 days, then 7–10 days, and then I worked my way up to a few 14-day water fasts. Each time I water-fasted, I experienced great improvement in my symptoms, but as soon as I started eating cooked food again, the problems would return.

We tried so many different diets, and most of them had certain things in common: they focused on whole foods and excluded sweets, white flour, fried foods and other junk. This is why they worked partially, yet none of these diets worked completely like the raw food-diet did.

When I first heard about the raw diet, the information resonated so deeply within me I couldn't put the it down. I completely woke up to this truth; it was like someone had turned on the lights. I was ready to go in this new direction wholeheartedly and I embraced it knowing that this would stop my suffering once and for all.

I changed to a 100% raw vegan lifestyle overnight. I was 21 at the time. What convinced me the most about raw food was that humans and their pets are the only creatures that get sick with degenerative diseases. They are also the only ones who eat cooked food.

I went to see and studied with many raw-food experts – something I am still doing to this day. I learned about the importance of rest, little or no stress, sunshine and exercise, and that a program that combines these essential elements with raw foods and periodic fasting enables the body to perform miracles.

When we start doing what's right to our body it starts healing immediately. It's amazing, really, how simple it all is. After six months on a 100% raw-food diet my condition started to change for the better and kept improving all the time. First I could walk without pain. Then for the first time, I could run. I gained 40 pounds over the next few years. This is what happens when the body is freed of mucus and able to absorb the essential nutrients on an enzyme-rich raw vegan diet. With patience and perseverance, coupled with forgiveness for the doctors and my parents, I was able to overcome what had seemed to be insurmountable problems.

Raw, organic food is a very important part of healing, yet without emotional healing, finding peace in your heart and forgiving everyone, you will not heal completely. But the 100% raw vegan diet not only got me better physically, mentally and emotionally; I also woke up spiritually. I have a deep spiritual connection now with Nature and with every person I meet on my path. I have to tell everyone starting on this path to get ready for a healing crisis and not to give up.

Today I am totally healthy, extremely happy and I can walk, run and climb just like anyone else. The only thing that is noticeable is that my right leg at the knee turns inward when I walk slowly. People do ask me at times if I've broken my leg or hurt my foot. I am working on that and soon it will be perfect, I know it will. The raw vegan lifestyle delivers on all levels and every year it just keeps getting better and better. I have been on this path for over 13 years now.

What this lifestyle has done for me is… actually, there are no words in the dictionary that can describe it. But if I had to pick some words I would choose 'beyond fabulous'! To stay on this path and feel like I do, one must eat very simply and get away from raw gourmet foods that cause health problems, cravings and all sorts of disorders.

It is very important to stay away from all the packaged and heated raw foods which cause you to crave wrong things. Eat plenty of fresh, organic fruits and vegetables – lots of leafy greens – and don't forget to throw in some wild foods such as berries and edible weeds. Add soaked raw seeds and nuts in tiny quantities and make sure they are organic and truly raw.

This way of eating can bring peace to your mind just as it brings peace to your tummy. It also brings clear thinking and love in your heart and soul.

It has definitely been a process of learning the hard way, but I wouldn't change anything. Now that I am well and strong, my calling is to help spread this health message, which needs to be heard all over the world, starting in kindergarten.

People sometimes ask me if I would ever go back to eating cooked food and I tell them that I would never do that. Why would I? Many people do not stick with raw foods and fasting long enough to reap the rewards, but my story is an example of what is possible. Through proper nutrition and fasting my body healed itself, and I believe these practices will do that for anyone willing to do the same.

Jesse Bogdanovich is a co-founder of The Cure Is In The Cause Foundation (thecureisinthecause.org). He is also the founder of The Whole Lifestyle, through which he supports individuals on their raw vegan diet, health, exercise, passion, happiness, peace, emotional aspects and home environment.

Cathy Francis, Australia

Since mid July I've gone from 92.3 kilos to 68.8 and I could not be happier. What inspired me was that I wanted to look awesome in my wedding dress.

In the past, fad diets and quick-fix 'lose 7 pounds in one week' crappy diets were only temporary solutions and ultimately resulted in dire outcomes for me. So I decided what my favorite exercise was and based my whole weight loss on that. I love walking, but preferred not to do it on a treadmill. When I walk I like to have a purpose and achieve something. So after doing some research and figuring out exactly how much I spend on public transport from work and how much a gym membership would cost me, I decided to start walking home from the city every night. It was 8 kilometers and took me an hour and a half at a solid good pace.

The first week was tough, but over time it got easier and the walk became a pleasure instead of a chore. As far as my diet, after doing that walk every day I didn't even want to touch junk/naughty food and found my diet changing so naturally to incorporate more fresh fruit, vegetables, and fresh produce. I also felt like I needed a lot of protein in the evenings, and had small evening meals after my walk, combined with at least 2 liters of water throughout the day to keep me hydrated.

The end result – over 20 kilos lost in a healthy, satisfying and ultimately long-lasting way. It's a complete lifestyle change for me. I save half of my monthly travel expenses. And I don't have to pay for a gym membership as I am starting to do exercises at home for toning (sit-ups, crunches, etc.). It's also made my relationship a lot better as my fiancé can see not only a thinner me; he sees a happier me. I still have a bit more weight to drop, but I'm not at all worried or stressed about it. And I still have the odd day here and there when I eat my fair share of chocolate and pizza!

Cathy got married in August 2012 and was able to fit into her dream dress and has still kept her weight off by embracing her new lifestyle.

Nicola McCarthy: my macro journey

Looking back, I was an extremely lazy child whose greatest pleasure was to sit in front of the TV eating sweets. I hated exercise and when I was written off PE permanently – because my allergies meant my skin would break out if I got too hot – I was overjoyed.

Given what I now know about the importance of diet, my childhood allergies, lethargy and low self-esteem could all be directly attributed to the sweets and chocolate that systematically stripped my system of any possibility of health and happiness. The deep-seated insecurities that tormented me as a child, I now realize, were the inevitable result of regularly sending my blood sugar haywire with yet another brightly colored mouthful of junk.

The frightening thing is, this is the story of the majority of childhoods: now and then. The upshot was that, from my teenage years, I was crippled with arthritis and taking large doses of medication. Plus my allergies had become debilitating: I couldn't even go out in the sun. If I did, my skin would erupt in huge, water-filled blisters. My childhood insecurities had blossomed into full-blown panic attacks that began to rule my life. I was a prisoner and my mind and body were the prison.

Fast-forward ten years: I am a mother of two. My PMT is so bad I have to write off ten days every month, my marriage is falling apart, and I exist in a haze of exhaustion and confusion. The doctor prescribes hormone pessaries that I gladly add to my hefty list of anti-inflammatories, painkillers, antihistamines and heartburn medicine, rounded off each day with generous dollops of junk food. Yes, to add to my woes, in my late 20s I am now also fat.

Moving forward again, my eldest child, Jack, was 6 when he was diagnosed with hyperactivity and dyslexia. In addition he had constant ear infections and general poor health. I was literally at my wit's end when a friend suggested he see a kinesiologist. I didn't realize it then, but I was about to change not just his life but the rest of mine. The kinesiologist prescribed a diet of simple food, excluding sugar, dairy and wheat. Jack transformed. The kinesiologist suggested I too change my diet. Sadly, I wasn't ready to give up the junk.

But something had sparked in me and in my mid-30s, as a result of what they had been able to do for Jack, I became fascinated by complementary therapies. I visited an iridologist who, by looking at my irises, gave a stunningly accurate appraisal of my health – or lack of it. I enrolled on a Natural Therapy course and found myself, for the first time in my life, completely comfortable in the presence of others. The people on the course were something I hadn't come across before: kind and gentle. And I literally gobbled up all the information I was getting. A door had opened for me: little did I know then that stepping through it would close the door to my old life forever.

I signed up for a foundation course in Anatomy, Physiology and Massage and, from that, went on to qualify as a practitioner in Reflexology and Reiki, and studied Homeopathy, Crystal Healing, Aromatherapy and Kinesiology. Yet, I still avoided studying the most fundamental healing tool of all: food.

Thankfully, this vital, missing part of the equation was soon to be addressed. David McCarthy had recently lost his son to cancer when he came to me for treatment. We got talking and he told me how he had prolonged his son's life to the astonishment of the medical fraternity: he treated Jonathan just by stripping his diet of everything toxic. As a pharmacist, he was acutely aware of how standard drugs affect the body, and his experience of Jonathan's illness and treatment convinced him that these drugs were not only, in the main, not effective but usually hastened death rather than preventing it.

David had decided to dedicate the rest of his life to searching for a natural cure for cancer and promoting a measure of health attainable for everyone. Using food.

A successful businessman, this life-changing decision had cost him his marriage. My own marriage, never strong, had been dealt a fatal blow by my increasing emotional investment in a belief system outside the norm. I had outgrown my old life, and the next phase with David would see it transformed beyond my wildest imaginings.

David could see immediately that all my health problems stemmed from my eating habits. He was becoming increasingly interested in the possibilities of macrobiotics in realizing his dream of naturally preventing and treating cancer, and together we gradually took the plunge and began to clean up our diet. We took some classes – learning how to turn all the weird and wonderful items we were faced with into tasty food – and within 2 weeks all the joint pain I had suffered for decades had disappeared. I could move my body freely: it's difficult to adequately describe what that meant to me. My allergies subsided, and in a short time they too had vanished. My anger and depression receded, and as my mood began to stabilize I was, for perhaps the first time, interested in life. My energy levels skyrocketed; my skin was clear and literally sparkled. It was like being reborn.

The next astonishing transformation was my weight. I lost 3 stone (42 pounds).

We signed up at the Kushi Institute of Europe in Amsterdam. Their 'Art of Life Program' combines food and cooking knowledge with life-enhancing philosophy. The course took several years and during this time we learned the importance of cooking classes in order to follow a macrobiotic way of life properly. Meals should be balanced correctly in order to get the most out of the food.

David and I have been extremely lucky. Just when our lives looked like they were about to crash and burn, we both rescued the possibility of a better life from the ashes.

Our macrobiotic lifestyle has given us immeasurable benefits. It isn't limiting, as many people assume; it is actually freeing. To live in harmony with yourself, with others and with the planet is to experience the best life has to offer. Our 9-year-old daughter Kerry has been macrobiotic from birth and, to finish this story where it started, is a living example of how it is possible to break the cycle of illness, depression and waste that is the sad hallmark of our culture. She is all the things I was not as a child: bright, healthy, happy, full of energy and yet completely centered.

Wouldn't it be wonderful if all children could be like this? Guess what, they can.

Nicola and her husband David run a macrobiotic & organic shop in Haywards Heath, East Sussex. They both also teach macrobiotic courses and have a successful online shop stocking very hard-to-find ingredients.

✓ macrobioticshop.co.uk

Star Khechara: how going back to my childhood helped me to regain my life

I started my holistic journey early on in life as I was lucky to have been born to a non-conforming mother who used to take us away each summer to a rustic retreat by a nature reserve beach to enjoy several weeks of barefoot walking, wild swimming, no-electricity, story-telling and communal chores. I still remember those holidays fondly and it made me realize that living a natural healthy life is not only good for us, in the traditional sense, but also really fun too, an adventure! Often we're fed images by the media that somehow caring for the environment and eating healthily is weird, or a mental illness or a boring ascetic way to survive (cue images of eating beige gruel in unheated houses while wearing a hairy jumper and waxing lyrical about compost toilets and the benefits of hemp).

During my childhood summer holidays, while on retreat, I would meet all kinds of interesting characters: boat people, hippies, gardeners, crafters, herbal experts and spiritual types; I learnt to sketch, make baskets, meditate, pick up jellyfish, sing around campfires, macramé, pick wild mint, and to also be part of a community who ate, slept and worked side by side. I ate a lot of homemade bread, marrow and Marmite and learned to like cold showers, candlelight and the sound of crickets.

Then I turned 14 and I was far too 'cool' to do the homespun life; I wanted the latest trainers, to fancy a boy and to have a Sony Walkman. I became super-addicted to sugar and this led to many years suffering from chronic hypoglycemia (long-term low blood sugar), I was always of a nervous disposition, and also suffered from IBS (although I didn't know it had a name back then). Sometimes it felt that no matter what I ate, I would spend the next hour on the toilet, then suffer a sugar low where all I could do was lie down and moan. As I hit my early 20s I experimented with drugs, namely marijuana and speed (amphetamine); I also tried MDMA (Ecstasy) and cocaine a few times. By this point I was literally living on cheap cake so I could spend my money partying. I felt tired and depressed all the time, my body was very thin yet flabby at the same time, even my eyelashes started to fall out with my terrible lifestyle. I couldn't hold down a job as I was too messed up so I was a drop-out benefit claimant. Throughout this time I constantly felt sad as I knew there had to be a better life for me, but I was so sick (mentally and physically by this point) I didn't know how to climb out of the hole I had willingly dug for myself. I knew there was more to life and I started borrowing 'self-help' books from older friends and attending spiritual circles to end my downward spiral. Slowly I weaned myself off the self-hate life and my awareness started to blossom – admittedly it was a faint glimmer at first.

I started becoming aware of the invisible toxicity around me, in my air, my water, my thoughts, my skincare, my diet and in the friendship choices I made. I realized that it was all connected and that it was up to me to detox each aspect of my life to become the truly joyful, happy person I wanted to be. It dawned on me that everything we do in life has only two outcomes: it either builds up health or destroys it. Nothing, it seems, is ever neutral. And by health I am not just talking about diet and fitness but about total vibrancy in every aspect of life. The words 'health', 'whole', 'heal' and 'holistic' are all related; to be healthy is to function at the highest level in every aspect of your life – mind, body and spirit; to have a healthy home, fulfilling job (life path), love connection, and to enjoy emotional balance.

For me the process started with beauty and skincare. I began making my own earth-friendly and skin-friendly products which would actually nourish my skin without containing any harmful chemicals. I made potion after potion for myself, for friends and for family. I trained in aromatherapy which taught me so much about how plants contain amazing natural properties and have the power to heal body, mind and spirit. Our sense of smell is closely linked to emotion and these natural essences are Nature's psychologists.

Around that time I found a book about raw food and thought, Wow! Isn't it funny how sometimes the most bizarrely 'out there' idea is actually really simple and logical when you finally take notice of it? I decided to study nutrition and became my own health expert.

I really believe that we are all the experts of our own bodies and that by becoming autonomous self-reliant beings we are allowing ourselves to really 'be'. I took responsibility for my life – out went the drugs, the toxic friendships, the cheap nasty food. I decided to make my health the number-one priority no matter what – an attitude I have kept since. I became selfish; I learned to put myself first and to not worry about what others thought of me. By being a shining example, I unconsciously inspire others to do the same – just as I was inspired by others along the way. The path to true health is not always easy but it has multiple rewards. My IBS and blood sugar issues disappeared when I adopted a low-fat, raw vegan diet. I no longer suffer with mood swings, depression, chronic cystitis, kidney problems, eczema, nervousness/anxiety and all those other minor niggles like joint pain, splitting finger nails, mouth ulcers and multiple allergies. It's such a relief to be able to go on a long walk without constantly worrying about whether I'll need a bowel movement or not – I honestly can't believe I suffered for so long at my own hands. However, I am glad of the path my life took; after all, I wouldn't be here doing exactly what I do now had it not been for the journey that led me here. I feel that I can be a better example to others having come through the swamp and emerged shiny and triumphant, reborn into vibrancy. I've come a long way in my 36 years and I feel blessed to have made it thus far.

'Appreciation' and 'gratitude' are two words that I now live by. I have created my dream life. Each day, I enjoy eating a rejuvenating diet abundant in delicious raw fruits; I have my dream career writing, teaching and helping others, and wonderful friendships with like-minded folk. Not bad for a girl from a council house and a broken home, so if I can do it, anyone can.

Dream it, live it, be it!

In beauty

Star Xxx

Star Khechara is the author of The Holistic Beauty Book *and runs the School of Holistic Cosmetology – teaching the science of professional organic skincare formulation. She is currently offering a free holistic anti-aging course at her nutrition website TheFaceliftDiet.com and also runs Fruitforbeauty.com.*

Magdalena Tamara Callea

In 1991, at the age of 41, I went into Casualty upon the advice of my GP at the time and was hospitalized. I underwent test upon test and was found to have a tumor in the abdomen on my left side. For years I had had inexplicable bouts of pain which was excruciating and caused me to withdraw from everything and everyone for days at a time.

In October that year I was operated on and the tumor was removed. When I went to see the surgeon, a month later, I remember vividly how he advised me to sit down and generally behaved as if he had something unusual to tell me. He let me know that the tumor he had removed was a low-grade malignant metastasis, meaning that the primary tumor was elsewhere; also the tumor was such that it could not be identified, so the specialists did not know where the primary tumor might be, what organ might have thrown this secondary one off. The tumor had been attached to the psoas muscle, on the back abdominal wall. He suggested I look into further treatment after the operation, like radiotherapy or chemotherapy. The feelings I had were of shock at hearing that diagnosis: I had joined the millions who had the big 'C' and it felt very peculiar. I remember going for a second opinion to the Royal Marsden Hospital in Surrey and very little emerging from that encounter other than that it might be the pancreas which had thrown it off... I remember thinking to myself how unsatisfactory all the investigation methods were and that I would be left to grow another one – not realizing much about the power of manifestation at the time.

I felt it would be useless to continue to worry about it, since it had been removed and I was feeling fine. So I went for a healing session, started taking homeopathy, went into doing lots of exercise and getting fit and generally getting back into good health. About 4 years later, I began to feel a twinge of pain again in the same area. I duly had a scan and nothing showed up. By 2000, the pain was back and I was having regular attacks again and taking codeine to alleviate the pain.

By this time, I'd begun working out that my left-sided pain might have something to do with my feminine side not being honored. Cancer might have something to do with allowing something inside to eat at me rather than externalizing how I was feeling. But the actual situation of the tumor remained a mystery to me. The psoas muscle had something to do with standing upright. It would be years later that the connection would emerge and make sense to me. How to remedy this? I had no idea. It was one thing recognizing these symbolisms and another putting them into action.

2006 saw me back in hospital with acute pain and the prospect of a nephrectomy – the removal of my left kidney, since the tumor seemed to have wrapped itself around it.

In the event, I was opened and then sewn up again as the doctor decided not to remove anything. When I came round from the anesthetic, he told me that he was not pleased with his operation as he had not taken anything out. The reason was that to do so would have caused too much damage to the psoas muscle and would have hindered my walking.

I remember thinking: Well, I guess it's up to me, now, to find a way of healing myself.

Mental, emotional and spiritual tools for healing the mind

After convalescing for a few months, I began earnest self-inquiry. I used The Work sheets of Byron Katie and wrote reams and reams of responses to the questions – www.thework.com.

I began a training in Systemic and Family Constellations which went on for some years and shed much light on the hidden dynamics both in my family of origin and in my relationships with my children – see my website www.love4miracles.wordpress.com for more details of my work.

In 2008, I finally consented to begin working with A Course in Miracles.

Physical tools for healing the body

Around the same time, I also agreed to start some physical cleanses. I had had three people suggest the liver flush to me and so I decided to do it, as I believe that if something comes up three times, it's time to pay attention. I went through the whole cleansing program as set out by Savannah Alalia – www.savannahalalia.com: salt-water colon flushes, kidney cleanse and liver cleanses. These began a process of clearing out old patterns and stuff held in the cellular memory of the body's organs. I began to shed pounds and pounds, but gently, and adjusted my eating habits, so that within four years I have dropped 2½ stone (21 pounds) in weight. Earlier this year, 2012, I started taking clinoptilolite zeolites from Pure Body and that has made an enormous difference to my physical wellbeing.

A Course in Miracles and then a few months later The Way of Mastery – www.wayofmastery.com – began to turn my mental attitude and beliefs around. I began to realize that there are only two possible ways of experiencing life: from Love or from fear. Fear contracts and poisons the body in the most extraordinary ways and causes all the body's illnesses. Fear in the mind causes judgment, blame, anger, jealousy, possessiveness, insecurity, and all the negative emotional states and these in turn affect the body chemically – and do I then try to be positive and avoid negativity at all costs? NO! It is vital to learn that all our states are self-induced. This means that I am 100% responsible for everything that happens to me because it is my reaction which causes an emotional state to occur within me. So, if I encounter someone who triggers anger in me, for example, it is important for me to enquire within what it is that this person has touched in me. At first this seems ridiculous. It seems so much easier to point a finger and blame. But eventually it becomes pleasing and exciting to actually do the detective work and find out what this person is showing me about myself that I didn't know. And what is being touched, or what button is being pushed is usually an old wound, a pattern, a belief that 'I am right' and something I therefore believe I have to defend. When I am defending, I am in fear.

The above is very important to explain how my healing process began. I first had to come to a point in my life where it became clear to me that I was treading on the spot. I had contorted myself this way and that, and had not gotten anywhere except to become ill and dissatisfied with my life. I was existing rather than thriving. My relationships were based on obligations and opportunism.

I had to arrive at rock bottom. I had to admit that I had lost control over my life and that fear was controlling me. Everything I did was out of fear. Until I chose differently. I left my job, I left the country, I went to live abroad with a loving friend. I changed my circumstances, but I took myself with me! And again, the old patterns surfaced. But this time, there was a difference in my responses. I had committed to finding healing and so to finding out the truth about my illness. I had the time and the support of true friends to do this.

My commitment was such that I surrendered to the process and so began a new part of the exciting journey of healing. I was able to go to Bali for a life-changing workshop with Jayem, the scribe of the Way of Mastery. I learned about the gain I had had in keeping myself ill. I learned about the beliefs that keep illness and fear of scarcity locked in the body so that they can just be triggered at any time, surprising me and keeping me in a state of victimhood. But here's the crunch: if I am 100% responsible for everything that 'happens' to me, how can I then also be a victim?

The answer is: I can't!

I learned that I held a belief about being inferior because I was 'just' a girl. This meant that I necessarily viewed men as superior – but was also deeply resentful of this because somewhere deep within I knew it was a lie! No wonder I was so vulnerable on my left side, the feminine side of the body. I did much work to let that belief dissolve and let myself find equality with men without having to compete with them. Now I am in a relationship with a wonderful man whom I can love without resentment or fear, thus also without any expectations, allowing him to be himself, where previously I would have sought to control and possess. I am in a relationship in which I am free to be myself.

My choice now is to ask myself: what would Love do? Do I choose to act lovingly, have loving thoughts, treat myself lovingly? Yes!

When negative thoughts arise, do I choose to love myself enough not to give myself a hard time over them? Yes!

Do I just allow them and let them pass? Yes!

Do I give myself permission to acknowledge and express them if necessary? Yes!

This way, I make sure that I get to know myself instead of being frightened of my feelings and therefore of myself. I become more and more comfortable in my own skin.

At the beginning of this year I had a scan. The scan showed that the tumor had noticeably reduced in size. I have had no more symptoms and know there is nothing there at all anymore.

All my relationships are now based on truthfulness and honesty and this for me is Love in action.

Anita Moorjani, who had a near-death experience while afflicted with terminal cancer, is now back among us, a picture of radiant health – www.anitamoorjani.com. I share with her the absolute certainty that it is gratitude and the celebration of life which helps us heal.

In summary, I have used a manifold approach to allowing myself to be healed. I have embraced all the aspects of being human, from the physical to the mental, to the emotional, to the spiritual.

I realize that this chapter may raise many questions. May these questions spur the reader on to find the answers within! The more questions, the better! Be curious; return to the wondering state of innocence, as in childhood. Remember the light in your eyes as you looked upon something that aroused your curiosity!

Above all, be blessed, grateful, joyous and happy, knowing that you are loved by the very fact of your existence!

When parents learn how to create children in accord with natural law, how to mold their bodies and their characters into harmony and beauty before the new life sees the light of day, when they learn to rear their offspring in health of body and purity of mind in harmony with the law of their being, then we shall have true types of beautiful manhood and womanhood, then children will no longer be a curse and a burden to themselves and to those who bring them into the world or to society at large.

These thoughts are not the mere dreams of a visionary. When we see the wonderful changes wrought in a human being by a few months or years of rational living and treatment, it seems not impossible or improbable that these ideals may be realized within a few generations.

Children thus born and reared in harmony with the law will be the future masters of the earth. They will need neither gold nor influence to win in the race of life- their innate powers of body and soul will make them vistors over every circumstance. The offspring of alcoholism, drug poisoning and sexual perversity will cut but sorry figures in comparison with the manhood and womanhood of a true and noble aristocracy of health.

Nature Cure Henry Lindlahr first published in 1914

PART 3

RETHINKING THE WAY WE PARENT – THE OTHER TOXIC PROBLEM IN OUR SOCIETY TODAY

Chapter 31

How Unhappy Childhoods Cause Unhappy Adults

None of us is born knowing how to be a parent, any more than we're born with knowing how to drive a car. When we decide to learn how to drive, however, we take lessons, read the manual, and practice - a lot - before we take to the road. But when we become parents, we're forced to hop into the driver's seat with no experience and - for many of our number - very little knowledge or skill. We're driving recklessly at best, blindly at worst, either way, we can endanger lives if we're not careful. It's important that we take the job of parenting seriously - seriously enough not to follow the easy road, seriously enough to consciously examine how we parent our children, seriously enough to change when necessary. A thoughtful, organised, calm approach - in which we slow down enough to identify our mistakes, and make adjustments to correct them - will keep us all from careening uncontrollably off the shoulder

Hidden Messages - *What Our Words And Actions Are Really Telling Our Children* - Elizabeth Pantely

When I first began writing this book, I was just going to write about the effects of toxins in our food, beauty products and the environment. It wasn't until I fell pregnant and became thirsty for knowledge about 'how to be a great parent' that it suddenly dawned on me that the *entire* subject of parenting, and the reality of what is happening in society due to either *bad* parenting or from the wrong type of advice, was impacting on the happiness and health of so many adults today. And that what people's childhood was like shaped almost *every* aspect of their personalities, their behavior and their future. I saw that because so many people had unhappy childhoods, this was now *another* sort of epidemic and that it was also very toxic to the world.

I strongly believe that we have not been bringing up enough children who are happy and well-adjusted. Many become deeply depressed adults and, when questioned about their pasts, many say that they were so unhappy with how their childhoods were. They didn't feel loved, felt ignored or not worthy and were therefore not able to develop healthy inner self-esteem, and this connected to huge problems later in life.

Many adults grow up with lots of emotional baggage, perhaps developing anger problems. They can also become addicted to drugs, food, shopping or sex and show all sorts of other signs of unbalance. These behaviors can also be quite toxic to a romantic relationship, and if children are created, of course these patterns will often get passed down to the new generations, continuing the cycle of chaos and unhappiness.

I could easily write another book about this subject because raising healthy and happy children is something that is *very* important to me. I think there is a major epidemic in the world of unhappy children, with terribly low self-esteem, who more often than not, will grow up into troubled, unhappy and unsure adults. It's a very vicious cycle. It's got to change. And it's so important to note that if *our* health is in dire straits, due to the enormous amount of toxic exposure we are facing, then it's blatantly obvious that our children are facing a problem many, many times worse than what we grew up with. And this is exactly why I have written this book. We've all *got* to do something about it.

Our children's future is pretty darn scary if they are to go through life without being protected from toxins and without being *nurtured* in the best way. It's a recipe for a pretty disappointing life. When I figured all of this out, I knew that I had to write a big section on all of these subjects, that there was so much to cover, and a great deal of change could occur if more people considered and implimented these things.

We must all realize that for the planet to progress in a good way, we are going to need children who grow up to be *amazing* strong adults, conscious and caring of their own health and the rest of the environment too. With the way things are going on in society, it's safe to say that we need to act *very* quickly in regards to this. Each child born on the planet has the capability to help change many things for the better. Unfortunately if we don't change in a hurry, we will be leaving a big mess for them to clean up (or not leave them anything at all!) so we need to make sure we support them on their journey through life.

A parent's job is really to love and nurture their children, so that they grow up to be successful, well-adjusted and confident adults. And 'successful' does not mean rich or famous; it means an adult who is healthy, empathetic, has good morals, is smart, is kind to others and has a desire to help people for the greater good. Adults like *this*, with all of these valuable qualities, will *really* turn the state of the earth around. We would begin to create close communities where we care about *all* people, rather than just our own immediate families.

If you are planning on having children, or are pregnant, right now I want to share with you some things that I have found to be very important for health and also for the emotional development - which may help you avoid problems later in their lives. If you don't have children, you will one day more than likely and still might find this information interesting. If you already have children then this information can still help, no matter their age. It's never too late.

There may be a few reasons why so many people suffer with depression later in life, but I think it may mostly be from how they were treated as a child, and the emotional baggage that is still affecting them. And this is not about automatically blaming each parent, because they may not have known any better and were just doing what their parents did to them. We *all* pick up things from our parents, whether we like it or not. This is about helping parents to not carry on harmful behaviour to new generations.

I am going to discuss some things that might seem a bit 'out there', but just have an open mind and hopefully you will see the sense to them, like I did. You don't have to do anything I say – it's always your choice – but I do hope you perhaps consider that it could work for some families and their children.

To have successful, healthy and happy children, for the benefit of socieity it's all about how we parent, so the pressure is on you (and *me* too) for this to happen.

Chapter 32

Attachment Parenting – A Way to Help Build a Lasting Connection

It must be clear from the baby's confusions about reality that the ego is not yet present. Until it is, the infant is totally dependent on the nurture and care of his mother. Although he may feel omnipotent, he requires constant care because he cannot act rationally in the real world. If his mother cares tenderly for him, he will acquire a sense of trust and optimism that lasts him through life. On the other hand, if his needs are not met or satisfaction is consistently delayed he will cry and rage, unable to bring about a realistic change. When this occurs, the child will grow up to become pessimistic and mistrusting in adulthood.[122]
Sigmund Freud, from the book *Childhood Development: A First Course*

This topic is something I only discovered when I found out I was pregnant. I want to share with you in case it appeals to you and is perhaps going to help you be a better parent. Now knowing that usually anything that is 'mainstream' is not always the right way for all, I had a feeling that how we are told to parent is not really going so well these days. And, looking around me at the people I know, and strangers in the street who struggle with their own happiness and their day-to-day life, I wondered: Where did this all start? Could this unhappiness and lack of self-belief later in life, often leading to depression, anger issues or addictions, be stemming from the earliest years of one's childhood?

The first year of an infant's life is absolutely crucial and shapes their *entire* future. What a parent does in this time really is *everything*. A child's personality may be formed by the age of 7, but their ability to be happy and to feel loved is formed by the tender age of 1. So you have a very short window to create this vitally important bond.

'Attachment parenting'[123] is a term coined for parents who wish to continue this bond so that their child still feels attached to them, for the purpose of bringing up children who feel truly loved, confident, happy, independent and secure. And if an adult comes from this type of healthy childhood then they are *less* likely to suffer from depression nor will they bring lots of emotional baggage into their future relationships.

Why is the attachment process so important?

In the womb, the baby hears the mother's heartbeat 24/7 as soon as he or she has developed this sense. This provides crucial comfort and security for the child. So in tune is the baby to the mother's heartbeat that it can also sense when she is stressed and unhappy. If she is in a great mood, then the baby will sense that; but if the mother is anxious and upset, the baby will sense that as well.

For 9 months this security and connection is all the baby has known, and now upon entering into the harsh reality of the world – the different sounds, temperatures, and new people – is often a very scary time for babies, to be in such a different environment.

The connection we have to our child is much deeper than we may think. He or she relies on the nurturing of the mother to feel safe and secure and this is required for a very long time until the bond that is created is long lasting and permanent. In this time of attachment, the child learns to *trust* that we will always be there and will always meet its needs. It's not about 'spoiling' but nurturing. With the right kind of love, a child can truly *never* have too much.

The amount of attention and time that a mother spends with her child, and how quckly it's cries are attended to is absolutely crucial to the way the child feels about its own security and will shape its view of itself and the world. In the book, *When You and Your Mother Can't Be Friends* author Victoria Secunda writes:

Infancy is a time of wondrous sorcery when we have no sense of ourselves as a thing apart from mother. The infant cries and is picked up, it's body shudders in relief, unaware of where it ends and the mother begins – they are, as far the child is concerned, still one. It is the most perfect of unions, every need met – shelter, protection, love, food – all suffused by physical closeness to mother, the warmth and comfort of her skin, the smell and taste of her milk, the soothing reassurance of her voice, her adoring smile and touch. Unless of course, the infant cries and is *not* picked up. Or is yelled at. At that awful moment, the baby, her body tensing, begins to be aware of something missing, even if she does not understand cause and effect; she continues to howl for some *thing* to ease her panic, the anguish of *not* being held, or fed or tended to. And if the mother, or her surrogate, does not 'rescue' the child, the world begins to be a dangerous place.

Attachment parenting is simply about teaching parents and caregivers, how to *avoid* our children experiencing that feeling of traumatic danger in their infancy.

Throughout the history of mainstream birthing, babies were taken away from the mother pretty quickly and whisked off to the nursery ward where nurses and doctors poked and prodded the child over quite a few days. They performed numerous tests on the baby to see if it was healthy. This literal 'ripping away' from the mother caused great distress not only to the child but also to the mother, as she was not able to bond straight away.

More and more scientific evidence is coming out now about the 'crucial hour' of bonding, which is immediately needed after birth. Today, many women undergo Cesarean sections, which can of course be lifesaving for the baby's wellbeing, but can cause problems long term for the baby's emotional life. It is now strongly recommended by most in the medical/birthing field, that the child should be taken straight to the mother's breast so that he/she can hear the heartbeat (and will therefore still feel attached and be instantly calmed) and will feel the warmth of the mother's skin. The baby will simply feel safe and start to experience the mother in this new way. Breastfeeding is usually able to happen immediately when mother and child are able to spend this important time together, quietly and calmly.

The hormones that both the mother and baby are exchanging and feeling at this time are ones of deep and profound love, which magically sets up this strong tie and 'attachment' for life.

When a baby is taken away and this bonding time is not allowed, it is thought to be detrimental long term. Some women who fall into postpartum depression (1 in 10 mothers) more often that not, experienced a Cesarean section, or a birth with lots of drugs and trauma, and were sadly not able to bond properly with their child, which in turn may lead to an awful bout of depression with feelings of guilt and frustration, both of which the baby can sense. If you have experienced severe pain and trauma from your baby's birth, it may impact how calm and happy you feel with this massive life change. This kind of intense stress can also lead to the failure of breast-feeding, which may add to a further lack of attachment, not to mention the immunity problems associated with bottle feeding.

Although this bonding time is always strongly recommended, many mothers have not been able to have a stress-free or drug-free birth. Lack of proper attachment does not happen with all babies born like this, so do not fear that if you did not have this bonding time that your child is not going to grow up happy. There is still *lots* a parent can do to create this bond.

Another form of un-attachment may be to do with our modern-day sleeping arrangements. When a newborn baby is a few months old (or for some babies just weeks), it is typically sent off to its own room, placed in a cot and left on its own for very long periods. The child goes from one extreme environment to another: sleeping close to the parents after birth, therefore feeling safe and secure, to an empty room, where it's suddenly all by itself. If you have had a child, you may be aware that children are highly sensitive and do not generally like being on their own.

This sudden shock can often be *very* stressful for the child, and at that small age, they *do not* have the skills to understand that you *will* come back to them later on and therefore cannot calm or self-soothe – that part of the brain has simply not been developed yet. With the regular crying fits, parents start to think that the child is 'being difficult', but the truth is, they just want to know you are *still* right there, that they are *safe* and not in any danger. When they are left in a cot on their own for any amount of time, they may not understand what is going on and feel intense fear, stress and become hysterical.

Also, perhaps consider this for just a moment: on an appearance level, if you were asked to describe what a cot looked like, what would you say it personifies? Maybe the word 'cage' or 'jail' springs to mind? I personally can see why some children find them very frightening.

When animals are placed in a cage it is clear to see that they feel distressed and alarmed and would do *anything* to get out of it. Most children can also sense this and tend to react terribly when first placed in a cot as they are also well aware that this is another form of un-attachment from their parents. After animals are newly born, they stay close to their mother at all times until they have developed the skills needed to become their own carer. Until those skills are developed, they require the nurturing and protection, constantly from the mother. Without it, they simply would not thrive and more than likely would die. Humans are no different and in actual fact *need* this nurturing more than the animals do.

If your baby sleeps in a cot and seems genuinely happy with that, then it's probably completely OK. The point to this chapter is to encourage parents to rethink what they are doing only *if* their children seem unsettled and 'troublesome' – these are the signs they give us when something is not right in their minds. If there are no signs, then chances are they are fine with what you are doing.

How today's society has caused a disconnection from our past

Typically, society has conditioned us to believe that for the parents' 'best interests' you should always put the child in its own room in a cot, and as soon as possible. You should not always pick a child up. You do not want your child to have you wrapped around their fingers. The child should 'learn the rules of life' from a very young age, and this means leaving the child to 'cry on its own until it learns to stop'.

I personally believe that we *must not* have this attitude. To make a child fit in with us is *not* right – they are unsure of the world, and so very sensitive, so the only thing that makes them feel safe is our constant *connection*. And once this connection has been removed, even if it's only temporary, they have no choice except to get very upset and stressed. To a small child, just like to a newborn animal, the parents - especially the mother, are their protectors. Without them the newborn animal will die, and in a newborn baby's case, if the parents are often absent, the child's *spirit* may die. And it can also do an immense amount of damage long term, something we should be much more educated about as young parents.

Victoria Secunda explains in her book *When You and Your Mother Can't be Friends:*

> One reason it is vital to respond to an infant's needs is that the baby feels it is the cause of it's own neglect, although this is not a conscious thought. Such narcissistic feelings pave the road to an infant's psychological and physical growth; since the baby senses no boundaries between herself and her mother, she 'believes' that her cries cause the mother to tend to her. And if the mother does *not* tend to her, the baby feels she created her own rejection by not being lovable, not worthy of care. It is a belief that haunts one's life.

Teaching them the ways of the world can come much later in life indeed, but while they are very young, children just need to feel safe and secure and this is purely down to the parents' actions. I have seen this with Lola, where she is perfectly fine, then if I walk out of the room only for a minute and she cannot see me, she starts crying with deep despair, which is immediately stopped as soon as I come back. She literally feels terrified that she cannot see me, or even if she can see me she is scared because I seem so far away. It's because, to her, I am everything; I am her protection from the world. It's not because she is being difficult or unnaturally clingy. It's a totally *normal* reaction. And it won't always be like this. When she is older, she will understand that I will come back and won't be upset at all. If I have kept her from feeling scared most of the time (it may be quite impossible to shield her from it all) during this crucial stage, then she will not have unnatural fears when older. She will have a much better ability to trust her surroundings and confidence in knowing everything is OK.

When you understand this highly important attachment process, this belief in 'controlled crying', or baby sleeping on its own - starting very young young, may not now sit well with you and you might not want to leave your child in the dark like that anymore. Perhaps you have tried this and found that every time you've walked out of the room and shut the door, your child usually immediately panics and begins to howl and scream, often for hours on end, night after night. If you are torn about sleeping arrangements, it may be a good idea to try and imagine what's going on inside your baby's body.

It feels so distraught, and in their mind, you are gone forever, and this deep emotional upset creates the dangerous stress hormone called cortisol to be released throughout the body. Often, after many times of this, the child will give up crying as it's either too tired and worn out or it simply thinks you're not going to come back to soothe its cries. Once the crying has stopped you may think, 'Great! That's a good boy or good girl', yet the sad truth is, the child has had no choice but to fall into a deep sleep due to the stress. Their 'good night' of prolonged sleep is more than likely from total exhaustion. And researchers have discovered that children who were left to cry for periods of time are *ten* times more likely to develop ADHD, as well as very poor school performance and antisocial behavior among their peers.[124]

I know personally just how *damaging* stress can be. Constant stress over many years (for as long as I can remember), also contributed to my fragile mental state. Stress raises the heart rate (and can actually cause damage) , puts pressure on the brain often resulting in splitting headaches, and can also seriously affect the digestive system, all the while triggering sleep problems such as insomnia. To have small children being affected by prolonged sessions of constant stress is really concerning to me and should be to *every* parent. Intense stress also *detrimentally* effects baby's brain development. Therefore, during infancy, it's vital to try to *decrease* these instances of high stress as much as possible and is again, why attachment parenting seems *so* important.

The adrenal glands - found just above the kidneys, secrete cortisol when the body is under stress. Cortisol breaks down fat and proteins so that it can then generate extra energy. It temporarily puts other regulatory functions such as the hormonal and immune systems on hold. The cortisol basically stops the body from functioning normally. The body is on high alert with the 'fight or flight' response in first place of importance. What this means is that over prolonged periods of stress the body will not be able to remain balanced, nor will it be able to regulate itself. Something which could cause lifelong problems.

Sue Gerhardt, author of the groundbreaking book *Why Love Matters – How Affection Shapes a Babies Brain* writes:

There is some evidence to suggest that high levels of cortisol might be toxic to the developing brain over time. In particular, too much cortisol can affect the development of the orbito-frontal area which as we have seen is responsible for reading social cues and adapting behaviour to social norms. Maternally deprived rats have been found to have reduced connections in this area of the brain. The hippocampus may also be particularly affected by early stress. With too much cortisol at a sensitive time of development, the number of cortisol receptors in the hippocampus can be reduced.

This means that when cortisol levels rise under future stress, there are fewer receptors to receive it and the cortisol can flood the hippocampus, affecting its growth. On the other hand, those who are touched and held a great deal in babyhood, who receive plenty of attention in early life, have been found to have an abundance of cortisol receptors in the hippocampus in adulthood. This means that they can cope more easily with the cortisol triggered by stress; when its level rises, there is somewhere for it to go.

Many scientists now realize that this constant stress experience can really damage a child long term. When a child is not given enough attention or nurturing, the child begins to learn that something (you) was missing from a very young age. They believed that their parents had abandoned them and were never going to return. The bond which was once formed in the beginning, with trust, may now be seen as broken and fear now sets in where the child sees the world as quite scary. This fear can stay with them for *life* but in a way where they do not recognize (or, of course, remember) how it all started.

Knowing that a small baby and child feels this pain and despair, and what can happen long term, I think is absolutely heartbreaking, and one we can avoid if we know how.

If this subject of attachment parenting appeals to you and you want to create a deep and long-lasting relationship with your child, then the following things can be incorporated into your daily routine:

1) *Breastfeeding* for as *long* as you can – at least a year. The World Health Organization actually recommends breast-feeding up until the age of 2 years, if longer.[125]
2) *Baby-wearing your child* in a sling as often as possible (used safely and correctly so that they feel your heartbeat like they

did in the womb).

3) *Co-sleeping in your bed* or in the room close to your bed so that you can attend to the baby quickly. Your baby will not feel the need to get worked up into a cry that produces cortisol. For those that worry about SIDS, many studies show that sleeping with a baby actually *decreases* the chances of this happening.[126]

4) *Attending to baby's cries* as soon as possible. Despite people thinking this makes a clingy child, the *opposite* is what is most likely to happen. When a child's needs are met, this safety and security makes them see the world as safe and secure and they feel that you are always there for them, so they have no need to behave in a clingy way. They tend to trust people (even strangers) more because they have learnt to trust you.

There are other methods in attachment parenting but these are the most important. For parents that have brought up children by the old method (and I would say a huge percentage of the Western world cultures do it this way - due to how *we* have been brought up and also what the magazines tell us), I realize that all of this new information may sound a bit shocking, and may even be slightly offensive as it may not be the way you have previously done things with your children. This is not about pointing fingers; it's merely to perhaps instill some new ideas into the way we can parent, to try and make it more *likely* that a child may grow up with better self-esteem because his or her needs were met as often as possible when small. Highly sensitive children respond very well to attachment parenting.

Look back and think about how parenting began many years ago and about the customs of tribes and people from continents like Africa and other very traditional societies, where they are kept away from mainstream culture – customs they are still practicing today. They only have their intuition to guide them with no rulebooks –

only generations of advice given to them. How do you think they parent? Pretty much the exact opposite way to us! They do not have cots or pushchairs or the latest gadgets. They carry their babies around all day, they breastfeed for a very long time, the children have constant companionship, and the entire community cares about everyone else's children. It's said that African children, brought up in this way, rarely cry at all. The amount of love the child is immersed in from the start ensures that the child knows, without a doubt, that Mum and Dad and a whole bunch of other people really care about them and that they are never truly on their own. They do not grow up to be needy, depressed or sad. For a child to develop well; love, warmth, food and attachment are all they need. Many parents of the Muslim faith also practice co-sleeping today, as well as many Indian families.

While it may seem that the old-fashioned ways don't belong in this modern world, the only thing I can say to that is, we *know* that things are going wrong with our children today – that much is more than obvious – so maybe we have to look at *alternatives* and reasons as to *why* happiness is such a big problem for so many people. All psychologists will agree that people's personalities and sense of self are shaped by their childhoods. And many are realizing that it may even be down to where a child sleeps:

We must ask ourselves here, whether in removing the newborn from his mother, as is customary in hospitals, and placing him in an open space of a bassinet or crib, we are not visiting a seriously disturbing trauma upon the baby, a trauma from which, perhaps, he never completely recovers? A trauma, moreover, which in the civilized world of the West, and those cultures that have been affected by the West's childbirth practices, is repeatedly inflicted upon the infant during the early years of his life. It may be that fear of open spaces (agoraphobia), or of heights, (acrophobia), or of sudden drops, may have some connection with such early experiences. It may also be that a preference for having one's bedclothes about one's body, rather than tucked in at the foot and side of the bed, reflects a desire to recreate the conditions enjoyed in the womb, in reaction to the lack of body support experience in infancy.[127]

Another benefit of attachment parenting is the smaller amount of items you will need to buy. If a baby is going to share your bed for at least a year or even longer, then you won't have to fork out for an expensive cot and all of the bedding that goes along with it. You also do not need to buy an expensive pram until the child becomes much heavier, even then you may not ever have to buy one. However, if you do want to get a pram, then I would suggest getting one that has a seat which can be swiveled to face you as you push it. That way, your baby knows you are right there.

If you can use a baby sling then I really suggest you give it a go. When you carry your baby around with you, the child learns to be in different environments and sits quietly, observing how the world really is. It's actually quite handy for a mother to carry her baby like that as it means you can do housework, travel and do most of the things you used to do. And there is no big heavy pram to push around either.

There are some reports that these baby slings are dangerous. Like most things, sometimes accidents do happen and I have read one story where a baby died while in its sling. You do have to make sure your baby is resting in it the correct way and is able to breathe at all times by not constricting the throat. Your baby sling should come with instructions on how to do this and there are also mothers' groups you can join where everyone uses the slings with their children. On an interesting note, kids that come from attachment parenting backgrounds and were carried in a sling generally learn to speak earlier and grow up to be more secure, independent and confident, despite what mainstream information would tell you.

The ERGO Baby Carrier is the best type I discovered – more on that shortly.

Isn't co-sleeping dangerous?

Often the media will say that sleeping with a baby is dangerous, and while it's true that there have been some tragic stories, they tend to leave out the important information about the parents being seriously overweight or that they had taken recreational or medicinal drugs that night, smoked or had a lot of alcohol or were extremely tired. All of the *common sense* rules must be applied here. You must *not* get into bed with your baby if you have even had the tiniest amount to drink. And even if you are on certain medications (sleeping pills or antidepressants) then you must be even more careful and not sleep with your child. If you are a super-deep sleeper then it's also probably not a good idea. And do not wrap up baby too much either; your body warmth most of the time is usually more than enough to keep the baby's temperature comfortable. Have a light duvet instead of a heavy one and make sure the baby's head is always uncovered and the duvet will not be able to go over it.

This is Erika Roberg's story about how co-sleeping worked for her family. She is a mother to three children.

I co-slept with all my children. I'm VERY glad I co-slept. The biggest reason I'm thankful is that my second son would go hypoxic (quit breathing and turn blue) for no apparent reason from birth. There were a couple of times I found him turning blue in his car seat and I would pick him up to arouse him enough to take a breath. Several times during the night, I felt or heard him quit breathing. I was right there where I could immediately pick him up, cradle and rock him, pat his back, etc. to get him to breathe again. Later we found out he was deathly allergic to many foods – some of which I had eliminated from my diet (because his older brother had been sensitive to those foods) – but he was being exposed to some that I wasn't aware of through my breast milk. He was actually having bouts of mild anaphylaxis during these episodes. I know my son would be dead if it weren't for co-sleeping. I was so in tune with him and his breathing that

I would wake easily when he was hypoxic.

Now, my kids are all SO well-adjusted, and don't have that big separation anxiety issue that I see other kids of their age having. They are nurtured when they need it most – at night, when they are most vulnerable – so that they can feel more confident about being more independent during the day. If you think about it, how many of us would like to sleep alone? Why is it OK for us to sleep next to our spouses but our babies aren't allowed to feel the comfort of someone sleeping close to them? I feel isolated and very alone when my husband is out of town or somehow separated from us during sleep time, so how can I expect my child to sleep alone and just deal with the feelings of isolation? That makes no sense. Every day of my life I'm thankful that I co-slept.

If the idea of having your child in bed with you does not appeal, or you can't do it for safety reasons but you still want to follow attachment parenting, you can purchase little cots that connect to the edge of your bed. The baby is pretty much on your level so she/he can see you and vice versa. This means that you can have your own space in your bed, but that your baby is still right next to you. It's so easy when you need to breastfeed as you don't have to get up out of bed to fetch the child. A popular brand that makes these infant beds is Arms Reach. If you are to purchase one of these, I do strongly recommend you getting a made-to-measure organic mattress because the Arms Reach mattress is made with the typical toxic chemicals which are derived from petrol.

Try armsreach.com, Google or even Ebay/Amazon. Or if your husband, relative or friend is a real handyman, they could build you one (out of recycled wood perhaps) and you could get an organic mattress.

The subject of co-sleeping is often very heated. Some parents think it's absolutely irresponsible for others to sleep with their child, but I think it makes perfect sense that we do. To me it offers a child pure protection if done safely. I can also understand, however, why some parents would never consider doing it due to the way the media has presented the stories that have happened when tragedies have occurred. But as previously explained, the deaths are related to people that should just not have slept with their child in the first place. I do very much strongly believe, though, that it is not beneficial for the child to be in its own room under 12 months of age, especially if they show signs of distress when you do leave them. Repeated hours of crying will show you if they are indeed distressed sleeping like this. You want to try and wait until your child understands that you *will* return even after they can't see you. This will be far less stressful for the child and also you, as you won't have to put up with crying fits as much.

What made me consider attachment parenting?

After reading only a little bit about it, the method automatically appealed to me as it just made such *sense*. When I also looked at how animals were brought up and also how other cultures parented their babies, it seemed obvious to me that we may have been doing many wrong things by our children. If society was much better than it was, with far less depression and problems with unruly teenagers, then I would not be thinking like this – but it's just so obvious to me that so many are struggling with life and feeling unloved. And I do *firmly* believe it can be directly related to our attachment. So for me, I set out wanting to try and follow this method as accurately as I could.

I also personally happen to know many parents who follow attachment parenting and their children are so vibrant, confident and happy and love to be around new people. They tend to be so easy to talk to and look you right in the eye and are not afraid of adults. They seem very well-adjusted and are often very mature socially for their age. My husband and I have always been really surprised at these kids because they seem so different from most of the ones we have met before.

Another reason for us wanting to consider this parenting style is that I also know many children who were brought up with the typical parenting methods, with controlled crying, formula feeding and unnatural births. These children tend to cry *a lot*, are quite clingy to their parents, are often ill, and do not seem to like being around new people. It's as if they don't *trust* anyone. It's exactly what the parents were trying to avoid in the first place. Strangely ironic, right?

My experience with attachment parenting

I gave birth to a baby girl, Lola, on the 11th of February 2012. I thankfully had a natural birth with no intervention and was able to have that crucial bonding time with her. Lola also breastfed immediately and I very luckily had no troubles afterwards with her latching on. After reading many books on the subject of attachment parenting, I had all these ideas in my mind about what I was going to do with Lola. We planned to co-sleep, breastfeed on demand, and carry her in a sling when out of the house, and one of us was always going to be with her, or at least nearby at all times. I did, however, relax a few of my initial ideals.

Sometimes when you read a book you want to follow their advice 100% and you plan to, yet when the baby is here, you do change your ideals due to practicality and just feeling a bit different about it all. Babies do tend to let us know if what we are doing is good for them, and if it's not, then they certainly let us know, and very quickly too. Lola certainly liked to be super-close to us and if she had a choice she would have been on either of our chests 24/7 as she found this the most soothing and comforting thing. But she was also very content when sleeping on a large cushion, as long as we were nearby. As soon as she woke up, I would immediately attend to her needs. This is the key – quickly giving your baby what they are wanting. It's not 'pandering' to them; it's simply providing basic necessities, avoiding stress and upset.

Ergo Baby Carriers

I intended to use a sling all the time, literally carrying Lola around in it all of the time when I was not in bed with her. But I had no idea how much it was going to hurt my back. After I gave birth, my back just wasn't the same; I had quite severe pain during the contractions that radiated at my lower back area. Throughout my pregnancy, I did not do anywhere as much yoga as I intended to, so my back muscles were very weak. I also have a very long spine – longer than the average person, it seems – as well as having bad backs in our family, so I think this contributed to the problem as well.

When Lola was born, I tried a whole bunch of different slings (and spent quite a bit of money!): the long 5-foot stretchy wrap ones, the ones that go on over one side of the body; we also tried a baby Bjorn and another carrier that was similar. All of them did not suit me; either Lola did not like being in them or they hurt my back no matter what position I tied or how I wore the slings. None of them seemed to distribute her weight evenly, which is why my lower back was always pulled in the same area.

I eventually came across the Ergo Baby Carrier and I believe that it is by far the *best* carrier on the market. These carriers are not only incredibly well-designed, they are just gorgeous too; some are made out of organic fabric, and some are available with the most beautiful patterns (or can be purchased completely plain, and more 'Daddy friendly' as well). They can be worn at the front and at the back like a backpack and even on the side so baby rests against your hip. They have wide, padded fabric straps which do not dig into the shoulders like many of the baby carriers can. There is also an attachment to go around the waist to help distribute the weight evenly. They have inserts you can put into it so a newborn can sit snuggly inside and there is a brilliant cover for the head, as well as extra bits you can purchase to protect the baby from rain and cold weather. They are not cheap, but are certainly worth the price due to the high quality and comfort factor, and second-hand ones can be bought off eBay. I think you can tell just by looking at them that they are going to be so comfortable.

Another benefit of the Ergo Baby Carrier is that they have been tested as a safe way to carry your baby in terms of hip dysplasia. It is reported that some slings are not the best for babies' spinal development and can negatively affect the hips and other joints. The Ergo Baby Carrier helps the child to sit in the correct seated position, allowing the development of the body to progress as normal. They come in a huge range of patterns and colors, and kids love sitting in these carriers because they are so comfortable.

Beware of counterfeit items; there are loads of people producing very good fakes but you don't want to get one that is not 100% legitimate. If they aren't made the way the company intended, how do you know that it will be the safest for your baby? If purchasing second hand, ask for a sales receipt as proof that they were bought from Ergo Baby. The following websites are trustworthy.

✓ store.ergobaby.com

✓ cleverclogs.ie

I hear that both the Patapum and Boba slings are also very good.

Despite attachment parenting supporting the closeness between mother and baby, some babies may not like being carried around all the time, and may perhaps prefer being in a pram, or sitting on their own and observing the world – you will know as your baby will give you signs as to what they like, so it's always wise to really pay attention to them rather than what you think they should do. Because I wasn't able to carry Lola like I intended, we opted to purchase a pram. It was either buy one or never leave the house, because how could I carry Lola without my back hurting? And staying in all the time is definitely not healthy so the pram won. We purchased one that has a front-facing baby seat so that Lola can always see us. When she grows and becomes a toddler she will sit facing away from us, but by that age she will have developed the ability to remember that we are right there. Personally, I love having a pram; going for walks in the country, and being able to put shopping underneath, is fantastic. But I do love being able to carry her in the Ergo Baby Carrier as well, it's like giving her a constant hug. It's also very cute seeing her dad carry her like this as I know it ensures their closeness too.

If we are going to go for a long walk in the country, the pram would be such a nuisance so a baby carrier of some sort in this situation is really necessary.

After 16 months (at the time of writing) of being a mum, I do personally feel that one of the most important aspects of attachment parenting, and ironically one of the most controversial, is by far co-sleeping. From what my husband and I have seen, Lola feels protected and comforted, on either side, due to sleeping in the middle. As soon as she wakes up, Lola sees either of us and feels safe. I think in the future, with her continuing to sleep with us until she wants her own room, nightmares or being scared of what's under the bed will be few and far between because she won't feel on her own. I love the co-sleeping because it's also so easy to breastfeed during the night; I have become so in tune with Lola's sleeping patterns that as soon as she starts to move I know it's time to start feeding her a little bit again, and we are both still pretty much half asleep. Now I don't really remember waking up properly during the night. I just love it and wouldn't have it any other way. Lola sometimes wakes up briefly and looks at her dad, then over at me, and goes straight back to sleep; it's as if she's checking, 'Where are they? Oh! They are right here! I can go back to sleep now – I am safe!'

At first, co-sleeping is a little bit tough to do; we as adults are used to drifting peacefully off to sleep and don't tend to get woken up by little noises. Babies are *not* always quiet, even if they are not crying. Lola would make noises (grunts!) that, although they were very cute, did keep us awake. You have to really commit to co-sleeping but I do feel the benefits pay off in the long run. Your child will simply feel secure in your love.

If we had used a bassinet or cot very early on, I definitely don't think she would have slept well at all, as she didn't even want to lie in-between us the first few nights; she had to have skin-to-skin contact as I think being out of the womb, and into such a foreign environment, was just too much of a shock to her. I am sure most babies are like this and need lots of cuddles and companionship. You will know from how easily your child falls asleep if how they are sleeping makes them happy.

One thing to keep an eye on is baby falling out of the bed. You do have to be very careful because as they get older, and once they can crawl around, or stand, they could fall off the bed, as they naturally want to explore. This happened to Lola when I was out of the room literally for two minutes. She fell off onto the floor, and while she was not hurt, she certainly was very upset. To avoid this, you can try and push your bed next to a wall and put a whole bunch of pillows around your baby so that they can't climb over them, but the safest option is to put your mattress on the ground so that your baby can't fall very far. Co-sleeping is truly wonderful; it's such a special way to bond with your baby, but you must use common sense too.

Preparing for parenting: the perfect time to learn all you can

I always say to people: If you started a new job, or were at university, you would have to study to know how to do the job or to pass the exam. You couldn't just 'wing' it and expect to do well. Becoming a parent is one of those times when you should try and learn as much as possible before the big day arrives.

It is often said that a child does not come with an instruction manual, but I firmly believe there *is* a lot of brilliant literature that can really help you have a much better idea about what to expect and what you want to do for your child. Don't just read one book either; read as many as you can! And most importantly *listen* to your intuition about what information sounds right to you; try to remove the not always helpful advice you have been given by the media or by your friends. They may not be right.

What other reason in life is better than having a child for learning as much as you can about what you can do to make that child thrive?

Obviously, each parent has the right to choose what style of parenting they want to do, and if what you are doing is working for you, and the child is happy, well-adjusted, confident, and you are all sleeping as well as can be, then keep doing what you are doing. But if things just seem too chaotic and too stressful, and you feel that something is up with your child, then perhaps it is worth looking into attachment parenting.

Please remember that attachment parenting is just a theory that can help some children to turn out better adjusted. It does not mean that if you don't or didn't follow it, your child won't be happy.

I have not even really touched the surface of what attachment parenting is all about, but if you do think it sounds interesting I can suggest some wonderful books: *Attachment Parenting* by William Sears MD and Martha Sears RN. Look out for their entire series on parenting, birth, breastfeeding and child development. Truly fantastic books with so much valuable information! I have provided the names of their other books; all are easy to read, and offer brilliant and helpful advice. Jean Liedloff, who wrote *The Continuum Concept,* originally made attachment parenting very famous. Although she has since passed on, her book is still read by many new mums today.

✓ askdrsears.com

✓ attachmentparenting.co.uk/

Another brilliant book (in my top 5 of must read books) on the attachment process, child rearing and development and how it can affect every aspect of a person's life is *The Manual* by Dr Faye Snyder. I recommend to *every* parent and person to read this book. Even if you don't have children now you can learn a lot about your own past, how you were raised and discover *why* you are the way you are and how to go about changing if you are not happy with yourself.

✓ drfayesnyder.com

Chapter 33

Breastfeeding and Why Nothing Else Will Compare

An infant's immune system has three aspects: her own immature, developing immune system; the small component of immunities that passes through the placenta during natural childbirth (and to a lesser degree with premature births and Cesarean sections); and the most vast and valuable, living portion that is passed on through mother's milk on an ongoing basis. Remove any of these components and you take away a vital support structure.[128]

Dr. L. Folden, author of *The Baby Bond* and 'The Deadly Influence of Formula' Study

There is a massive problem in regards to breastfeeding today and it's affecting children's lives in many ways that is not given enough attention to. I am going to tell you as much as I can about the subject. From the information I have read, breastfeeding is absolutely crucial to a child's *entire* life. It doesn't just protect them from illness when they are young, it sets up the foundations for healthy gut function which is vitally important to someone's general overall health. Unfortunately mothers today simply aren't doing it: a) at all- breast-feeding rates are lower than ever or b) for anywhere long enough. And this is *directly* causing harm to our children's short-term and long-term health.

It really shocks me that, in days gone by, mothers were advised *against* breastfeeding; even the doctors were against it and would encourage mothers to dry their milk up so that they could get their bodies back to normal. Mothers used formula instead, and no one was telling them what a bad idea that was for their child's short-term and long-term health. It's also clear to see that many today think it's also no big deal if you don't do it - that there isn't 'that much difference between breast milk and formula'.

This view of formula as more than OK and as 'close to' breast milk
came about when companies started to realize just how many
children were being born every day and how much money they
could make if everyone's child were having their product. This is
how the multibillion-dollar infant formula empire began and also
how the public fell for all of their marketing ploys and promises that
formula is better than or 'close to' mother's milk. We now know, due
to overwhelming scientific proof, that this promise was and still is an
outright lie. What is in these formulas simply cannot compare, no
matter what they claim, to the magical qualities of breast milk. Even
mothers in Africa who are not eating regular meals (and are
seriously malnourished) provide their baby with *better*-quality milk
than any formula can provide, simply because formula cannot copy
the nutrients that breast milk provides. And most parents don't ever
really know what is in their child's formula.

'If anybody were to ask "which formula should I use?" or "which
is nearest to mother's milk?", the answer would be "nobody
knows" because there is not one single objective source of that
kind of information provided by anybody,' says Mary Smale, a
breastfeeding counsellor with the National Childbirth Trust
(NCT) for 28 years. 'Only the manufacturers know what's in their
stuff, and they aren't telling. They may advertise special
"healthy" ingredients like oligosaccharides, long-chain fatty
acids or, a while ago, beta-carotene, but they never actually tell
you what the basic product is made from or where the ingredients come from'.[129]

This is pretty concerning indeed. For many infants, formula is *all*
they get from birth, or not long after - *I* would certainly want to
know what is in my child's receipe.

The World Health Organization suggests breastfeeding for up to two years, and even *longer* if mother and baby are happy to do so. This will help set your child up with a very strong immune system which is only a *very* good thing for their future health. The longer you breastfeed, the better the immune system is for longer term – some experts, such as Hilary Butler, say for life.

> Breast milk is NOT just food. Breast milk has functions which go far beyond nutrition. Breast milk has a dramatic and long-term effect not only on the immune system development, but gut flora, allergy, brain development, and other health parameters. Breast milk is an immune regulator, a hormone conductor, a bone density wizard and a genetic blueprint scanner. It is a gene methylator, and two years of breast milk lays, stabilizes and solidifies the core genetic manual of health for your child, for that child's whole life.[130]

Unfortunately, it seems normal these days just to breastfeed for the recommended minimum of 6 months (or even far less and most worryingly not at all), then it's time to put baby on cow's milk formula (which tends to give children lots of mucus and other allergies) or, even *much* worse, soy-based formulas. Sadly, this is *not* the best option for baby whatsoever.

Back in the old, traditional days, babies were always breastfed for up to at least a few years. Now, when women want to breastfeed longer than the standard 6 months, they are often ostracized by the public or even their friends and family, and made to feel like they are irresponsible mothers for continuing on longer, yet the truth is the *exact* opposite. It's horrible to think that by doing the best (which is also *scientifically* proven) for your child, the mainstream will tell you that you are doing something wrong! Yet countless studies prove that formula does not even come close to having even half as much benefit for a child's health. Nature is *incredible* and gave us the gift of being able to breastfeed. There is *no other substance* on the planet that can even come close to comparing, so let's take a closer look as to why it just is so amazing.

These are some of the many benefits of breastfeeding:[131]

- provides a bonding with the mother due to the physical contact
- the 'colostrum', which is the first thick breast milk, contains a high amount of nutrients and antibodies – something formula is lacking
- can prevent ear infections
- helps to prevent obesity
- prevents diarrhea
- can prevent allergies
- breast milk changes its nutrient profile depending on how old the child is and what time of the day it is
- is said to prevent diabetes
- prevents the risk of SIDS
- some studies have shown that breastfed babies are more intelligent than formula-fed babies.

Mother benefits:

- provides important and close bonding with the baby
- is reported to prevent breast cancer
- is said to prevent ovarian cancer
- allows more time to rest as no bottle preparation is needed.
- can aid in weight loss. Due to the calories needed to produce the milk, mothers find they burn them off quite quickly, and the uterus also contracts due to breastfeeding so the stomach regains its pre-pregnancy shape very quickly.
- may prevent cardiovascular disease
- breastfeeding is free!

Compared to the benefits of bottle feeding:

- can provide the baby with certain vitamins
- allows the baby to bond with the father as he can feed

Mother benefits:

- watching the diet is no longer necessary
- anyone can feed the baby allowing the mother to have more time for herself
- the baby can be fed anywhere without having to expose the breasts

It's clear, isn't it, that breast milk wins hands down and is always going to be the best choice, when taking responsibility for your child's health. I stress the importance of breastfeeding because I know that its crucial to long-term health. I want mothers out there to know that you must do all you can to feed your baby this way.

How about a little bit of poison in your baby's formula?

A little-talked-about yet extremely concerning fact about formula is that most brands contain high levels of aluminum.[132] Both cow's milk and even more so soy-milk formulas have fairly high levels of aluminum in them. And if you are adding poor-quality water that contains many toxins in it, then it's just creating a very unhealthy start to life. This 'nourishment' is anything but.

Formula also contains worrying levels of lead and other heavy metals, and pesticides too, compared to the levels found in breast milk. If our cows are in fields and eating grass (those are the lucky cows!) then they will be eating grass tainted with heavy metals from pesticides sprayed nearby and from dust and air particles falling on the grass. And in their water too – there will be toxins in that also – and all of this goes into your child's formula.

Of course by now you know that we are all so toxic these days that even breast milk contains toxins, but as we have discussed in Chapter 13, you can minimize the levels and it's *always* better to breastfeed no matter what. My point here is that formula is not quite what you think it is. There are far *more* ingredients lurking inside, and truly unhealthy ones, than what is actually listed on the tin.

I think it's clear that the benefits of formula feeding seem to only be good for the mother (much easier) and not at all for the child. Formula is missing so many nutrients, such as the vital antibodies, and it is a big part of why kids are struggling with their health these days. Nature gave us the ability to breastfeed and it has also cleverly made the milk to contain everything a child needs. It also has the incredible ability to change its level of nutrients for a particular time of the day/month. If your child is sick, somehow the mother's body knows to produce more powerful antibodies which will help your child recover more quickly.

Below is some information about the different types of milk that the breasts produce.

1. Colostrum

- Colostrum is the first stage of breast milk, which occurs during pregnancy.
- It lasts for about 3–6 days after the birth of your baby.
- This milk is high in fat-soluble vitamins, minerals, proteins, and immunoglobulins. Immunoglobulins are antibodies, which are passed from the mother to baby. This provides immunity for the baby.
- This immunity acts as a shield in protecting the infant from a wide range of viral and bacterial diseases.

2. Transitional milk

- Transitional milk is produced immediately after colostrum

and lasts for nearly 2–3 weeks.
- This milk is found to be rich in water-soluble vitamins.
- It also contains lactose and high levels of fats.
- Transitional milk has much higher amounts of calories than colostrum.

3. *Mature milk*

- Mature milk is the last or final milk produced by the mother.
- It is made up of 90% water which helps in maintaining the hydration of the infant. The other 10% contains nutrients like the carbohydrates, fats, and proteins. These give vital energy to the infant and also help in the growth process. There are two types of mature milk: fore-milk and hind-milk.

4. *Fore-milk*

- This type of milk is produced during the first few minutes of feeding. It contains vitamins, protein, and water.

5. *Hind-milk*

- This type of milk occurs immediately after the initial release of milk. It contains high levels of fat. This is the milk helps the infant to gain weight. Both hind-milk and fore-milk are required for the baby. Therefore, mothers must ensure that the baby is receiving the required nutrients for proper growth and development.

And guess what happens with formula? Absolutely *none* of this – it stays the same nutrient type night and day, week after week, as it *cannot* be created to mimic breast milk. Human beings cannot even replicate it, so what does that say? That there is some pretty special stuff inside mumma's milk. I hope I now have you completely convinced you of the wonders of breast milk.

When Lola was sick with her first cold (the only one she has had at the time of writing), I will admit, I was worried. I still didn't really 'get it' that these little viruses were a good thing for her to go through, that my breast milk alone was truly going to be like medicine for her. I just didn't want her to suffer, but guess what? She didn't even seem to know she was 'sick'. She had a runny nose, a slight cough, but no fever and was not disgruntled in anyway. I marveled that she instinctively knew to feed more, and within a few short days her symptoms had disappeared. However, I caught her cold and was much worse. The magic of breast milk is, without a doubt, the incredible effect from the antibodies. It is the best kind of nutrition for your baby, and it is not stressed anywhere enough that formula is lacking in these antibodies. When a child is sick and is being fed with formula, the antibodies are missing and it means that the child is more likely to have symptoms that are far worse and the parents are more likely to reach for Calpol and other toxic medications. And if the baby is already so young and being treated like this, it will mean that illnesses in the future are likely to be a lot more virulent, rather than being just a mild cold.

I try to suggest to mums to breastfeed for as long as possible (and at least a full year) and avoid going down the formula route at all if possible, or to be very aware that if they do use formula, to choose a good one, and that their child's immune system is going to need lots of natural boosters to help it develop into one that will be as strong as possible. The longer you breastfeed, the longer the immunity will be stored inside the child's body.

The reason I personally think we should breastfeed for much longer is that in today's toxic world, children are getting struck down with illnesses that not that long ago were never found. Now we are hearing of small children being diagnosed with diabetes and arthritis and other un-typical problems. Children's immune systems are simply not functioning well and if they do not work well in these precious years, then that points to a pretty scary future for their health. The building blocks of good health must be created in childhood. Because breast milk is full of antibodies and formula is not, it makes sense to me to keep a child on mother's milk for much longer so that the immune benefits can be passed on to the child, and the parents will not have to resort to using typical medications when the child is sick, because they more than likely will not need to – mother's milk is that amazing!

One of the most famous studies on the health and death rate of formula-fed infants versus breastfed babies is the 'Deadly Influence of Formula in America' article which was compiled by Dr. Linda Folden Palmer. In the USA, if you feed your baby formula the risk of infant death is automatically doubled.[133] The information in the study presented was shocking and I am only going to share with you here a small part of these important findings. Various studies showed that the risk of infant death occurred up to 3 *times* more in formula-fed babies, and in regards to SIDS, formula feeding was found to increase the chances of SIDS occurring up to 5 *times* more than in breastfed babies (even partially breastfed babies). Heart, circulatory and respiratory failure was also studied and one study reported that more than half of infants with congenital heart disease lost oxygenation during bottle feedings, while none did so while breastfeeding.

In regards to childhood cancers, a joint study between the United States and Canada on neuroblastoma, a common childhood cancer, revealed a doubled risk for children who did not receive breast milk for more than one year. This study is consistent with several other childhood cancer studies in other nations, with results ranging from *1.45 to 4 times* the risk for developing various common childhood cancers for formula-fed babies.

Dr. Linda Folden Palmer's website is truly wonderful for any mother, old or new:

  ✓ thebabybond.com/

I also think that what we should be promoting is perhaps *partial* breastfeeding combined with formula if a mother cannot give her breast milk all day. For example, you could express (or breastfeed) 125 ml of milk a day and use formula for the rest of the milk feeds. This way, at least the child is getting some antibodies from that one bottle of breast milk. I think this could be very powerful as opposed to just using only formula, and would be less stress on the mother. Milk only stops being produced after 3–5 days of stopping breast-feeding, so there should be no problems with doing it once per day, and if anything, milk should come out very easily, making expressing fast.

Breastfeeding for the working mum

I know this may be hard for many mothers to do, especially if they have to go back to work during the day, but you can try using a breast pump at work, then freezing the milk to take home with you to use later on. Many offices are becoming much more 'mum' friendly and won't cause a fuss when you need privacy to do this. There are even laws in place now in the UK so that a company must support you with this, and for however long you decide to continue it. The Workplace Regulations and Approved Code of Practice require employees to provide suitable facilities for pregnant and breastfeeding mothers to rest.

It will take motivation and commitment to continue breast-feeding when you go back to work, but if you can do it, your child's health will *really* thank you for it. And you won't have to take as many days off because your child is not so likely to fall ill.

Although some formulas seem to be really advanced these days, saying they are packed with vitamins etc., they all are missing many vital ingredients – up to 100, which is a lot when you consider how powerful one vital nutrient is capable of being.

Comparing ingredients

Breast milk contains more than *100* nutrients that the formula industry simply can't duplicate. For example, breast milk is full of antibodies that protect babies from illness and help them develop their own immune systems. Some other key differences between the ingredients in breast milk and formula include the following:[134]

- Formula has a higher protein content than human milk. However, the protein in breast milk is more easily and completely digested by babies.
- Breast milk has a higher carbohydrate content than formula and has large amounts of *lactose*, a sugar found in lower amounts in cow's milk. Research shows that animals whose milk contains higher amounts of lactose experience larger brain development.
- Minerals such as iron are present in lower quantities in breast milk than in formula. However, the minerals in breast milk are more completely absorbed by the baby. In formula-fed babies, the unabsorbed portions of minerals can change the balance of bacteria in the gut, which gives harmful bacteria a chance to grow. This is one reason why bottle-fed babies generally have harder and more odorous (stinky!) stools than breastfed babies.

Breastfeeding may not always work for some mums, but not as many as we think

Actual inability to produce enough milk is rare, with studies showing that mothers from developing countries experiencing nutritional hardship still produce amounts of milk of similar quality to that of mothers in developed countries.[135]

Some women, but actually only a very *small* percentage, have real physical trouble breastfeeding and this is very tragic both for the child and for the mother. If you have had lots of help, and discovered this has happened to you, and there is nothing you can do, please don't beat yourself up and feel guilty; sometimes we cannot change what our body is or is not doing. The main thing is just to *try* as hard you can – don't give up after a few weeks; try everything until you really know in your heart it's just not going to work. Being a new mum is extremely exhausting and taxing on the body. It's very easy to get into a stressful situation when you aren't getting enough sleep, and if you aren't eating too well or drinking enough fluids, all of this can impact on how easy it is for you to produce milk.

During this period of trying, if problems are really occurring, you may need to use formula (the best kind you can find) as well as expressing your breast milk until you can work the problem out or decide that you have to use only formula.

Many new mothers get mastitis, and more often than not, due to the horrible pain, they will unfortunately give up breastfeeding and have to use formula. But ironically, the advice from many lactation specialists is, you just have to keep persevering to get through it – and that feeding *more* often may actually improve the condition. You may need to have treatment for the infection (most doctors will prescribe antibiotics which can cause problems for the child as the medication is passed through the milk, giving the child thrush and immune problems – so if this happens please increase your amount of high-quality probiotics, and include in your daily diet a bowl of miso soup (organic and fermented, mixed with warm water to preserve the life force of the miso, which is super-high in probiotics) but more often than not, you *can* get past the mastitis, and soon breastfeeding will be much easier. It's all about persevering, if you can, through the tough times.

I highly recommend the brilliant *The Breastfeeding Book* by Dr. Sears and Martha Sears. This is an entire book dedicated to everything you need to know about breastfeeding. It has the most amazing and valuable information for every mum, and there are great tips and solutions to any problems you may encounter with breastfeeding. This book shows that with a little know-how, you may actually be able to breastfeed successfully when you originally thought you couldn't.

I personally hope that in the future we bring back 'wet nurses'; these are nannies who can breastfeed your children for you when you just can't. It would be ideal for working mums who have to go back to work ASAP after giving birth. This is what happened in the past, and it kept children from falling seriously ill before medicine came along.

> The prophet Muhammad had a wet nurse. So did Napoleon, Alice Roosevelt, and Luciano Pavarotti. After the future King George IV was born, in 1762, his wet nurse, Mrs. Scott, became a minor celebrity.[136]

I know it might sound odd, but I would rather have someone I trusted and knew, who was healthy, feed my child than use an inferior product out of a tin that's more than likely full of bad sugars, GMO ingredients, heavy metals, and non-organic ingredients.

Could you donate your own breast milk?

I was thinking recently that when I slow down with Lola's milk feeds, I would like to see if I could donate some milk to a local mother, who perhaps gave birth to a premature baby and cannot feed her baby herself. The hospitals recommend breast milk at all costs for these tiny babies (and others who have health complications) and will try and source it from another healthy mother if possible, rather than using formula. I thought, what could be a better way to help a new life? To donate healthy milk to a child whose poor mother was unable to feed would be such a *wonderful* thing to do, and I could easily pump at least one or two bottles a day for a child who really needed it.

In the UK there are milk bank organizations which source donations to local hospitals. There are certain requirements the mother must pass, though, i.e. she has to be of a certain level of health, cannot have any alcohol or cigarettes in her system or certain medications, and must have a blood test to see if the milk is healthy:

✓ ukamb.org

In the USA/North America you can check out this website:

✓ hmbana.org

I hope that if you do have the ability and time to do this that you will consider it. I think it's vitally important for us to try and help other mums wherever possible.

What about using formula?

If you have no other option and have to use formula, research the brands as *much* as you can, to find out what the best formula is for your child. *Avoid* all of the soy-based ones as they are *not* based on ingredients that your child should ever have. Many brands have terrible and toxic ingredients (as well as including GMOs) that make your child gain too much weight, increase the likelihood of catching more viruses, and are not the best at all for their delicate immune systems. It's ironic how mums often think that weight gain from formula is a sign their child is healthy, but sadly it's because of the ingredients that the child appears this way, but long term, this 'chubbiness' could actually develop into obesity. A very chubby baby, while it looks so cute, is not always healthy.

Another alarming problem with using soy-based formulas is what happens to girls when they are older, and it directly relates to so many women these days who suffer with uterine problems.

> Women who were fed soy formula as babies were 25 percent more likely to develop uterine fibroids ... The link between uterine fibroids and soy formula is thought to be a response to the isoflavones (naturally occurring estrogen-like substances) in soy, and in particular, the high exposure at an early age in women given soy formula during infancy.[137]

Here is another reason *not* to ever use soy-based formulas:

> It is estimated that infants fed soy formula have 13,000 to 22,000 times the amount of estrogen in their little bodies than infants fed

other types of formula or who are breastfed. In fact, infants fed soy formula take in an estimated three to five birth control pills' worth of estrogen every day, depending upon the particular batch of formula and whether your baby is a big eater.[138]

As you can see, this shocking amount of hormones *cannot* be OK for a young woman to develop properly later in life.

I want to share with you just how untrustworthy and downright *evil* some formula companies can be – they sometimes act as irresponsibly as pharmaceutical companies do. The FDA admit that they don't have a law which says formulas and their ingredients must be approved first by them before they are marketed.[139] This is truly alarming because it means the manufacturers can make any claims about their products and can produce TV and magazine advertisements to say whatever it is they want the consumer to believe. And the chances are, you are unknowingly feeding your child one of these brands. In 2008, six infants died in China and more than 300,000 became sick because the ingredients in the formula of one popular brand, Sanlu (which also had ties to Nestlé – more on them later) was found to contain a toxic chemical inside called melamine.[140] Melamine was sneakily used to make the formula appear like it had more protein in it. But melamine is never to be used as a food item; it is actually an organic compound (not meaning 'organic' as in healthy, but as in a gaseous, liquid, or solid chemical compound whose molecules contain carbon) that is often combined with formaldehyde (a cancer-causing agent) to produce 'melamine resin', a synthetic polymer which is fire resistant and heat tolerant. When there were reports of very ill children being connected to this formula, the company also tried to cover up the problem for a long time before it was too late to stop the infant deaths and sickness. The case went to court and two of the company's executives involved were tried and *sentenced to death* and were executed in 2009.

Isn't it shocking to know that this toxic chemical was actually put on *purpose* into formula designed for *babies,* just to make more *money* for the company? And that children actually unnecessarily died as well, as did the CEOs who were responsible for their careless decisions? This is not the first shocking case to do with formula linked to Nestlé either, who are one of the most powerful and highly lucrative companies in the world. They own many brands under the 'Nestlé' umbrella.

Their first scandal began in the late 1970s, when the brand was promoting formula as 'better than breast milk' and many mothers in Third World countries were conned by the marketing schemes and fed their children formula from the first moments of their child's life. They saw the healthy pictures of 'First World' babies on the tin, cute and chubby-looking, and thought that by feeding them this formula, they were doing the best by their child. But many children soon became unwell due to the inadequate formula not providing nearly enough nutrients and because they also contained other nasty ingredients. When the media picked up on this, people who were outraged and disgusted began to boycott Nestlé; this lasted for decades, with the campaign going strong still, to this very day. Nestlé used dirty tactics to make massive amounts of money, again putting children's health at risk.

Nestlé encourages bottle feeding primarily by either giving away free samples of baby milk to hospitals, or neglecting to collect payments. It has been criticized for misinforming mothers and health workers in promotional literature. Nestlé implies that malnourished mothers, and mothers of twins and premature babies are unable to breastfeed, despite health organizations' claims that there is no evidence to support this. Evidence of direct advertising to mothers has been found in over twenty countries such as South Africa and Thailand. Instructions and health warnings on packaging are often either absent, not prominently displayed or in an inappropriate language. All of these actions directly contravene the Code regulating the marketing of baby milk formulas.[141]

According to some, it's still going on in Third World countries.

> It's estimated that Nestlé kills approximately one baby every 21 seconds. In Africa they're sending sales reps into hospitals to convince new mothers that formula is medicine. It costs a family an entire week's wage to feed one baby for 7 days, these families are given just enough milk to stop the mother's own milk from coming in. The instructions are not written in the native language but, even if they were, they don't have the electricity needed to sterilize or heat the bottles and with not enough money to buy it, they're watering it down and using dirty water. Add to this the fact that breastfeeding helps to space children; without it the mother quickly becomes pregnant again and has ANOTHER baby to buy milk for, convinced that her own milk is not good enough, or that her body will never make enough. In most cases this is just not true, even a mother who is malnourished and under stress can still produce enough milk for her baby.
> Jane Tindall

How disgusting and downright evil! I also suggest *completely* boycotting Nestlé and its umbrella companies (Nestlé holds about 50% of the world's breast milk substitute market as well as nearly 50% of the cosmetics company L'Oreal, so definitely *not* a good company to spend your money on) so find out who owns the formula you are using currently (or are considering using). There are simply too many horrible stories that are tied to this brand, and they don't deserve a penny (or cent!) of your money.

Not all formulas are made by unethical companies like this, but *please* use legitimate non-GMO *organic* formulas, ones based on goat's milk rather than cow's milk, and those that are recommended by natural healthcare specialists. If you go into a pharmacy or even talk to your doctor, they won't know about these other, far better brands. Chemists and doctors get targeted by formula sales reps too and will promote a certain brand just because someone has been to see them to tell them about it. It certainly doesn't mean it's the best for your child, just because your doctor has said so. I would personally use goat's milk formulas for they contain properties which are far closer to human breast milk than those in cow's milk.

Also, try and avoid the formulas that are advertised on TV and in mainstream baby magazines; these ones are not necessarily the best. Just like the big beauty brands which advertise their products due to having a huge marketing budget, so too do the formula companies.

Despite this information I have shared with you about formulas and how they are nowhere near as good as breast milk, they can at times literally be a life-saving food. Children who suffer from major allergies and gastrointestinal upsets can often depend on these types of 'elemental formulas' which were developed especially by scientists so that their stomachs would not violently react like they do to most foods. In this case, formula does have its place, but I do urge that it's the last resort and not the first option.

For those of you that want to learn all you can about breast-feeding, please check out this wonderful website aimed at helping mums make it a priority and educating them when there is a problem:

✓ babygooroo.com

What I recommend formula-wise

When you have to use formula, here are a few brands that I recommend. Nanny Care Goat Milk is said to be one of the best for older babies (+6 months). Goat's milk has a higher uptake of certain minerals compared to cow's milk such as zinc, calcium and iron. Studies have shown that goat's milk not only prevents loss of bone demineralization but also helps to prevent iron deficiency. Nanny Care goats are bred to produce milk that is soft and more digestible, which is easier on infants' tummies.

✓ vitacare.co.uk

Holle Biodynamic Infant Formulas

If I had to feed Lola formula, this is the brand that I would choose. Holle has been around since 1933 and has created a whole range of formulas and infant foods, made from organic and biodynamic ingredients. They have several different formulas, one which can feed a newborn (although I hope no one needs to use it as early as that) and others which are for the next stages of growth. There is even an organic goat's milk formula for children older than 6 months. This is the best-quality formula brand I have come across. I am sure there are others out there that are good, but so far I haven't seen any. Goat's milk would be my preferred type because aluminum does not seem to be found in goat's milk as opposed to fairly high levels in cow-and soy-milk formulas.

holle.ch/

If you are interested in making your own formula, so you know *exactly* what goes into it, then you can use the following suggested recipe:

2 cups whole milk, preferably unprocessed (raw) milk from pasture-fed organic cows

1/4 cup homemade liquid whey (see recipe for whey, below)

4 tablespoons lactose*

1 teaspoon bifidobacterium infntis**

2 or more tablespoons good quality cream (not ultra-pasteurized), more if you are using

milk from Holstein cows

1 teaspoon regular dose cod liver oil or 1/2 teaspoon high-vitamin cod liver oil*

1 teaspoon expeller-expressed organic sunflower oil*

1 teaspoon organic extra virgin olive oil*

2 teaspoons organic coconut oil*

2 teaspoons Frontier brand nutritional yeast flakes*

2 teaspoons gelatin*

1/4 teaspoon acerola powder*

1 7/8 cups filtered water

Add gelatin to water and heat gently until gelatin is dissolved. Place all ingredients in a very clean glass or stainless steel container and mix well. To serve, pour 6 to 8 ounces into a very clean glass bottle*, attach nipple and set in a pan of simmering water. Heat until warm but not hot to the touch, shake bottle well and feed baby. (Never, never heat formula in a microwave oven) Note: If you are using the Lact-Aid, mix all ingredients well in a blender.

Recipe c/o Westen A Price Foundation sourced from Mercola.com

Supplements to Take When Formula Feeding

If you have no choice and have to resort to using formula, then of course, please use a good brand as I have mentioned above. If you do use goats milk-based formula's (highly recommended over cows-and-soy milk ones) you may need to look into supplementing with extra folic acid due to the lower amounts found naturally in goats milk. However, goats milk contains more calcium than cow's milk (13 %) and also 25% more vitamin b-6, 134 % more potassium, 27% more selenium, three times more niacin and four times higher in copper. It also has 47% more Vitamin A. I would also check if there are sufficient Omega 3s in the formula you choose as well. If not, you may need to add extra to the formula mixture. Deficiencies in Omega 3s are causing children's brains to have difficulties with developing in the way they should. This can impact the way that they learn. Many learning disabilities are being diagnosed and whilst a lot of them could be stemming from toxicity, it still makes sense that if they are being fed with inferior foods (as we know that formula will always be inferior) then supplementing with the vital nutrients at this crucial time in their life is highly recommended. You could use the Wellspring supplement from Touchstone Essentials as that contains a very good blend of different organic oils, and because they are food grade, it's safe to give to your child. You can find information about them through my website.

The following website shares valuable information about children and the importance of Healthy Fats in their diet.

✓ durhamtrial.org

Chapter 34

The Vital Importance of Healthy Food for Children

The connection between food and behavior is so basic that it is being overlooked by parents, the school system, counselors, and most of the medical professionals. Ask any hyperactive child, depressed, angry teenager, violent adult, or criminal what they eat, and you'll find they 'live' on junk food – sweetened boxed cereals, candy, carbonated drinks, potato chips, and fast food. Junk food abuses the mind, undernourishes the body, and negatively affects behavior.[142]
Barbara Reed Stitt, author of the book *Food and Behavior*

Due to the alarming rate of childhood obesity, behavioral and learning problems, we can tell that something is going very, very *wrong* with how we feed our children. It's not only affecting their weight, but also affecting their *minds*. What parents don't often realize is the connection between food, behavior, *and* illness, and the impact on their long-term health, including their mental state and choices in life.

The World Health Organisation published a report from their Commission on the social determinants of health - which stated that:

Research now shows that many challenges in adult society – mental health problems, obesity/stunting, heart disease, criminality, competence in literacy and numeracy - have their roots in early childhood.

A healthy diet in early infancy and childhood is just *so* important. Quite often, a young child will 'appear' to be healthy, so parents just assume that whatever they are feeding them is absolutely 'fine'. At a young age, the body can have a marvelous way of staying vibrant and indeed it's usually not till later in life that problems start to show – and sometimes only on an appearance level too. But on an emotional and cognitive level, if we look hard enough, we can notice changes in our children, and quickly after certain foods are eaten. One only has to give a sugary drink or food to a child, and you can see within minutes how it negatively affects their mood and behavior.

We need to *always* remember that food is *fuel* for the body and brain, and even more so for a child. Nutrients and vitamins play the *most* important role in creating a strong immune system and brain function, and if we are feeding our children many chemical-based foods, then it is certain to cause a chemical *reaction* in their brain and body. If we feed kids well from the start, it makes sense to assume that they will be smarter, more active, and happier people in the long run as their brains and bodies are getting exactly what they need to function at their best.

What *really* concerns me is most parents' *idea* of what healthy food actually is. I see so many parents constantly feeding their kids white bread, white pasta and lots of dairy, which are three of the *worst* things you can feed a child. White bread and white pasta does nothing nutritionally and dairy is a highly *allergenic* food, and because it has been pasteurized, the goodness it did have has been heated right out of it, yet still leaving behind the pus from the cows. Intensively farmed cows tend to suffer with chronic mastitis, often for their entire short lives, from being constantly made to act like nursing mums, sometimes for years and years on end. They are then given antibiotics to treat the infection and they also get given different types of hormones from the countless vaccines that they receive.

There is more than just this lurking in milk too. In recent studies, carried out by Spanish-Moroccan scientists, it was found that there can be up to 20 different painkillers, growth hormones, and antibiotics in a *single glass of milk*.[143] The scientists analyzed 20 different samples of milk, coming from goats, humans and cows, and were shocked to discover a chemical cocktail of ingredients added to the animals' diet prior to milking or from contamination through feed on the farm. Some of the contaminants found in trace levels included florfenicol, used as an antibiotic, triclosan (an anti-fungal medication) and something called 17-beta-estradoil which is a sex hormone. Other medications found in these milk samples were pyrimethamine which is used as an anti-malaria drug. There were 20 in total found in this study, which was published in the *Journal of Agriculture and Food Chemistry*. There are too many of them to list here, but I am sure you are getting the picture. Factory-farmed milk, which is not organic, is *not* a health food, and if anything it is a *drug*.

Too much dairy (and of the non organic, pasteurized kind) is said to make children prone to lots of coughs and colds, due to the mucus it creates in the body. And it's now also being linked to causing asthma. And despite us thinking that dairy contains lots of calcium for 'strong healthy bones', all of the countries who consume the most dairy also have the *highest* rates of osteoporosis.

25% of sixty-five-year-old women in the United States are diagnosed with osteoporosis. For a person technically to qualify for this label, it means she has lost 50–75% of the original bone material from her skeleton. That is 1 out of every 4 women of sixty-five years old has lost over half her bone density! Today, more deaths are caused by osteoporosis than cancer of the breast and cervix combined. I used to believe that bones lost calcium only if there was not enough calcium in our diets. The National Dairy Council is the foremost spokesman for this point of view, and the solution they propose, not all that surprisingly, is for us all to drink more milk and eat more dairy products. In fact, the dairy industry has of late spent a great deal of money promoting this point of view; and it does seem logical. But modern nutritional research clearly indicates a major flaw in this perspective. Osteoporosis is, in fact, a disease caused by a number of things, the most important of which is excess dietary animal protein![144]

Regarding the increase of childhood illnesses rarely suffered from years ago, there is a strong case for them being triggered by a cow's-milk allergy:

According to Alternative Medicine, up to half of all infants may be sensitive to cow's milk. As a result, symptoms of an underlying milk allergy may start as early as infancy, only manifested as eczema, a symptom that may remain later on in childhood and adulthood. Furthermore, in addition to asthma and eczema, an underlying milk allergy may manifest as bronchitis, sinusitis, autoimmune disorders, frequent colds and ear infections and even behavioral problems.[145]

Research also shows us that needing to have high levels of calcium for strong bone density is just not true. According to Nathan Pritikin who studied at length the current medical research on osteoporosis, there is no truth to the Dairy Council's viewpoint:

African Bantu women take in only 350 mg. of calcium per day. They bear nine children during their lifetime and breastfeed them for two years. They never have calcium deficiency, seldom break a bone, rarely lose a tooth ... How can they do that on 350 mg. of calcium a day when the (National Dairy Council) recommendation is 1200 mg.? It's very simple. They're on a low-protein diet that doesn't kick the calcium out of the body.[146]

You can get *far* better bio-available calcium (meaning calcium that is much more easily absorbed by your body) in higher forms from things like almonds, spinach, cashews, whole grains and many other whole foods. A better alternative to cow's milk is goat's milk and many shops are now selling it these days.

If you don't want to stop giving your children or yourself milk then try and source *raw* milk – as it's far better for health and in fact does contain many valuable nutrients not found in heat-treated milk. In the United Kingdom, it's quite easy to get hold of raw milk (some producers even deliver) but in the USA, unfortunately, not so much; in fact, it is deemed illegal in many states, which is *crazy* because there are rarely any illnesses stemming from raw milk. If it's produced in a clean factory with healthy cows, and stored well, then it simply *cannot* be dangerous, if consumed within a few short days. There is a lot more illness (possibly tens of thousands times higher rates) associated with consuming too much *pasteurized* dairy rather than with raw... If most of the beneficial nutrients have been killed, then how can it still be classed as a health food?

The medical and food industries always say how dangerous it is due to something that happened in the past. One would think that thousands of people had a bad reaction to raw milk. But in actual fact, it's only ever been on a very small scale. The, minuscule amounts of fatalities are why the *entire* world seems to be scared of raw dairy, and it's thanks to the media for continuing to spin this story. Lots of health authorities (mainstream doctors) think it's highly dangerous though, and are all for pasteurization due to what they were taught in medical school. We must remember that doctors do not receive much nutritional training at all when attaining their degree.

As recently as 2011, the CDC (Centers for Disease Control) has admitted that there has not been one death in 11 years associated with the consumption of raw dairy:

The US Centers for Disease Control and Prevention (CDC) refuses to acknowledge that, based on all available statistics, raw milk produced on clean, small-scale farms is actually far safer than pasteurized milk from factory farms. But the agency did admit earlier this year, after being pressed and warned of a potential Freedom of Information Act (FOIA) request if it failed to comply, that not a single person has died from raw-milk consumption in over a decade.[147]

When looking at the nutritional value in raw milk as opposed to pasteurized milk, the difference is chalk and cheese, night and day. The two simply *cannot* compare in health aspects. And it's how we drank milk (with the cow we had at home that we milked in the barn!) before the big factory-farming industry was created.

It has also been said recently that Queen Elizabeth supports the drinking of raw milk:

A writeup on raw milk published in *The Globe and Mail* back in 2010 explains that Queen Elizabeth personally drinks raw milk, and that when her grandsons Harry and William were students at Eton College, she went out of her way to smuggle it in for them as well. The Queen apparently recognizes some value in raw milk beyond what health authorities are willing to admit.[148]

It's not just health concerns that have made raw milk a big no-no. The majority of the dairy industry, which is made up of mostly pasteurized and UHT milks, in 2005 was said to be worth $27 billion alone and today it has increased to $37 billion per year.[149] Think about the financial impact that it would have on the dairy industry if everyone suddenly stopped wanting to consume pasteurized dairy products. It would mean total collapse for the farmers and all of those involved in the dairy industry. Even the US government would suffer. It makes sense that so much bad information is put out into the world so that people think that raw milk is bad, and that pasteurized is the only way we should consume our dairy.

For raw milk and other raw dairy products in the UK which are home delivered I love:

✓ hookandson.co.uk

For raw milk in other countries, you may have to do a lot of digging around or even start asking local farmers to see if anyone is selling it. In the USA you can use this website to see where it's being sold:

✓ realmilk.com/real-milk-finder

The same website also has lots of international information about raw milk and the industry.

In Australia there is a company which stocks raw milk called 'Cleopatra's Bath Milk'. Raw dairy seems to be illegal for sale in Australia but this company very cleverly markets it as bath milk, and not as a food or drink. They also deliver Australia-wide. To check it out please visit:

✓ angelfire.com/folk/raw milk

No matter what milk you drink, if you just can't give it up, *always* try and get an organic kind. There will be far fewer traces of pus, hormones and medications in the organic source.

Another aspect of childhood nutrition which concerns me is, the length of time children go on having poor diets and the eating habits they take with them to adulthood. When poor food is being eaten at a young age, before the brain has really developed, the effects can only be negative. In my own experience, I ate *very* badly for decades and the older I got, the *worse* my moods and energy levels got, not to mention how bad my stomach felt. I never really took notice of eating something 'bad', then seeing how I reacted, because really, everything I ate was generally chemical- and sugar-based, so it happened constantly. It's only now that, if I have a naughty moment and eat say a piece (or two!) of chocolate cake that is high in sugar, I will see very quickly how my moods change. Even my husband will notice and say, 'Hmm, have you had sugar, Anna? You're super-grumpy!' It's quite interesting to see it happen to yourself, when you know what signs to look for. But when children have regular chemical-based foods, then their behavior may constantly be so erratic that the parents tend to just think the child is being 'difficult' and are not able to make the connection between what *they* had actually chosen to feed them with.

One of the most important things to do for your child is to feed them with organic *whole foods* as much as possible, and to keep them off junk, sugary things and foods with artificial sweeteners in them. I have discussed things like aspartame in the food chapter (Chapter

10) and that it's highly important to make sure children don't eat anything that contains that ingredient (a proven poison).

It is also very concerning to go outside and see parents feeding their small children McDonald's and other fast foods and labeling it to them as a 'treat'. It was certainly very cleverly advertised as one, so that's why people do see it as something special, a 'reward' perhaps for good behavior. Food that is full of addictive chemicals (which can't be processed at all easily by a tiny body) should *not* be used to make a child think it's a novelty or special. When they hear that it is a treat, they tend to want it often when they are older, and once able to buy themselves this 'special' food, it becomes a regular addition to their diet.

Don't forget that children are very smart and also very empathetic at certain ages, and when adults explain to them about *why* this type of food is bad, not to mention the cruelty aspect and the destruction to the environment, they tend to not want to eat it at all. So if you really don't want your child eating this kind of food, be honest and tell them exactly why it's not good; don't just say it isn't good. Tell them how the animals are treated and that many harmful chemicals are added to the food to make it appear to taste good and to also make people become addicted to the foods.

Shocking sugar

Not only do we have to worry about artificial chemicals in our children's food; we also really need to worry *more* about plain old sugar. Why? Sugar is seen by the body, literally, as a poison. It serves no useful purpose and studies are showing some very worrying things. If a child is brought up on a sugary diet, and maintains this through their life, chances are they will end up having problems with alcohol and/or drugs. Simply because sugar affects the same part of the brain as drugs like cocaine, heroin and even alcohol do. Sarah Best, investigative journalist wrote about this in her report, *Shocking Facts About Sugar:*

We all know that refined sugar is the leading cause of tooth decay and diabetes, but that's just the tip of the iceberg. Few realize that sugar also weakens our bones, ages our skin, damages our liver and all of our other organs, and wreaks havoc with every system of the body – most notably the nervous, digestive, endocrine, circulatory and immune systems. What is even less widely understood is that it can cause anxiety, depression, brain fog, mood swings and, in those especially sensitive to its effects, even a state of intoxication, erratic behavior and/or violent outbursts. And just like any other addictive drug (make no mistake – that's what sugar is), if taken regularly, in sufficient quantity and long term, its effects on physical, mental, emotional and spiritual health are eventually devastating.[150]

This is shocking, right? Well, guess what, you can hear it from me that this connection makes sense. I personally developed a drug problem and would drink a lot as well, when I was older, and I grew up eating loads of sugary things. Sugar is so *very* addictive; we just need to have a tiny bit of it and it alerts both our brains and our stomach that we want more, and immediately. It never keeps us full for long and always makes us hungrier. Bread is a nasty culprit for this reaction too as it converts to sugars in the body very quickly, which is why bread is so addictive as well. Wholegrain breads, for some people, are suitable for their diet, but for most of us, we really need to go without, or search for a gluten-, wheat-free substitute, and it's certainly not good for children to be given lots of bread. And by all means, try and avoid white bread altogether – you may as well feed them cardboard.

It is highly worrying to see what sugar does to children's brains and in only a short amount of time. If you have ever been to a kids' party and seen how hyperactive they become after eating sweets and junk food, you will know exactly what I mean. I witnessed it myself only last year, when I had to look after our plumber's 2-year-old twins for a few hours. We were in my room sitting on my bed and the father came in and gave them some food because I had said they were hungry. I was absolutely horrified at what he brought back to give them for a snack. It was red cordial (a 'sugar free' with aspartame in it) and a packet of Doritos cheesy chips (containing GMO corn *and* MSG among other unsafe additives). Unfortunately, I didn't know this man well enough to say, 'Don't you know this stuff is so dangerous for them?' so I felt that I had to give the kids this food. It was *torture* for me, but now I look back and I think I was meant to see it, so that I can tell you about what happened.

Within 15 minutes of having these snacks, both the kids' personality and behavior *significantly* changed. The little girl, who was once very shy and sweet and had been lying down, became *very* aggressive, very loud and actually tried to hit me! Her brother became super-aggressive as well and they both started physically fighting with each other. Shortly afterwards, they both quickly became very tired and very grumpy. The father took them away, but it gave me time to think about how quickly a young body responds to these types of chemicals.

Sadly, I could tell when I first met these children that they were not at all healthy. They didn't have any energy or 'light' behind their eyes; both kids' eyes were bloodshot, murky and not at all clear or white. They were only 2! And the father was certainly not abusing them as they were dressed well and treated well, but another still highly worrying *form* of abuse was coming from feeding them this type of diet. I dread to think what they were fed at night? Was it a struggle for them to wake up, with lots of tears and causing Mum and Dad to get angry? And how they behaved at night after a day's worth of food like that – did they sleep OK? (Highly unlikely!) And how did they wake up in the mornings? It seems *very* unfair that children are fed foods that create *massive* personality changes which can then cause them to become erratic and misbehave, then are yelled at by their parents, deemed as troublesome and difficult, yet it was the *parents'* fault in the *first* place because of what they fed them! Doesn't that seem so hypocritical and completely unfair to these kids?

It was very sad spending time with those kids. I sat and wondered how their lives would turn out just because of the damaging effects from eating food like this over their lifetime. And it hasn't been the last time I have seen this. Whenever I go on the Tube, or into the city, there is always a parent feeding their toddler absolute rubbish. I find it very hard not to go up to them and beg, *'Please stop. To you it's just food, but to your child, it's changing their brain chemistry and setting them up for a lifetime of health concerns.'* But I can't interfere and have no choice but to walk on.

The sugar industry is worth even more money than the dairy industry. So it's in the best interests of certain companies and also some pharmaceutical companies to have the public believe that there is no proof that sugar really does affect the minds of children. I think you can just do an experiment on yourself, and that is to monitor how it affects you after you have eaten a huge amount. If it affects you, then imagine what it's doing to children who have a much smaller weight ratio.

What *can* you use to sweeten foods then?

Some much better alternatives to white sugar are organic:

- maple syrup
- date syrup
- brown rice syrup
- coconut nectar
- coconut sugar
- apple puree
- fruit purees
- Xylitol

'Raw' cane sugar, despite its healthier-sounding name, is still not a good form of sugar as it is also heavily processed. But with all types of sweeteners, moderation is the key here.

I recently discovered the joys of making desserts and other sweet treats with recipes that use only fruits. You can make amazing cakes and muffins, jellies and other yummy things where the only sweetener required is from fruit juice or mashed fruit. So instead of adding any honeys or syrups, you can use for example 1–2 mashed bananas and add cocoa powder, vanilla, gluten-free flour and other typical baking things. It's changed my life really because I keep some homemade cookies nearby so that when I do want something sweet, I can reach for them and not for processed biscuits or chocolates. And it will be great when Lola is older and I can give her these after school instead of the typical unhealthy snacks. After testing out a few recipes, I was amazed at how great they tasted; the much less sweet taste means you can taste the other ingredients. They are simple to make, and will impress even the most fussy cake lover!

A fantastic book that I highly recommend is *Sweet and Sugar Free: An All-Natural, Fruit-sweetened Dessert Cookbook* by Karen E. Barkie. You can find this on Amazon and it's very inexpensive as it was first written in 1982. It's now one of my food-making bibles.

Prepackaged baby food

Be very cautious of buying prepared baby food as well. You may think it's healthy and safe 'because it's for children', but many test results show that there is still quite a lot of chemicals in the food from the pesticides. These detrimentally *harm* your baby's brain development. The EU has tried to regulate this, but the truth is, many brands have up to *33 times* the amount that is actually legal. And even more worrying are the chemicals the companies put in their food. In some brands you can find 'fragrance' listed as an ingredient, and while this may seem harmless enough, it is certainly not. The fragrance is man-made from diethyl phthalate (DEP); studies have shown that liver tumors appear in mice which have had a regular dose of this DEP.

Another scary ingredient is DMDM hydantoin, and just to confuse you even more, this chemical has up to *15* other names which mean the exact same thing. Dimethylol and hydroxymethyl are the most typically used names. DMDM is said to be an antimicrobial formaldehyde releaser which is pure poison for the immune system. It's used as an embalming agent for dead bodies. Formaldehyde is something you don't even want around you to breathe in or put on your skin, let alone in your child's food. Absolutely disgusting and downright evil that this is in common baby foods!

Methylparaben is also used in baby food and something that is often found in beauty products as well. It is used as a preservative and is very cheap to buy, which is why the manufacturers are big fans of it. Studies have shown that this food additive mimics estrogen, which can negatively affect reproductive glands – something you do not want happening when your own child's reproductive glands have not even formed properly yet, and if they are already having soy-based formulas this extra addition of more estrogens is just not good.

Retinyl palmitate, which is more commonly known as vitamin A retinol and palmitic acid, is another ingredient in baby food. We have been led to believe that anything with 'vitamin' in the name must mean that it's good for us, right? Not in this case! Vitamin A, when exposed to sunlight and UV rays, breaks down, while releasing free radicals in the body. This has been shown to damage DNA *and* cause cancer. Twenty-five studies have been published proving this vitamin's dangerous effects. Studies are also showing that vitamin A causes skin tumors to form and is appearing as skin cancer. You wouldn't think this vitamin A was in sunblocks then, would you? Well, think again, it is, and is actually one of the most common ingredients added to sunblocks.

All of these ingredients are in beauty products and even things such as baby wipes. This is scary enough, as whatever is put on the skin affects the inside of the body, but why the heck is it being put in children's food? It is beyond disturbing and about time parents wised up to what they are giving their children. Please do the research and don't trust the mainstream's seductive marketing.

Below is a list of food additives and preservatives from the foodmatters.tv website:

Additives

- 102 tartrazine
- 104 quinoline yellow
- 107 yellow 2G
- 110 sunset yellow
- 122 azorubine
- 123 amaranth
- 124 ponceau red
- 127 erythrosine
- 128 red 2G
- 129 allura red
- 132 indigotine
- 133 brilliant blue
- 142 green S
- 151 brilliant black
- 155 chocolate brown natural color
- 160b annatto (in yoghurts, ice creams, popcorn etc, 160a is a safe alternative)

Preservatives

- 200–203 sorbates (in margarine, dips, cakes, fruit products)
- 210–213 benzoates (in juices, soft drinks, cordials, syrups, medications)
- 220–228 sulphites (in dried fruit, fruit drinks, sausages, and many others)
- 280–283 propionates (in bread, crumpets, bakery products)
- 249–252 nitrates, nitrites (in processed meats like ham)
- Synthetic antioxidants – in margarines, vegetable oils, fried

foods, snacks, biscuits etc.

- 310–312 Gallates 319-320 TBHQ, BHA, BHT (306–309 are safe alternatives)
- Flavor enhancers – in flavored crackers, snacks, takeaways, instant noodles, soups 621 MSG 627, 631, 635 disodium inosinate, disodium guanylate, ribonucleotides

(Table compiled by Sue Dengate, author of the bestselling book and film, *Fed Up: Understanding How Food Affects Your Child and What You Can Do about It*.)

* * *

If you do buy non-organic fruits and veggies, check the shopping list previously mentioned and purchase things with the least amount of pesticides on them. And always wash and scrub them thoroughly. You can use baking soda and a bit of hydrogen peroxide to clean them as effectively as possible.

Just so you know, strawberries and other thin-skinned fruits are some of the worst for pesticide levels, yet usually are a favorite among children. These simple methods of intensive cleaning can at least help a little bit, so it's such a terrible shame that some parents don't even do that. I've seen parents give their kids unwashed fruit and it's been very hard not to shout out and say, 'Stop! Pleeeease wash it!' If there was a cup full of the toxins that the child was to eat and absorb in one day, no parent would give their child that cup to drink! So it makes no sense to me why people ignore simple ways of reducing these chemicals by washing.

And please don't *ever* microwave their food or bottles! The plastic containers/bottles will heat up (despite what the company says!) and the particles will drop into their milk, and settle in their tissues, and over the long term will probably disrupt their hormones. Not to mention that microwaving means the nutrients will mostly be pretty much completely destroyed anyway, leaving your child to eat or drink nutritionally deficient foods. Children are precious pure beings and need to be fed foods that are pure.

For a high-quality prepared baby food in the UK you can try Ella's Kitchen or HIPP Organics.

In the USA, 100% organic brands Plum Organics and Sprout Baby Food look very good. Earth's Best also have some great-looking meals, but I can see that some of their formulas use too many concerning ingredients such as soy oil, corn syrup and other sugars. I would buy their food if I couldn't make it fresh myself, but not their formulas for my child.

Here is an eye-opening piece which shows how upside down our current relationship between the medical and food industry is. Written by John Robbins who wrote the foreword for book *The China Study:*

If you are like most Americans today, you are surrounded by fast-food chain restaurants. You are barraged by ads for junk foods. You see other ads, for weight-loss programs, that say you can eat whatever you want, not exercise and still lose weight. It's easier to find a Snickers bar, a Big Mac or a Coke than it is to find an apple. And your kids eat at a school cafeteria whose idea of a vegetable is the ketchup on the burgers.

You go to your doctor for health tips. In the waiting room, you find a glossy 243-page magazine titled *Family Doctor: Your Essential Guide to Health and Well-being.* Published by the American Academy of Family Physicians and sent free to the offices of all 50,000 family doctors in the United States in 2004, it's full of glossy full-page color ads for McDonald's, Dr Pepper, chocolate pudding and Oreo cookies.

You pick up an issue of *National Geographic Kids,* a magazine published by the National Geographic Society "for ages six and up," expecting to find wholesome reading for youngsters. The pages, however, are filled with ads for Twinkies, M&Ms, Frosted

Flakes, Froot Loops, Hostess Cup Cakes and Xtreme Jell-O Pudding Sticks.

This is what scientist's and food activists at Yale University call a *toxic food environment*. It is the environment in which most of us live today.

Chapter 35

Safe Skincare for Children

More than half of children's bath soaps, shampoos, lotions, and other personal care products tested by the group Campaign for Safe Cosmetics (CSC) were found to contain 1,4-dioxane and formaldehyde, according to a report released today. Both of the chemicals are considered probable carcinogens by the Environmental Protection Agency. Because they are not intentionally added by manufacturers, there is no requirement that product labels list the chemicals when they are present. There are also no federal restrictions on allowable levels of the chemicals in body care products, but several other countries do not allow the chemicals at any level.[151]

Report: 'Toxins Common in Baby Products'

When we see baby products in the shops or on the TV, they are generally advertised as safe and gentle, yet often the truth is the opposite. A large percentage of baby products are *completely* unsafe due to their shockingly high chemical content. Let me get straight to the point: you must *only* use safe skincare products on your children. As you now know, the skin is the body's largest organ and the easiest way for toxins to get into the body. There are loads of companies who make products for children and babies and a large percentage formulate them the way they do for adults – with a list a mile long of toxic chemicals. And don't be fooled by the brands you have grown up with and seen on TV; they are some of the worst!

Recently Johnson & Johnson came under fire for using the ingredient formaldehyde in their 'no tears' baby shampoo.[152] As previously mentioned, formaldehyde is an alarmingly unsafe ingredient and a known carcinogen. This chemical is used in many things but, most shockingly, as an embalming fluid in morgues. Totally *not natural* and not something you would want anywhere near or on your baby's skin. The company are now changing their formula due to public demand, but they have said it's going to take up to 2 *years* for this to happen. This is a real worry, as one would think it would just take a few days to sort out a new ingredient to replace it and this could be implemented ASAP. Goodness knows why it will take them this long. And for a company that has been around for decades, you would think they would know better than putting in dangerous chemicals in the first place, but the truth is they always have used them. It's a cheap product, affordable to even low-income families, and this is why the company uses inexpensive and poor-quality ingredients.

So this means having to do a bit of research into what you buy. Do not use mineral- or petrolatum-based brands, even when they claim to contain lavender and other natural-sounding ingredients.

The reason why I think it's much more of a necessity to buy safe products for children is because a baby's skin is 5 *times thinner* than an adult's, so this means they are absorbing even more chemicals – and far more quickly too. And when a toxin enters a baby's body, because of their low birth weight compared to adults, it's going to be a much larger amount in comparison. You do not want these avoidable toxins harming your newborn baby or small child. With the high rate of infant eczema and other skin problems later in life, it makes sense to really treat your baby's skin as precious (because that's what it is!) and only deserving the best and safest ingredients. It's not as expensive as you think either.

When I was getting ready for my own baby's birth, I had some home visits from midwives from the local hospital. While the care they give expectant mums, for me, was more than great, it was also very alarming to see the type of 'free' stuff that gets given to mums-to-be. In my 'care' pack, I saw only mainstream brand things like nappies, nappy cream, wipes, even some food items and personal care things for myself such a facial cream. What was immediately obvious to me was that it was the common and easily available cheap stuff I had seen in the shops and I recognized that it was also *very* toxic! Not *one* thing in the pack could be deemed anywhere near truly healthy or safe. And this stuff was approved by the NHS whose employees were supposed to be looking after our health?

This is how the big brands get into the *minds* of the mums. The mothers use their products, which were recommended by a healthcare system that they think they can trust, in the first stages of the newborn's life and then they tend to keep buying them because they are the most popular brands and of course cheap. You must *always* trust the hospitals and the medical system, right?

All of this marketing and manipulation starts at day one. You also get given lots of free magazines which, again, advertise all the toxic products that are just so common in the shops. In one of the magazines I was given, there were only *two* things in the there that were safe: an organic baby towel and an organic mattress. This was better than nothing, of course, but it was still so shocking to realize that from day one of a newborn baby's life all of the personal care items that are recommended, from the clothing to the bottom wipes, were *all* toxic. And really, the *entire* magazine should have been full of healthy and safe things – it seems very wrong to me that no concern for toxicity is found in these magazines. But, by now, we *do* know why – it's because there is little to no regulation, and people are pretty much blinded to how severe a problem toxicity is to human health. Not enough people are speaking out about it.

Common problems such as nappy rash affect many babies, but the toxic baby wipes that are used often *do not* help keep it at bay – in fact I think they would probably make it *worse*. Most wipes contain very harsh ingredients and can dry and irritate the skin, as well as adding more toxins to the body. I sometimes had to use baby wipes when I did a photo shoot if I had to clean my makeup off. I was always horrified at how they made my skin feel, and when I looked at the packets, I could see that the formulas were almost entirely chemical-based.

Then there are the nappy rash creams which also contain toxic chemicals, so you get a double whammy each time you clean your baby's backside, and as any new mother knows, you may do that up to 12 times a day. And what is even worse is that you apply these products to the most *private* parts of a tiny baby's body. Nappies are also toxic too and made with plastics and dioxins.[153] It blows my mind that companies can make products like these and do not care that they contain poisonous ingredients. Many of these companies also have countless mums write to them or phone up about the reactions their babies have had to chemical-based products – but the media hardly ever report on just how many.

What about the mums who don't know better and continue to always use them? Well, that's just down to the evils of marketing and the very cheap price point. When people see advertisements on TV and remember that their place of care was telling them to use this or that, then of course most people are going to trust them! A hospital giving unhealthy advice? Surely not!

If you are planning to get or are pregnant, then it's highly important that you keep as many toxins out of your body, for they will affect your unborn child.

Developing embryos and fetuses are exquisitely sensitive to hormonal variations. Chemicals polluting a mother's body can cross the placenta, leaving the fetus exposed to chemicals in the mother's blood. For instance, bisphenol A (plastics) has been found in amniotic fluid, confirming passage through the placenta.[154]

I think most people assume that these big companies and our governments always do what is best for the people, especially in regards to children, but the lack of testing and ridiculous lack of regulations shows this is just *not* true. It's the same with doctors and the medical industry – most people automatically trust their doctors (which they *should* be able to, by the way) yet do people really know that they mostly just prescribe toxic drugs these days to cover up a symptom and do not actually *know* how to treat the root cause?

I get really concerned when I hear that people take their child to the doctor at the first sign of any illness and always walk away with prescribed drugs; then the child starts to get continuously sick as the drugs do not help with building a healthy immune function and if anything they *lower* it so that they are more likely to catch every other virus around them. And then they are not given *any* advice on how to counteract the drug's side effects, nor are they talked to about diet and nutrition.

In the highly recommended and very famous book, *How to Raise Healthy Kids in Spite of Your Doctor*, Robert S. Mendelssohn MD educates readers to try and *avoid* visiting the doctor's surgery by doing all you can at home first. This book is absolutely brilliant for giving mums (and dads) vital knowledge about signs and symptoms that are *normal* and can be treated easily, and the warning signs that *do* warrant a visit to the doctor or the ER. From his many years' experience as a pediatrician, Dr. Mendelssohn learned that far too many children were being piled with unnecessary medications which led to more problems in the future. He truly was a pioneer for children and natural health with minimal intervention.

In regards to safe skincare, thankfully, there are now many affordable products that really won't cost an arm and a leg at all. To give you an idea, I have mentioned a few good brands in the resource section at the back of the book which you can use instead. You can even find them at most chemists and some supermarkets these days. It's vital to use skincare that contains very simple and gentle ingredients. My personal favorite brand is the entire Weleda baby range. Every single product is nothing short of fantastic. I also love to use organic raw shea butter on Lola's skin as a moisturizer. It is simply fantastic and can be purchased in bulk sizes so it is long lasting and fairly inexpensive. Something the whole family can use.

Please remember: while it's *so important* for you to make sure you don't use toxic beauty products on yourself, it's even *more* so for children.

"An activist is someone who cannot help but fight for something. That person is not usually motivated by a need for power, or money, or fame, but in fact driven slightly mad by some injustice, some cruelty, some unfairness - so much so that he or she is compelled by some internal moral engine to act to make it better." Eve Ensler

Chapter 36

Vaccinations – The Hidden Dangers Posing Great Risks to the Health of Your Child

The Golden hopes of scientific medicine have, with some notable excep-
tions, failed to deliver the promise of a disease-free passage into an ever
youthful old-age. Nor have the hopes for high-tech conjugated vaccines
materialized, as the equivocal experiences with HiB, Men C and
Pneumococcus show. The killer infectious diseases of yesteryear have
been replaced with chronic ill-health. Over seventeen million adults in
Britain suffer from chronic diseases such as arthritis, diabetes and
asthma. Modern drugs, for all their benefit, are not the panacea either
when they directly cause one in seventeen of all admissions in this
country. In such a climate, doctors become disillusioned, patients desert
orthodox medicine for complementary therapies, and all the while
health costs soar astronomically. It is no wonder that governments are
desperate to cling to whatever apparent successes they have achieved.
Immunization seems to offer a solution at a modest price with central
budgetary and administrative control. Doctors who advise the
government on vaccination policies have often spent their whole careers
working with vaccines and immunization. It would be painful and
concerning for them to learn that their lives' work was of less value
than they had hoped.[155]
Dr. R. Halvorsen, *The Truth about Vaccines*

I will warn you right now: this chapter and its controversial subject
may be the most *difficult* one in my book for you to digest – as it was
for me when I first heard about this 'other side' to vaccination many
years ago. I was brought up in a medical family and I believed for a
very long that medicine was *always* good in every situation, and
especially that of vaccines. But when I saw such alarming and
compelling evidence, it caused me to question them, and before I

knew it this opened a very wide door into a *very* deep rabbit hole.

This chapter is going to be the longest one in my book because it *deserves* deep attention as the subject has so many concerns to discuss.

Most people have made up their minds about vaccinations *before* they have *really* looked at *all* of the information that is available to them and therefore they automatically think that vaccinations are *always* necessary for health, are very *safe,* that they always work, and that if you do not have them, then you are risking your life and others around you. And that you must be a highly unintelligent and 'irresponsible' person if you choose to not have your children vaccinated. People also tend to think that the unvaccinated kids will spread the disease, or are more likely to catch the disease and suffer terribly. They think that being unvaccinated is way more of a risk than suffering from the dangers of being vaccinated. That was certainly what I thought too and why would we not believe this? The media and our doctors have told us all of these things for years. Yet the problem is, vital imformation *is* being kept from the public and kept from the doctors.

The topic of vaccines is also the most highly emotive subject today; it can cause people to become extremely angry if anyone even *suggests* that what we originally thought about vaccination is perhaps very far from the truth. I remember the first time someone said to me that their 'childhood vaccinations caused them harm' and I couldn't help but think that the lady who told me must have been absolutely crazy. What a funny and ignorant thing to say, I thought. These *life-saving medicines* were supposedly harmful? How ridiculous!

But after continuing to hear more about this other side, something in me made me sit up and take more notice. *I wanted to learn why so many people thought this way.* There were just too many parents, doctors and scientists writing and speaking out about their concerns. And surely if there was nothing to worry about, that vaccines were so safe and so good - then *why* would anyone be concerned? Why are hundreds and thousands of parents opting out of having their children vaccinated? Are they all irresponsible and unintelligent?

I began to put my own view aside and soon realised I didn't actually know very much about them at all. I then allowed someone to show me some things about the history of vaccinations. I learnt the shocking fact that the disease eradication charts all over the world showed that the vaccines were *always* introduced *after* the disease started to decline naturally. I learnt that most doctors had never even seen these charts themselves, they just thought that they showed the opposite. I learnt about what sorts of chemicals were in the shots, how many vaccines these days children are supposed to get compared to when I was young, and that many of them are for diseases of no concern these days – which seemed totally pointless to me. I quickly discovered that they were risking *more* chances of developing an injury associated with the enormous amount of toxins being given to them via vaccinations. And I was also *very* concerned after reading about how many pharmaceutical companies make an enormous amount of money from these shots (billions!) and that *none* of them were ever tested for safety long term on humans (or at all).

Quite alarmingly, I was also completely shocked to know that there have *never* been any properly funded, *official* studies under-taken on the comparison between unvaccinated and vaccinated children to prove that a) vaccines do work, they do protect against these diseases and b) that having them makes children *healthier,* with a better immune system.

What was *another* big clincher for me that vaccines may in fact be far more dangerous than what we are told, was discovering that some of the most lucrative and famous pharmaceutical companies have been sued for *massive* misconduct and fraud when it came to the information and 'proof' that they provided in their *self-funded* studies. I felt pretty quickly that there were *far* too many concerns regarding this matter than could be ignored. And that a lot of time would need to be spent looking into all of this.

I know what you may be thinking: this all sounds totally nut bag *crazy*. It was hard for me not to immediately dismiss all of these things too, for how could any or all of this possibly be true? But as my own curiosity got the better of me I began to look much deeper into the issue. Many of the same subjects came up time after time again from people who researched from all different angles. There were so many books published on vaccine concerns, and none that I had ever seen on a doctor's book shelf. And there were also many documentaries that had been made which I started to view. I never saw any of these on mainstream TV channels. And the information I was reading and viewing was not from a 'dodgy' source; it was coming from *highly* acclaimed doctors and scientists – who, ironically, were highly acclaimed *before* they questioned these issues, but didn't always remain so *after* they voiced their concerns. When they tried to bring attention to the dangers surrounding these vaccinations, they received intense ridicule; many have since been threatened, some have lost their jobs, and some have even had their medical licenses completely removed, or had lucrative funding pulled from their proposed future studies into the safety of these vaccines.

Isn't *real* science supposed to be about *always* continuing to work on finding the proof and the truth to everything in this world, and *especially* in regards to the health of our children? If you were a vaccine maker, wouldn't you *want* to prove without any doubt that your vaccines are safe, effective and actually do indeed make children healthier? Wouldn't a properly conducted study showing these results, which would ensure people trusted your vaccine, be worth putting your money into?

If a vaccine company does *not* want to do this (to date, *zero* vaccine makers have come forward to say, 'Yes, let's prove once and for all that our vaccine does all of this'), then what does this make you think – knowing that out of all of the companies who make billions and billions of dollars each year from their vaccines, none of them have come forward to say, 'We believe in our product because we have 100% proof.'

The real problem is, they already *know* that most people automatically trust the entire medical world and therefore them - the vaccine makers, that they are producing safe and effective vaccinations.

When it comes to pharmaceutical vaccine and drug scandals, there have been *so* many. Just recently in 2012 GlaxoSmithKline (GSK) was sued for a whopping US $3 billion dollars for promoting drugs for unapproved uses, which resulted in deaths and suicides. Another case, also involving GSK, was brought to our attention by the Argentinian Federation of Health Professionals who reported that up to *14 children* died after receiving an experimental GSK vaccine called Synflorix.[156] What is tragic and equally disgusting about this case is that it's said GSK *'deliberately misled participants and pressured impoverished, disadvantaged families into enrolling their children in clinical trials of this experimental vaccine.'* GSK of course – surprise, surprise – denies the charges. And Merck are under investigation for vaccine fraud too (which we cover a little further on).

If I were to tell you about all the other cases involving scandals like this, it would take another huge book. And even if you knew all of the stories involving, quite often, young children who are forced to take toxic medications – and if they don't want to take them, they are *forced* to have them through tubes sewn into their stomachs – you probably wouldn't even believe me. You probably wouldn't even believe me that homeless people and the very poor are often used as guinea pigs to test drugs on. And that the people of Third World countries are often trialing new drugs, yet they aren't *told* before hand that they are. The least expensive way to do a trial is on real people, especially the poor ones, right? Honestly, the way these companies act makes me want to throw up, and because it's happening on a massive level, I feel even worse knowing just how many people are involved in using and harming others this way, just because of profits.

I also find it odd that most people (doctors included) realize that drug companies can be very unethical and say, 'Yes, we know that this drug was taken off the market' (for example the scandal involving the drug Vioxx which killed about *100,000* people and the drug Thalidomide which caused countless babies being born with severe birth defects), yet they mostly think that vaccines are *always* safe. And that anyone raising concerns is trying to discredit a 'sacred cow'- one we must hold up in high regards like that of a god. I find this way of thinking odd and illogical. When I discover a company or brand has done very unethical things, (and in the case of GSK what can be more unethical than committing fraud by harming and killing children) I wipe them, *completely.* I don't just stop using one of their products, I refuse to use any at all. How can I trust *any* part of their brand?

It seems vaccination has turned into a *'religious science'*, just like in many religions you can't question if God exists, and you can't question in the medical world if vaccines are safe or effective.

My main aim in this chapter is *not* to make your mind up for you, but to *encourage* you to start doing your *own* research, and to be very *careful* of where you get your information from. Many organizations are tied together financially (and especially the government/medical websites that most parents only stop to look at) so it's in their best interests to have you, the public, believe that vaccines are believed to be safe and are *essential* for health.

In this chapter you won't just hear what I think, you will read articles from doctors who have now publicly started questioning the lack of safety of these shots, their lack of effectiveness, their dangerous ingredients, and why they have now turned their back on the curent mainstream belief. You will also hear why parents have chosen not to vaccinate and sadly you will also read the heart-wrenching cases of parents who did vaccinate their children, without being *fully informed*, and what has now happened to their kids, after the vaccines injured them.

Before we go any further, it's also quite important to keep remembering who has the most to gain *financially* out of the public believing that vaccines are safe and effective. Is it the people who are trying to bring attention to the public regarding the dangers of vaccines? Is it the doctors that lose their jobs after they have got proof that these vaccines were harming children? Is it the scientists who undertook a study and found alarming results implicating that a chemical used in vaccines is deadly to humans and may cause cancer? Are these people making billions of dollars each year and are they all making this stuff up purely for financial gain? No, of course not.

It is the *pharmaceutical* companies who sell these vaccines, the *doctors* who receive financial bonuses on how many people they vaccinate, the *governments* who make deals with pharmaceutical companies and the charities like the Bill and Melinda Gates Foundation who get big tax deductions for creating a 'generous' vaccination scheme in poor countries like Africa. Yet these charities won't invest the same sort of money for providing food, clean sanitation and other more necessary things for these people. They just invest in giving them vaccines. And as you wil see further on, the Bill and Melinda Gates Foundation also test new vaccines on these poor children without giving them *all* of the information, the risks, the fact that it may be a new vaccine and that their children are being tested on – this is *highly* unethical and evil.

In regards to *any* company listed on the stock exchange – it's important to know that they owe their *shareholders* the promise to always strive for *more* profit. Which means if something *really* big jepordises this, (and questioning how safe a drug is is pretty big) then their *entire* company could fall apart. So it's very easy to understand that throughout history when things like smoking were questioned, they did *whatever* they could to have the public believe for as *long* as they could that there was no harm being done. Until of course, they could deny it no longer. It's very hard to believe that not that long ago, smoking was declared as *'healthy'* by the Government, and encouraged to do by the doctors who promoted them and of course by the tobacco companies. We need to see that these blatant lies, are still *very* much a huge part of how our society operates today.

The Graphs Tell The Real Truth

A very easy way to see for yourself if vaccines are truly *the* miracle on planet earth and for all of humankind is to check some graphs which have collated information and statistics about when a disease started causing deaths, when it increased, when it declined and when the vaccine was *introduced* for that disease.[157] It's plain and quite shocking to see that the diseases were decreasing on their *own*, quite a few years *before* the vaccines were introduced. Yet when you say this to a doctor, they just wont believe it themselves, yet they have not seen the actual graphs. Author Jock Doubleday of the vaccination book, *"Into The Labyrinth'* shares his experience:

I have talked to many doctors about these raw, unaltered numbers and the charts based on them. None of them have seen these numbers. None of them have seen the charts based on them. When I email them the graphs, they say, 'These numbers must be wrong.' Doctors who willingly admit that we have no long-term studies on vaccination are absolutely unyielding on the issue of epidemiology. And understandably so. They have been taught – they have had it drilled into them – that the history of modern civilization is the history of the triumph of artificially induced immunity.

So they are put into a corner, and they come out fighting: 'These charts are wrong! The numbers they're based on must be wrong!' But the numbers are not wrong. These are the only numbers we have. They are the government numbers – raw data from many different governments.[158]

You will have to make a decision one day – be informed now

While some of you reading this may not have kids right now, you probably will in the future. And if you do have kids, then it's *very* important you really know the real risks and hidden dangers of this subject. If you decide you don't want to vaccinate but your husband or partner does, then you may end up in court with your child being forced to have these injections that you know are highly likely to be dangerous. It's imporant you are armed with the right information

Later on in this chapter, I also share valuable information on how to reduce the risks of vaccine damage if you do still decide to vaccinate, or feel pressured to in the future.

We are now going pretty deep into this subject and I ask you now to have an open mind, to think logically, and to also think about how the human body has been designed – and that is, when it is fed well, is brought up in a clean and sanitary environment, has regular exercise and healthy sun exposure, then it is meant to be able to look after *itself*, to fight viruses and to not suffer from disease.

Logic kicked in very early for me, during my investigation – that due to the overwhelming evidence, that children are being born *already* toxic with traces of highly poisonous industrial chemicals, it really made sense to me that we must try to help them *avoid* other ways of absorbing toxins as much as possible, and not to purposely give them large amounts of others. So much sickness and disease is occurring because of *accumulation* of dangerous toxins. And this evidence comes from all different types of exposure. Overwhelming research already pointed to the fact that there was great harm being caused, simply by putting products on our skin, eating toxic foods and breathing in fumes from our home and from outside. I couldn't therefore imagine that it would be OK to be injected with industrial toxins – whatever the amount. Yet, our vaccines I discovered, actually contained far *worse* things – and this was the real clincher: they had *never* been adequately tested for safety, or over a long period of time. If I was going to give *more* chemicals to my child, I would at least want to know without a doubt that they were proven to be 100% safe. Does my, or your child for that matter, deserve anything less?

And what could these concerns mean for our children's health as a society?

As previously mentioned, we know that our babies are being

born with approximately 200 different chemicals inside their tiny precious bodies, including heavy metals, which are quite possibly going to wreak havoc in the near future or later in life.

Surely, I thought, if we want our children to thrive throughout their formative years and to avoid developing many of the now far too common autoimmune disorders/diseases later on in life, we must encourage their immune systems to develop in the way that Nature intended, and not force them to have to deal with, at times, *many* viruses at once? Children today can quite often get injected with between *5 and 9 different viruses* in one day. This to me was *nuts*. And not at all natural – no one ever catches a whole bunch of viruses at once. *If the medical community thinks that the human body is so strong and indestructible that it can handle having up to 9 viruses suddenly being forced into a child's body, then why does it think this marvelous body can't handle dealing with one virus that the person catches naturally?*

Of course, a healthy body will respond better to dealing with viruses, but that's the point here: how can we make a body healthy by injecting it with known *neurotoxins* and *cancer-causing agents*?

After starting to look into this subject further, it almost became an instant obsession of mine. One disturbing fact led me to another, and still does, to this day. More and more information is coming out, from studies that have shown disturbing results that vaccines have actually *spread* the disease amongst highly vaccinated groups of children, caused paralysis among many victims due to a new vaccine which clearly did not go through enough testing, and caused a large number of infant deaths, (not only in the preliminary studies, but also in the public) which are rarely reported by the mainstream media, nor have they reported on the countless miscarriages linked to them and that vaccines may be the cause of triggering many cancers and autoimmune disorders.

It's *impossible* for me to tell you everything that I have discovered because it comes from reading detailed books, viewing documentaries, and spending hours perusing articles and finding recent and old studies. It takes a *lot* of time to really look into this and to come to a conclusion such as this. Sadly, what I have found is that the parents who have now got vaccine-injured children did not do any research of their own, before their poor child became so damaged. Their biggest regret now, and one that racks them with guilt, is that they did not look outside the information they were being told by the medical world and government bodies. Two powerful organizations which are always tied together. And two that will never admit there may be a problem with a vaccination or, if they do, it may take years and only when *many* children/people are injured by a certain brand of vaccine. Only then will it be taken off the market and quickly replaced with something else. There are no further discussions on what was in the vaccine that made these people sick. They just assume that it was a bad 'batch'.

Pharmaceutical companies have also done some very disgusting things with vaccinations that were once deemed as safe, yet caused great harm among people (men, women and children included), pressuring these companies to take them off the schedule in certain countries, only to send them to other countries and pass them off as safe. Yes, this is very true. Take for example an MMR vaccine which was used continuously in several countries at different times, and under different names. In Canada it was called Trivirix which was produced by the notourisly unethical GlaxoSmithKline (known at that time as Smith Kline Beecham) pharmaceutical company – as we have seen previously, they are well known for doing such unethical things.

In 1988, after seeing that Trivirix was causing many cases of aseptic meningitis among some children, Canada withdrew the licenses and took it off the North American market. Yet in the very *same* year, the UK JCVI (Joint Committee on Vaccination and Immunization) went right ahead and introduced the *same* proven-to-be-dangerous vaccine, yet *renamed* it (to Pluserix and Immravax) and *added* it right into the UK vaccine schedule.[159] As soon as it was introduced to the UK and given to children, quite a few kids developed... guess what! The *same* reactions to this MMR shot which caused aseptic meningitis among Canadian kids were now happening to UK children. Surprise, surprise! After four years, it was eventually banned here in 1992. Thank goodness! OK! Problem solved, right? Um… unfortunately, no. You would think by now that this awful situation which had happened in two different countries would mean that this brand of vaccine would be thrown straight into the bin, incinerated never to see again the light of day, or never again to hurt the lives of small children. Here is where you might want to put down a drink if you have one in your hand.

Nope, these *same* dangerous vaccines were shipped right off to Brazil. Why? Simple. There is far too much money at stake to just throw away these vaccines which were worth billions of dollars to the pharmaceutical companies which make lucrative deals with governments and also with institutions like the NHS. They just can't throw away billions of dollars.

Unfortunately this true story is, tragically, not one that is by any means rare. Even the organizations that are meant to protect us have been involved in many scandals surrounding vaccines and quite a few are coming to light recently.

Are we being told everything we should be told about vaccines?

Most of the people in the USA will do whatever they are told. We are encouraged not to think for ourselves. We are programmed to place blind faith in our physician and the Medical Establishment. We are taught not to ask questions. The sad fact is that most Americans simply believe in vaccinations, although it is likely that they have no idea what is in them. Decades of studies published in the world's leading medical journals have documented serious adverse effects from vaccinations, including death.

Dozens of books written by doctors and researchers have revealed serious flaws in immunization practice and theory. Yet, incredibly, most pediatricians and parents are unaware of these findings. Believe it or not, most pediatricians don't even know what's in the vaccinations they are administering. Don't believe me? Just ask them ... and be prepared to see a perplexed look on their face ... right before they get mad at you for daring to ask questions or threaten you if you don't submit to their policy of mandatory vaccinations![160]

Ty Bollinger, author of *Cancer – Step Outside the Box*

One of the main problems with regards to vaccinations is the subject of *informed consent*. Are we being told anywhere near enough about the risks by our doctors, before our children (or we ourselves) get vaccinated? Are we being told about the types of ingredients in them, and what they can do to some babies, children and adults? The answer, it seems, 99% of the time is, *no*. Parents are simply *not* being told about the real risks from vaccinations; if anything they are being downplayed because the *doctors* themselves are *not* educated about the real risks or ever see the full scope of injuries which are occurring due to only 10% of vaccination problems ever being reported. The FDA have even stated this themselves. So that means that the duty of care which doctors are actually obliged to follow, which is to give all patients *informed consent*, is just *not* happening. And no one in power above them is making sure they give this informed consent. So we can't always blame the doctors, they only do what they get told, and if they aren't told, then they aren't going to be telling you about it.

In the UK a scandal involving government experts covering up vaccine hazards was reported by Lucija Tomlijenovic:

Here I present the documentation which appears to show that the JCVI (Joint Committee on Vaccination and Immunization) made continuous efforts to withhold critical data on severe adverse reactions and contraindications to vaccinations to both parents and health practitioners in order to reach overall vaccination rates which they deemed were necessary for 'herd immunity', a concept which with regards to vaccination, and contrary to prevalent beliefs, does not rest on solid scientific evidence as will be explained.

As a result of such vaccination policy promoted by the JCVI and the DH, many children have been vaccinated without their parents being disclosed the critical information about demonstrated risks of serious adverse reactions, one that the JCVI appeared to have been fully aware of. It would also appear that, by withholding this information, the JCVI/DH neglected the right of individuals to make an informed consent concerning vaccination. By doing so, the JCVI/DH may have violated not only International Guidelines for Medical Ethics (i.e. Helsinki Declaration and the International Code of Medical Ethics) but also, their own Code of Practice.

The transcripts of the JCVI meetings also show that some of the Committee members had extensive ties to pharmaceutical companies and that the JCVI frequently co-operated with vaccine manufacturers on strategies aimed at boosting vaccine uptake. Some of the meetings at which such controversial items were discussed were not intended to be publicly available, as the transcripts were only released later, through the Freedom of Information Act (FOI). These particular meetings are denoted in the transcripts as 'commercial in confidence', and reveal a clear and disturbing lack of transparency, as some of the information was removed from the text (i.e. the names of the participants) prior to transcript release under the FOI section at the JCVI website (for example, JCVI CSM/DH (Committee on the Safety of Medicines/Department of Health) Joint Committee on Adverse Reactions Minutes 1986–1992).[161]

Truly disturbing isn't it? The financial ties these organizations have to each other are not at all new. We all know that governments receive donations from big and powerful companies so that the government will do what the company wants them to do (which means usually protecting them from being sued, allowing them to label things however they like and letting them self-regulate). It happens in the food industry too, and in regards to the drug industry, *it* pays the government the *most* amount of money out of *all* the other industries to these politician's campaigns. In 2012, just in the one year, the pharmaceutical industry paid as a whole *US $69.6 million dollars* lobbying in the first 3 months.[162] This factor alone is one that I think *should* make parents sit up and take note of what the vaccination industry really benefits from the most.

In the USA, and it's said also here in the UK, pediatricians and GPs make quite a bit of extra money from giving vaccinations. They receive incentives from the pharmaceutical companies, if they reach their 'targets'. According to Dr. Robert Sears, it happens more than anyone would think:

I recently talked with two physicians in different states that told me the HMO plans that they contract with do chart reviews and patient surveys at the end of each year. If their office scores high enough on these reviews, the HMO plan gives them a several thousand dollar bonus. This bonus varies depending on the number of patients the doctor sees. One of the requirements for a patient's chart to pass the test is that they are fully vaccinated... So, why not give their doctors a bonus for meeting this goal?

Here's why. This policy gives any doctor who contracts with such HMO plans an incentive to NOT want any unvaccinating families in their practice. Maybe a few such families wouldn't make them fail the chart reviews, but if they have too many, there goes their year-end bonus.

I've always wondered why so many doctors are so adamantly hardcore about demanding all their patients fully vaccinate, and why they kick patients out of their office who refuse. I'd always just assumed it was because the doctors felt that the vaccine protection was so important that they don't want any children to be at risk, so they draw a line in the sand for the good of the child (in their minds). BUT some doctors, especially those large groups who rely heavily on large HMO contracts, may actually be doing this because of money. Do they have the right to do so? Of course. But is it right? I don't know. The American Academy of Pediatrics Committee on Bioethics makes it very clear that the official AAP policy is that doctors NOT kick patients out of their office over this issue. But when money talks, some people don't listen... I thought you'd find it interesting to know why you might be having a hard time finding a vaccine-friendly doctor.[163]

I don't know about you, but I find it *very* disturbing knowing that my doctor would make extra money by vaccinating my child so that he meets his 'quota'. Doesn't this mean that money goes higher in his priorities than the safety of my child?

I know, I am not a doctor, but I have, however, read many studies and articles and countless books that were written *by* doctors, who know how to research and check the studies for accuracy and more importantly, for *ethical* conduct. And there aren't just GPs speaking about this issue; there are doctors from all areas of medicine such as neurologists, nephrologists, immunologists, who are all *very* concerned and desperately trying to educate people about what they have come to know.

Taking the emotion away, no matter what your belief in vaccination is, these shots do *add more* toxic chemicals to the child's (or anyone's for that matter) body. These so-called (by the doctors) 'insignificant' amounts will and *do* accumulate in the body, especially when it's already being bombarded with other toxins through the different pathways, and if the body is receiving lots of medications that add even more toxins and are not helpful to the development of the immune system, then perhaps you can see why alarm bells are ringing for so many people.

Mercury, which is otherwise known as Thimerosal, is known for being the *most* toxic ingredient (as we know from Chapter 3, mercury is a neurotoxin and classed as one of the most dangerous substances on earth) – but each shot contains *many* other chemicals – the common ones of which are listed later on in this chapter. Aluminum seems to be the second most dangerous chemical and, as you know already, is linked to neurological disorders such as Alzheimer's disease and, as you will soon discover, has higher than legally safe levels of the chemical in each shot. Vaccines simply *cannot* be made safely and have to contain toxic additives for them to stabilize and preserve the virus.

And now that the vaccine schedule is increasing every few years, the more shots that are injected, this means the more likely the child's immune system is going to become compromised much sooner, resulting in even more injuries, because it now has to deal with all of the additives and preservatives that are used in the shots. Back in 1984, there were 10 different vaccines given to children. In 2010, there were currently between 36 and 38 vaccines recommended, with most parents giving their child all of the ones that are suggested, despite the fact that some of the diseases have actually long been declared eradicated and are not a threat today.[164]

There are many more vaccines in the pipeline and we have to ask ourselves, where do we draw the line?

Many of these vaccines are not single vaccines either but can be a '5 in 1', which means that it's carrying 5 different viruses – this is a lot for a delicate immune system to deal with in one day. It's interesting, and important to note, that when a disease is caught naturally, you will never ever encounter 5 viruses at once. So why would the body be able to handle having 5 *injected* into the bloodstream?

Thimerosal is said to have been removed from the majority of vaccines so many parents think that this means they don't have to worry about the mercury problem anymore. Yet *most flu shots contain mercury*, and flu shots are recommended for children to have each year, and from the age of 6 months. So this problem, which most of us might think has gone away, is still right there, and in fact *far worse* because these shots are recommended to be given each *year*.[165]

Young children are recommended now to have many shots, given quite close together, starting at much younger ages than ever previously given, and some will even be given quite a few on the same day. I have read that sometimes a child will have 9 *shots* in one day. I have also discovered that countless children over the years have died just *hours* later, after developing a bad reaction to this massive assault on their immune system from all of the chemicals [166]. And why is this surprising when you know what's in the shots and what these ingredients have actually been proven to do to the brain and body?

When you break down what is in these shots and add up the amounts of heavy metals together and what the FDA states is 'safe', it will truly shock you that these vaccines are still allowed and marketed as necessary and completely safe. For example, take aluminum – this proven dangerous heavy metal is used in vaccines as a preservative. The FDA states that a toddler can have up to 63.8 mcg of it in their bodies and this is a 'safe level'. But if you were to give your 6-month-old child (who is a lot younger and lighter in body weight than a toddler) say 5 shots in one day (which is quite common if your child has been sick and needs to 'catch up' with the schedule) and you added up the aluminum in all of those shots, it would come to an amount *far greater* (some say *1000 times greater!*) than that safe level which was recommended by the FDA – whose job it is to approve medicines for the safety of the public's use. If you need to, please go back to Chapter 3 and have a read about aluminum again and see what it does to the brain. If not, the below information will put it all into presepective for you. Dr Russell Blaylock, Neurosurgeon writes:

> The amount of aluminum in vaccines is tremendous, especially in such vaccines as the anthrax vaccine, hepatitis vaccine and tetanus vaccine. Since many American children are being exposed to multiple doses of aluminum-containing vaccines by the time they are 6 years old, one would expect very high exposures to

injected aluminum. A recent study by Lucija Tomljenovik and Chris Shaw found that a newborn receives a dose of aluminum that exceeds FDA safety limits (5mg/kg/day) for injected aluminum by 20-fold, and at 6 months of age a dose that was 50-fold higher than FDA safety limits. Aluminum at this young age will accumulate in various tissues and, with new vaccine recommendations, children and young adults may be exposed to many more aluminum-containing vaccines every year throughout life. With the ability of aluminum to displace iron from its protective proteins, we may not only see a dramatic increase in breast cancer, but also other iron-related diseases, such as liver degeneration, neurodegenerative disease, diabetes, heart failure and atherosclerosis. No one is addressing this very real danger.[167]

Below is a list of the common vaccines and their amounts of aluminum given to most newborns and small children.

- Hib (PedVaxHib brand only) – 225 micrograms
- Hepatitis B – 250 micrograms
- DTaP – depending on the manufacturer, ranges from 170 to 625 micrograms
- Pneumococcus – 125 micrograms
- Hepatitis A – 250 micrograms
- HPV – 225 micrograms
- Pentacel (DTaP, HIB and Polio combo vaccine) – 330 micrograms
- Pediarix (DTaP, Hep B and Polio combo vaccine) – 850 micrograms

(List sourced from askdrsears.com)

If you have vaccinated your children, or are still considering it, have a look at the recommended schedule (or check the book where you have recorded what your child has already received), use this list and add up what types of vaccines your child had on one day where several vaccines or even just a single was given. Now, have a think about what you just read in the previous paragraph regarding what the FDA states is a *safe* daily limit for a toddler (*hint: 63.8mcg*). Read the total of what you have added up and try to think reasonably about how this should be OK for your tiny child's body.

OK, is your mouth hanging open? I hope it is – it darn well *should* be! Here we have the FDA stating the 'daily safe level' of a single heavy metal (and we aren't even talking about the *other* dangerous chemicals in them and what the FDA's safe level is for them) yet there is no *regulation* on the amount of heavy metals from vaccines that a child can have in *one* day. The FDA are talking about aluminum which is ingested through food, by the way. They haven't released any 'safe' levels for injected aluminum. Isn't it *far* more dangerous to have it injected into the body? Dr Robert Sears of the The Vaccine Book writes:

> As a medical doctor, my first instinct is to worry that these aluminum levels far exceed what may be safe for young babies. But then my second instinct is to assume that this issue has been researched and that studies have been done on healthy infants to determine their ability to excrete aluminum rapidly. My third instinct is to go looking for these studies, and so far I have not been able to find any. It is likely that the FDA feels the kidneys of healthy infants work well enough to excrete this aluminum rapidly before it can circulate through the body, accumulate in the brain, and cause toxic effects. However, I can't find any references in the FDA documents that show that using aluminum in vaccines has been tested in human infants and found to be safe.[168]

With what we know about toxins such as aluminum, how can we expect a tiny baby (who may not weigh more than a few kilograms) to cope with all of this toxicity, and the *other* hundreds of chemicals it already has in its body since birth? How does this make sense that it makes someone healthy long term? Does it not add to the logic that it could be why so many children suffer with health concerns that weren't even an issue 50 years ago?

We only need to look at the rate of autism these days; it's absolutely skyrocketing and is increasing dramatically each year. Mainstream science does not want to officially link it to vaccines, but from what I have seen, and more importantly from the mothers of autistic children I have spoken to, it's only a matter of time before they simply *cannot* deny the link any longer. With more vaccines being pushed onto children, there will be far more injuries that cannot be hidden.

Here is a list of the most *common* ingredients in vaccines, and yes, these are all true!

- aluminum hydroxide
- aluminum phosphate
- ammonium sulfate
- amphotericin B
- animal tissues: pig blood, horse blood, rabbit brain, dog kidney, monkey kidney, chick embryo, chicken egg, duck egg
- calf (bovine) serum
- betapropiolactone
- fetal bovine serum
- formaldehyde
- formalin
- gelatin
- glycerol
- human diploid cells (originating from human aborted fetal tissue)
- hydrolyzed gelatin
- monosodium glutamate (MSG)
- neomycin
- neomycin sulfate
- phenol red indicator

- phenoxyethanol (antifreeze)
- potassium diphosphate
- potassium monophosphate
- polymyxin B
- polysorbates 20
- polysorbates 80
- porcine (pig) pancreatic hydrolysate of casein
- residual MRC5 proteins
- sorbitol
- sucrose
- thimerosal (mercury)
- tri(n)butyl phosphate,
- VERO cells, a continuous line of monkey kidney cells
- washed sheep red blood cells

(List sourced from mercola.com [169])

These ingredients are so alarming that, quite often, most people think it's a joke when they hear what's in these shots. Monkey kidney cells? Aborted fetal tissue? Animal by-products? Anti-freeze? Formaldehyde? Am I serious? Yep – these are *all* in there and floating around your body if you have had shots and floating around inside your child's if they have had any vaccines. And the more a child has, the *higher* the levels will be and the more likely they won't be a truly healthy child long term.

Here are some more disturbing facts about vaccines

- Most vaccines go virtually untested and success rates are based strictly on results from testing animals in a laboratory.
- Many vaccines contain Thimerosal, a preservative made with methyl mercury, which is extremely toxic to the central nervous system.
- Many vaccines contain chemical adjuvants, like squalene, and aluminum which cause inflammation of the central nervous

system.

- Autism is a neurological disorder. Vaccine ingredients break down peptides in the body which regulate the CNS, severely disrupting specific high cognitive functions and processes all characteristic of autism.
- Rates of autism have doubled in the past decade.
- More than 1 in every 60 children in the US are diagnosed with autism, which is the highest rate of any population in all of history.
- H1N1 vaccine greatly enhanced health risks for the elderly, children, and those with heart disease, breathing issues and diabetes.
- The main group of scientists who convinced the World Health Organization to declare the H1N1 a 'pandemic' had financial ties to the drug companies that profited.
- Australia banned flu vaccines in children after reports of seizures, and Finland banned H1N1 vaccines after linking them to narcolepsy in children.
- Injecting genetically modified bacteria and viruses runs the risk of causing a cytokine storm in the body, which is an exaggerated immune system response to a highly pathogenic invader. When a cytokine storm occurs in the lungs, fluids and immune cells accumulate and eventually block off the airways, often resulting in death.

(Sourced from '25 Amazing (and Disturbing) Facts about the Hidden History of Medicine' – Natural News.com)

Most people think vaccines did not harm them, so they are OK for their kids

In the 1930s the average child only received three vaccines in their young life. Many vaccines are added to the schedule over the years, with an increase in the 1980s and with three vaccines added to the schedule in 1991 alone. The current vaccine schedule calls for 31 vaccines in the first 18 months of life, 48 with full flu vaccination (occurring every year) by 72 months of life.

Many say, 'I had all of my shots when I was young and I am fine' – especially people in their 50s quite often say this to me. Yet they *don't* look fine to me; most of the time they are overweight, are super-tired, have bags under their eyes (sign of kidney trouble), have regular colds and flus, and will more than likely get cancer or something pretty bad at some stage, proving that they are not 'so healthy' after all. I always try and point out that when they were young, there were only a small amount of vaccines that had been developed and were given routinely – even less than the 10 that were on offer back in 1983 when I was young. Nowadays that amount has *tripled* with more vaccines being invented every year. I try and explain that the heavy metals and toxic chemical exposure that the adult had faced years ago when they were young was far, far less than what our young children are being exposed to today, and guess what? Children's health today, and the rate of autism, is *way* worse than it was ever years ago! But it's very difficult to get most people to think, 'Oh, this sounds alarming – I might go and look into it.' All that they do usually is say, 'Well, the doctors and government say that we have to do it and I trust them.'

In regards to autism, it is a *neurological* disorder, and heavy metals and chemicals affect the *neurological* function of the brain. I really think if people stopped and had a think about this very fact, and used a logical mind, they would realize that the amount of vaccines given today is of *huge* concern. If a child already has a neurological disorder, please don't give them any more chemicals that may cause them more neurological damage. Your GPs and pediatricians are *not* experts in the field of toxicity. Why are we allowing them to inject our children with ingredients they don't know much about?

Some things carry warnings: why don't vaccines, or *do* they?

When someone buys a pack of cigarettes, it is required by law to have a warning on it e.g. 'Smoking can harm your baby,' or 'Warning: smoking kills', so why do we not have warnings on vaccinations? Actually we *do* have warnings, but they are on the vaccine insert inside the pack, which a parent *never* gets shown *before* a vaccine is given to their child. It's only after an injury occurs that parents take the time to find out what was in that shot that harmed their child... And when they read it, they are absolutely horrified. It is clearly written in every insert, the reported side effects -what these shots *have* done in the studies, and therefore what it *can* do to your child.

You know, we can't always blame the doctors; they are not evil people here – they genuinely believe that vaccinations are essential for all of us to avoid getting ill, particularly our small children. They are not wanting to make us sick on purpose; they genuinely worry that we will all catch disease if we are not vaccinated. One of the reasons they do feel so strongly about vaccination is that when they go through medical school, they see videos of the *worst possible cases* of diseases, which *are* truly very shocking – I have seen a few of them myself. It's not at all pretty Because of what they have witnessed, they then believe that if anyone catches the disease, they will get it in the worst possible way like they saw on the video and perhaps die. Indeed, little babies who have caught whooping cough do look absolutely awful – it is very frightening to see, and of course, no one wants to see an innocent baby sick like this. Some doctors also see real cases in hospital of very sickly babies catching something that they feel would have been avoided by vaccination.

Yet what we must realize is, diseases are only severe, if an immune system is *weak*, and as we have seen with the studies already done on particular chemicals, they can't possibly improve someone's immune system. A toxin is a poison. Back in our grandmothers' era, measles was so common and most healthy kids caught it and were able to get through it easily. The people who did succumb to measles were sickly in general beforehand. It's like the flu – some people who are fit and have strong immune systems will suffer from a very mild case, and it will not harm them at all, and if anything will make their immune systems naturally stronger so that next time that particular virus comes into contact with them they will not recognize it as a new one. But for some, and this is *key* here, who already have a very *weak* immune system, that flu virus may cause them much greater harm, and in some instances they *will* die. Elderly people who have many other health problems may be in a very fragile state and recent contact with the flu virus may be what it takes to finally end their lives. It's the same for children with a poor immune system; they are more than likely to catch a disease or virus because their own health is not strong enough to fight it. Sadly, it's these immune-compromised children that are always targeted the most by vaccine schedules. When looking at the issue of vaccination logically, do we really think that by giving someone who already has a weakened immune system (or one that is not yet fully developed, like that of babies and small children) injections of toxic ingredients which have been shown to *directly* affect, in a negative way, brain function and immune function, that these shots will make an immune system stronger? The answer is NO; it *cannot* possibly do that.

If people are scared of getting a virus or catching a disease, then they must make their own immune system naturally strong, through diet and lifestyle changes, not through toxic drugs.

Which one makes more sense to you? Yet which makes more *money* for powerful organisations?

Vaccinated people spread the disease itself through the 'shedding' process

While many parents feel safe knowing that their child has been vaccinated, they do not get told that their child is now actually able to *spread* the virus that they were injected with, in particular around the first 6 weeks after vaccination. Shocking, yes, but makes sense really, doesn't it? Just like catching measles naturally is contagious, and certain people will catch it from a child, so too is it able to be contagious when it's injected into the body, and probably more so because it hasn't actually been caught naturally.

I will give you an example. In India, despite the government hailing the programs as a complete success for wiping out polio, the use of the OPV (Oral Polio Vaccine), which was given to millions of children through mass immunization programs, has actually left hundreds of thousands of children paralyzed *with* polio - because of the *vaccine* itself. This means that the virus given to them did not react mildly; in fact, it 'took over' the child's body and made them very sick and/or severely damaged and gave them the virus in a very virulent form. And in a country like India, where poverty and poor hygiene prevails, it makes sense that their little bodies were not able to treat the virus in the way that we get taught vaccines should behave.

It was hoped that following polio eradication, immunization could be stopped. However the synthesis of polio virus in 2002 made eradication impossible. It is argued that getting poor countries to expend their scarce resources on an impossible dream over the last 10 years was unethical. Furthermore, while India has been polio-free for a year, there has been a huge increase in non-polio acute flaccid paralysis (NPAFP). In 2011, there were an extra 47,500 new cases of NPAFP. Clinically indistinguishable from polio paralysis but twice as deadly, the incidence of NPAFP was directly proportional to doses of oral polio received. Though this data was collected within the polio surveillance system, it was not investigated. The principle of primum-non-nocere was violated. The authors suggest that the huge bill of US$ 8 billion spent on the program is a small sum to pay if the world learns to be wary of such vertical programs in the future.[170]

In the case of the polio vaccine shedding, it is not the only vaccine to have done this; studies are showing that *all* vaccines are capable of causing the disease to spread, and not just to what you would think is in the unvaccinated public, but the outbreaks are actually occurring in *highly* vaccinated areas:

In 1984, the Morbidity and Mortality Weekly Report (MMRW) of the CDC reported a late 1983 early 1984 Illinois high school/junior high measles outbreak. The total student population was around 400, and ALL of them (100%) had complied with Illinois State Law requiring the complete MMR schedule.[171]

And here are more cases:*

- In 1871–2, England, with 98 percent of the population aged between 2 and 50 vaccinated against smallpox, experienced its worst ever smallpox outbreak with 45,000 deaths. During the same period in Germany, with a vaccination rate of 96 percent, there were over 125,000 deaths from smallpox. (*The Hadwen Documents*)

- In Germany, compulsory mass vaccination against diphtheria commenced in 1940 and by 1945 diphtheria cases were up from 40,000 to 250,000. (Hannah Allen, *Don't Get Stuck*)

- In the USA in 1960, two virologists discovered that both polio vaccines were contaminated with the SV40 virus which causes cancer in animals as well as changes in human cell tissue cultures. Millions of children had been injected with these vaccines. (*Med. Jnl of Australia* 17/3/1973, p555)

- In 1967, Ghana was declared measles free by the World Health Organization after 96 percent of its population was vaccinated. In 1972, Ghana experienced one of its worst measles outbreaks with its highest ever mortality rate. (Dr. H. Albonico, MMR Vaccine Campaign in Switzerland, March 1990)

- (http://www.naturalnews.com/027203_Chi_vaccination_va ccine.html)

* Natural News.com

According to Christina England:

> On December 20, 2012, a vaccination tragedy hit the small village of Gouro, located in northern Chad, Africa. According to the newspaper *La Voix*, out of five hundred children who received the new meningitis vaccine MenAfriVac, at least 40 of them between the ages of 7 and 18 have become paralyzed. Those children also suffered hallucinations and convulsions. Since this report, the true extent of this tragedy is coming to light, as parents of these vaccinated children have reported yet more injuries. The authorities in the area are shaken, as citizens set fire to a sanitary administration vehicle in a demonstration of their frustration and anger at the government's negligence. 'We wish that our children would get their health back,' shared the parent of a sick child.

And Christina continues:

> Mr. M., the cousin of two of the vaccine-injured children, who currently remain critically ill and hospitalized, explained that many of the children reacted within 24 hours of receiving the vaccine. He said that at first the children vomited and complained of headaches, before falling to the floor with uncontrollable convulsions while bent over with saliva coming from their mouths. He shared that on December 26, 2012, the Minister of Health and the Minister of Social Security visited Gouro, bringing with them two Members of Parliament. He said that after some discussion, they decided to evacuate approximately 50 paralyzed children to a hospital over three hundred miles away in N'Djamena, the capital city of Chad. He added that the government responded to the tragedy by paying the parents money in a desperate bid to silence them, further stating that many of the parents are traumatized and confused.[172]

How absolutely *disgusting* that these parents were paid off to keep their mouths shut! Where was the proof this vaccine was previously tested for safety? Oh wait, that's exactly what this *was* – using these poor African people as guinea pigs for a vaccine that was hoped to have been used in other countries. But after what I have shared with you before, chances are this vaccine may end up in some other country anyway.

Even though many people and children will *appear* to not have any health problems associated with vaccinations, we cannot possibly rule out that they are not being harmed *long term* as no studies have been ever conducted to test this theory out. It is said that chronic fatigue and MS and many other auto-immune problems are caused by the aluminum in vaccinations.[173]

What if you do vaccinate and your child dies? Will YOU be to blame?

Here is where the rabbit hole goes even deeper. The following story is something parents rarely consider in relation to childhood vaccines: Lorraine Allen was accused of murdering her baby in 1998. Lorraine gave birth to a healthy baby boy whom she named Patrick. At four months of age, Patrick died, two days after his third set of vaccinations. Within hours Patrick had started having the sniffles and by 11 pm that night he seemed to have a lot of trouble breathing. Lorraine knew something was wrong so phoned her doctor who came around, checked the baby and said that he was 'fine'. Patrick was put to bed and then checked on one hour later after the doctor had left. He was limp and floppy and clearly not 'fine'. Lorraine called an ambulance and her son was taken to hospital. Poor Patrick died the next day, but this terrible ordeal had really just begun for Lorraine.

Because Patrick had bleeding behind the eyes, and blood was found over the surface of his brain, the doctors began to think this was a case of 'shaken baby syndrome', for they could not make the connection that some of the ingredients in the vaccine actually caused the hemorrhaging. Lorraine was arrested and charged with Patrick's murder, and from 2000 spent five years in jail. Even more tragic is that while in jail, Lorraine gave birth to another boy, Joshua, who was quickly taken away from her and put into care. In 2005 her sentence was ended after medical experts doubted that Patrick's death was indeed a genuine case of shaken baby syndrome. Twelve years after this ordeal, Lorraine is taking her case and requesting compensation for the loss of her life, her son, and spending time in jail for a crime she did not commit. If she wins, it will be a landmark case in UK history.[174]

Don't be fooled into thinking this sort of case is rare. Many concerned are suggesting that the numbers of SIDS which are either reported as related to parents' fault, or just to some 'unexplained' reason, may actually be *directly* caused by the effects of vaccine reactions. This makes perfect sense to me. If you give a tiny baby doses of extremely toxic substances that are over the safety limit set by the FDA, then no wonder there are chances of the baby having a heart attack or just dying for 'no reason'.

Some vaccines *are* directly connected to SIDS (Sudden Infant Death Syndrome), says Dr. Joseph Mercola:

Routine use of the hepatitis B vaccine for all newborns began in 1992, and according to the Vaccine Adverse Event Reporting System (VAERS), operated jointly by the CDC and FDA, there were 36,788 officially reported adverse reactions to hepatitis B vaccines between 1992 and 2005. Of these, 14,800 were serious enough to cause hospitalization, life-threatening health events or permanent disabilities. And 781 people were reported to have DIED following hepatitis B vaccination – and this is likely an underestimate because only a fraction of the serious health problems, including deaths, following vaccination are ever acknowledged due to a lack of public awareness about how to recognize signs and symptoms of vaccine reactions.

Vaccine adverse events are substantially underreported –

some estimate by as much as 90 percent – even though the National Childhood Vaccine Injury Act of 1986 mandated that all doctors and other vaccine providers report serious health problems, including hospitalizations, injuries and deaths following vaccination.[175]

In the USA, a man by the name of Alan Yurko, like Lorraine, went to jail for allegedly killing his newborn son (also named Alan), when in fact it was later proven that the death *was* caused by his son's DTaP vaccination.[176] Alan spent several years in jail trying to fight for his innocence. After doing some investigating about what was written on the autopsy report and from what kinds of medications the hospital gave baby Alan when he was brought into hospital, Alan knew that the vaccine his son had recently had was the *real* cause of his sudden death. He found doctors who provided the proof needed to build a case for his innocence. Alan spent years trying to overturn his sentence and was released from his life sentence back in 2004. You can watch the movie *Vaccine Nation*, available on YouTube to learn more about this truly shocking case.

In a recent and explosive interview between Christina England and a retired police officer from Queensland, Australia, Christina uncovered that police officers are trained to 'never question vaccinations could be causing harm' and that if SIDS happens they must automatically think it was probably the parents' fault and never that it could perhaps be because of recent vaccinations.

According to Sergeant Christopher Savage of the Queensland Police Service:

The police officer is a member of the pro-vaccine brainwashed society and joins the Police Service where the SIDS mindset is already held. When he or she is tasked to attend a baby death, not only does the officer believe SIDS is real but they are also trained to look for signs of abuse and assault and manslaughter. So there is brainwashing on SIDS pushing the officer away from looking at vaccines and their training is to find evidence of foul play, which includes side effects of vaccines. The parents are too traumatized to think rationally and when the police start asking them questions about the other parent they become frightened, paranoid and defensive. The body is taken to a doctor for an autopsy to find out why the baby died. So there is another problem.

Doctors receive more pro-vaccine training than the public and so they won't think of the vaccines as being the cause. The police also don't want to rock the boat. They want to finalize the file. So in the absence of corroborating forensic evidence the police and doctors will most likely describe the case as SIDS.

Christina England of Vactruth.com writes:

Sergeant Savage has given me a copy of a signed statement, which has been countersigned by JP N. Newbury (Qualified Number 10175) of the Gympie Magistrates Court office, stating his belief that vaccines are the cause of many cases of Sudden Infant Death Syndrome (SIDS). He believes innocent parents are also being blamed and are being falsely charged with manslaughter when babies die.

The statement identifies clearly and succinctly a variety of cases in which babies appear fit and healthy on the day of their vaccination but deteriorate after they received the vaccine. He has revealed a clear catalog of cover-ups used by the police force and the medical professionals. He has exposed the fact that every case is treated as if it were a case of manslaughter and newly bereaved parents and parents of critically ill children are being interrogated as prime suspects and potential child abusers. Their homes are being ransacked for clues and precious possessions such as sheets, mattresses and medications are being bagged up as forensic evidence. Their homes are being treated as possible crime scenes.[177]

These stories are all like something out of a movie, aren't they? But it's not a movie; this is real and stories like this are being found all over the world. It's just very rare that people connect the dots, or hear about it in the first place in mainstream media.

Real stories I found far too easily

I now want to share some stories with you about what *can* go very wrong with vaccines. I have found all of these people *just* from my network on Facebook, and it was quite alarming to find out just how many people and their children were affected in my circle of 2000 friends. If I did a little more searching, I could *quickly* find many more. I found real, and truly heartbreaking, stories way too easily, notifying me of how huge this problem truly is.

Sherrel's story about her daughter Deborah and the HPV vaccine Cervarix

My perfectly healthy, academically bright, fun-loving, sporty, active 13-year-old daughter, Deborah, who enjoyed doing typical teenage things had the HPV vaccination Cervarix, the first dose in September and the second dose in November 2010. She did not follow up with the third vaccine.

Like every parent, I wanted to protect my daughter from cervical cancer. I read the leaflet, looked up the NHS website and spoke to the school nurse and her superior. 'It's safe,' I was told. *But was it?*

Now one year on, I look back at my daughter's life of pain, suffering, misery, doctor, A&E, hospital, rheumatologist, podiatrist, physiotherapist and hydrotherapy appointments. The sleepless nights, the worry and my guilt! Because, yes, I do feel guilty that I *did not do more research* before I agreed to let my very precious daughter have the HPV vaccine.

More than one year of our lives wasted. I am questioning the safety of this vaccine. *How safe is it?* Every parent should question the validity of this vaccine and its safety record.

One by one Deborah's activities stopped: judo, roller bowl,

cycling, badminton, basketball, guitar, piano and PE, to name but a few. Stiffer and stiffer she got. Unable to rake leaves in the garden or hoover the sitting-room floor or open a bottle of water! Unable to go for walks on the beach or in the woods with our two dogs. Her enjoyment of life RUINED, taken from her.

Panicked by the realization that I thought she had some type of paralysis, I had started taking her swimming every day before going to school. A girl who was once agile and able to swim 64 lengths was reduced to doing two lengths using a float. Day by day we attended the swimming pool, building up the lengths. Until one day out of the blue, at school, she collapsed. She had abdominal pain. Rushed by ambulance to hospital, she underwent an emergency operation for the removal of her appendix. She had acute suppurative transmural appendicitis with peritonitis. This was followed by two infections. She missed 10 weeks of school. Whether the appendix was associated with this I do not know for sure, but I do wonder as it nags at the back of my mind.

Despite the removal of the appendix, Deborah was becoming sicker. She walked with the aid of a walking stick and could hardly put one foot in front of the other. We got special insoles for her shoes to absorb the shock, similar to what the police wear. We bought a memory foam bed to help comfort her aching joints. She had to wear dark glasses because of light sensitivity. This is so NOT COOL for a little girl of 14.

Then we watched a video by Grace Filby about mineral water. It seemed at first unbelievable that perhaps a simple mineral water could help. But I was desperate for a remedy.

Why mineral water? Well, it is rich in silica and silica is an antidote to aluminum poisoning. Aluminum being a *neurotoxin* contained within the HPV vaccine. I had to try it. Twenty-eight weeks ago my daughter started drinking 1.5 liters of a specific mineral water each day.

Twenty-eight weeks ago we were in the depths of despair. But gradually we saw improvements. After 3 weeks of just little things like small movements, I could feel hope coming back into my life. I started researching foods that contained silica. It was in everyday things like potatoes, cabbage, onions, cucumbers, porridge, cereal, strawberries. The improvement continued. I worked hard – mineral water, foods, exercises, swimming, tiny walks, kept her motivated when things were bad – and she was determined to keep up with her school work.

Now she's back in school with all teachers recently reporting how well she has done after missing 10 weeks of school. She's not fully recovered. She can't do PE. But she can play the piano again and she swims a lot. But we are not out of the woods yet. We still have a lot of problems, obstacles to overcome like the fatigue, but I have faith. We take each day as it comes.

So, parents – after reading our story would you call this long list of illnesses a coincidence? Or would you question it as possibly a very severe adverse reaction to the HPV? Please think very carefully, think twice, research from independent sources, and ensure that when you make this huge decision, it is the right one for your child.

(By Sherrel Halliday, Nairn, Inverness, Scotland)

April Boden's story of what happened to her son Aydan who is now severely autistic

Last night I woke at 3:30am. I do this frequently, but last night my visions kept me awake until sunrise. I saw my son at age 12 months, on his birthday, standing on the bed at a hotel in San Diego near Legoland. Watching Elmo. This episode, Elmo was talking about hands: 'Hands are clapping, and hands must be washed before you eat...' With a bright beautiful smile and a look straight in the eye, Aydan clasped his hands together and said with conviction 'hands'.

One month later he would receive the MMR and chicken pox vaccine in one day. Although he is now aged 6½, I have not heard the word 'hands' come from his mouth again.

A year later, waiting in the doctor's office, Aydan sang the 'Itsy Bitsy Spider' song – sort of. The doctor came in after about an hour.

I should've just left, I should have walked away and taken the sign, but I didn't. I asked the doctor if I should be concerned about Aydan's speech loss, but he'd just sung 'itsy, bitsy, spider...' She said not to worry, we'll look again in six months. He was vaccinated that day and I never heard 'itsy bitsy spider' again.

Fast forward a year later: Aydan had been diagnosed, was receiving treatment and was starting to get better. He had just learned the names of all of the farm animals on his favorite puzzle. At 3 he received yet another set of vaccines in order to enter school. He has never said the name of those farm animals again.

Needless to say, my heart remains broken. I am haunted by these images. Painfully aware that if we had stopped sooner, if we had just skipped one round, he would be better off today. Aydan is considered on the severe end of the spectrum; he remains pre-verbal.

Today I am reading the Bolen Report which, on 10/04/11, started publishing part 1 of this 3-part groundbreaking series that declares the CDC has known since at least 2002 that Thimerosal(mercury)-containing vaccines contributed to the rise in autism. Not surprisingly, after Danish researcher Dr. Paul Thorsen fled the country with millions of dollars in stolen research money, his study would turn out to be a complete fraud. Lies, withheld data and more have been revealed, proving what so many of us have known for years. Vaccines cause autism!

So isn't this what we've been waiting for, fighting for, screaming for? Can't we all sleep well, knowing that the truth has come out and lives will be spared? So why do I feel worse than ever? Because the truth is, through all my rantings and carrying on, through all my fighting of the good fight... I just want my son back.

I would gladly sacrifice the knowledge of any of this to hear my son speak, to see him write his name, to have him run up to me after school and ask if his friend can come over for a play date. I just want my boy. I don't want to be smart, or insightful or clever or wag my finger and say, 'I told you so.'

I want my boy, *I want my boy, I WANT HIM!* I just want him! I want him healthy; I want him to feel good. I don't want to watch him slapping his head because the inflammation causes chronic headaches. I don't want to see him at age 6 still walking on his toes and flapping his arms, or screeching for no apparent reason – or to do yet another round of anti-fungals, for yet another yeast overgrowth, for a still-distended belly, caused by more constipation.

I watch him as he watches his older brother run down the stairs with his friends and around the apartment complex as they go riding their scooters. Aydan and I pray every night that one day that will be him. But here we are, age 6½, and progress remains slow.

I wonder if I hold on to this pain because I fear that if I let it go, I will be letting go of my recovery dream.

Each day I try, try, try again. Fighting the school over an apraxia speech therapist. Time to test the kidneys to make sure he's ready for chelation. More magnesium cleanses, anti-fungal parade, more probiotics, more vitamin supplements, antioxidants, Relationship Development Intervention, evenings spent giving Mustgatova massage, occupational therapy brushing protocol. Can I have a moment for myself or am I neglecting a potentially groundbreaking teaching moment?

So someone tells me the other day she is worried about talking to people about vaccines because she wants to be taken seriously. Will this new information allow us to be taken seriously? Will it allow the mainstream to stop their nonsensical, unscientific rantings about the safety of vaccines? I don't care. I don't care what the mainstream media says; I don't care what the government does. I just want my boy. I just want my Aydan.

I won't return to the government (who caused the problem), looking for an answer or an apology. I won't ask the mainstream media who has denied us acceptance for years. Like returning to an abusive boyfriend who claims to change but never will, I will not return to my abuser in anticipation of a new outcome. I don't care to be taken seriously. I just my want my son. I want Aydan.

I want him back. I want time, I want just one, just one of those days to be erased from our history. The rest of this life, and the next, and the next after that, I give back to you, God, if you can give me my boy – if you can return him to his healthy state, if he could just be that carefree child that I know he longs to be when I see him watching his brother and his friends.

I commend us all, the parents of the vaccine-injured, who throw off the shackles of fear and speak openly and truthfully. Horribly painful stories I have heard. I sympathize and usually empathize, but in the end, I just want my boy. I want Aydan. I want him back.

Will the acknowledgment of the truth change the past? Can I have my son back now? If I remain a hard-working devoted mother and a good little activist will he come back to me? Will he?

Oh, and please don't give me pity; please don't compliment me for my bravery or tell me all the lives I will save or the people I have spared this pain. Don't get me wrong, I care… I care about them all. I want a different world more than anyone can imagine; I want to save my son for a purpose. I do not see the logic in bringing up a well-adjusted child to a maladjusted world. I am profoundly grateful each time I hear a new parent questioning vaccines and I am more than willing to share my story for the cause, at any given opportunity.

I know there is a greater light, a higher power … of this I am certain, but I wonder if in this life I will ever be able to have a conversation with my son, play hide and seek. Will he want the keys to the car when he turns 16? This is my dream, this is my desire. That is the truth!

✓ aydansrecovery.blogspot.co.uk
✓ blogtalkradio.com/truthertalk

Amanda's story about her niece Bella who had a series of shots in one day

Bella, my niece, was born May 2010. She was a C-section birth and when I first saw her I thought she looked red and swollen and nothing like her brother who was also a C-section birth – he came out looking plump and clear-skinned. Her mother said when the doctors were taking Bella out of her that they were quite forcefully pushing on her (the mother's) ribcage. It took a few weeks until Bella began to look like herself and look like her big brother. Bella wasn't breastfed for long; this was something that upset her mother but she found breastfeeding too painful to do.

At 8 months old Bella was beginning to find her voice. She was becoming a vocal little girl that wanted to be heard, and when others were chatting together she would shout out as if to say,'Look at me!' The last time I saw Bella before she got sick she was shouting and giggling; it was a delight to see. Her mother mentioned Bella had had her vaccinations that day and not cried at all when she got them. But, I was told later, that evening Bella started to have seizures and was taken to hospital. They did lots of tests to try and discover what was causing the seizures but couldn't pinpoint it to anything. I asked my brother if it could have been the vaccinations but he said no, the doctors said they were not the cause. I wondered then, how they would know they were *not* what caused her seizures? Bella was sent home when her seizures had stopped.

Then a day later they started again. The local hospital didn't have the resources to treat Bella so she was then taken to the sick kids' hospital where they specialize in neurological problems. They gave Bella almost every anti-epilepsy drug, but nothing worked – the seizures would be continual – until they discovered they would have to sedate Bella. As soon as Bella woke up she had another seizure, but they couldn't always sedate her as there was a limit to the amount of the drug they could give her. So we watched her heart rate go up and her oxygen levels go down and thought she was going to die so many times. As the days went on, Bella began to stop expressing any emotion; she would just stare into space. She did, however, begin to roll herself over onto one side while she was in her hospital bed. But this all stopped within a few weeks. After every anti-epilepsy drug was tried, the doctors then decided to give her steroids – which made her huge, bloated almost beyond all recognition, plus the steroids also gave her pubic hair – which she still has. It was truly horrific to see this sweet little baby be experimented on in this way. The doctors did lots of tests and scans and finally (although they had no idea what caused it or how to treat it) gave a name for her disease: 'Partial Migrating Epilepsy'. There are a few hundred babies over the world that have this rare form of epilepsy and it usually results in death. Babies usually develop it within the first three months and generally don't make it beyond their third birthday. I pleaded with my brother to see a chiropractor and homeopath but he refused, instead choosing to trust the medical profession even though there was nothing they could do but sedate her. I was exasperated and one day I sat my brother down and with tears streaming down both our faces I begged him to at least try the chiropractor. He said he would but not until Bella got out of the hospital as the doctors might 'get put out' if they saw a chiropractor coming in!

After 3 months of being in the sick kids' hospital Bella was indeed sicker than ever but was now sent to a care home for children. They had all the specialized equipment needed for Bella, and the care home was closer to her family so it was a better place for her to be. Bella got her first adjustment with the chiropractor and looked interested in what was happening to her. She slept well afterwards but nothing too startling happened. During her third adjustment Bella raised her arms over her head; this was amazing as she had not moved her body for months. We were all overjoyed – my brother and his wife were delighted – although they said they didn't want to have false hope and get too carried away... Unbelievably, they never got any more adjustments for Bella after that. I don't know what happened. I tried to find out and got responses that made no sense. For example, they said that the chiropractor's clinic was too far away or it wasn't really doing much to help her. (?!) I couldn't believe this was happening! I can only assume they spoke with a doctor and were advised not to continue with the chiro.

I also contacted a friend who is a homeopath; she came to visit Bella and her mother. Bella was given a remedy but her mother never actually gave it to her. I realized there was nothing more I could do and I had to back off from visiting as it was just far too upsetting to see. Bella is now 3 and still unable to move very much – she can't sit up unaided, she's blind, doesn't speak, cries a lot and very, very rarely smiles. She is fed through a contraption that's stitched to her stomach with a tube as she has difficulty swallowing. In the winter months she has infection after infection and is treated with antibiotics which of course weaken her little body further. I am heartbroken about what has happened to Bella and unable to discuss this with my own family as they get angry when I question what has gone on, and is still going on. They believe as they were told by the doctors that this condition is something Bella was born with and that they can't do anything about it. Bella is back home now four days a week as my brother has had his house adapted to suit her needs – she still has regular seizures and is still on medication to sedate her every day.

I wish this story had a happy ending. Maybe one day her parents will wake up and see that the vaccine given that day was the only thing different that logically makes sense as to why she has this condition now, and they will start to look for other ways to support Bella's body and energy. But until then I will keep sending them all my love. I ask whoever reads this to do the same.

Marcella's story about her daughter Rachel, now 18

My name is Marcella Piper-Terry. I am the mother of a child who was injured by vaccines. I am also an independent researcher. I have a master's degree in psychology and have extensive experience reading and critiquing research articles from the peer-reviewed literature. I have participated in the design and implementation of original research studies and am listed as author in studies that have been published in the scientific literature. I have worked as a family therapist, neuropsychological evaluator, educational advocate, and biomedical consultant for families whose children have been diagnosed with autism spectrum disorders, ADHD, learning disabilities, and such psychiatric disorders as bipolar disorder, obsessive-compulsive disorder, and schizophrenia. In August 2011, I became one of the founders of the non-profit, VaxTruth.org. VaxTruth will also be submitting a statement to be included in the record.

This is my personal statement. This is the story of my daughter.

Rachel was born in the spring of 1994. However, the story of her lifelong battle begins many years prior to her birth. As someone who has researched a lot about neuro-developmental disorders, including autism, Asperger's Syndrome and ADHD, I have come to understand there is something different about our children. There is something that makes them more vulnerable to vaccine-injury than other children.

Rachel's increased vulnerability to vaccine-injury begins with my childhood. I was born in Los Angeles and grew up in Southern California. During the 1960s & early 70s, I attended an elementary school where the playground was situated on an embankment of the 55 freeway. Prior to 1978, lead was still present in gasoline. At that time school children still had multiple recesses each day. When we arrived at school (during the time of the morning rush hour) we were outside running around on the playground for 20-30 minutes before school began. We had a 15-20 minute recess in the morning and another in the afternoon. We also had P.E. every day. So, we were running around on the blacktop and on the field playing dodge-ball, kickball, tether-ball, 4 square, etc... for a total of approximately 90 minutes per day, 5 days per week.

The reason children are so vulnerable to the effects of lead fumes is because kids run around a lot and when they are running, they breathe deeper and more rapidly, which increases the amount of lead they take in. I attended the same school from first through sixth grade. At 90 minutes per day over six years, I (and my peers) spent more than 2,000 hours breathing in fumes from leaded gasoline.

My family moved to Mississippi when I was 12 and we lived in a home that was built in 1875. There were many layers of lead paint in the house. I lived there until I graduated from high school, and then moved back and lived there again after my divorce at age 23. During the times when I lived in that house, there were intermittent episodes of "home improvement" going on, many of which included the sanding of lead paint. (This was well before graduate school, or working in a neuropsychological private practice, and I didn't know any better. None of us did.)

Here is what I now know about lead: It mimics calcium from a structural standpoint and it displaces calcium in the body. When one is exposed to lead, it circulates in the blood for a while and then deposits in bone and soft tissue, where it is stored for decades. It accumulates. The more one is exposed, the more it accumulates. Because lead mimics calcium, it is very easily passed from mother to the developing fetus in utero, and in breast milk, particularly if the mother has a calcium deficiency. Like mercury, lead damages the brain and virtually all biological processes in the body. The effects are systemic.

When I became pregnant with Rachel, I had already had two back surgeries and been diagnosed with degenerative disc disease (most likely due to mineral deficiencies and connective tissue problems because of the lead). I had what was deemed a "spontaneous" DVT (deep vein thrombosis) at the age of 30 and spent 10 days in a drug-induced coma in neuro-intensive care because my blood pressure was so high and would not respond to medications. (What I have since realized is that my "spontaneous DVT" occurred within 2-3 weeks after I received a tetanus shot and a flu shot.) Ultimately I recovered, but I had to wear TEDs support stockings and take Coumadin for nearly a year afterward. I was told that if I ever got pregnant it would most likely kill me.

At the age of 33, I got pregnant. My husband was in the Air Force and I received prenatal care through the obstetrics department at Keesler Air Force Base in Biloxi, Mississippi. Due to the history of previous DVT, I was started on heparin injections (another blood thinner), which I administered to myself every 8 hours throughout the pregnancy.

My blood-type is O-negative and I have the Rh-factor incompatibility issue. I received two Rhogam injections during the pregnancy with Rachel. Both contained Thimerosal.

At 25 weeks gestation, I started contracting and threatened miscarriage. I was hospitalized for a week, started on Terbutaline (a medication given to forestall pre-term labor) and sent home on bedrest for the duration of the pregnancy. I was still giving myself heparin injections every 8 hours. At 33 weeks, the Terbutaline started making me sick and I had to be taken off of it. One week later, my daughter was born.

Rachel was tiny and beautiful. She was also lethargic, would not latch on to nurse, and wanted to sleep all the time. We spent 11 days in the hospital, partly because she was losing weight, and partly because I had to be switched over from heparin to Coumadin. When we were finally discharged she weighed 6 pounds, 1 ounce. She continued to be lethargic and was very slow to gain weight. Trying to nurse her was difficult, and after 3 weeks and a whopping episode of breast impaction, I had to start her on formula. She had already had difficulty keeping down what little breast milk I could get in her, and when switched to formula she started having episodes of projectile vomiting. We went through multiple formula changes and then she was put on soy formula. She stopped puking up everything and started to sleep a little better. In hindsight, I know now that the soy formula she consumed was a source of very high levels of manganese. Exposure to high levels of manganese is known to cause mitochondrial disorder and neurological problems.

Because Rachel was born in 1994 and because she was fully vaccinated, she received a considerable amount of Thimerosal (mercury) at a very young age (beginning in utero with the Rhogam injections). She was always beautiful, and always a joy, even though she had terrible problems with her digestion, couldn't tolerate milk, and almost never smiled or made eye contact. She met all of her motor milestones on time, but she was clumsy and uncoordinated. Her language appeared at the proper time, though it was very minimal and she had a terrible time with stuttering as a toddler. She was also extremely late in teething. She didn't cut her first tooth until 11 months, and her second didn't come in until she was sixteen months old. I now realize the reason she was so late in teething was because her minerals were dysregulated because of the lead she got from me, and because of the mercury she got from vaccines.

The ear infections started within two weeks of her four-month vaccinations. They continued almost constantly for the next four years. It generally took 3 rounds of different antibiotics to get her over each infection, and then she would get another one within a week to ten days after stopping the last round. Finally, she was put on prophylactic antibiotics for six months. When we took her off the antibiotics, she developed another ear infection within two weeks. Ultimately, she had two sets of tubes surgically implanted, the first at age two and the second at age four. She also had several bouts of conjunctivitis, two episodes of stomatitis, and more than a dozen odd illnesses consisting of high fevers ("of unknown origin"), mysterious rashes, upper respiratory infections and what was thought to be gastrointestinal viruses with vomiting and diarrhea. At four years of age she was diagnosed with hepatitis A. Shortly after, the whites of her eyes turned yellow and they stayed that way for the next seven years.

She ate virtually nothing and was diagnosed with "Failure-to-Thrive" – meaning that she was consistently below the 10th percentile in weight for her age. Because my husband was in the Air Force, we saw Air Force doctors, and because we moved from Ocean Springs to Washington D.C., we saw several different military doctors. When my husband retired from the Air Force, I requested and received a copy of all of our complete medical records. It was upon review of those records that I learned I had been suspected of child abuse, and at one point had been in danger of being referred for mandatory nutritional counseling because my daughter was not gaining weight.

While we were in D.C., Rachel was seen by the head of Developmental Pediatrics at Bethesda Naval Hospital, and was diagnosed with ADHD, combined type (the most severe kind). It was suggested that she be put on stimulant medication. I resisted and wanted further testing. She was evaluated by the Chief of Child Behavioral Psychology at Walter Reed Hospital. Results of testing confirmed the ADHD, combined type, and Expressive Language delay. She was also having absence seizures and auditory processing problems. When she started kindergarten (after another round of vaccinations that contained Thimerosal), everything was magnified. At the first meeting with her kindergarten teacher, she was labeled, "My Flower Child" because she was so slow to transition. She seemed to not have a clue as to what was going on around her. Mrs. Smith said, "When the bell rings for lunch, and everyone else is already in line to go to the cafeteria, I have to physically go and touch Rachel on the shoulder to get her to stop what she's doing and come line up." Ultimately, I gave in and we started her on stimulants for ADHD. We saw immediate improvement in her attention, but we also saw increases in anxiety and tearfulness, and more aggressive behavior – to say nothing about what it did to her appetite and sleep. Soon she was also taking Zoloft, prescribed to help mediate the side-effects of the stimulant. Next came the Clonidine for sleep.

In addition to her medical problems and her struggles with inattention and impulsivity, Rachel did not seem to "connect" with kids her own age. She was more interested in drawing and doing projects than in playing with the other kids in the neighborhood. She loved animals and would play for hours with our boxers, Annie and Theo. She nagged and nagged us about wanting a horse. When she was six she started riding. She was so tiny and thin and those horses were huge! But even as little as she was, she displayed a confidence and sense of control I had not seen in her previously. It was amazing.

At the time of the 9/11 attacks, we were living on Andrews Air Force Base in D.C. That day was a nightmare. My husband frequently worked at the Pentagon and I worked in Silver Spring; 45 minutes away. My children were on base, and it was four hours before I knew if Steve was alive. I was unable to get home until 7:30 that night because of the gridlock – and the fact that once I got to the base it took more than 3 hours to get through security. Every day for months, whenever we left the base or returned, we went through rows of armed soldiers on either side of the car. Rachel saw all of this, because her school was just outside the gate of the base. It was at this time she developed tics – rapid eye-blinking and head-rubbing. She also started getting sick more often with strep infections, and by "more often" I mean repeatedly, over-and-over again. She was diagnosed with asthma and allergies and was prescribed medications for both. By the time we left the military and moved to Indiana, my daughter was in 3rd grade and was taking five different prescription medications on a daily basis.

I thought things would get better with the move. I had never been to the Midwest, and I had envisioned a place that was big and open, with lots of fields and farms. I was right about that, and initially I loved it here. We moved here in the fall and within a week, we had our first snow. However, in the spring, when the temperature started going up, the sky turned gray and Rachel started breaking out in hives. She continued to have recurrent strep infections and our physician here kept prescribing antibiotics and steroids – which were in addition to the Strattera, Adderall, Zoloft, Zyrtec, Clonidine, Albuterol and Flovent she was already taking. Her diet was extremely limited and she was still so small and frail. Her eye contact was fleeting; she never laughed or smiled, and rarely spoke, though she was extremely emotional and cried often. It was almost like she couldn't get the words out unless they were fueled by extreme anger or upset. In addition to her earlier diagnoses of ADHD and OCD, we added PANDAS (Pediatric Autoimmune Disorder Associated with Streptococcus) and Asperger's Syndrome.

The gray sky, I soon learned, was from the smokestacks of the coal-burning power plants that are so prevalent in the Midwest. We live in the lower Ohio Valley. This is "The Coal Burning Power Plant Capitol of the United States." There are more coal plants here than in any other place on earth (with the exception of China), and our air quality shows it. The by-products of coal burning include lead, mercury, arsenic, antimony, cadmium, manganese, and other heavy metals. As sick as my daughter was in D.C., she got even sicker when we moved here. The hives continued to be more frequent and worsened in their presentation. By October of her fifth-grade year, we had to pull her out of school because she was sick virtually ALL the time and we felt the only way to help her get well was to decrease her exposures by getting her out of the classroom. It wasn't hard socially because she really didn't have any friends anyway. It's hard enough to make friends when you're the "new girl" in a small town; it's even harder when your auditory processing is so poor you only "get" about every 3rd or 4th word that's said. It's really hard when you tend to jump, flap, and rock when you're excited or upset. Third, fourth and fifth grade girls can be exceptionally cruel, and the isolation and ostracism she endured no doubt was another factor in the damage to her already fragile immune system. This was a bleak time. I will never forget my beautiful daughter, lying on her bed with her entire body covered in horrendous red patches, her lips swollen so big she could hardly talk, and her eyes swelled up like she'd been on the losing end in a prize-fight, with tears rolling onto her pillow. Her question, "Why does God hate me?" and her decla-ration, "I wish He would just let me die" are things I hope no other parent ever has to hear from their 11-year-old child.

I had had enough. I started researching and made a vow that if there was any way, I was going to figure out how to help my daughter. Over the next five months, I put her on a regimen of vitamins, minerals, probiotics, digestive enzymes, cod liver oil, and other supplements that were reported to help children with ADHD and other neuro-developmental disorders. It was expensive, and it was a slow process, but gradually I was able to wean her off of all of the prescription medications she was taking. Her hives disappeared, her eye-contact improved, she started gaining weight, she became more social, the jumping and rocking decreased dramatically, and – best of all – she laughed. And she smiled. And I cried. And I kept researching.

I attended a Defeat Autism Now! conference and I realized that what I had been doing with Rachel was called Biomedical Interventions for Autism. I got involved with Defeat Autism Now! because I had already seen it work. I started recommending things to my clients in the psychiatric practice in which I worked – and they started getting better; many of them got better to the point that some children were being weaned off their medications completely. Others were able to reduce the amount of medications they were taking. (This didn't go over well with the psychiatrist in who's practice I was employed, and I eventually left by mutual agreement.) I became a biomedical consultant and attended my second Defeat Autism Now! conference, and was allowed to take the clinical training. I established my own company and was building a client base that was steadily growing. Rachel was also doing well. She did have a couple of seizures, beginning when she was twelve, but after adjusting her supplements and increasing her B6 intake, she was seizure-free and stayed that way for more than two years. She continued to have struggles in some classes, particularly in math, due to ongoing issues with her memory and processing speed, but overall, she was holding strong. She had a few good friends, was playing drums in the school band, and was looking forward to getting her learner's permit. Her health had improved to the point where instead of

being in the doctor's office every week, we actually had a period of two years when she was never sick!

Everything changed in April of 2010. Rachel attended an Earth Day Celebration at Wesselman Woods Nature Park and while she was there she was bitten by a brown recluse spider. I had been bit by a brown recluse a few years prior, and had treated my own bite successfully, using salves and natural anti-bacterials. I applied the same methods to treat Rachel's bite. This worked for a while, but then the bite started to get worse. It was on a weekend, so I took her to the emergency room to have it checked. Immediately, I was asked if she was up-to-date on her shots. I replied that she was, and the nurse cautioned me that if I was unsure, Rachel needed to receive a tetanus shot. We passed on that. The E.R. visit was followed by a visit to our family physician, who prescribed a different antibiotic because the first one was not working. After another E.R. visit, another push for a tetanus shot (also declined), and a third antibiotic, we ended up back in our family doctor's office, where I was told that not only did she have a brown recluse bite, but she had developed MRSA at the site of the bite. Once again, a tetanus shot was recommended and once again, I declined. This time, my family doctor pushed the issue. This time, I caved. I gave consent.

Brown recluse spiders are nasty critters. Their bite can cause necrotizing of the skin and can result in the need for skin grafts and amputations. Some people die. MRSA is equally nasty, causing many of the same horrific outcomes including limb amputations and death. So when our doctor said she had to have the tetanus shot, I very reluctantly gave the okay. I knew in my gut it was a mistake, and I had refused twice previously in the emergency room, but I just couldn't take the chance of anything else happening to her.

Three hours later I was in the kitchen and Rachel was upstairs with an ice pack on her rear end (at the injection site). Everything was quiet until I heard a loud thud and then the horrible rhythmic banging of her head on the hardwood floor. I ran up the stairs and yelled for my other daughter to call 911. When I got to her, Rachel's eyes were rolling back in her head and she was gasping for breath. I knelt on the floor and held her head in my hands. The seizure went on for about two minutes. As I watched her struggle, she stopped breathing and I knew that it was my fault. I had killed her because I gave consent for the vaccine. Within a matter of seconds my neighbor came bursting into the room and took over. Thankfully, we live across the street from a fire-fighter/EMT and he had heard the call go out over his scanner. The ambulance was there in less than three minutes and she was on oxygen and IV's within minutes. This was one of the times when, despite everything else, I was very glad to be living in a small town in Indiana. I can only imagine how long it would have taken for help to arrive if we lived in a larger town, or in a metropolitan area. I fully believe Rachel would not be alive today if that had been the case.

I messed up. I gave in to pressure for the vaccine because I was afraid. That was my first mistake. My second mistake was in not making sure that she was only getting the tetanus shot. I assumed that's what the doctor was ordering, since that's what he said she needed. It was only later that I learned she got the Tdap, and that the vaccine she was given contained 1,500 micrograms of aluminum; a known neurotoxin. I also later learned that Rachel's seizure, three hours after vaccination, is a frequently reported adverse reaction to DTaP and Tdap vaccines.

Since the Tdap vaccine, Rachel has suffered a series of setbacks in her health. We have lost a great deal of the ground we had worked so hard over the years to regain after her early years of vaccine-injury and illness. She has had multiple seizures and has had two additional battles with MRSA. Her memory, while never great, has deteriorated significantly. In the fall of 2010 she came down with mononucleosis and was sick for several months, during which time she was unable to focus on school or anything else. All she wanted to do was sleep. I quit my consulting business so I could be home with her. In the spring of 2011 she was diagnosed with a Primary Immune Deficiency Syndrome. She has chronic Epstein-Barr virus that has invaded her central nervous system. Once this happens, there is "nothing that can be done" from the standpoint of traditional Western medicine. Because her immune system is so damaged, she is unable to fight off bacterial and viral infections. She is very prone to bleeding problems. Children and young adults who share Rachel's diagnosis most often succumb to severe bacterial infections or hemorrhage, if not to leukemia or lymphoma. The prognosis is frightening. But, just as we did not accept that there was nothing we could do when she was eleven, we are not accepting that there is nothing we can do now. We are working to recover the level of health she had, prior to the Tdap. Once again, it's a slow, expensive process. Rachel is a trooper, though. In the last few months she has taken her G.E.D. and passed with flying colors. She also recently took the ACT and scored high enough to qualify for entrance at our local community college. She finally got her driver's license and is looking forward to starting college.

The reason I have chosen to share Rachel's story at this time and in this amount of detail is because two years ago, my daughter looked like a healthy 15-year-old. She had improved so much with the intensive interventions we employed over the years, and she was functioning at such a high level that most people would never have suspected she had ever received her earlier diagnoses. All of that went down the drain because of one vaccine.

My daughter is part of a sub-population of children that are at increased risk of vaccine-injury. What I have described in this statement, and what I have observed in my work with countless families of children with ASD diagnoses, is the result of epigenetics. (Please see the work of Dr. Martha Herbert.) I always believed that my prior exposure to high levels of lead contributed significantly to her health problems, including her diagnoses of ADHD and Asperger's Syndrome. It wasn't until she was much older and I did a timeline of her medical records that I saw the connection with vaccines. From infancy, every time she was vaccinated, her health deteriorated. I wish I had researched the connection earlier. Even when I started going to the Defeat Autism Now! conferences, I was still convinced that it was lead and not vaccines that had harmed my child. By the time I was faced with the decision in our doctor's office in May 2010, I knew vaccines were a big part of Rachel's neurological and immunological problems. I was pressured and I was scared. My decision almost killed my daughter, and as a result of the further damage to her immune system, it still may.

There is nothing else in medicine that is prescribed, or in the case of vaccines, mandated for 100% of the population, without regard to individuality. That's because there is no medical procedure that is safe for everyone. To say that vaccines do not cause autism in some children because they do not cause autism in all children makes no sense.

When it comes to the epidemic of autism (and other developmental neuro-immune disorders), if we only consider individual exposures or individual environmental factors, or just the genetic component, we will never find the truth. I was grateful to hear Mr. Kucinich discuss the contribution of mercury from coal-burning operations. I also agree that exposure to lead from gasoline is a contributing factor. I agree that age of the parents may be contributing factors for some families; particularly if the aging parents live in areas of the country where there are high amounts of environmental toxins; more years exposed to toxins equals higher toxic load in the parent and more mutations in DNA as a result of cumulative exposures (including mercury, aluminum, formaldehyde and other toxins in vaccines).

I agree there is a genetic predisposition. However, we need to reconsider the terminology. Our children are not predisposed to "autism." The are predisposed, by virtue of epigenetics, to vaccine-injury. Those who already carry a high load of toxic metals in their systems will pass those toxins to their offspring; either directly (from mother to child) or indirectly (through mutagenics affecting DNA in the sperm). Children who are born to parents who have high exposures to environmental toxins will be more likely to have severe reactions to additional sources of environmental toxins; including those that are injected through vaccines. The childhood vaccine schedule has never been studied for synergistic effects or interactions when multiple vaccines are given simultaneously and over time. This must be done. The interactions between exposures to environmental toxins and those contained in vaccines must be studied. Until these things are accomplished, the entire vaccination program has to be recognized for what it is: medical experimentation.

Our children are not all the same. They have different genetic make-ups and they have been exposed to different environmental toxins. They MUST be treated as individuals when it comes to their medical care. It is not acceptable to sacrifice those, like Rachel, who are part of the susceptible group, in the name of "the greater good."

Sara's story who was given the Gardasil vaccine when she was 13

When I was 13 years old, on October 17, 2006, I received the first and only Gardasil HPV vaccine; the first vaccine in a series of three injections. Before I get into the aftermath of receiving Gardasil, let me describe myself before the vaccine.

I was healthy, active, and full of life. I was always out in Nature, swimming, biking, and just being a kid. I had no history of serious illness. The only thing that I had was allergies and I received allergy shots from ages 6 to 11. After the Gardasil, that all changed. Since I had allergy shots as a kid, I was never afraid of needles. Once I was administered the Gardasil vaccine by my general practitioner (GP), fear took over me for the first time ever when receiving a shot. I was uncontrollably screaming and crying. The pain felt like a metal bat slamming into my right arm repeatedly. I didn't stop crying for a half-hour.

Two weeks later, my arm was still hurting as bad as it did the day I got the vaccine. My mom then called our GP and explained the pain I was still having. The doctor said that this tends to happen with this vaccine, but it should go away and not to worry about it.

A couple of days after talking with our GP, I started to feel dizzy, light-headed, and had frequent nosebleeds. Most of the symptoms I was experiencing could be explained away, it seemed. My allergies were acting up so I was getting nosebleeds. I played basketball in gym that day, my muscles were probably just tight, and that's why the right side of my neck and arm hurt.

Then I became fatigued along with all the other symptoms and started to come home early from school. I took naps more often, which I never used to do. The pain traveled up the right side of my neck and started to cause nerve pain. Soon we couldn't explain away my symptoms anymore.

I woke up to go to school one morning and I couldn't move my neck and needed an X-ray. It showed that my neck vertebrae were too straight where there should be a slight curve. I was then sent to get an MRI of my neck and nothing showed up. Due to the severity of the pain I was having, we decided to get a MRI for my arm as well. It showed a deep pocket of inflammation where I had the injection. The doctor suggested we look into brachial plexus neuritis because the nerve pain in my arm and neck could be coming from a pinched nerve.

Brachial plexus neuritis affects a collection of nerves that extend from the spinal cord into certain areas of the upper body, including the shoulders, chest, hands, and arms. Symptoms of brachial plexus neuritis are severe pain, arm weakness, and decreased sensation.

My mom and I went to several specialists, but the pain soon traveled down my other arm, which ruled out that diagnosis. We always asked every doctor we saw if the Gardasil did this. The answer was always no.

That April, my right knee swelled up to three times its normal size. I was immediately taken to the hospital. The doctor said he needed to run some blood tests to see if this was an autoimmune issue. He then sent me to a rheumatoid arthritis specialist. My blood test showed that I had an Rh factor, and that I had juvenile rheumatoid arthritis (JRA). I had my knee drained to make sure the fluid wasn't infected and it wasn't.

Throughout the year 2007, I saw two different rheumatoid arthritis specialists that put me on many toxic medications, such as Prednisone, Methotrexate (chemo: first pill form, then injection), Enbrel, Remicade, Tramadol, Mobic, and Celebrex. I was on each of these medications at different times for about six months. I soon enrolled into homeschooling because I was so sick with extreme nerve and joint pain throughout my entire body.

During November, I went through a Methotrexate overdose and couldn't keep any food down or medicine. I then learned what a heroin addict goes through during withdrawal pains and symptoms. We found out during that period that Tramadol was a derivative of morphine. I was only 14 years old at the time. I stopped all the above medications, except for Prednisone, and I slowly weaned myself off Tramadol.

I later did antibiotic therapy: one week of intravenous antibiotics, and then pill form. A week later, I stopped walking. I was screaming and crying all the time. I had food sensitivities to corn, wheat, gluten, dairy, soy, nightshades, and peanut butter. Six months later, I was 15 years old and looked like a concentration-camp victim. I was at death's door. My organs/systems were shutting down. I was in excruciating pain every second of every day.

The naturopathic doctor I had been seeing led me to Dr. Bruce Shelton Homeopath/MD in Arizona. I was there for 3 weeks doing homeopathic and biomedical treatments that I will break down in later posts. Dr. Shelton saved my life and helped put me on the path of natural healing.

✓ sarashealingjourney.wordpress.com/

Kash's story

(As told by his mother Kerri)

On June 23rd, we took our son into the pediatrician's office to receive his one-year vaccines. We were getting ready to go on vacation and we wanted to get it over with since they were already late. Just like most other parents, I dreaded these appointments. I couldn't stand taking my sweet, smiling, cheerful child into the doctor to have him poked and prodded, but I didn't know I had a choice. I ran a home-based childcare facility and I thought immunizations had to be current for that, as well as future schooling, camps, etc. Kash is the youngest of 5 siblings, all of whom have been vaccinated, and we never had issues, so unfortunately, I didn't put much thought into doing any of my own research.

Kash was immunized, I got him dressed, and we both left the doctor's office in tears. The next morning I was cuddling with Kash when he first woke up, and he began to vomit. When he finished, I turned him over and tried to get him to communicate with me, or even respond, and I got nothing from him but a blank stare. His body was limp, he was staring off into space, and he wouldn't even acknowledge his own name. Knowing something wasn't right, we took him to the closest ER, which was about five minutes away. After evaluating him, the attending physician told us that more than likely Kash had suffered a seizure due to 'system overload' from his vaccines the day before. We were told to take him home, let him rest, keep an eye on him, but that everything SHOULD BE OK.

A couple of days later we left for our family vacation. Eight hours of driving and Kash screamed all the way. We couldn't figure out what was going on because he was always such a delightful and passive child, and this was completely out of the norm for him. Over the next week, Kash was extremely fussy, broke out in a rash, and ran a fever. With any change in his personality or health, I called back home to his pediatrician who instructed me to treat him with Benadryl and Tylenol. After a week of being on vacation with a fussy child and not in our own environment, it was time to make the long trip back home. Once again, eight hours in the car, and eight hours of Kash screaming. By the time we got home, we were all exhausted and decided to go to bed.

The following day, July 4th 2010, Kash woke up fussy and running a slight fever. I got up with him, gave him a dose of Motrin, and since we had a big day of celebrating ahead of us, I decided to lie down and take a nap with Kash. I took him into my room to nap with me while my husband and our other children went about their day. About an hour later, I was awoken by the most horrifying sound that I've ever heard ... it was my baby screaming and convulsing at the same time. I shook him and screamed his name several times, neither of which he responded to. I didn't know what to do, so I screamed for my husband to help, grabbed my baby and began to run up the stairs with him.

I got about halfway up the stairs before my husband met me. Both of us have some medical knowledge and we know that seizures shouldn't last long, so we stood in the kitchen holding Kash, trying to comfort him, saying his name, trying to do anything to get him to come out of the seizure, but he didn't. After a couple of minutes we decided it was best for me to stay with the other children while my husband took Kash to the nearest ER, which thank GOD is only about 5 minutes away.

(Cody's narrative – Kash's father)

On July 4th Kash and Kerri had awoken early so they took a nap together. About 45 minutes after they went down I heard my wife scream my name along with the word 'Help!' I met her halfway up the stairs with Kash in her arms and he was convulsing and unresponsive. I know this sounds terrible but at the time it seemed best and it was the decision I made – I put Kash in my lap and drove as fast as I could to the ER (about 5 miles from our home; I really felt I could get him there faster than an ambulance could arrive at our home). The drive to the hospital felt like hours and I spoke to Kash... yelled a few times to try and get him to come to. We arrived at the hospital and I jumped out with Kash and ran in through the ambulatory entrance where the receptionist started to tell me that I would need to enter through the front door but I interrupted her with all I could get out: 'Help – my son is having a seizure...'

No time was wasted; we were in a room and had three nurses and the doctor that was on duty in the room with us right away. I remember thinking that I felt guilty about all the other patients that were going to have to wait because we demanded all the attention for something that would have probably resolved itself (odd thought-process and I was WRONG). We had to estimate his weight for medication because the seizure was too violent to get a good weight using the scales. The staff tried to get a line in but couldn't because his veins were too small and, as I previously stated, he was convulsing, violently, so the doctor informed me that they would have to 'drill' a small hole into his shin. I remembered arguing with him that it would be too painful for him and the doctor told me that in his current state he wouldn't feel a thing. So with the hole drilled and the line started, they pushed the first dose; the drug was something similar to Valium. The doctor told me the drug would work very fast and he would come out of the seizure quickly. At this point of the visit, Kash had been seizing for about 12 minutes, and 5 minutes later the doctor whispered something to a nurse and she quickly left the room. The doctor turned to me and told me that the medication didn't work and that they would have to administer another dose and then told me something that didn't register because I was distracted by the nurse that had just left the room returning with the crash cart. This is all a little fuzzy but I know Kerri was still home waiting for someone to come for the other kids and my mom had just arrived when I asked why they brought the crash cart in. The doctor told me for the second time that this second dose of medication would stop his breathing… Once again I argued with the doctor, 'Don't give him the medicine then', and the doctor told me that seizures should never last this long (we were now at the 20-minute mark) and the longer he remained seizing, the higher the chance of permanent neurological damage. So the second dose went in and he stopped breathing.

This is the part of the story that I usually stop talking at, when the lump in my throat gets too big to talk through and I know if I blink a tear will fall. I hadn't noticed the large man, that looked more like a bouncer than a respiratory specialist, who had entered the room until he began bagging my son. Kerri arrived right around this time and so did my realization that Kash wasn't coming home today as I finally inventoried my surroundings and noticed nurses were beginning to cry.

Sorry this is so long. Obviously, this is a story I get very involved in telling, but I will fast forward for you.

Kash spent the next ten days in a coma and it was during this time that we began educating ourselves on the risks of vaccines. Bad timing considering we were too late to do anything now and we got to learn that IF Kash ever woke up he faced certain brain damage and could be a vegetable. That was IF he woke up.

Kerri was my rock. I know I should have been that one, but when it comes to my kids I am soft, cotton-ball soft. Kerri is also soft when it comes to the kids but she is a much better actor than I am. How can someone be so tough but have such a soft touch? She left the hospital twice, once to shower (then she found out she could use the showers there) and the second time she left to take the other kids to dinner (Kash was in the pediatric intensive care unit – where kids are not allowed).

It was in the PICU that we met several other very ill children and their families. There were some great stories of recovery that we got to watch as we waited for Kash to wake up… there were also some very sad stories that we were on the same floor with. In the PICU we learned about the hand plates, the same hand plates that you remember making and may still have from your childhood or maybe hand plates with your own children's palms on them. These hand plate kits were there for the children that would not make it home. They were there to make a hand print for you to take home after your child had lost their fight. The same day we learned about the hand plates the hospital chaplain came by, and I remember I got very angry because on TV they only come by to bless or baptize the dying. Again, I was wrong. I asked Kerri, 'What the hell is he doing here?' and she informed me that he had been by every day to pray with Kash.

FAST FORWARD and Kash woke up. He battled seizures for the first several days until they got him on an appropriate dose and schedule to keep the seizures at bay. Kash had reverted back to a newborn. He had no muscle strength or control (couldn't even hold his head up) and had lost the words that he had begun to say before the seizure. BUT OUR KASH WOKE UP AND CAME BACK TO US.

(Kerri's narrative)

FAST FORWARD. A year later Kash is 2 and still doesn't have many spoken words; he can actually sign more than he speaks. Kash is running, laughing, smiling, crying and gives us kisses. He did wake up a little different from before and not just with the loss of speech, or the left-sided weakness, but he NEVER gave my husband kisses before the seizure, just myself. Now, my husband and I get more kisses than we can manage with one face. Kash has speech therapy every week, has a state-funded therapist that comes out an additional two times a month for speech, PT, and OT, sees a neurologist, and also goes to a spasticity specialist. We are also in the process of getting him into see a pediatric stroke specialist because, during his coma, Kash also suffered a stroke that has left him with left-side weakness. With Kash turning 3 in May, he will also begin his adventure in school, and will be placed in a special needs education class. With all that Kash and our family have been through, looking at his face is a constant reminder of the second chance of life that we have been given. Kash is living proof that God still performs miracles. I will NOT be passive in my journey with a vaccine-injured child. I will use this as a chance to educate other parents, future parents, grandparents, and anyone else that will listen.

(Story originally published on the vactruth.org website)

The Story Of Johanna

On September 28, 2011, my three-year-old daughter, Johanna, was diagnosed with type-1 diabetes, an autoimmune disorder. As there is no history of type-1 diabetes in my or my wife's immediate family, we couldn't establish a genetic link, leading us to look for external factors. At Johanna's diagnosis, an A1C test was performed, measuring her glucose levels over the past three months. When comparing the A1C results to the onset of symptoms as expressed by behavioral signs, it became evident that the onset of Johanna's autoimmune disorder and the administration of vaccines matched.

I have been screened for positive auto-antibodies and none were found. My wife has been screened for positive auto-antibodies and none were found—neither of us passed diabetes on to our daughter. My parents have no signs of type-1 diabetes, and neither did my grandparents. I have four brothers and sisters; none have type-1 diabetes. My wife's parents have no signs of type-1 diabetes, and neither does her brother. Her grandparents never showed signs of type-1 diabetes.

There's no genetic link; therefore something must have overcome Johanna's natural resistance to type-1 diabetes. Numerous medical articles suggest that vaccine adjuvants (by definition, an adjuvant is an ingredient intended to aid in the effectiveness of the vaccine, substances such as aluminum and mercury) can cause autoimmune disorders. Shaw Tomljenovic, from the National Center for Biotechnology Information states: "experimental evidence shows that simultaneous administration of as little as two to three immune adjuvants can overcome genetic resistance to autoimmunity."

Vaccines caused my daughter to develop an autoimmune disorder— possibly for the rest of her life. And they have no doubt caused other children to suffer from type-1 diabetes and other autoimmune disorders. Research shows that when one part of the immune system is over-excited, the others may not function adequately, and the one targeted is likely to react excessively and ineffectively, such as in the case of allergies and autoimmune disease.

Whenever Johanna was vaccinated, signs of allergies appeared. We could never quite figure out why she had so many allergic reactions. The signs of allergies became mild a few weeks after the vaccines were administered, and disappeared after we stopped vaccinating our children completely. But now she suffers from an autoimmune disease. Why? Because her immune system reacted excessively and ineffectively to the vaccines she was given.

My research journey took me to Germany, Israel, and the US. The deeper that journey led me into vaccine safety, the more emotional this research became as I realized that I had needlessly harmed my child by having her vaccinated. I found pediatricians, general practitioners, and scientists falling victim to confirmation bias—only looking for, or only accepting, research that supported their pro-vaccine arguments. As I have listened to many of the pro-vaccine arguments given by pediatricians to persuade concerned parents, I was astonished that a simple search at the National Library of Medicine provided me with an abundance of credible research articles showing the harm vaccines can do.

In a research article conducted by the Department of Medicine at the Ottawa Hospital Research Institute, the researchers concluded, "There are significantly elevated risks of primarily emergency room visits approximately one to two weeks following 12- and 18-month vaccination." The researchers found that for every live vaccine given, there's one high-risk event to be expected for every 168 twelve-month-olds vaccinated, and one high-risk event for every 170 eighteen-month-old children vaccinated. Doctors expect to see twenty seizures for every 100,000 children vaccinated. Slowly it became evident to me that vaccinating our children is a shot in the dark, like playing the lottery using our children's lives.

I wonder why it was that as a parent, I hadn't been informed in greater detail that vaccines had the potential of causing incredible harm to my children. Why was it that pediatricians and pediatric nurses, the people to whom we had entrusted our children's health, didn't engage us in a dialogue, pointing out the potential adverse events in order for us to make a well-informed decision?

Why was it that any drug commercial on TV informed me of most possible, even unlikely side effects, but only a few were mentioned as far as vaccines were concerned?

Had I known that vaccines could cause unpredictable damage in children and that adjuvants used in vaccines had the potential of causing the immune system to attack its own cells (as in type-1 diabetes and other autoimmune disorders), I would have never exposed my children to vaccines, and I am convinced that I would have spared my daughter the torture of a life-long autoimmune disorder.

Markus Heinze is the father of Johanna and author of the book *VACCeptable Injuries* vacceptableinjuries.com

* * *

Thank you to Sherrel, April, Amanda, Sara, Markus, Marcella, Kerri and Cody for allowing me to use their children's tragic stories. These are just a few of *many cases*I have come across and, as tragic as they are, there are even far more severe stories out there. One lady I personally came into contact with, lost her newborn son Ian. After Ian was born, he wasn't very well and suffered with a compromised immune system, and was treated for various conditions. He got better, but before he was allowed home, the parents were told he had to be given a hepatitis B injection. The vaccine immediately gave him a very bad reaction. He eventually fell into a coma and died days later. The parents had no idea this could happen to their baby – they weren't informed of the risks beforehand.

People who hear about these so-called rare stories may ask their doctors if the reactions are something to be concerned about. Their doctors usually say, 'Of course, there are always some people who don't respond well to vaccines, but it's such a small, insignificant tiny number.' But the *real* truth is that reactions are happening every day, on a *much* larger scale.

Here is why you don't know about it. The problem is, rarely are they *officially* recorded, *because the hospitals and doctors will hardly ever admit (or even think) that the vaccine actually caused the injury.* Remember, its said that only 10% of reactions are properly reported, which means the real numbers are far, far greater than what we are being told. So for trusting parents, it is easy to go away thinking that the reactions occur in only a few 'unlucky' children. And try telling Sara, Deborah, Bella, Aydan, Johanna and Kash that they were just 'unlucky'. Does that make it any better for them?

Here is something to think about: why don't people get tested *before* being given shots to see if they are going to have a reaction to certain chemicals? Like the recommendation from Dr. Natasha Campbell-McBride, why don't children get tested to see how their gut function is behaving *before* they get vaccinated? After all the deaths and injuries related to vaccines, shouldn't there be measures in place to test for safety before these problems happen? Shouldn't there be long-term studies on the entire vaccine schedule performed over decades? Considering that vaccines have been around for at least a hundred years by now, it is *very* odd that this has not yet happened.

People who are concerned about vaccine safety are certainly not alone, and in fact on social networking sites such as Facebook there are thousands of people joining groups such as the 'Vaccination Information Network' (VINE) which had 36,250 members at the time of writing. The Refusers Facebook group had 18,034. I predict that by the time my book comes out, the numbers will be far higher. These groups have open discussions on studies, injuries and why they are concerned about vaccinating their children. And they're full of *educated* parents who have *done their research* and have genuine questions that the medical profession are not able to answer satisfactorily.

Despite so many speaking out about the dangers of vaccines, many are not 'anti-vaccine'. They are, instead, hoping for *safer* ones, or that the medical authorities will now recommend giving vaccines to children spread out over time and to also not give so many vaccines when an infant is very young.

Why don't vaccines openly carry the warnings, when there are health warnings about certain foods?

I find it *really* odd that children who have peanut and other food allergies have concerned the health world so much that the food manufacturers have to label their products with certain warnings, yet when it comes to the hundreds of thousands of vaccine injuries, including the many deaths, vaccines are still classed as totally *safe for all* – and that these reactions are thought to be 'minor' and 'very rare'.

Far fewer children have died due to peanuts than to vaccines. And the news that the medical authorities plan to add *even more* vaccines to the already heavy current recommended schedule means that there will be *even more* reactions in the future. This is a sickening guarantee.

Please also be aware that the multiple-shot vaccines have *never* been properly tested for safety, or they have been tested in general for way too short a time, and there have also *never* been tests for safety on the *entire vaccine schedule*. So the 38 or so vaccines your children are supposed to have by the age of 4 have not gone through the rigorous testing you would expect with such *serious* medications.

For more real vaccine-injury stories, which are something to not be ignored, please visit

✓ www.followingvaccinations.com

What makes a doctor speak out about vaccines?

A growing number of highly trained doctors and scientists, now in the thousands, are beginning to speak out about vaccine safety and efficiency. It's interesting to note that they originally very much believed in them and would administer them to children and adults and would think that non-vaccinating parents were totally irresponsible. Why, then, are so many starting now to question them?

Below is Dr. Donegan s story, which poses a lot of questions we should all be asking.

Dr. Jayne Donegan's story

Having trained as a conventional medical doctor, qualifying from St. Mary's Hospital Medical School, University of London, in 1983, all of my undergraduate teaching and postgraduate experience in Obstetrics & Gynecology, Family Planning, Child Health, Orthopedics, Emergency Medicine and General Practice led me to be a strong supporter of the Universal Childhood Vaccination Program. Indeed, I used to counsel parents in the 1980s who didn't want to vaccinate their children against whooping cough – which was regarded as the 'problematic' vaccine in those days. I used to tell them that there were, indeed, adverse reactions, associated with the vaccine – I was not one of those doctors who would gloss over such unpleasant details – but that we doctors were told that the adverse reactions that might occur after the pertussis vaccine were at least ten times less likely than the chance of getting complications from having the disease, and that, essentially, the point of giving their child the vaccine was to prevent them from getting the disease.

Indeed, I used to think that parents who didn't want to vaccinate their children were either ignorant, or sociopathic. I believe that view is not uncommon among doctors today. Why did I have this attitude? Well, throughout my medical training I was taught that the people who used to die in their thousands or hundreds of thousands from diseases like diphtheria, whooping cough and measles – diseases for which there are vaccines – stopped dying because of the introduction of vaccines.

At the same time, I was taught that diseases like typhus, cholera, rheumatic and scarlet fever – for which there are no vaccines – stopped killing people because of improvements in social conditions. It would have been a logical progression to have asked myself why, if social conditions improved the health of the population with respect to some diseases, would they not improve their health with regard to them all, but the amount of information that you are required to absorb during medical training is so huge that you just tend to take it as read and not make the connections that might be obvious to someone else. It was a received article of faith for me and my contemporaries that vaccination was the single most useful health intervention that ever been introduced, and when my children were born in 1991 and 1993 I unquestioningly – well, that is to say, I thought it was with full knowledge backed up by all my medical training – had them vaccinated, up as far as MMR, because that was the right thing to do. I even let my 4-week-old daughter be injected with an out-of-date BGC vaccine at a public health clinic. I noticed (force of habit – I automatically scan vials for drug name, batch number and expiry date) that the vaccine was out of date and said, 'Oh, excuse me, it looks like it's out of date', and the doctor answered matter-of-factly, 'Oh don't worry, that's why the clinic was delayed for an hour – we were just checking that it was OK to give it, and it is', and I said, 'OK', and let her inject it… my poor daughter had a terrible reaction, but I was so convinced that it was all for the best that I carried on with all the rest of them at 2, 3 and 4 months.

That is where I was coming from – even my interest in homeopathy didn't dent my enthusiasm for vaccines; so far as I could see, it was the same process – give a small dose of something and it makes you immune – no conflict. So what happened? In 1994 there was the Measles Rubella Campaign in which 7 million school-children were vaccinated against measles and rubella. The Chief Medical Officer sent out letters to all GPs, pharmacists, nursing officers and other healthcare staff, telling us that there was going to be an epidemic of measles. The evidence for this epidemic was not published at the time. In later years it seems that it was predicted by a complicated mathematical model based on estimates and so might never have been going to occur at all. We were told, 'Everybody who has had one dose of the vaccine will not necessarily be protected when the epidemic comes. So they need another one.' 'Well, that's

OK,' I thought, 'because we know that none of the vaccines are 100% effective.'

What did worry me, however, was when they said that even those who had had two doses of measles vaccine would not necessarily be protected when the epidemic came and that they needed a third. You may not remember, but in those days there was only one measles vaccine in the schedule. It was a live virus vaccine, so it was like coming in contact with the wild virus, just changed slightly to make it safer and leading to immunity. Since then, of course, the pre-school dose has been added because one dose didn't work, but in those days there was just 'one shot for life'. And now we were being told that even two shots of a 'one shot' vaccine would not protect people when the epidemic came. At this point I began to ask myself, 'Why have I been telling all these parents that vaccines are safer than getting the disease and that basically, having the vaccine will stop their children getting the disease – with the risk of complications – it's not 100%, but that's basically what they're designed to do – when it seems that they can be vaccinated, have whatever adverse reactions are associated with the vaccine, and still get the disease with whatever complications may be associated with that, even when they've had two doses of the "one shot" vaccine? So what was the point? This doesn't seem right.'

If you are wondering how come anyone would have had two doses of the 'one shot vaccine', it is because when the MMR was introduced in 1988, many children had already been vaccinated against measles, but we were told that we should give them the MMR anyway as it would 'protect them against mumps and rubella and boost their measles immunity'. We were also told that the best way of vaccinating was en masse, because this would 'break the chain of transmission'. So I thought, 'I wonder why we vaccinate all these small babies at 2, 3 and 4 months? Why don't we just wait two or three years and then vaccinate everyone who has been born in the meantime, and "break the chain of transmission".'

So some things just didn't seem to quite add up. However, it is very hard to start seriously questioning whether or not vaccination is anything other than safe and effective, especially when it is something that you have been taught to believe in so strongly. The more medically qualified you are, the more difficult it is, as in some ways the more brainwashed you are. It's not easy, or at least it wasn't then, to start going down a path that might lead you in the opposite direction to all your colleagues and the healthcare system in which you work. I read some books that could be described as 'anti-vaccination'. They contained graphs showing that the majority of the decrease in deaths from and incidence of the infectious diseases for which we have vaccines occurred before the vaccines were introduced in the 1950s and 60s, for example with whooping cough, and in the late 1960s with measles. I decided that I couldn't just accept what these books were telling me, especially as the message was the opposite to what I had learned up until now. I needed to do some research. The graphs in my textbooks and the Department of Health Immunization Handbook (the Green Book) appeared to show that the introduction of vaccines caused precipitous falls in deaths from vaccinatable diseases.

I decided that if I were going to seriously question what I'd been taught at medical school and by my professors, I would have go and get the real data for myself. Accordingly, I called the Office for National Statistics (ONS) and asked them to send me the graphs of deaths from the diseases against which we vaccinate from the middle of the nineteenth century, when we started keeping records, until now. They said, 'We don't have them – except for smallpox and TB; we suggest you try the Department of Health.' Which I did. They didn't have graphs from the nineteenth or early twentieth century either. They said, 'You'd better try the Office for National Statistics.' 'I've already tried them,' I said. 'They were the ones who advised me to contact you.' It seems to be getting rather circular, so I called up the ONS once again and told them my problem. 'Well,' they said, 'we have all the books here from when the Registrar General started taking returns of deaths from infectious diseases in 1837; you can come along and look at them if you like.' There was nothing for it.

I had to go the Office for National Statistics (ONS) in Pimlico, London, with my two young children aged 6 and 4 in tow, to extract the information myself. The girls were very good – they were used to traveling/following me around – and the library staff were very nice; they kindly gave my daughters orange juice to drink, and paper and crayons to draw with and amuse themselves, while I pulled out all the mothy old books from 1837 until 1900, after which, thankfully, there was a CD ROM that could be bought at vast expense and taken home. It was the most user-unfriendly piece of data storage that I have ever come across, but it was better than having to physically be there day after day. So I went home with all my notes and the CD Rom and eventually produced my own graphs. I was startled to find that they were similar to the graphs in some of the books that I had recently read. I was astonished and not a little perturbed to find that when you draw a graph of the death rate from whooping cough that starts in the mid nineteenth century, you can clearly see that at least 99% of the people who used to die of whooping cough in the nineteenth and early twentieth century had stopped dying before the vaccine against whooping cough was introduced, initially in the 1950s and universally in the 1960s.

I also realized that the reason the Department of Health's graphs made the vaccine appear so effective was because they didn't start until the 1940s when most of the improvements in health had already occurred, and this was before even antibiotics were generally available. If you selected only deaths in under-15-year-olds, the drop was even more dramatic – by the time whooping cough vaccine was part of the universal immunization schedule in the early 1960s all the hard work had been done. I now began to realize that graphs such as those featured in the Department of Health Green Book were not a good or clear way of showing the changes in mortality (death) and morbidity (incidence of disease) that occurred before and after vaccination was introduced against these diseases.

Measles is similar: the Department of Health Green Book features a graph that does not start until the 1940s. There appears to be great drop in the number of cases after the measles vaccine was introduced in 1968, but looking at a graph which goes back to the 1900s you can see that the death rate – death being the worst-case complication of a disease – had dropped by 99% by the time the vaccine was put on the schedule. Looking specifically at under-15-year-olds, it is possible to see that there was a virtual 100% decline in deaths from measles between 1905 and 1965 – three years before the measles vaccine was introduced in the UK. In the late 1990s there was an advertisement for MMR which featured a baby in nappies sitting on the edge of a cliff with a lion prowling on the other side and a voice-over saying, 'No loving parent would deliberately leave their baby unprotected and in danger.'

I think it would have been more scientific to have put one of the graphs using information from the ONS in the advert – then parents would have had a greater chance of making an informed choice, rather than being coerced by fear. When you visit your GP or Health Visitor to discuss the vaccination issue, and you come away feeling scared, this is because you are picking up how they feel.

If all you have is the 'medical model' for disease and health, all you know is that there is a hostile world out there and if you don't have vaccines, antibiotics and 100% bactericidal handwash, you will have no defense at all against all those germs with which you and your children are surrounded. Your child *may* be OK when they get the measles, but you can never tell when disaster will strike, and they may be left disabled or dead by the random hand of fate. I was like that myself, and when the awful realization began to dawn on me that vaccines weren't all they were cracked up to be, I started looking in a panic for some other way of protecting my children and myself – some other magic bullet. My long, slow journey researching the vaccination disease ecology involved learning about other models and philosophies of health and the gradual realization that it was true what people had told me all along, that 'health is the only immunity'.

We don't need to be protected from 'out there'. We get infectious diseases when our body needs to have a periodic clean-out. Children especially benefit from childhood spotty rashes, or 'ex anthems' as they are called, in order to make appropriate developmental leaps. When we have fevers, coughs, rashes, we need to treat them supportively, not suppressively. In my experience, the worst complications of childhood infections are caused by standard medical treatment which involves suppressing all the symptoms. What is the biggest obstacle to doctors even entertaining the possibility that the Universal Childhood Vaccination Program may not be the unmitigated success that it is portrayed to be? Or that there may be other ways of achieving health that are better and longer lasting? Possibly it is the fear of stepping out of line and being seen to be different – with all the consequences that this can entail, as I know from personal experience.

As George Bernard Shaw says in his preface to 'The Doctor's Dilemma', 1906 : 'Doctors are just like other Englishmen: most of them have no honor and no conscience: what they commonly mistake for these is sentimentality and an intense dread of doing anything that everybody else does not do, or omitting to do anything that everybody else does.'

Dr. Jayne L. M. Donegan MBBS DRCOG DCH DFFP MRCGP MFHom

Holistic GP and Homeopathic Physician

Here is some very interesting information regarding Dr. Donegan, and why her authority on vaccines should be paid attention to, simply because the medical world actually did. In 2002 Dr. Donegan went to the High Court as she was involved in a case where two mothers were fighting their ex-partners about their children's vaccinations. The mothers did not want them to be given to their children under any circumstances, for fears of causing irreversible harm, but the fathers did, so a controversial court case ensued. Dr. Donegan had been writing publicly about vaccinations and natural ways of keeping children healthy so she was asked to be an expert witness by the mothers. She gave her opinion that the safety and efficacy (how well they work) of vaccines has not been well studied and that there were other ways of achieving health than vaccination for these children. The case proved very long and extremely stressful. At times it was under very unfair circumstances where she would be given hardly any time to get documents together, despite the opposition having double the time to prepare theirs. Due to the information she was providing in court, (which went against the typical mainstream medical advice), the Appeal Judges called her evidence "Junk Science" and the GMC (General Medical Council) - the organisation that regulates doctors and tells them how to practice - targeted the doctor herself. Dr. Donegan ended up being accused of 'serious professional misconduct' which could have eventually ended Dr Donegan's entire medical career. They served her official papers in 2004. but it took three long years of writing reports and going through hundreds of medical documents and studies before the case was finally heard in 2007. The allegations are below:

"That you (Dr. Donegan):
6a. Gave false and/ or misleading impressions of the research which you relied upon, 6b. Quoted selectively from research, reports and publications and omitted relevant information, 6c. Allowed your deeply held views on the subject of immunisation to overrule your duty to the court and to the litigants, 6d. Failed to present an objective, independent and unbiased view;
7. Your actions in head 6. above were, 7a. Misleading, 7b. In direct contravention to your duty as an expert witness; unprofessional, 7c. Likely to bring the profession into disrepute; And that in relation to the facts alleged by you have been guilty of serious professional misconduct."

As I am sure you can appreciate reading this, these allegations were incredibly serious. They basically said that the testimony Dr. Donegan provided in court was made up, that she was giving harmful advice, which could damage the entire medical profession and had allowed her personal views to come into the case. Over the next three years Dr. Donegan had to prepare her defence, answer letters, go through stacks of evidence and collate documents which made it very difficult to look after her family or carry on her professional life as a doctor. She also had to cope with having her legal team withdrawing from the case, six weeks before she was originally due in court. Dr. Donegan then managed to find Mr Clifford Miller, a lawyer, who was exceptionally well read on the subject of vaccination. Not only was Mr Miller very good with the law, he was also a scientist having attained a BSc in physics. He had an in-depth knowledge of the scientific method, what constitutes scientific 'proof' and how this is very different from what is *accepted* as 'proof' in a court of law. This case had started out with almost impossible odds, yet after almost three years of legal wrangling and a three-week hearing at the by the GMC panel in Manchester the GMC came to this conclusion:

"The Panel were sure that at no stage did you allow any views that you held to overrule your duty to the court and to the litigants.

You demonstrated to the Panel that your reports did not derive from your deeply held views and your evidence supported this. You explained to the Panel that your approach in your report was to provide the court with a alternative view based on the material you produced in your references. That material was largely drawn from publications that were in fact in favour of immunisation.

It was clear from your evidence and the evidence of your witness that your aim is to direct parents to sources of information about immunisation and child health safety to help them to make informed choices.

You told us that there are many books by doctors and others in this and other countries who seriously question vaccination and they cite a lot of history, proofs and medical papers to support their arguments. You did not use any of those publications because you did not think that the GMC would regard those as satisfactory support or references for your recommendations. You largely used what was available in refereed medical journals.

The Panel is sure that in the reports you provided you did not fail to be objective, independent and unbiased.

Accordingly, the Panel found that you are not guilty of serious professional misconduct."

The case between Dr. Donegan and the GMC was very much like that of David and Goliath, and was another rare example of David actually winning.

I would like you to have a really *serious* think about this trial, the claims that were made, the eventual outcome and what it might mean about the *entire vaccine industry*. Dr. Donegan was called upon as a witness to provide evidence that children *do not need vaccines to be healthy* and that many are unnecessary and unsafe. She presented her evidence against a very tough opposition involving many QCs and a very expensive legal team, yet Dr. Donegan and her much smaller team WON the case. What do you think it means about the evidence she provided and the fact that this medical council could not prove her wrong? What does this cause you to think about vaccines now?

This shocking outcome with its unlikely win - surprise surprise, never really made it into the media. When Dr. Donegan was first accused of serious professional misconduct it did, but after she won, there was hardly any media attention at all. Yet wouldn't you think the public deserved to know this outcome? Dr. Donegan was asked after her GMC enquiry ended, what had she learnt from this experience:

'Perhaps it is that if a parent says, "I'm worried about the safety of vaccination," they are told, "You don't understand, you're not a doctor." However if a doctor says, "I'm worried about the safety of vaccination," they are told, "We're charging you with serious professional misconduct..."

You can find the details of this case and much more information in general about vaccines on her website http://www.jayne-donegan.co.uk/

Can we always trust the drug companies who make the vaccines?

It seems the answer is a resounding no, as was recently uncovered in the early part of 2012. Merck, who make many of the vaccines given to people all over the world, are being taken to court due to serious allegations:

Scientists sue Merck: allege fraud, mislabeling, and false certification of MMR vaccine

by Suzanne Humphries MD

Vaccinationists tell us we don't understand science. Well, maybe they are right. 'Science' in the world of vaccines could mean: throwing out results that don't fit the desired outcome, throwing out the evidence before the FDA comes to inspect, offering bonuses to scientists to deliver the necessary results ... I was the head technician in a biochemistry lab for two years prior to medical school, yet I never saw science carried out like that. Maybe Temple University was just a bit behind the times in its evolution of 'science'.

This is the story of the MMR vaccine and two Merck scientists who filed a lawsuit in 2010 over Merck's efforts to allegedly 'defraud the United States through Merck's ongoing scheme to sell the government a mumps vaccine that is mislabeled, misbranded, adulterated and falsely certified as having an efficacy rate that is significantly higher than it actually is'. Merck allegedly did this from

2000 onwards in order to maintain its exclusive license to sell the MMR vaccine and keep its monopoly of the US market.

In the complaint, the scientists outline in great detail exactly how Merck manipulated the efficacy results in order to be able to say they had a 95% effective vaccine so that they could meet the fairytale goal of vaccine-induced 'herd immunity by 2010'. Well, it turns out that the vaccine could not meet the goal that CDC projected to eradicate mumps by 2010, BECAUSE the vaccine in its current state cannot reliably confer immunity, and is in fact a dilute version of what it once was when Maurice Hilleman invented it using the virus of his five-year-old daughter. The same viral mumps strain has been in use in every mumps or MMR vaccine Merck has made since 1967.

In order to mass-produce live but non-infective vaccine virus, the 'wild' virus from 1967 has had to be 'passaged' through different cells or animals over and over and over. In that passaging, mutations take place that render the virus non-infective or 'attenuated' but also, those many years of passaging the same original viral strain has lowered the antigenicity, or the antibody-stimulating capacity of the virus.

When testing was performed to show the efficacy (neutralizing antibody provoking potential) of the forty-year-old virus strain, for use in the newer combination mumps vaccines, Merck's scientists could not produce a 95% efficacy rate.

Merck got the old virus to pass its new tests by doing three things. First they tested efficacy on the vaccine strain virus and not the wild virus as had previously been done. The testing is done by vaccinating children and testing the ability of their blood to neutralize the virus before and after the vaccine. There should be a marked difference between the two tests. For the new testing method, the children's blood was tested for its ability to neutralize the virus, using the vaccine strain virus, instead of the wild-type strain that is much more infective, and the one that your children would most likely catch. By using a weaker virus, the old vaccine strain virus allowed the neutralization to occur much more easily.

But still it was not 95% effective.

In order to make the blood pass the test, antibodies from rabbits were added. The addition of rabbit antibody increased the efficacy to 100%. But that was not the end, because the test has to be done on pre-vaccine blood and post-vaccine blood. Just the addition of rabbit antibody made the pre-vaccine blood go from 10% positive to 80% positive and that was such an obvious sign of foul play that yet another manipulation had to be made. The desired end result is to have very low pre-vaccine viral neutralization and 95% or more post-vaccine viral neutralization.

So... yet one more change in procedure was made: The pre-vaccine 'positive' tests were all recounted. None of the post vaccine tests and none of the post-vaccine negatives were recounted, just the pre-vaccine positives. According to the Merck scientists, they did this by fabricating the 'plaque' counts on the pre-vaccine blood samples, counting plaques that were not there. The test is called a 'plaque reduction neutralization' (PRN) assay. Plaques are areas on cell culture dishes where a virus attacks cells, demonstrating viral activity and lack of immunity. Because the rabbit antibodies were used in the pre-vaccine tests, there was positive PRN meaning that the pre-vaccine blood looked immune, or that there was plaque reduction. This is not desired when wanting to show that the vaccine is what led to the immunity, where you would only want the post-vaccine samples to have positive PRN – or a reduction in plaques. So, the pre-vaccine positive PRN assays were recounted because there were not enough plaques to show the desired result – that virus was active in the pre-vaccine tests. According to the scientists, plaques were counted where there were none. This allowed a mathematical dilution of the pre-vaccine positive PRN tests, turning them negative. The complaint says that 45% of the pre-vaccine samples recounted were revised.

According to the complaint, the plates used to recount the pre-vaccine positive PRN tests were discarded just before the FDA arrived to inspect.

While this alleged fraudulent activity was occurring in Merck's labs, two courageous scientists voiced their objection. They claim to have been told that if they called the FDA they would be jailed. They were also reminded of the very large bonuses that were on the way after the vaccines were certified.

If what these scientists claim is true, the net result of Merck's questionable activity was epidemics and outbreaks. It is known that the mumps component of all MMR vaccines from the mid 1990s has had a very low efficacy, estimated at 69% (Harling 05). The outbreaks started in UK and Europe in 1998. USA's outbreaks began in 2006.

These mumps outbreaks have already been proven NOT to be the result of failure to vaccinate, but vaccination failure … and now it looks to all be a result of Merck's cooked books, used in order to maintain a commercial monopoly to generate increased revenue from increasing numbers of boosters.

You can read more from Dr. Suzanne Humphries here:

✓ vaccinationcouncil.org/

Concerned and informed parents on why they won't vaccinate their children

The following is a selection of quotes by parents found in various groups on Facebook. I was inundated when I asked for people to submit their opinions. While I don't know many at all personally, they all seem to be from educated backgrounds, not what people usually think, i.e. not from low socioeconomic groups or people who could be seen as 'uneducated and irresponsible parents':

As I had had a severe reaction to a vaccine as a child, my husband and I were keen to do lots of research before giving any vaccines to our child. We were aware that all vaccinations were toxic before our research, but we were both shocked just how many additional chemicals and additives they actually add to each vaccine. We were also concerned about the decision to combine multiple diseases in single vaccinations to ensure they vaccinated as many children as possible due to poor uptakes in the past. No wonder our research kept highlighting long lists of terrible side effects. We also found out that most vaccines often don't offer full immunity and that any immunity gained is very short-lived.

We were also surprised when looking at the history of vaccines to see that statistics actually showed that vaccination programs were ineffective at stopping the spread of disease and in fact contributed to the spread in many cases as many children develop the disease from the vaccines. Looking at the government statistics you could clearly see these were cleverly manipulated to get their pro-vaccine message across and we started to question why the government would need to do this if the vaccines were as safe and effective as they suggested. Together with the government's vaccination compensation scheme it was clear that even the government didn't believe the vaccines were truly safe. After a lot of research we decided we wouldn't risk the dangerous side effects of a vaccine that might even give our child the disease itself and would only offer very short-lived, if any, immunity, and we would instead rely on our baby developing his own immunity by more natural means such as breastfeeding.

Amy Crumpler, New Forest, UK
Age 28

Injecting a baby with toxic substances to protect their health doesn't make any sense to me. I want my baby to have a strong immune system and to me that means limiting all toxins, giving him the best diet, lots of water, fresh air, sunlight and exercise.

Joanne Thompson, Liverpool, UK
Age 34

I have one fully vaxed, one partially vaxed, and one unvaxed child. They are all breastfed and healthy children. However, my youngest is by far the healthiest. I changed my mind after doing the research required to make an informed decision. The reactions to vaccines (although I believe they are significantly fewer in ebf children) scare me. The ingredients (MSG, mercury, aborted fetal cells, monkey organs...) are against many of my beliefs and standards. Having friends with vaccine-injured children began my quest to really find out what we were injecting into our children. What I found wasn't pretty.

MarthaLynn Albritton Manterfield

From the long list of potential side effects including death and the poisons used in them, as well as the fact that some of them are cultured in aborted fetus tissue... I am a strong Christian woman and I do not believe abortion is acceptable so I would never inject my child with something that was made that way. There are plenty of natural alternatives and my healthy daughter has thrived because we do not vaccinate.

Nicole Cartland Davis

My number one reason is the Hep B vaccine. What possible reason could there be for giving a newborn baby, who is only a few hours old, a vaccine against a sexually transmitted disease? If I can't trust the very first shot a baby will ever get, why should I trust any of the others?

Kimberly Odasso

Probably every doctor or nurse you go to will tell you that 'vaccines are 100% safe' – to assume that vaccines are safe for everyone that is born into this world doesn't make sense to me... we can't even all eat the same exact foods without some of us getting sick... why are vaccines looked at differently??

Denessa Rose

I initially started looking into vaccines when I realized that many of them had fetal cell tissue. As I was looking more into them, I became more concerned with the way they worked. Since my family already lives a fairly natural lifestyle, it was fairly easy to see how a naturally strong immune system is so much better than an artificial one that is weakened further by the toxins and chemicals that are used to irritate the immune system, therefore making the vaccinations 'work'. That, and the increased SIDS risk from all the toxins pushed into little systems and all the problems that can be triggered by the chemicals and stress... it was easy for me to risk worst-case scenarios with the illnesses compared to knowingly risk the worst-case scenarios from vaccines.

Sarah Warren, USA

My husband (a doctor) and I simply did a little research. It was easy enough to find all the hype for vaccinations, and even easier to find the ingredients and search what they were. Just knowing that some of those ingredients are known human carcinogens (known to cause cancer in humans) was enough to never inject my children. They are happy and never had more than a common cold. More importantly I can say my kids are truly healthy. Do any vaxxing moms have kids that ask daily for their vitamins and would rather have apples over fries? Not generally.

Melissa Roberts Redwine, USA

I have made a conscious decision to take personal responsibility for my child's health through breastfeeding, organic vegetarian diet, healthy sanitation practices, and rejection of processed foods. This is all one really needs to fight disease and infection.

Stephanie Erickson

There are three unvaccinated children in my home. Vaccines are unsafe, ineffective and responsible for the spread of disease such as polio and pertussis. The diseases on the schedule do not intimidate me and with a healthy immune system can be fought off without complication. If someone doesn't have a normal immune system, vaccines aren't for them either. I feel SIDS is a cop-out and reclassification of uncompensated vaccine injuries for the majority of cases. The dangers and side effects are the real concern. Not only will injecting your child with a virus (or viruses), aborted fetal cells, toxins and heavy metals NOT make them healthier, it may damage them forever or even kill them. Furthermore, we measure the rate of public health not by the instance of infectious disease but by the rate of chronic illness; by these standards we are failing our children and society. Autism, epilepsy, asthma, allergies, ADHD, obesity, cancer, diabetes, and the epidemic of ear infections. Health comes from clean air, water and nutritious food; none of which are provided by super-corporations or government regulations. It is our responsibility to claim our children's health, because there is a reason you cannot insure against vaccine injury. It's prevalent and nobody's stepping in.

Brittany Sheehan

I am a nurse and a mother of four. I had my oldest daughter when I was young, uninsured and horribly uneducated. Because I was uninsured, my daughter's doctors offered me the chance to enroll her in a vaccine study. By taking part in the study, her Well Child visits would be paid for, including the vaccines, and she would receive $300. All I had to do was keep a journal of her temperature, temperament, appetite, etc. for a week following her injections. I was given the impression that the vaccines were safe and the only difference in these vaccines was that they were combined and she would be getting fewer shots but the same amount of viral protection. I thought it was a win-win situation. It saddens me to think about how many other moms are being taken advantage of the same way. Then I went to nursing school. We were taught where to give and how to give injections, what diseases they prevent, but nothing about delayed schedules, refusals or vaccine injury. I had another daughter after finishing nursing school and she was vaccinated as well. I began working as a school nurse at a pre-school for children with developmental delays and disabilities soon after my daughter was born. I had parents who told me that their children were completely typically developing to a certain age and then just changed. They had pictures and videos of children that were fine before their shots. That's when I actually started looking into the dark side of this system. But I never thought it would happen to my own children.

I knew that children would not be allowed to attend preschools or public school without them, so I knew there was a risk of injury, but in my mind, it was a small risk. Until it wasn't such a small risk. My second daughter was 14 months old when she had her last round of shots. Within 2 hours, her fever was at 102 °F, she was screaming uncontrollably, and inconsolable. I called the doctor, who told me it was normal. I called my husband to come home because I was terrified. I was so afraid she was never going to be the same kid. This is what those other moms told me happened with their kids and I didn't listen. My second daughter is now 5 and will never receive another vaccine. I also have 3-year-old boy/girl twins who have never been vaxed. I fight with the doctors every time we see them (which is very rare), and have been threatened with being fired from their clinic for vaccine refusals. They also wanted to do surgery on my son for recurring ear infections in his first year (he had a kink in his eustachian tube from being mashed in the womb with his sister) but chiropractic care was the better option and worked quickly.

Tasha Tankersley-Hankins

My son would not be vaxed if not for my hubby. Hubby is pro vax, I am not. We compromised. We got selective ones (two as of now and two more later, after our son is 4 years old). I am against because I feel that the potential side effects are much more dangerous than the disease process of which most are very mild. I am opposed to using our children as guinea pigs (with very little testing done prior to injecting into humans). The mere fact that no one investigates or even ENTERTAINS the thought that vax could have detrimental side effects (like autism, ADD, ADHD, arthritis, cancers, etc.) on humans is a very pompous way to think. And if someone (or multiple people) think that, and those people are the pushers of vax or makers of such... Well, then I laugh and mock those people. Because to be pompous is to be ignorant. I am my son's guardian, protector, advocate until he has sense enough to make his own decisions. If he decides to get them at an older age, that's fine. But his body and brain are growing MUCH TOO RAPIDLY, cells turn over so fast, and blood/brain barrier plus kidneys are not fully functioning yet... So who am I to inject aluminum, formaldehyde, etc. WHEN IT'S NOT EVEN 100% guaranteed! Do you see how many vaxed kids get the actual disease?! Do you see how sick our children of America are as a whole?! Gah. Wake up, America, stop being little sheep. Make your decisions for your children but make your decisions 'educated' ones by reading, researching, and reading some more before you say 'Yes' – ignorance is an epidemic in America in everything from birthing (C-sections sky high), food (processed garbage), parenting (no structure/discipline), vaccines (blindly following doctors' advice when it's driven by money/quotas/big pharma) etc.

Crystal McSwiggen Caccamo

None of these comments sound like they are coming from uneducated, irresponsible parents, do they? In fact, don't you think they all seem to know a lot of facts that perhaps you may never have thought or heard of? Pro-vaccine people always dismiss those like me, and the people above who are concerned with the real dangers of vaccinations, as stupid, evil and dangerous. From what you have just read, do you think this is true about *any* of the parents? I certainly don't!

If viruses are always so deadly, then why did entire countries/populations not perish before vaccines were introduced?

This question poses some *very* valid reasons for thinking about what we did hundreds and thousands of years ago to stay alive, long before vaccines were introduced. While we can't deny that there have been some very serious viruses throughout history, causing massive amounts of deaths, we cannot assume that they killed *everyone* that the virus came in contact with because – they didn't. Many people died, yes (and why – I cover below), but many *more* survived. Otherwise we would not be here today. And how did individuals *not* get sick when others would seem to fall ill so very easily? What factors made someone more likely to catch a disease and someone else not contract it at all?

The answer always lies with... you guessed it. The state of their natural *immune system!* If someone had a stronger immune system, their body could fight the virus on its own, the way their body was *naturally* designed to. And when someone was *not* able to fight the virus, it was because something had previously happened to their own immune system to become weakened and not be able to recover. What were these factors? Vital things such as: living in poverty, not getting enough sunlight, having access to only dirty water and not having enough food; these were the main causes of a weakened immune system. Completely logical stuff, right?

The very rich and royalty were able to live longer lives compared to the very poor people because they could afford to have regular meals (which were all organic!), had access to clean water, and were able to live in much cleaner homes. They weren't always immune to disease of course, but it was few and far between compared to others who lived the other way – in filth. When the Black Plague occurred back in the mid 1300s, it did indeed wipe out millions of people, globally; however, it was generally happening in people who were living in absolute slum-like conditions – the very poor, who had no access to clean water, toilets, food or sunlight. They were literally living in s**t. What hope does someone have to kick any virus living like that? So why do we feel more fearful and extremely scared of viruses today, when the countries which vaccinate the most have the *highest standards of living*?

Let's now look at the present day. Why do we think that the poor people of Third World countries have such terrible health? Why do we think they catch viruses and die early deaths? It's the *same for them* as it was back in the 1300s – they too cannot afford what most of us can afford today – and that is the *basic* necessities of a clean life.

Florence Nightingale, the world's most famous nurse, wrote the following in *Notes on Nursing*, in 1860 what she had come to know about infection:

> Diseases are not individuals arranged in classes, like cats and dogs, but conditions, growing out of one another. Is it not living in a continual mistake to look upon diseases as we do now, as separate entities, which must exist, like cats and dogs, instead of looking upon them as conditions, like a dirty and a clean condition, and just as much under our control; or rather as the reactions of kindly nature, against the conditions in which we have placed ourselves? I was brought up to believe that smallpox, for instance, was a thing of which there was once a first specimen in the world, which went on propogating itself, in a perpeatual chain of descent, just as there was a first dog, (or a first pair of dogs) and that smallpox would not begin itself without there having been a parent dog. Since then I have seen with my own eyes and smelled with my own nose smallpox gowing up in first specimens, either in closed rooms or in overcrowded wards where it could not by any possibility have been 'caught', but must have begun. I have seen diseases begin, grow up, and turn into one another. Now, dogs do not turn into cats. I have seen, for instance, with a little overcrowding,

continued fever grow up; and with a little more, typhoid fever; and with a little more, typhus, and all in the same war or hut. Would it not be better, truer, and more practical, if we looked upon disease in this light (for diseases, as all experience shows, are adjectives, not noun-substantives):

True nursing ignores infection, except to prevent it. Cleanliness and fresh air from open windows, with unremitting attention to the patient, are the only defence a true nurse either asks or needs.

Wise and Humane management of the patient is the best safeguard against infection. The greater part of nursing consists of presesrving cleanliness.

Wow. Here we have the most famous nurse in the world, who changed the way nursing and healthcare was carried out in Britain and who also advocated the same for the people of India was saying all those years ago; that *germs do not create disease*. Florence over the course of her career, would have been around hundreds, if not thousands of people suffering from diseases like thyphoid, small pox, cholera, and typhus - yet she herself lived till the ripe old age of 90. If she was wrong, and that the 'germ' was something to fear, then *why* did she survive for so long? After she began to believe that the *dirty conditions* caused disease, she campaigned for cleaner hospital conditions and better living conditions for all people in general. She impacted the medical industry so much that each year on May 12 (her birthday) nurses from all over the world, celebrate International Nurses Day.

My point here is that in regards to the 1300s when plagues broke out, there were *no vaccines*, yet many people who came in contact with a virus were able to *beat it*, with little to no medical help.

Today, we are *made to feel very scared* by the medical world about viruses, that 'we will all catch this or that if we don't have the vaccine', yet most people today are *living in better conditions than ever before*! Why do we need to be giving our children approximately 42 vaccinations by the time they are 4?

It's also very valid to think about the topic of 'fearmongering' and perhaps that's how vaccination became so popular – just like advertising makes a product popular; people rushed out in their thousands to get vaccinated because they were told 'everyone would die' if they did not.

This fearmongering continues more than ever today and also happened quite recently, yet the fear was completely unfounded. Let's look back to the 'swine flu pandemic' of 2009. For the entire year (and they have been trying recently again to scare us that it's back!) we were all being told that 'millions of deaths' were going to occur and that we must run out and get the (incredulously poorly tested) vaccine. Millions of people were highly frightened indeed and not a day went by where stories weren't written about this 'deadly virus'. Yet, *nothing really happened*. There were far *more deaths from the yearly seasonal flu* than the swine flu. And the people who did die from the swine flu had underlying medical conditions, so the swine flu itself was *not* the cause of their death. And in the case of the swine flu vaccine, those people were actually *11 times* more likely to end up in hospital.

Now it looks as though the H1N1 scare of 2009 will go down as one of the biggest government and pharmaceutical scams ever, renewing a healthy, and necessary, skepticism about government fearmongering, the swine flu vaccine and the dubious dealings behind the implementation of worldwide mass-vaccination programs.

It started last month when British and French media began saying the H1N1 pandemic has been 'hyped' by medical researchers to further their own cause, boost research grants and line the pockets of drug companies.

Ontario health officials have also declared H1N1 a 'dud' pandemic, stating the huge government investment made so far may have been unjustified. And now, a new study by researchers at Harvard University and the Medical Research Council Biostatistics Unit in the UK is finding that this 'pandemic' was never a cause for alarm.

After analyzing H1N1 deaths in the United States in the spring, then projecting outcomes for this past fall, they found the flu season should have been no different than a typical flu season – and possibly even milder than average![178]

With so many parents now questioning vaccine risks, it appears we are facing a huge backlash. Many of us just want to be able to talk to people of authority about these issues, to bring up our concerns, to talk about the studies and the ethics of the vaccine companies, to try and get *something* done about these problems. Yet most of us are squashed before a reasonable conversation has even begun. In some USA states, vaccines very soon, may be forced upon children without parental consent. This is *totally* against human rights. Healthcare workers who don't want to get certain vaccines may (and some already have) lose their jobs. And journalists who write articles about these concerns also may face losing their positions. What the heck ever happened to free speech?

Barbara Loe Fisher, president of the Not for Profit National Vaccine Information Centre spoke in a video titled *Desperate Times for Vaccine Risk Denialism* in May 2013 on her website concerning these issues. This is the transcript:

These are desperate times for those denying vaccine risks. We know it because we are witnessing so many acts of desperation being committed by doctors determined to shut down the public conversation about vaccination and health. Vaccine-risk deniers are working overtime to restrict public access to information, cover up vaccine injuries and deaths and violate the human right to informed consent to medical risk-taking.

No Flu Shots? No Employment.

2013 was only a few days old when public health agencies and medical trade groups called for veteran nurses and other healthcare workers to be fired for refusing to obey orders to get annual flu shots – no exceptions and no questions asked. It did not matter that the risky and notoriously ineffective influenza vaccine turned out to be almost useless in preventing infection with the most prevalent influenza strains circulating in the U.S. this year.

Proposed State Legislation to Force Vaccine Use

This was followed by the introduction of legislation backed by public health officials and Pharma-funded medical trade groups like the American Academy of Pediatrics in states like Texas, Oregon, Arizona and Vermont. Their goal is to remove or restrict non-medical vaccine exemptions in state laws so doctors have more power to force vaccine use by children and adults - no questions asked and no exceptions.

Institute of Medicine Report: Where Is the Good Vaccine Science?

In mid-January came the eye-opening Institute of Medicine committee report acknowledging that only 37 scientific studies have examined the safety of the current U.S. vaccine schedule for newborns and children under age six, which now totals a stunning 49 doses of 14 vaccines compared to 23 doses of 7 vaccines recommended in 1983. The lack of enough good scientific studies meant the committee could not determine whether the numbers of doses and timing of government recommended vaccinations is - or is not - associated with development of chronic health problems like seizures, autoimmunity, allergies, learning disabilities and autism in the first six years of life.

New U.S. Autism Prevalence Statistic: 1 Child in 50

CDC Study Fails to Confirm Offit's Claim 10,000 Vaccines Safe for Babies

On Good Friday, April 1, during Easter and Passover observances, a study conducted and funded by the Centers for Disease Control was released by the *Journal of Pediatrics* declaring that "increasing exposure to antibody stimulating proteins and polysaccharides in vaccines is not associated with risk of autism" and, therefore, vaccines don't cause autism. It was a pathetic attempt to validate a Machiavellian hypothesis forwarded in 2002 by pediatric vaccine developer Paul Offit claiming that an infant could safely respond to 10,000 vaccines given at any one time.

However, an eighth-grade science class student with an elementary understanding of health research methods, the bioactivity of various vaccine ingredients and the difference between naturally acquired and vaccine-acquired immunity, could figure out that the absence of an unvaccinated control group meant the study was fatally flawed. It proved absolutely nothing about the potential relationship between administration of multiple vaccinations in early childhood and the development of autism among genetically diverse children with and without increased biological susceptibility to adverse responses to vaccination.

Pediatricians Label Social Networking Parents "Nonconformers"

On April 15, *Pediatric News* published an online survey stating the obvious: a person's knowledge, values and beliefs, as well as the opinions of friends and families in social networks, strongly influences decisions about vaccination. Parents, who expressed doubts about vaccine safety and used alternative vaccine schedules for their children, were pejoratively labeled as "nonconformers".

Pediatricians commenting on the survey suggested that nonconforming parents did not base their vaccine decisions on "rational logic" and "scientific evidence" because they were influenced by non-conforming friends and misleading information on nonconforming websites. Apparently, there was no consideration given to the fact that nonconforming parents found the poor science and empty rhetoric buttressing one-size-fits-all vaccine policies entirely unconvincing.

Journalist & Magazine Attacked for Article Questioning Gardasil Safety

April was also the month that a veteran journalist and radio show host was personally attacked by pediatricians and public health officials in Buffalo, New York for daring to write an article questioning the safety of Gardasil vaccine and urging parents to make informed vaccine choices. Outraged doctors threatened to financially ruin the magazine that published the article by destroying the magazine's paid advertising base unless the article was retracted.

Offit Plays Class & Race Card to Demonize Smart Nonconforming Parents

By the end of April, a CNN reporter quoted doctors blaming outbreaks of whooping cough, measles and mumps on unvaccinated people in developed nations, who spread their vaccine safety doubts on the Internet and jeopardize the health of people around the world. Crassly playing both the class AND race card, the magical thinking, attention seeking Dr. Offit offered the opinion that "It is the upper middle class, well-educated Caucasian parents who are shunning vaccines. They have generally gone to graduate school, are in positions of management and are used to being in control," he said flatly.

Doctors playing the blame game apparently disagree about whether nonconforming parents asking questions about vaccines are simply stupid and irrational or are just over-educated, rich white folks refusing to acknowledge the intellectual superiority and infallibility of those with M.D., PhD or MPH written after their names regardless of the color of their skin or how much money they make.

Doctors like Offit, Halsey, Plotkin, Omer and others denying vaccine risks are blaming everyone but themselves for the miserable statistic that 1 child in 50 in America develops a type of brain and immune dysfunction labeled autism when it used to be 1 child in 2000 before they dumped three times as many vaccinations on babies.

Regression Into Poor Health After Vaccination: A Universal Experience

What doctors drowning in denialism refuse to accept is that, today, everybody knows somebody who was healthy, got vaccinated and was never healthy again. That pattern of regression into poor health, that universal experience of suffering after use of a pharmaceutical product that has a long, well-documented history of risks and failures, is why the public conversation about health and vaccination in the 21stcentury must and will continue. It will continue until doctors, who are pushing more and more vaccines on children and adults already more highly vaccinated and sicker than ever, come up with a much better explanation than it's "bad genes," "better diagnosing" or all "a coincidence."

Vaccine Makers and Doctors Shielded from Liability Have Ethical Duty

In the U.S., vaccine manufacturers are shielded from product liability in civil court and doctors promoting and administering vaccines are also shielded from vaccine injury lawsuits. Doctors without legal accountability have an even greater ethical duty to encourage patients and parents of minor children to become educated about all risks and honor the vaccination decisions patients or parents make, even if the doctor does not personally agree with the decision made.

"Freedom of thought, speech and conscience are deeply valued and constitutionally protected rights in America. The public trust in the integrity of public health policies is destroyed when defensive doctors unwilling to share decision-making power fail to respect the human right to informed consent to medical risk taking and behave like schoolyard bullies instead of compassionate healers committed to, first, doing no harm."

References for this article *Desperate Times for Vaccine Risk Denialism* can all be found here: nvic.org

What to do when you do vaccinate your child

For some parents despite knowing all of this new information, might still decide to vaccinate their children. I have included some essential information for you below so that you can prepare yourself for vaccinating in a way that may cause them the *least* amount of harm.

First, please ask your doctor before you go ahead on the day, these 8

important questions:

1 Am I or my child sick right now?
2 Have I or my child had a bad reaction to a vaccination before?
3 Do I or my child have a personal or family history of vaccine reactions, neurological disorders, severe allergies or immune system problems?
4 Do I know the disease and vaccine risks for myself or my child?
5 Do I have full information about the vaccine's side effects?
6 Do I know how to identify and report a vaccine reaction?
7 Do I know I need to keep a written record, including the vaccine manufacturer's name and lot number, for all vaccinations?
8 Do I know I have the right to make an informed choice?

I would also strongly recommend that you ask to see the vaccine insert *before* you vaccinate, read the small print about *all* of the warnings, and take it home and keep it somewhere safe.

For those who do not want to vaccinate but feel they are being forced/pressured to and cannot seem to get religious, spiritual or medical exemptions, the following disclaimer is highly beneficial to give to the doctor and nurses who are going to be administering the shots. It has been prepared by a team of lawyers in London care of What Doctors Don't Tell You, 4 Wallace Road, London, N1 2PG.

Child's Name:

_____

I give my consent for my child to be vaccinated with the vaccine(s) subject to the following conditions:

That the information which has been supplied is fully accurate both as to the safety and the efficacy of the vaccine.

That the doctor or nurse performing the vaccine, the Health Authority, the manufacturer of the vaccine and the Department of Health will accept full joint and several responsibility for any injury caused to my child as a result of the vaccine being administered.

That in the event of any such injury being caused, my child will receive full compensation, assessed in accordance with the normal principles of English Tort Law.

If these conditions are not acceptable, the vaccination should not take place.

Date:

Signed:

This consent form is courtesy of the book *The Vaccination Bible* edited by Lynne McTaggart.

Type, then print some copies out on A4 paper and take them with you to get signed, leave them a copy and photocopy the one you have and keep it somewhere safe.

Things you can do to help reduce the risk of a vaccine reaction

Dr. Russell Blaylock, who is a highly esteemed neurosurgeon, has compiled this helpful list of things to take if vaccinating to try and avoid an unwanted reaction.

1 Take a cold ice-pack to put on the injection site immediately afterwards – this will block the immune reaction. Keep it on the site as much as possible.
2 Take a high-dose Omega oil – Eicosapentaenoic acid (EPA) is one of the Omega oils found in fish oil which will help to reduce a reaction to the adjuvants used in vaccines. Take the dose 1 hour prior to the injection being given.

3 Take flavinoids such as Curcurmin which is also found in Wellspring by TouchStone Essentials. Take an hour before injection.

4 Take vitamin E, but the natural form which is high in Gamma-E, not the synthetic version.

5 Vitamin C at a dose of 1000 mg 4 x a day between meals. It is anti-inflammatory and must be taken in a buffered form, not as ascorbic acid.

6 Astaxanthin is highly recommended to take – as it's anti-inflammatory. Children that have died due to vaccines were found to be deficient in carotinoids such as astaxanthin.

7 A daily dose of zinc is also highly recommended.

8 Avoid taking any immune-stimulating supplements such as mushrooms, whey protein and beta glucan.

9 Take a multivitamin + mineral every day – ones that do not contain iron. Choose one that is full of B vitamins and selenium – this is very important as it fights viral infections and reduces the inflammatory response to vaccines.

10 Magnesium citrate/malate – 500 mg of elemental magnesium, 2 capsules three times a day.

11 Vitamin D3 – recommended to get pure source, from the sun, or take (for children) 5000 units a day for first 2 weeks after vaccine, then down to 2000 units a day. Adults are to take 20,000 units a day after the vaccine then down to 10,000 units a day.

12 Take calcium supplements as well because the vitamin D3 will work more efficiently in conjunction with the calcium. Adults to take 500–1000 mg a day and children under 12 are to take 250 mg a day.

13 Avoid all mercury-containing seafood.

14 Avoid oils that suppress immunity and increase inflammation e.g. corn, safflower, sunflower, soybean, canola and peanut oils

15 Drink strong organic white tea, four times a day. This can help

prevent abnormal immune reactions.

16 Drink 8 ounces of organic parsley and celery juice each day. (This list was sourced from clareswinney.wordpress.com)

Why I strongly recommend the use of Pure Body Zeolites when vaccinating your child

Another supplement I *highly* recommend using if you do decide to vaccinate is Pure Body Zeolites. Two weeks before the vaccination, start giving your child some drops of Pure Body Zeolites. Depending on their age, you can give between 1 and 4 drops a few times a day. Adults' dosage is on the back of the bottle – 4 drops 3 x a day. If not buying from my site, whoever you purchase these from will be able to tell you the right dose. Give your baby/child *plenty* more water; if breastfeeding, feed more if possible. The zeolite needs plenty of fluid to travel around the body with. You can use zeolites even during your pregnancy, and after the birth for the baby (and it's beneficial for yourself too) if you underwent a birth that was assisted by drugs. It's a good idea to get those drugs out that they used in the hospital, especially if you are going to breastfeed. Whatever goes into your body goes out through your breast milk too, and into your child's body.

There goes that chemical circle of life again.

Zeolites are tasteless when put in juice, or even water, so kids won't know they are drinking something other than what they think is in the glass.

There is more information about Pure Body Zeolites of which we have previously discussed in Chapter 13.

* * *

If you *are* interested in learning more about the pros and cons of vaccinations, and reading about the studies which are rarely talked about in the media, please look out for *The Vaccination Bible* that is listed at the end of this book in the vaccine resource section. It answers so many questions that many people always have, whether or not they really eradicated polio or smallpox, and if the herd immunity actually works, how dangerous each shot is statistically, and whether or not vaccines do provide lasting immunity. If you are someone that wants your 100% backed-up-by-science proof, then this book provides you with that.

I have also compiled a list of vaccine websites/books/documentaries in the resource section of this book for you to continue researching. There are certainly thousands of them to read. That's all I ask of you, that you keep learning more about this *highly important* subject.

I also want to drive home that if you don't vaccinate your kids, it *doesn't* automatically mean greater health. It's far easier for them to achieve it yes, because they won't have all of those toxins in their bodies and brains, affecting the strength and function of their immune systems, but parents *must* also know how they can help encourage a healthy immune system. If you feed your child bad food, don't breastfeed, use formula and use lots of medications when your child is sick, then yes, your child may be more susceptible to suffering from illness, more severely and regularly. And if they do catch measles or mumps then it might be much more stressful for them than it needs to be.

What I want to discuss in this next chapter is *how* to build a strong immune system through trying to avoid pharmaceutical medications and using natural supplements instead.

✓ The informedparent.co.uk website is a great place to start when looking into vaccines
✓ If you know of anyone with an autistic and/or vaccine damaged child please send them over to generationrescue.org

I'm now going to leave you with this last quote on the subject of vaccination dangers that certainly poses food for thought:

The chief, if not the sole, cause of the monstrous increase in cancer has been vaccination.
Dr. Robert Bell, once Vice President, of the International Society for Cancer Research at the British Cancer Hospital

Chapter 37

Natural Ways of Healing Your Child

At least 90% of the drugs prescribed by pediatricians are unnecessary and a costly risk to the child who takes them. All drugs are toxic and thus dangerous per se. Beyond that, excessive childhood use of prescription drugs may generate the belief that there is a 'pill for every ill'. This may lead the child to seek chemical solutions to emotional problems later in life.[179]

Dr. Robert Mendelssohn, author of *How to Raise a Healthy Child in Spite of Your Doctor*

When it comes to treating childhood illness, many parents immediately resort to pharmaceutical medicines to treat their children's common illnesses. At times, its all they know, due to constant advertising and, of course, listening to their doctor's and chemist's well-intended advice. Things like Calpol, a paracetamol-based liquid for pain relief, are frighteningly popular to use amongst even very young children. It can have a sedative effect so, many parents view this as a godsend when the child is not well. As it can quickly calm the child down and helps them sleep, it must be a good thing, right? What many parents do not realize is that paracetamol is not exactly kind to the liver; in fact, it can be downright dangerous and if it's used regularly, it can be detrimental to the development of the immune system. Which means, the more you use, the worse your child's immune system may be.

The overuse of Calpol has even hit the mainstream news. According to the Medicines and Healthcare products Regulatory Agency (MHRA): 'Parents are giving their children more than what is necessary' and 'giving high doses over a longer period can, in rare cases, lead to liver damage'.[180]

Just recently the makers of Calpol have been advised to change their 'suggested dose' levels and these should now be cut by *half*. So that means for years, most parents have been *overusing* the drug, due to the *incorrect* advice of the company, yet now they have had to release new information saying that at those previously suggested levels, it was in fact quite dangerous. How many parents have used the old 'standard' dose on their children, and over many times? And again, we put *so* much trust into these brands and companies – yet are *they* always certain how safe their product actually is? Judging by this recent and dramatic change, then the answer clearly is plain to see – no.

A recent Danish study, which included 336 children who were followed from birth to seven years, has added more concern regarding the overuse of paracetamol-based medicines for children.[181] The researchers found that regular use resulted in children being more likely to develop asthma before they started school. Scientists believe that the drug may cause changes in the child's body which leaves them more susceptible to allergies and inflammation. And the damage is mostly done in the infant's first year of life. While it's not proven to cause asthma, it is still linked to contributing to the development of this very common problem in children today. Senior researchers have advised parents to only use Calpol, and other medications like it, when fever is very severe.

In regards to fever, we really need to lose our fear of it. A fever, most of the time, is a good thing because it means that the body is trying to fight whatever is affecting its immune system. So it may be the worst thing to do to try and *suppress*. Hippocrates, the 'father' of modern medicine, was reported to have said, 'Give me a fever and I can cure any ailment.' Fevers rarely reach dangerous levels, yet most parents will suppress the fever at its first appearance. A fever is *good* for the body because it promotes fasting, sleep and sweating. When it's artificially suppressed, the defense system of the body won't be fully activated, and the real problem is most likely to be unknown. Calpol, and other medications like it, suppress fevers and therefore suppress the root cause. And with repeated use, these medications weaken the immune system, so in the future, a fairly mild illness will cause the child to suffer much more than is necessary. A fever is OK to a certain point. When a fever gets up to around 104 °F (40 °C) that is when there is a real problem and you need to seek help immediately from a doctor. Obviously, when dealing with an illness, keep testing your child's temperature to keep an eye on the fever.

Another study also linked other common pain medications, such as naproxen and ibuprofen, to causing children to be more likely to develop asthma. And an international study involving 300,000 teenagers from 50 countries showed that regular paracetamol users were being found to suffer from eczema and allergic nasal problems.[182]

When out with Lola in the shops recently, I picked up a bottle of Calpol as I wanted to see the ingredients for myself. I was absolutely horrified. This 'sugar free' version had about five E numbers (food additives) in there as well as maltitol which is a man-made sweetener, derived from corn. Although this ingredient is not as bad as aspartame, it still is *not* a safe sugar and, more alarmingly, would probably also be made from GMO corn which is just awful to think about.

What to do when your child has a fever

- Use homeopathy to help – find a remedy that suits the child's illness (e.g. not just treating the fever but the cold).
- Get your child to have sips of spring water, or mix this with some fruit juice, and give light vegetable soups.
- Encourage lots of rest.
- Let them tell you if they want to be kept warm or cool.
- If they are upset, tell them the body is working hard to make them well.
- Bring down high fevers with cool baths, fans and homeopathic remedies, such as Belladonna 30c which is very effective.
- Get urgent medical attention if the child has a seizure.

- Do not give any aspirin, or sugary or processed foods. Don't force a child to eat if they don't want to.

(Sourced from homeopathyworld.com)

Other concerns with popular infant medications

Many of the chemist-bought teething gels contain chemicals such as benzocaine, lidocaine and prilocain – all are anesthetics which, in some cases, can cause such severe reactions that you may need to take your child to the ER. The statistics for this are very minute, but is it really worth the risk when natural and safe options are out there? All of these types of mainstream drugs are toxic too so while they may have some short-term benefit, long term it is not good for them to be used regularly. And that's common sense. It must also be said that if your child is not responding to anything, you must take him/her to the hospital immediately. Sometimes there are serious things wrong and you do need medical intervention. Your intuition will tell you when it's more than just a little problem.

For teething problems, you can use homeopathic 'teething crystals' or Chammomilia 200cc. We use it when Lola is having pain and it's absolutely *incredible* how quickly it can work. You can also use a tiny amount of pure organic clove oil on the gums that are affected. This will numb the area and won't be toxic to the body.

Here is Leian's story in which her daughter had a reaction to a very common eye product:

A few months ago my youngest daughter Mikayla had a case of very mild conjunctivitis which only lasted a couple of days. I boiled up water and used that, gently wiping her eyes every few hours. This healed up very quickly and again was mild.

Bella (who loves touching and playing with her younger sister) catches it and immediately I could tell it was much stronger than the infection I had to worry about with Mikayla. I started wiping Bella's eyes and by the next day I found it hard to open her eyes and realized she needed something else to help clear it up than just my rinsing method. Al, my husband, takes her to the doctor for me and comes home with some drops called Chlorsig.

The drops didn't make a scrap of difference and in fact it just continued to get worse and we took her straight back to the hospital and they said, 'Keep using the drops – it will work shortly.' So we followed their instructions and continued to wash and medicate the eyes as we were told and the next day when we got up, it took me 2 hours to get her eyes open; they were swollen shut as well as glued shut by the pus. The 2 hours was spent rinsing gently to get her eyes open and during the day they were not getting any better so I rang our private health insurance medical advice line and even the doctor advised me to continue what I was doing!

I was very distressed and told Al, 'We have to go to the hospital – I can't keep washing her eyes and putting these drops in', and by this time her eyes are again swollen shut. We got to the hospital and the doctor pressed on her eyes to open them up and she had so much pus just pouring out of her eyes just at the slightest touch. In just 3 hours her eyes had worsened times 2. The doctor admitted her and had to put steroid drops in her eyes. We were told that the Chlorsig drops are the first kind of drops everyone is given; they are the preferred doctor's choice kind of thing... but apparently a lot of people have trouble with them also like Bella. She stayed 2 days in the hospital having flushes and other drops and thank God her eyes reopened 24 hours later.

I had never seen an eye infection this bad. I didn't know what to do and turned to the doctors for help. I thought I wasn't doing the right thing with my methods and I was to blame. But I now realize a common eye drop you can get even without a prescription, and recommended by a doctor, nearly caused my daughter permanent eye damage!

Facts about Chlorsig, an antibiotic used for eye infections

Possible side effects

Blood dyscrasias have been reported in association with the use of chloramphenicol. Chloramphenicol is absorbed systemically from the eye, and toxicity has been reported following chronic exposure. Local irritation with the ophthalmic form may include subjective symptoms of itching or burning.

More serious side effects:

- Anaphylaxis
- Angioneurotic oedema
- Fever
- Urticaria
- Vesicular and maculopapular dermatitis

Chlorsig is supposed to be a simple medication that is used on children, but personally, after reading these side effects and hearing Leian's story, I would much rather avoid using something like this and search for something far safer that has zero to low side effects. Why risk things with our children? Makes sense, right?

* * *

A *natural* and harmless way to treat an eye infection could be with the following:

- a cold compress soaked with Euphrasia officinalis – use a teaspoon of the herb in a cup of hot water which is then cooled.
- clean the eye from the inside (near nose) with moist tissues and water. Use chamomile tea to remove drainage.
- rub a tiny amount of pure aloe vera on the inside of the upper and lower lids.

Homeopathy

When children are sick and crying, no parent wants to just sit and do nothing. So what is there for a parent to do when you don't want to always use pharmaceutical medicines first? Thankfully, there is a *lot* you can do with a bit of knowhow. There are many natural ways of healing that are not at all new. In fact, some of these treatments have been around far longer than modern medicine.

Homeopathy is said to be one of the best methods for treating children's illnesses (and of course adults too) and can even treat serious things like pneumonia, measles and other troublesome health problems. Obviously I can't say that you should never contact a doctor at all – that is not what I want to drive home here – but in *most* cases, you probably won't need to.

Homeopathy is the oldest form of medicine in the world. It was developed in the 1800s by Samuel Hahnemann who discovered the healing ability through the 'Law of Similars' or 'like versus like' which meant that to cure a disease or virus, one would need to give the patient a very small dose of something that gave the same symptom. In a healthy person, giving them this pill would make them come down with some of the symptoms of the virus, but in a sick person it would actually *allow* their body to heal. Interestingly, the British Royal Family have long since been advocates of this natural form of healing. Although mainstream medicine tends to say that homeopathy does not work, millions of people attest to the fact that it does. One of the benefits of homeopathy is that you cannot overdose on the pills. So minute is the concentration in the tiny sugar pills that it cannot overload the system. So, even if a small child was to get hold of a whole bottle of them, there would be no need to rush to the emergency ward. My little dog Coco actually ate an entire glass jar of homeopathy pills and was completely fine, although was in a slight bit of trouble from me!

Even babies can take these pills as they are very small, very sweet and pleasant to the taste. I encourage all mums to try homeopathy. I see many who seem scared of it, despite it having no side effects and no toxins in it, yet they are fine with giving their children pharmaceutical stuff, which can and *does* cause harmful reactions. Again, it's all down to previous conditioning and seeing all of the advertisements, listening without questioning doctors' advice and hearing all of the other mums who tell them to take it. Many people dismiss homeopathy, saying it's a placebo effect, but when it comes to children and babies it *cannot* possibly be 'just placebo' because they do not have the thought processeses to think, 'It's going to work.' But let me assure you, as a parent who at the time of writing has used nothing (apart from one night) but homeopathy on my daughter when she was screaming from teething, it *does* work. Within minutes she would be fast asleep. You just have to try it really yourself, to see what I, and hundreds of thousands of others, have seen. Before there was allopathic medicine, homeopaths and herbalists were in pretty much every village and town. Our grandparents, and their parents would have more than likely used homeopathy and herbs when they were sick.

Luckily there are still many practitioners who are homeopaths and I highly suggest getting in touch with one before your child is born. You can even take certain things during the pregnancy and in preparation for the labour to make things easier.

Homeopathy is also very *inexpensive* to use and you can get a kit made up with remedies for the typical ailments such as colds, flus and common viruses. It can also treat emotional and anger problems as well. There are many remedies available, although at first it may be a bit daunting to figure out what to use. To help you get started, here are three homeopathy items that you can purchase which will treat many symptoms:

Ferr Phos 6x – to help those who suffer from infections
It is also good for inflammation, an early fever, and tiredness. You can also use it for diarrhea, when a cold is coming on, or if you have a boil or sore throat. Take it at least three times a day; it can gently

minimize the problem and may even stop it quickly if taken early enough.

Mag phos 6x – the pain reliever

For pain that is comforted by warmth Mag phos 6x is wonderful. And, for a grown-up, if you have period pains which are lessened by using a hot water bottle, then Mag phos 6x will really help. An extra trick is to put 4 pills into a cup of hot water and sip every 30 seconds or so. This remedy will also be wonderful in treating leg cramps, and people have even reported that it helps with hiccups.

Nat mur 6x

If you get a cold that starts off with lots of sneezing and mucus, quickly start taking Nat mur 6x. This is so helpful when fighting off a cold. The sooner you take it, the better! If you are sensitive to chemicals such as smelly (toxic!) perfumes or cigarette smoke, take Nat mur 6x every few minutes when first exposed to these fumes. If you have a bee sting, the reactions can be lessened with Nat mur 6x. The more bothersome the exposure is, the more frequent the dosing should be.

* * *

In the UK I personally see Kay Wesley who is a brilliant homeopath. Here she shares some fascinating case studies from her patients:

> I love the magic of homeopathy! It can easily be used at home to treat most first-aid situations and the emotional blips of childhood, but it's also fantastic for treating deep physical, mental, emotional and spiritual disturbances. And it's great for treating autism.

Treating common childhood ailments

Children are so very clever! When healthy, their bodies are able to 'throw' a good, strong and fairly quick fever to release any toxic build-ups or emotional strain, to boost their immunity and to support a growth spurt or developmental milestone. This is often accompanied by a release such as a runny nose or a bit of a cough, and a couple of lethargic days.

Frank, a sweet little boy of 3 was very healthy. He wasn't vaccinated, and had never been given antibiotics or Calpol so his immunity was given the chance to develop naturally. Most times if he had a cold, and his mum offered homeopathic remedies, he would refuse them ... he must have known that he was OK and that his body was doing what Nature had intended. One day Frank's mum called me (I was already treating Frank's brother for deeper issues) because he had asked for a remedy from Kay! ... he must have been struggling. After some disruption at home from renovations and a busy time generally, Frank had a fever which wasn't terribly high and had been lingering for a couple of days, he was lethargic, moody, his face was ruddy, he didn't want to eat and was not a happy boy! I suggested that he take a dose of Belladonna 30c to help his fever along; his fever peaked within an hour and then dropped to normal, he had a runny nose for a few hours which didn't bother him, and was back on his feet, playing, laughing and causing havoc of the best kind! And without the need for any toxic, suppressive medications. The Belladonna simply gave Frank's body the energy it needed and a little reminder of the natural and necessary process of fevers.

Belladonna is a must for any first-aid kit, helping fevers to complete and drop. In addition, Aconite is a brilliant remedy to take as soon as the first signs of a 'cold' come on, Chamomilla is a must-have for teething pain, for calming cranky and irritable children, Pulsatilla for earaches and clinginess, and of course Arnica for bumps and bruises.

An alternative to antidepressants...
I spend quite a bit of time in my practice, de-toxing the effects of

antidepressants, anti-anxiety and sleep medications from patients, and from their children (when taken before conception, during pregnancy or during breastfeeding and passed on by default). While there may be times when they are truly needed for the safety of the individual, often they're more damaging than helpful. I feel they are overprescribed and have a massive impact on the body, leaving quite a disturbance physically, emotionally and energetically. Rather than addressing the deep issues, they often mask the problem so that the person can 'get by', but 'getting by' isn't thriving and eventually the issues need to be addressed or our physical health is affected. I'm always thrilled when individuals reach for other alternatives. The case of Susan is a fantastic example of this.

Susan came to see me after what she referred to as a 'meltdown'. She had a difficult childhood with a dominating father and a lot of stress at home and a history of severe stomach aches from stress. She was six months into therapy and her doctor had prescribed antidepressants which she decided not to take. She suspected that the therapy sessions had 'stirred things up' and it was all too much. She was signed off work, was experiencing severe stomach and chest pains, was extremely anxious and more so with pressure of any sort, and she was exhausted. She really disliked her work and was thinking of leaving. She blamed herself for anything that went wrong and tried very hard to please others while not recognizing and fulfilling her own needs. I prescribed homeopathic remedies to help to boost her confidence, to heal her relationship with her father, and to help her to speak her truth.

I saw Susan for a second consultation two months later. She had been taking the homeopathic remedies prescribed, had been on holidays, taken time away from work and had continued her therapy sessions. Susan was beaming when she walked through the door, her eyes were shining, she had the widest grin and looked happy, such a contrast to when I first saw her. She had returned to work and realized that it wasn't the problem... she actually liked her work. She had forgiven her father and realized that he had done his best. She also realized that she hadn't been taught to love herself and hadn't been speaking up for herself due to childhood conditioning; her stomach aches were greatly improved and were only experienced when she obviously wasn't speaking her truth. She recognized that, particularly with men, she was a 'pleaser' out of fear that they might leave ... something that her father had threatened often. She didn't understand how, but she felt so much better. That made me a very happy healer! And of course I sent her off with more remedies for some deeper healing.

A case of severe hay fever...

Hay fever is a sign that our naturally very clever immune system has gone haywire! And this doesn't usually happen of its own accord. The case of Dee is a great example of how our natural processes can be disturbed by toxicity.

Dee had the most severe hay fever I have come across. She couldn't function without taking a cocktail of drugs and anti-histamines (most intensely for the past 6 years) and she had been suffering with it since she was around 4 years old, so for 25 years! Dee came from a culture which used medication widely; most families had a medicine cabinet full of drugs at home and would take them freely for any symptoms that arose, so her parents most likely took several medications before conception and during pregnancy, plus her mum smoked during pregnancy. As a child Dee was vaccinated and later in life was given travel vaccinations; she had taken the contraceptive pill for 8 years and had surgery in her teens, so she had quite a toxic load and her immune system simply hadn't been given the chance to do its job.

Emotionally Dee had suppressed quite a bit of anger as a child when her parents separated and as an adult she often experienced anxiety.

I prescribed for Dee homeopathic remedies to lighten the load, to cleanse her body of the physical and energetic imprint of the medications, to support her liver and to gently clear the emotions held. After 5 days, I received an email from Dee:

'It's a miracle – I haven't had a single blocked nose since Friday and I have only sneezed 5 times! ... The cleansing process is seeming to combat the hay fever symptoms (and who knows what other positive things are happening!). So thank you.'

A case of the measles...

Measles is one of those good old childhood illnesses which is a gift... parents always report that the child moves forward in leaps and bounds physically and emotionally after a stint of measles (as is the case with mumps and chicken pox). It shouldn't be feared but certainly should be treated with care in order to avoid complications.

Children who have contracted measles should be kept very warm and away from any draughts; bright lights should also be avoided so curtains and windows should be closed and kiddies rugged up. The fever of measles is essential and shouldn't be suppressed by medication or by cool compresses; without the fever more complications can arise – it's the body's clever way to burn the virus off. Plenty of liquids are also essential. And it's important to keep the child rugged up and away from strong light for a week or two after the fever subsides. So what can be done for measles? Each child might react differently and have different symptoms so the best approach is to provide a warm, draught-free environment with plenty of fluids and to consult your homeopath.

I received a call from 3-year-old Ella's mum... Ella had a fever and some raised red spots on her chest; she hadn't been vaccinated and her mum suspected that she had measles. I advised her to keep her very warm and to totally avoid draughts, just giving her liquids and to let me know how she progressed. The next day, Ella had been sleeping mostly and she had a cough, very dry lips and was very thirsty. I advised her mother to give two doses of Bryonia 30c from the family's homeopathic first-aid kit and to let me know how she was later in the day. Ella's mum reported that since the Bryonia, her cough had cleared and her spots were spreading down her body very quickly (the remedy had helped the spots to progress); she still had a fever and was drinking well. The following day Ella's fever was dropping and her skin was clearing, she was complaining that her legs were aching, and she was lethargic. I suggested a dose or two of Gelsemium 30c. A few days later Ella was up and playing indoors and her mum had promised to keep her warm and indoors for a further week while her immune system recovered.

CEASE therapy to clear vaccine toxicity...

A substantial part of my practice has evolved to treating children with damage from vaccines (or other toxicity). It's such a shame to see these sweet little beings in such a state as a result of receiving a shot of toxins mixed with viruses. Everyone who receives a vaccine is affected, our immune system is suppressed, our body needs to deal with the toxic load, and who knows what subtle changes have resulted, plus we carry the toxic burden and energetic imprints for a very long time (I often treat the effects of vaccines 20 or 40 years after they've been given in order to help people to heal and move forward). For some, unfortunately, the effects are more severe than for others: layers of vaccines on top of already poor gut bacteria, possibly genetic weaknesses, issues at the time of conception and during pregnancy, antibiotics, formula feeding, the introduction of poor foods at weaning and then... that last vaccine received tips the boat over!

I've found CEASE therapy to be invaluable in treating any ailment that's caused by a toxic load, in adults and in children – whether that be autism spectrum, depression, liver toxicity, nerve damage, digestive disorders... there's a long list! CEASE was developed by Dr. Tinus Smits who treated many children with autism spectrum symptoms. It combines a specific protocol of homeopathic remedies alongside supplements and lifestyle changes to clear the layers of toxicity and bring the body back to a state of health. This case is a great example...

Little Alex came to see me with his mum at 2 years and 10 months of age. His mum had noticed changes at 15 months of age; prior to that his development had been good – he was babbling and saying mumma, he was also very sociable with adults and children. Alex had received the usual childhood vaccines plus the hepatitis B vaccine at 1 month, 4 months and 12 months of age. Soon after the MMR vaccine, he completely stopped speaking, he no longer made eye contact and didn't respond to his name. I noticed that he was very 'babyish' – he looked like a baby in bigger boy's clothes; he also had large dark circles under his eyes, looked congested and had a terrible dry rash on his belly. I prescribed two months of homeopathic remedies to detox the vaccines received, homeopathic remedies to treat his stunted development and improve digestion, alongside some dietary changes and supplements.

Alex's mum called after the first dose of the vaccine detox remedy to say that he had started to kick a ball and couldn't do that before – she was very pleased. Two months later we caught up and Alex looked so grown up! He no longer looked like a baby, the dark circles under his eyes had cleared, he was very active playing (during the first appointment he just sat and stared), he was now speaking but only repeating words spoken by others, and the rash on his belly had cleared. Alex's mum reported that he was eating really well, more than before.

With four further prescriptions focusing on detoxing the vaccines layer by layer and healing/re-balancing Alex's system, nourishing his brain and digestive organs, he spoke more and more, he engaged with others and was ready to start school. He still had a little way to go as he had difficulty sitting still and concentrating for long periods of time but I feel confident that in time he will be just fine!

To find out more about CEASE therapy, go to www.cease-therapy.com
    I hope these examples will inspire you to add a homeopathic first-aid kit for your home and office, and to seek help from a homeopath if you feel your issues or the issues of your child run deep.
    ✓ kaywesley.com

If Lola ever gets really ill to the point where we need to involve a doctor, we will be contacting Dr. Jayne Donegan who is an experienced GP and has also trained extensively in homeopathy. And as you have read previously she's also an expert on the subject of vaccinations. With her expertise in modern medicine and natural medicine, we will know when it's OK to stay and treat Lola at home and when to go to hospital.
    ✓ jayne-donegan.co.uk
    For learning as much as you can about homeopathy, a wonderful book to read on homeopathy and natural healing for all sorts of ailments and concerns is *The Organic Pharmacy: The Complete Guide to Natural Health and Beauty* written by Margo Marrone, CEO and founder of the Organic Pharmacy.
    If you need a bit of extra help (but don't think you need to visit the ER) and you still think homeopathy may be the best option to use, you can get professional advice through calling this number from the homeopathy helpline website:
    ✓ homeopathyhelpline.com/consultations/telephone
    I highly recommend purchasing a homeopathy kit for children (which adults will be able to use too) so that you have the most popular remedies for the most common ailments.
    You can purchase homeopathy from these websites I recommend:
    ✓ theorganicpharmacy.com

✓ helios.co.uk

✓ nelsonsnaturalworld.com

✓ nealsyardremedies.com

Some websites I personally find very helpful are:

✓ joettecalabrese.com

✓ homeopathyworld.com

Bach Flower Remedies

Another much loved way, also with great success, of treating children with natural medicine is with 'Bach Flower Remedies'. These flower extracts are infused in a solution of brandy to preserve and keep the extracts active. They also taste pretty good so children won't screw their noses up when they get a few drops in their mouth. The story of how Bach Flower Remedies came about is quite remarkable.

Dr. Edward Bach began his career in the early 1900s when he was training to be a doctor. With a very impressive medical background, he was also a pathologist, bacteriologist and started out researching vaccines in his own research laboratory. During the war, he worked on wards looking after injured soldiers who had been fighting in France. Unbeknown to him, Dr. Bach was about to become very ill himself. One day he passed out and was rushed into the emergency room and operated on. His colleagues sadly discovered a tumor. They removed it immediately but felt that he was not going to live very long. They gave him only three months to live.

Dr. Bach did not want to waste any time before he passed away. There was far too much work he needed to carry out. When he was well enough, he returned to his laboratory. What was surprising to him was that he seemed to get stronger and stronger as time went by. The three months soon passed and he felt that he was better than ever. He realized he was living a miraculous life and that he was meant to continue on his life's purpose.

He continued researching vaccines, but something in him felt unhappy with vaccines being based on 'diseases' and not on the health of the whole person. So much was ignored and not taken into consideration. This caused him to aspire to become a holistic doctor. He was offered a post at the Royal London Homeopathic Hospital where he immersed himself in the homeopathic world.

He soon began to notice the strong parallels between his own work on vaccines and the meaning behind homeopathy. He adapted his vaccines and created a series of seven homeopathic 'nosodes', a much more gentle and toxic-free approach to injected vaccinations. These nosodes are used widely today, especially in the treatment of animals and in people who want to build up immunity to a particular disease that they are concerned about.

He had such success with these nosodes that he soon became quite famous in homeopathic circles. Some even nicknamed him the 'Second Hahnemann'.

Dr. Bach had been working with bacteria but wanted to find remedies that would be much less reliant on 'disease' and would also be purer. He began to look into the healing powers of plants, and in particular, flowers, which was the most developed/concentrated part of the plant.

He was so excited by this new direction his work was heading in that he completely gave up his popular Harley Street clinic and home, and moved away from London. He also moved away from typical scientific methods, laboratories and 'reductionism'. He began to rely more on his own natural gifts, allowing his intuition to guide him to using the right plants.

It took him many years, through lots of trial and error, with preparations of literally thousands of plants, but he soon discovered, one by one, the remedies which worked. He had discovered a new way of looking at health. He would aim a remedy at a particular emotion or mental state. In his testing, he saw that when he treated someone's emotional concerns, e.g. unhappiness, anger, sadness, shyness, their body would become free of the distress this caused and their own body's healing ability would come into effect.

He would travel according to the seasons, to places where he could study the different flowers when they were at their best. Dr. Bach became so in tune with his work and with Nature that he would often suffer himself from a certain emotional state and this would give him the inspiration to keep searching for the right flower to solve the problem. Dr. Bach ended up passing away in 1936, but this was 20 years longer than the doctors had given him when they first discovered his tumor.

His work lives on today and his Bach Flower Remedies have since become world famous. You can even visit The Bach Centre at Mount Vernon where Dr. Bach used to work and live. If you are interested in learning more about Bach Flower Remedies you can download some free eBooks from the following website as well as purchase any remedies.

What I love about this story is knowing how much intelligence and skill has gone into the discovery of these. Dr. Bach was obviously a truly brilliant man, who started out researching vaccines which would have been a highly lucrative area of medicine in his time. To know that he felt, even back then, that something was not quite right with them is very interesting, to say the least.

✓ bachcentre.com

You can also purchase Bach Flower Remedies from:

✓ nealsyardremedies.com

Australian Bush Flower Essences

As previously mentioned, because I am Australian, I *was* very intrigued by this range. I always knew that Australia is home to some of the most incredible plants and wildlife because the native Aborigines have been singing their praises for thousands of years. And they are some pretty wise and special people who know how to live out in the bush in such extreme conditions. But I hadn't really ever looked into exactly what these plants and flowers could do for people, including what could they do for children's health and wellbeing. Australia is home to some of the oldest and highest number of flowering plants which are extremely powerful.

Australian Bush Flower Essences was created by Ian White, a fifth-generation herbalist, who spent his childhood growing up in the outback. His grandmother, like her own mother before her, would often take him walking through the bush and point out which plant or flower could heal this or that ailment. Ian had this wisdom in his blood and became fascinated by what he knew and what he could discover through further study. With 30 years of research and after traveling all over the world, Ian created the now very extensive Australian Bush Flower Essences range.

Australian Bush Essences, like that of Bach Flower Remedies, work on helping balance and correcting mental and emotional functions, which will then free the body of illness, fatigue and general disharmony. Both Chinese and Ayurvedic medicine say that 90–95% of illness stems from emotional and mental imbalance. This sort of approach, using pure extracts from flowers and plants, has been used for thousands of years.

Through the use of these essences, many people have found that they help to improve strength, bring courage, and enable high levels of intuition, improve self-esteem, encourage creativity, and bring out the ability to give and receive love. You can also use these essences in treating children's health and wellbeing.

The range consists of single essences, oral sprays, and combinations of different essences. There are essences to help deal with stress, feeling fearful, being sad, feeling angry, and to encourage a calm nature, to help with jet lag, to help women cope with their mood swings, to help with sexual problems and to clear negative energy in your immediate surroundings. For children, they can help with feeling shy, being grumpy, being too hyperactive, and can also help when suffering colds, viruses and other health conditions.

Ian and his company Australian Bush Flower Essences try to encourage people to learn as much as they can about the range so, if interested, you can undertake a correspondence course to help you understand in great depth how these remedies work. The

Emergency Oral spray is a must-have for your children's health kit. Ian has also written five books on his essences and one in particular, *Happy Healthy Kids*, which is for children.

The topics covered in this wonderful book are:

- How the Essences work
- Preparing for pregnancy
- Pregnancy and your baby's birth
- The first few days
- The first year
- The toddler years
- Your child's spirit
- Common childhood infections and illnesses
- Toddlerhood to childhood
- Starting school
- Knowing your child
- Choosing Bush Essences
- Using Bush Essences
- A–Z of conditions and treatments
- Individual Essences
- Combination Essences

I have only just discovered this exciting range, but I am thinking about doing their courses in the near future. You can learn how to use their remedies professionally or personally through the international courses they offer.

Please visit the Australian Bush Flower Essences website to discover more:

✓ ausflowers.com.au

Probiotics: Nature's antibiotics

As we have covered previously, healthy gut function is *so* important for anyone's health but *especially* for young children. And it can easily be upset and put off-balance. So you will want to avoid the use of prescription antibiotics as much as possible. When a child has these in their system at a young age it can wreak havoc on their delicate immune system. It is also being reported that many children are now being born without the correct levels of healthy flora in their stomach and that the mother can pass on toxins through her placenta and into the baby's body.

In a vaginal birth, a newborn swallows what will become its first healthy intestinal micro flora as it passes through the birth canal. This is Nature's incredible way for mothers to inoculate their babies and also provides them with healthy bacteria for their future health. If the mother had to have a C-section, then the natural bacteria which is passed on to the baby through the vaginal passage misses out on being able to strongly protect the child from viruses. This means that when the child does *not* receive this, it is more susceptible to catching things and the immune system will already be struggling.

If a virus is caught then typically the doctor will prescribe antibiotics which will also wipe out the remaining good bacteria. Long term, this is such a worry and may mean your child is affected by lots of colds and coughs and other viruses regularly. And as Dr. Natasha Campbell-McBride has discovered, this unhealthy gut function may increase the greater likelihood of having a vaccine-induced reaction.

So how do we avoid this? Using regular doses of probiotics is a good starting point. You should even start taking these during (or before!) your pregnancy; if your own stomach flora is healthy then your child's will more than likely be healthy as well. Breast milk contains many immune system enhancers so for this reason I urge you to do this at least until the age of 1 year – preferably for up to two years. But if you cannot, after the age of 6 months you can give your child probiotics, especially formulated for them. The good ones will contain billions of different types of healthy bacteria so that the gut will be able to stay strong and healthy and will act as a 'white knight' to your child's immune system.

It's important to only use a reliable brand and to stay away from products that are piled with sugars and additives. It's quite concerning that the media again have manipulated mums into thinking that the probiotic drinks sold in supermarkets are healthy. The truth is, they contain dairy extracts that are often the 'rejected' milk and are piled with sugar and other additives to make them taste good. Sugar is not good for healthy flora in the stomach and in fact will 'feed' the bad bacteria which may end up being in a higher ratio to the healthy bacteria. Once this sets in, allergies and other problems can begin.

A brand I personally really trust is Optibac. They have a probiotic for children that is recommended from the age of 6 months. It's in a sachet form with no sugars or additives. If you are breastfeeding you can take it yourself and pass on the effects to your baby. If you cannot get hold of Optibac, you can always ask your local health food shop what they have on offer; just make sure that it's additive free and that the person advising you really knows what they are talking about.

The Organic Pharmacy also make a fantastic strawberry-flavored probiotic which you can give to your child.

You can also purchase some fantastic probiotic prodicts from rawliving.eu

Eat your probiotics

Another way to have regular probiotics is from eating organic miso soup. Miso is made from fermented soy beans and koji, which is a culture starter and turns the soybeans into a living food. The fermentation process causes healthy bacteria to grow which is vital for a healthy body.

The amazing benefits of miso:

- Reduces risks of cancer, including breast cancer, prostate cancer, lung cancer and colon cancer.
- Provides protection from radiation.[183]
- Immune strengthening.

- Antiviral – miso is very alkalizing and strengthening to the immune system, helping to combat a viral infection.
- Prevents aging – high in antioxidants, miso protects from free radicals that cause signs of aging.
- Helps maintain nutritional balance – full of nutrients, beneficial bacteria and enzymes, miso provides: protein, vitamin B12, vitamin B2, vitamin E, vitamin K, tryptophan, choline, dietary fiber, linoleic acid and lecithin.
- Helps preserve beautiful skin – miso contains linoleic acid, an essential fatty acid that helps your skin stay soft and free of pigments.
- Helps reduce menopausal complaints – the isoflavones in miso have been shown to reduce hot flashes.

It's super-easy to make and you can even just put a teaspoon of miso in some warm water and consume it as a delicious hot drink. You can even give a watered-down version to babies from 6 months old. You *must*, however, buy non-GMO organic miso as the majority of soy beans are unfortunately genetically modified. For a delicious soup recipe that will impress the most fussiest of eaters, please see Chapter 19 for Frank's healthy miso soup.

Fermented foods

Fermented foods are becoming so popular these days, and for good reason because you can make them yourself, fairly inexpensively, and because they are full of billions of beneficial bacteria. You probably won't even have to take any store-bought probiotics if you regularly eat this kind of stuff. You can ferment vegetables, make 'kefir' (a very thick yoghurt-type drink), 'kombucha' (a fermented drink that tastes a bit like a soft drink but without the horrible chemicals), and yoghurts and cheeses can even be made 'raw'. Fermented foods can also taste truly delicious. The websites below will guide you through making your own fermented foods at home.

✓ nourishingdays.com

✓ nourishedkitchen.com

Herbs for healing children

Another type of healing comes in the most used form in all of history – herbs! Up until the last 100 years, it's safe to say that most people, mothers and grandmothers especially, knew to go out into their garden to find wild herbs to heal themselves and their loved ones.

Today, mainstream medicine too is still derived from plants and herbs. But getting your doctor to admit that natural supplements are powerful is very hard because they are taught at medical school that processing and synergizing pharmaceuticals in a laboratory is what makes the best medicine for us. It's unfortunate that these medicines tend to have severe toxic side effects too, often requiring users to take another drug to counteract those effects.

Many pharmaceutical companies go to beautiful and wild places like the Amazon, to discover what the ancient tribes used for healing and then remove the chosen plants and herbs (sometimes with force and causing destruction to the rain forests), bringing them back to recreate the effects synergistically, so that they can market this 'new wonder drug' that will bring them huge amounts of millions of dollars in revenue.

For natural healing to be spreading at such a rate the way it is today is deeply worrying to these big companies, because for them it means that people are not buying their medicines, nor dying of cancer which, coincidentally, also makes many corporations lots and lots of money. And as they can see, the companies that do sell natural herbs make far less money than these big and powerful pharmaceutical companies do. In a world where profit and sales targets have become so important, more so than people's lives, herbs and their healing ability get pushed under the carpet by modern medicine and also the media.

But, again, we must look at things *logically*. We were given this incredible planet that really worked very well until us greedy humans came along. We have tried to change Nature so much and this also includes medicine. To have things growing wildly in the ground with such power and proven healing abilities suggests they have been put here for a reason – for us to use in times of ill health. Herbs can help with minor illnesses such as colds and flu, insect bites, rashes and also can be used for more severe and chronic conditions. Even arthritis, liver and heart problems can quite often be treated with certain herbs. If there is a problem with the autonomic nervous system, herbs can help normalize and balance the symptoms. The beauty of herbs is that rarely do they have side effects *if used wisely*, nor do they become addictive.

If you spend a bit of time researching on the effects of herbs, you will understand that they too can be very, *very powerful* and, if taken in conjunction with some pharmaceuticals, you could have a very unwanted and sometimes dangerous reaction. I had one of those years ago and, boy, did it make me realize how strong the two can be together. I mixed antidepressants with a herbal liquid (bought to help me sleep) and it was very scary indeed. I got severe heart palpitations and became very scared that I was going to pass out and die! Luckily everything was OK, but it really made me aware to be super-careful about mixing anything with herbs. The man in the health food shop even warned me to not mix the two but I remember thinking, 'Oh, it's only herbs – what harm can they do?' Typical me needing to learn the hard way!

Nature most certainly nurtures us well indeed, but we still need to be smart about what we are taking. It is *not safe* to buy a whole lot of things and take them without knowing what their effects could be. Correct dosage is *very important (especially in regards to children)* and you must follow the advice from a trained herbalist for how to include them in your family's lifestyle. It's also suggested that taking herbs each and every single day is not necessary either. You must use them when needed only. I guess that saying, 'Too much of a good thing is not good', very much applies here also.

It's important to know that herbs *must be organic*, and be wary of any that come from India and China. These are reportedly very high in heavy metals from the pesticides which are used during their growing process. Always ask where the herbs are sourced from.

There are many guide books available for how to use herbs. I cannot recommend highly enough the following book: *The Family Herbal: A guide to Natural Health Care for Yourself and Your Children from Europe's Leading Herbalists* by Barbara and Peter Theiss. It really is a herb bible and was written by health experts who actually had a background previously in pharmaceuticals. Back when they owned a chemist, they saw their customers getting sicker and sicker and began to realize that the medicines they were giving were not really helping them get truly better. They started to look into the healing effects of herbs and began selling and prescribing them in their pharmacy.

The Family Herbal covers subjects such as how to handle and prepare herbs, how to make herbal baths, as well as instructions for herbal teas, and how to make tinctures. There is also invaluable information on detoxing the body and what different types of herbs do this. There are recipes and advice on how to bring down a fever, which can be very common in young children, as well as other ailments and common problems. You also learn how to plan and grow your own herbs in the garden!

What to do when your child is sick: helpful advice from Dr. Jayne Donegan

- Get fresh air – open the window; during mild weather, lie outside if you can. At night, make sure that the window is open even if only a little.
- Avoid dairy produce – no milk (including soya) yoghurt, cheese, eggs until well on the mend. Dairy increases mucus, upsets stomachs and may increase fever.
- Drink plenty of clear fluids – for example, water with Rescue Remedy (a very popular calming tonic available from most health food stores), half-diluted apple juice.
- Ginger (fresh root grated or chopped, one good pinch), honey

(2 tsp) and lemon (¼ squeezed) in a mug plus boiling water, stir and sip hot stock. Ginger helps to sweat the fever *out* unlike paracetamol and ibuprofen which reduce fever but push it *in*, often making the illness last longer. If giving squash (pre-mixed cordial), make sure it contains no aspartame or saccharin. No orange juice.

- Fluids are best taken frequently; small frequent sips are more useful than occasional large gulps, especially if there is vomiting.
- Give no food unless hungry – this is *very* important.
- Do not force your child to eat if they are not hungry. When any fever is down, and they are hungry give them light food – starch, minimal fat, and advise them to chew it well.

Examples:

- peeled sliced apple
- organic wholemeal toast scraped with Marmite or organic honey
- mashed potato made with cooked potato, boiling water and a pinch of salt,
- vegetable soup, homemade, hot tomato juice with a squeeze of lemon +/- a little Tabasco/cayenne pepper (for adults and older children)
- fruit or cooked vegetables

(all in very small quantities)

- Give raw organic honey on a teaspoon – this is very good for sore throats and stops harmful bacteria from multiplying. (Government Health Warning: not for infants less than 1 year of age)
- Lots of rest– this is *extremely* important; most adults only get infectious diseases because they are tired and need a rest – if they had adequate rest first, they probably wouldn't get the infection.
- Wear loose clothing – made of soft, natural fibers.
- No TV/computer/books – listening is OK, so radio is OK, but

no ipods plugged into ears.

- Room temperature – try and keep it between 15 ºC and 18 ºC.
- Eat no meat, fish, fatty food or dairy until two days after better; up to a week if after diarrhea and vomiting.
- If dairy or normal diet is introduced and symptoms start again, especially after diarrhea and vomiting, go back to fasting or light diet until symptom free.

Dr. Jayne LM Donegan MBBS DRCOG DCH DFFP MRCGP MFHom
Holistic GP and Homeopathic Physician
  ✓ jayne-donegan.co.uk

Chapter 38

Creating a Safe Home Environment for Your Child

When babies are inside the womb, they feel safe and protected. Once they come out into the world, their senses go into overdrive. They can taste things and smell things and also can become easily upset if a chemical is near them; this may even give them a headache, causing them to scream and cry for no apparent reason. We covered the shocking amount of toxins that are in our houses in Chapter 7 so I won't repeat myself too much here. However, this subject is even *more important* for a newborn or child.

When a baby is born, it's always exciting to decorate their nursery and that usually means everything is new – new carpet, new paint, new toys, new clothes, new wallpaper and new cot and bedding. We rarely think that these shiny and new items are actually introducing enormous amounts of toxins into the environment our children will take comfort in.

If you are pregnant and are thinking of decorating a room for your baby, please consider buying as many non-toxic items as you can. That is, products that have been made with little to no chemicals. I recently went into a famous UK baby store to see what they sold in their shops. I was absolutely horrified that this big-name brand sold *nothing* at all that was safe to use. There were no organic clothes; all were made out of polyester or cotton with synthetic dyes and stitching and so much plastic was used in making everything else. I walked out of there knowing that I would never buy anything from that shop. There are far easier and even less expensive ways to buy safer items.

Something *very important* to buy is a non-toxic mattress. Baby mattresses (and all mattresses in general) off-gas so much due to the polyurethane foam which is made from petrol. This chemical has been linked to causing serious allergies, problems with the reproductive system, and can harm the immune system.

> While bed mattresses of 40–50 years ago were made mostly from untreated natural materials, the majority of mattresses and beds today are made using a variety of petroleum-based chemicals, foams, plastics and controversial flame retardants. Unfortunately, these are not stable compounds and continue to evaporate into the air and are then inhaled hour upon hour by the person sleeping on the bed. Research and personal accounts suggest people can become ill after repeated and continuous exposure to these chemicals while sleeping.[184]

Off-gassing can cause a great deal of upset to your child, both physically and mentally. These typical mattresses are filled with highly poisonous toxins, and it may well be the reason for one of those crying episodes where you just don't know what's wrong. Some also believe that the these toxic mattresses can contribute to SIDS as well, due to the off-gassing and the fact that the mother is not there.[185]

You can purchase organic mattresses which may have a bamboo covering (also antibacterial) or organic cotton and the inside may be made out of wool and/or coconut fibre. All of these are natural fabrics and far safer than any man-made materials. Wool is naturally fire resistant too.

I purchased an organic mattress for Lola, and also our own mattress from Abaca Organics which is a UK-owned and made company which produces safe and non-toxic high-quality organic mattresses, bedding and pillows. We have a king-size mattress from this company which has been brilliant and also our daughter now has a special made-to-measure organic cotton and wool mattress which fits her 'Amby Nest' hammock bed perfectly. We co-sleep at night but use this hammock bed during the day when she is sleeping and I need to do some housework. Abaca Organics have brilliant customer service and their products are second to none. The mattresses for children start at £45.00.

✓ abacaorganic.co.uk

You can try and find organic mattresses no matter where you live so just use google to find out where.

Paints used on the walls and ceilings in homes also off-gas an incredible amount and continue to do so over many many years:

CSIRO studies have shown that occupants of new Australian homes may be exposed to up to 20 times the maximum allowable limits of indoor air toxics for up to ten weeks after completion. Further CSIRO measurements in 27 suburban Melbourne residences more than a year after construction identified 27 airborne toxics. These included the carcinogens benzene, formaldehyde and styrene, and a cocktail of methanol, ethanol, acetone, toulene, dichlorobenzene plus a number of less well-known toxics, most of which are found in paints. Mineral turpentine (used as a thinner and solvent) may contain up to 20% benzene, which is a confirmed carcinogen and mutagen in chronically exposed workers.[186]

Many paint brands are now including solvent-free or low solvents into their range. This means that there will be little to no off-gassing and will be much safer than regular paint. When painting with them, you will hardly smell any scent whatsoever, unlike the older paints that smelt so toxic and usually give you a headache.

Also try and stay away from synthetic bedding and blankets. Non-natural fabrics actually have chemicals sprayed onto them and throughout their manufacturing process. These will seep into your baby's skin and can cause irritation and may even be a reason why your baby could cry a lot, or suffer with eczema. Many baby and children's clothes are sprayed with flame retardants too which are incredibly toxic.

Organic cotton, bamboo and organic cashmere are wonderful fabrics to wrap baby in. A bit more expensive to buy, but remember, check out Ebay for bargains; there are many second-hand and brand-new items to be found. As long as you can wash things then there is no need to be cautious about using second-hand items.

It probably goes without saying that toys are highly toxic as well. Despite being fluffy and cute, the materials used to make the toys are highly dangerous (made with dirt-cheap materials too) and are sprayed heavily with flame-retardant products. When a child starts to develop motor skills, they put everything they can into their mouths. So, in goes the toy through the mouth as does the flame-retardant chemical and other ones used to produce the item. Plastic toys are some of the worst culprits so try and avoid using them if you can.

When your friends want to bring you a present for your child, ask them to bring something organic. Perhaps tell them you realize that organic things can be more expensive, so if this is the case, it's OK not to bring anything, or perhaps bring a nice plant to add to your house. Tell them that you are concerned about the toxins in the products. Good friends will understand. Ebay is a really great place to buy organic things. I recently purchased about 40 items from Ebay second hand, and some were new as well; it cost me about £60 for all of them which is a total bargain! I think the pressure to buy all new things has to change; we must re-use what is already out there. I wish someone would set up a website with a network of mums who all pass on things which don't fit anymore to someone they are connected with through the site, a mum who has a child a few months younger.

I purchase the majority of Lola's toys from The Organic Toy Company and Myriad. Both stores stock certified organic toys and Myriad offers parents an enormous range of old-fashioned simple, wooden toys, for all ages, which help the child to use their imagination to play. Many toys today do not have this quality.

✓ otoys.co.uk
✓ myriadonline.co.uk

OK, what if your nursery/child's room is already made and you can't exactly rip everything down and start again? Well, I suggest the use of Mother-in-Law's Tongue and other healthy-air plants to be in your child's room as close to the cot or bed as much as possible. You need a mixture of healthy plants because you need both types to clean the air at night and to clean the air during the day. We moved house again in 2012 and it had recently had new carpet and new paint. This was horrific to me but we had no choice to move in because where we live, ideal places to rent don't come up that very often. So I had to make sure that we had enough healthy-air plants in our rooms to absorb as many as these chemicals as possible. I also make sure we open the windows every day to get some fresh air circulating through.

As previously mentioned, the Mother-in-Law's Tongue plant cleans the air at night by producing oxygen and during the day it produces CO_2. If you have a good balance of day and night plants, it will keep the air healthy by absorbing many of the toxins floating in the air, and coming off carpets, paint and furniture.

Remember that these types of plants absolutely thrive on toxins, and will actually look better, the more they suck up chemicals! Isn't it wonderful that Mother Nature has provided us with all of these things to keep us healthy? Also, you should always keep on top of dust as much as possible by vacuuming and mopping the floor very regularly. This is an easy way to remove air particles that are often contaminated with chemicals.

To clean wooden floors you can purchase a steam mop, which means you don't have to use any chemicals at all. Some steam mops are so advanced you can clean the bathroom and kitchen, windows, cloths and even mattresses and upholstery, all with just using water.

Please stay away from using any antibacterial products which are always advertised on TV and in magazines. Ninety-nine percent of children (apart from those with severe life-threatening allergies) need to be around germs; it is the only way they develop their immune system. The more we keep everything super-clean, the worse it actually is for their health. We have again been conditioned to think that we must always be 100% clean to be healthy – not so.

According to a new study from the School of Public Health at the University of Michigan, Triclosan, which is often used in these types of products, is a chemical that has been linked to asthma, allergies and a weakened immune system. Triclosan is an EDC – endocrine-disrupting compound – which disrupts the hormonal system. The study also showed that these products are no more effective at keeping germs away than normal soap. So what would you rather use: a toxic product that doesn't even do its job, or one that is gentle and safe?[187]

In the kitchen, most of what kids drink and eat out of is made from harmful plastics. When hot food is placed in these items, it can cause the plastic to leach in minute amounts, which is of course not so good for your child. While you can get a lot of BPA cutlery, cups, plates an bowls, it's still made out of other types of toxic plastics. You can use stainless steel, glass and ceramic items to eat and drink out of, but bear in mind they are heavy and of course the glass can still break if dropped on the floor.

I recently came across a great company, 'Beco things', who make a whole range of kid, pet and planet-friendly items. For the kids you can buy cute designed plates, bowls and cups that are all made from natural fibres such as bamboo and rice husks. They are very durable (just as tough as plastic), come in great colours and are ergonomically designed. You can also choose cute potties for toilet training (a matching step can be purchased too) which are made out of these same materials, as well as kids' clothing hangers. 'Beco things' also sell toys for pets and also drinking and eating bowls.

A very fun range, innovative, high quality and inexpensive.

✓ becothings.com

Chapter 39

Building Your Child's Self-Esteem to Last a Lifetime

The way we speak to our children becomes their inner voice.
Peggy Omara, author of *Adventures in Tandem Nursing*

Sadly, one of the biggest problems in society is the majority of people's lack of self-esteem. It's a *massive* problem and I would say that most of us have battled with feeling inadequate at one stage in our lives (or sadly, for some, for their *entire* lives). This can lead to problems later in life: depression, anger, drugs, other addictions, crime and even in the extreme and tragic cases, suicides. You only have to read the news to know that teenagers *are* committing suicide at an alarming rate. In fact, in America, suicide is the leading cause of death, increasing by 15% in the last ten years. We really have to do something about people's emotional suffering and very quickly.[188]

So, where does self-esteem begin? Well, parents, it starts with us and the *way* we encourage it. And we have to start building it as *early* as possible. Self-esteem is entirely shaped by the way we speak to our children and the messages that we give them. It's so important not to belittle or criticize them at all, but unfortunately, kids tend to grow up with both forms, no matter how much we think we are doing it for their own benefit.

Kids are like sponges and words *really* hurt, much more than what you may think at the time. Children will hold on to words even if spoken only once and it may be from that *one* instance that these deep messages begin to form, and stay with them for life. Parenting is *very* tough, especially in this department, because if you yourself don't have strong and healthy self-esteem, how will you know how to make sure your child will be able to have it?

Here are some tips from the brilliant Dr. and Martha Sears in *The Discipline Book* which can help to instill essential healthy self-esteem in your children.[189]

1. Practice attachment parenting

As we have covered, attachment parenting allows the child to feel safe and secure because all of its needs are met very quickly. The child learns to feel loved and has no need to suffer with loneliness or stress – which is where self-esteem problems can begin.

2. Improve your own self-confidence

It's so important what we tell our children about ourselves. We must not criticize ourselves in front of them (complain about our weight, our intelligence or our looks); if we want our children to be confident and happy with themselves, we must appear to be that way too. Parenting is the perfect time to try and heal our own old wounds. You can be the parent that you wished you had by learning from the mistakes and also using the positives that you learnt from how you were brought up. I was a very naughty child, but I was also very polite and I love that my parents instilled great manners in me.

3. Be a positive example

A child will not only worry about what you think of her/him but also about how others think towards them. If you give your child constant positive affirmations and also say that she is fun to be around and that her opinions, behavior and her 'whole being' pleases you – then she is more likely to feel internally pleased with herself.

4. Play with your child as often as you can

Interestingly, children will find being in your company, while playing, much more stimulating than playing with other people or children. More learning takes place when you interact and when the child chooses what to do. This also increases their self-esteem.

5. Encourage the child's talents

All children have a talent and all are capable of doing many things well. It can be very simple things from keeping toys tidy or a certain type of activity. The key is noticing what they do well and praising it. Children when at school may be gifted with sport or maths and may not be good at both. You can instill positive enforcement by saying that everyone has a gift and that it's OK to not be perfect at everything.

6. Have a wall of 'fame' in your house

Dedicate a wall or area in your home that displays your children's artwork, trophies and other achievements. Even if they aren't 'pretty' it doesn't matter; if you put them up, it shows your children that you are proud of what they have done and that you are also proud for everyone to see them too.

7. Find out what's going on in school

Sometimes, no matter what you do, sending your child to school can be absolutely devastating for their self-esteem. It's therefore important to find out what's going on. Is your child being bullied by anyone, students or even any of the teachers? Find out if your child has lots of friends, or is sticking by themselves all the time. Are they willing to join drama classes and to do a type of sport? Or do they just seem too shy? As a parent, you will want to protect your child from any upset due to school life, but the answer is not to wrap up your child in cotton wool. Parents must not be too over-protective either; the key is getting the balance just right.

Find out as much as you can about what is going on in school and consider ways to sort the problem out. A good teacher will be able to give you lots of advice on what is going on with your child and their classmates. Remember, you can use Bush or Bach Flower Remedies to help with shyness and other personality traits which may be holding your child back from being truly happy.

8. Treat your child like an adult and give them jobs to do

When children are little they take great pride in helping parents to do things. If you are folding the washing, or cooking, they are more than likely wanting to help you, even if they are too young to do much actual 'help'. At the appropriate age, give them tasks to do and say that you could not have the house run smoothly without their great help. This gives them praise and also the desire that work is a good thing. You can start between the ages of 2 and 4. This is not about creating little slaves, by the way; it's merely to get them into the routine of contributing to family life and feeling like they have a purpose.

Building better body image

This subject could not be more important. Self-esteem issues to do with appearance are a massive problem these days, more than ever before in society. So many children are battling with poor body image and many end up being diagnosed with 'Body Dysmorphic Disorder' later in life – where they simply cannot see themselves as attractive in any way, shape or form. Anorexia and bulimia are also rife these days, and are affecting even the very young.

While we can definitely blame the media and the governments for not trying to help protect our kids better *from* the media, the child's first view of their own body image comes from the parents. And how we make them feel about themselves, will last a lifetime and as many of us relate, this may mean a lifetime of pain and unhappinesss – where we feel we never quite measure up to our parents expectations. And as we have discussed previously, if the parents' have self-esteem issues, they more than likely will pass on those same feelings to their kids if they don't recognise what has happened to them.

Ask any psychiatrist or psychologist what problems they find their patients encounter the most and it will be lack of self-esteem and feeling unworthy. They may be in their 40s or 50s and *still* feel this way, despite having a successful career, lovely home and family of their own. As most research is pointing too, the first 6 years shapes our lives, our health and our happiness and self-esteem. As a parent myself, its alarming to know that it's virtually impossible to get parenting 'right' that it is inevitable we may do something in our child's eyes, that they say years later, they wished we had done differently. It's all about trying to minimise how serious these wishes may be. We can certainly try very hard to understand our children better, to take the time to really *see* them and to try to problem solve around their concerns or behaviors. And we can of course try to solve our own issues so we don't take them out on our children. This is the key and I can't emphasize it more, we must be able to handle our *own* issues so as not to let our children suffer from them. We must try and instill healthy self-esteem as soon as a child can speak and can understand what you are saying. It's very important to praise many different parts about a child, rather than saying, 'You look pretty' or 'You are beautiful'. Try to encourage them to see their body parts as unique and that you love every part of them. For example, if your child loves dancing, you can say, 'You are so good at dancing – you have very strong legs and move so well.'

I sing to Lola all the time my 'Lovely Lola Song'. I sing (very badly I admit) that I have a 'lovely baby with lovely eyes, she has a lovely chin, lovely legs, a lovely mind, and lovely arms' and so forth, so that I tell her that everything about her, to me, is lovely. When she is older and able to understand the words, I hope this will be very powerful in helping build her self-esteem.

I am also going to put affirmations on her walls (wall stickers) so that she sees those words constantly. Phrases like 'Twinkle, twinkle, little star, do you know how special you are' so that they will help 'program' her mind into powerful ways of thinking so that she knows we really do love and think highly of her.

It's worth noting that instilling self-esteem comes from the way *both* parents interact with their children. Females are at a *huge* risk of having 'daddy or male issues' if their own fathers did not take the time to instill strong messages of acceptance and validation in their daughters. And if they feel they don't measure up or they don't think their fathers think highly of them, it can cause a very destructive path ahead of them, often ending up with drug & alcohol addictions, self-harm, bad relationships and just a life of unhappiness and even ill health from all of the stress. Author Suzanne Fields, writes in her book *Like Father, Like Daughter – How Father Shapes The Woman His Daughter Becomes:*

Fathers have long been the forgotten parents, daughters the forgotten offspring, says Dr Michael Lamb of the University of Utah, one of the most important researchers in the field of father-daughter relationships. And yet, a girl's first perception of the opposite sex comes through her daddy; he forever colours the eye through which a woman sees men. He shapes her expectations of male behaviour. Did he hold our hands when we took our first faltering steps? Did he care when he watched us struggle through the multiplication tables? Was he comfortable showing us affection? Did he hold us close when needed to be hugged, roughhouse with us when we wanted to play, punish us when we secretly yearned to be disciplined? Did he care how we looked? When our bodies began to change did he notice – or pretend not to? Was he pleased when we appeared in the living room all dressed up for a boyfriend? Whether at school, with our mothers, or with our first boyfriends, could we count on him to see us through those early, agonizing crises? As we got interested in the world around us, did he freely share his knowledge and perception?

I'm sure many females can remember how their childhoods were in relation to their fathers, and that there was probably much more disappointment and critical discipline rather than loving memories where they felt protected and accepted by their fathers.

The mother-daughter relationship is also equally as important, if not more so and of course this also relates to the effects on sons as well as daughters. Each child, regardless of their sex, has a distinct need from either parent to enhance their self-esteem and the implications of *not* receiving it, can, and does impact people's entire lives.

Obviously these are *huge* subjects and ones that cannot be delved into here properly or at all adequately, I can however, point you in the direction of some wonderful books that can help the way you see yourself, and how to be better towards your children in relation to their self esteem.

Please, never tease a child about anything as they may hold on to what was said for a very long time, perhaps the rest of their lives! Even if it's 'just a joke' it may not be seen as one by them. If they are sensitive kids, then you should know that they probably won't find jokes funny that appear to put them down. Be attuned to their personality type and be sensitive to them if they aren't as strong as others. Try not to compare them to other children as well. You want your child to see that they are special just the way they are.

Children will naturally compare themselves to other children, and once they get to school they may even get teased – and yes it may be well be out of jealousy but that does not make it any easier for the child to handle. While we see it as a rite of passage it can *easily* get very out of hand, very quickly.

I never knew that anything was 'wrong' with my own appearance until I started school. It wasn't until someone called me 'Big Nose' that I started to look in the mirror obsessively many times a day. That teasing was with me until I was 30 and only went away when I changed my nose with plastic surgery – a really extreme way to deal with it and a way that is becoming so common these days for others to deal with their dislike of their own appearance.

I really think many children don't have self-image problems until they are teased. They've felt OK about themselves until their peers picked faults, with them. And if you see this happen, try to put a stop to it; if it's other siblings doing this, they must know that it is not allowed. And if it is happening at school, see if there is something that can be done to stop it. If my child was being bullied so much and the school could not do anything about it, I would seriously consider homeschooling my child. As previously mentioned, bullying is at another level these days; due to social networking such as Facebook and Twitter, kids are getting abused in ways that are most worrying, and now quite often, ending in their deaths. As well as teenage suicide, there are now more cases of even younger children taking their own lives, and it's usually all down to severe bullying. Our schools are dealing with so much that it seems almost impossible for them to sort this massive problem out.

If parents have done a great job at instilling self-confidence from a young age, the child is more likely to let the negative comments slide off their back, rather than affecting them for years to come.

This issue of building self-esteem covers a lot more than I have just discussed here. I really *urge* you to take much more time into learning about this vitally important subject for the sake of your child's life, health and also the impact this will have on society. As I mentioned, a really wonderful book which expands on this subject is *The Discipline Book* by William and Martha Sears. They advise parents on how to deal with a child's anger, how to get them to express their feelings and so much more. It's not just for small children but also covers how to help teenagers deal with life, their view of themselves and the world. Truly brilliant and a must-read.

Australian author and Psychologist Anthony Gunn, has also written a real gem- *Raising Confident Happy Children – 40 Ways To Help Your Child Succeed.*

Another great book many parents swear by - is *How to Talk So Kids Will Listen and Listen So Kids Will Talk* by Adele Faber and Elaine Mazlish.

Chapter 40

The Importance of Immersing Kids in Nature

Scientists have termed 'Biophilia' as an instinctive bond between humans and all living things – which basically means that we need to be around nature to be at our best. According to Erich Fromm who first discovered this connection, he describes a psychological orientation where humans are inherently attracted to all that is alive and vital. Edward O. Wilson, who wrote the book *Biophilia* also uses this term and suggests that biophillia describes 'the connections that human beings subconsciously seek with the rest of life'. He suggested the possibility where deep affiliations humans have with Nature are rooted in our biological makeup. The exact opposite of phobias, in which people have fears towards things in the natural world, philias are the desired attractions and positive feelings that people have toward certain habitats, activities, and objects in their natural surroundings.[190]

Since many of us live in big cities these days, it's rare that we have our own gardens. This means that children are not being around Nature as much as they should and need to be. They are missing out on the importance of breathing in healthier, fresher air, walking on the bare ground, and also being close to the healing powers of plants. This disconnect is causing all of us detrimental affects, but more so for our children.

Looking back in history, most children were brought up on the land and were able to play outside for hours each day, using their imaginations and the wonders of Nature to keep them entertained. Nowadays, children rarely ever even play outside; the weather is either too miserable or parents are too busy to keep an eye on them, not to mention the unfortunate safety issue – we simply cannot leave our children on their own outside of the home. So it seems easier to sit them in front of the TV or to keep them occupied with video games. Just like the school system teaches them to always keep their minds busy with constantly being told what to do, so do the TV and computer games. This is another reason why children are losing touch with their ability to be creative, and also to find their true purpose.

Even more worrying is the impact to their health; children brought up in big cities are at a greater risk because they are exposed to much pollution, EMFs and just the general stress that city life brings.

In recent studies, children who live in smoggy cities have been found to have (among other things) xenoestrogens in their bloodstream, which they are absorbing through the air, due to the high level of petrol fumes. Xenoestrogens are industrial chemicals which negatively affect the hormone levels in the body. It has been studied that children growing up in developed cities usually have heavier body weights compared to those who live in the country and it's said that it could be directly contributed to these xenoestrogens.

It's quite concerning to learn that as well as contributing to excess fetal growth, xenoestrogens have been linked to worrying problems such as obesity, hyperactivity, early puberty, cancers of the lung, breast and prostate, as well as fertility problems, later in life. This really worries me because our children already have so much toxicity to deal with; they are generally being born with hundreds of pollutants in their bodies and, combined with the lack of high-quality food, and the typical short time of time being breastfed, it's quite worrying that living in a city too is only adding more to this toxic overload.

It's also suggested that a child should literally 'get dirty' and this involves being outside and playing on the grass and getting exposed to outside germs. Today, we have been led to believe that all germs are bad and that we must always wash our and our children's hands with antibacterial soaps. This is one of the worst things we can do for health because we are not allowing our bodies to develop their own immunity. It is also said that children who are always keeping clean may even be more likely to contract allergies or asthma later in life too. If anyone is concerned about the risk of contracting tetanus, it is wise to always check where your children are playing and make sure it's a safe area. And if your child does get cut badly, you can learn to clean the wound in such a way that it will heal without a risk of tetanus occurring. Please refer to the *Vaccination Bible* by Lynne McTaggart for instructions on how to do this.

There are so many benefits of being around Nature and one of these is being relaxed. In a study led by environmental psychologist Frances Kuo, from Illinois University, it was shown that children who suffer with hyperactivity disorders tend to display a huge improvement in their behavior after only 20 minutes of being outside. This supports the suggestion that humans need to be around Nature to be calm and happy.[191]

And of course, children who grow up around the countryside or go to parks often tend to have a much lower, healthier body weight compared to those of a city. Children need to move often; not only do they produce a lot of energy at that age, but it's also a fun part of childhood, running around and being active. Sadly, due to diet and toxic burden, more and more children are having energy problems and becoming overweight. It's truly worrying – if there is a weight problem now, then the future is quite concerning.

After knowing how toxic city life is, I do realize that it's not so easy for families to up and leave. City life usually brings bigger pay checks for a family, so I am not suggesting we all pack up and move away, but there are things you can do to help bring this connection back to your children.

One of the many benefits of visiting the countryside, beach, forest or mountains is the difference in air quality. When you get away from pollution from cars and trains, the air will be much cleaner, especially in an environment surrounded by trees. If you can visit the countryside, beach, forest or mountains as often as you can, then this will really help you and your children on a physical, spiritual and emotional level, not to mention it's fun!

If this is hard for you to do, just say you live very far from Nature, one tip I can share with you again is to place as *many* healthy-air plants in your home as you can afford to at least create a healthy-air environment. This will add a great deal of healthy oxygen that your child and entire family will be able to benefit from. Even if your house starts to look like a jungle or rainforest, at least you can all rest easier knowing that your home contains air that is of a high quality.

I recently had some painting done at our last rental house (our landlord wanted it done) and the painter unfortunately did not use any non-toxic paints. I quickly placed a few of our healthy-air plants around the painted areas and marveled at how quickly the smell dissipated and how much perkier the plants looked! Plants also add lots of beauty to a house and you will find your guests will comment on how lovely the house looks and feels. One of my close friends (Lola's godmother) has many plants in each room of her house, big and small, and it always feels so wonderful when we visit. Everyone else that visits also notices that house has such a positive energy.

So, whenever you can, hopefully every day if possible, take your children to a park, or a forest or to the beach. Anywhere that is near Nature. It will not only be good for them health wise, it will also make them happy. Kids love going to the beach or park for more reasons than it just being fun; I think their intuition knows that this is where they are meant to be. The more they are around Nature, the more it becomes normal for them and even in adulthood they will often prefer the countryside than big cities.

We are directly connected to Nature, and we also become far healthier, develop a stronger immune system and become less stressed by being outside. As you can see, this is vital for our children. Explain to your kids the wonderful power of Nature and that plants and trees are very special, and the fresh air makes us smarter and healthier!

Chapter 41

Encourage Children to Remain Creative and Watch Them Thrive

Creativity is not merely the innocent spontaneity of our youth and childhood; it must also be married to the passion of the adult human being, which is a passion to live beyond one's death.
Rollo May American Existential Psychologist

I don't know anyone who can't remember with fondness, when they were young, playing with sand, painting, cutting out shapes, sticking things together and drawing. It's a part of most children's formative years and, for some, it's when they were at their most creative. Kids are naturally highly inquisitive and imaginative when they are little, but sadly, with time, they lose this due to entering the regimented schooling system and of course, our ways of society. They go from having the freedom to be as messy as they want to be, that there are no 'rules' with what they are creating, that being perfect is not what it's about. And once they reach a certain age, that freedom of both expression and thought now has lots of boundaries and rules, which often can involve putting a stop to a child's creative outlet.

As they go through school, the 'system' focuses on classes involving reading, science and maths etc. and does not really focus on keeping the child creative, or not for nearly long enough. Even art classes take up such a short period of the school day compared to the other subjects. This is very tragic because lots of enjoyment and happiness comes from being artistic. For some it is the most enjoyable aspect of their life and a way to connect with themselves. Art and other forms of creativity are often used in therapy sessions and are said to be very healing. Art is also very relaxing and can really help with stress levels.

What the school system does not recognize is that many children are not academic by nature and when their much-loved creative outlet is cut off, they switch off from school lessons and tend not to pay any more attention, therefore failing and often ending up being bored and highly unhappy adults who have *no clue* about what they want to do with their lives. They were usually not given enough of a chance when young to find out what they truly loved doing, and so begin many years of frustration and boredom, as well as bad grades in school and disappointed parents.

To avoid this from happening when your child is young, and also right through the teen years, try and keep your child doing fun and creative activities – even if the schools don't encourage this. Teach your children the beauty of art, singing, cooking, performing arts, dancing and playing. This is so essential for developing a healthy and confident self-esteem. If you join in on activities when your child is young and continue to do this, it will become such a habit to them that they may feel that they need to do something creative in their spare time, avoiding video games and TV! Lola and I go to playgroup together and I have already started to learn how to make inexpensive crafts from natural materials such as pine cones, sticks, flowers, and non toxic paints. Whilst Lola is not old enough at the time of writing this book to join in, I have so many unique activities I can do with her when she is. I think its very important to really give your child full attention as much as possible and doing artwork together is such a great way to achieve this.

Childhood should be full of wonderful happy memories and by doing lots of interesting things with them, its not only a bonding process for your relationship but may impact the career path your child will follow.

Whilst some activities can certainly add extra expense to your budget, there also many things that are of no cost to you, find out online what is available nearby.

Here are some ideas for having fun with your kids

- Learn to surf – doing this together is a great way to experience nature, learn something new and create special memories.
- Ride a horse on the beach – kids love animals, especially horses. Take some lessons together
- Dress up day – Your kids will think you are the bees knees if you dress up with them. Be a kid again and become a pirate or even a mermaid
- Camp on the beach – kids love the beach and camping so when you combine the two, you are onto a winner.
- Cook with the kids and teach them how to respect fire and to be safe when making food.
- Grow veggies in your garden – or grow things in small pots at home if you don't have much room. Get them to have the responsibility of watering and pruning if they are the appropriate ages.
- Beach games – there is so much you can do at the beach – build sandcastles, have running races, swimming and digging competitions, count how many birds/crabs/fish you can all find.
- Go Beachcombing – when you are at the beach, you can turn your experience into many types of games – go find shells and sticks and whoever finds the most, wins a prize.
- Visit a Zoo – if you can find a zoo that treats their animals really well (decent sized enclosures that are clean where the animals look healthy and well fed) then your children will absolutely love this.
- Create a Nature Table – use a table or even a drawer to store things in that you find when out and about in nature. Keep that interesting shell, nut, rock, stone and for the super creative, make plaster-cast moulds of footprints that you find in the forest. When you have built up a collection, take them out and get your kids to remember what they know about the object.

- Make a cubby/den in the woods/garden – kids absolutely love making things and pretending. Making a cubby house with them will be a highlight. And if you are super creative, try and make a real wooden cubby house in the garden. Much cheaper than buying and more fun.
- Go Bird Watching – if you live near where birds often frequent, you might like to take your kids out with a pair of binoculars and look for pretty and special birds. They might have to be quiet though so if they aren't too good at keeping silent, this might not be the best activity for noisy kids.
- Go on a 'City Safari' – if you live in the inner city and can't get out to nature as often as you like, you can go on a walk and show your kids the nature that you do find. Keep an eye out like a detective for any wildlife/animals you see. You will be surprised at what you will find, even in a big city. This teaches kids to keep their eyes open as to what is all around them.
- Help build your kids a stage – kids usually love performing, singing and dancing, so if you ask them to put on a show, they probably will! All you need is a sheet to make for a curtain and some other items you might have around the house. This can keep them occupied for hours!
- Go to a theme park – kids absolutely love going to theme parks, it can quite often become the highlight of their year and become a very fond memory later on. If they don't like roller coasters thought, don't make them go on them. Let them choose what they want to go on.
- Play a game in the garden or at your local park – kids need to exercise more than ever because they just aren't as active anymore. If you can play games with them, they are more than likely to want to do this regularly. Play cricket, soccer or just make up your own games. You could even have a sports day where you give out prizes. Doing this with cousins and your kids friends could make it a really fun event.
- If you live in a cold country like the UK or Canada you can

still play ball games inside (if you have a big house that is!) you can use a scrunched-up ball of paper instead of a real ball so if it hits anything it wont break.

Teach Your Children About Saving The Planet

You're a conscious parent right? So you naturally want your own kids to understand what it's all about, and *why* it's so important. Kids are often naturally very sensitive to things when they understand the big picture.

Another way of having fun with your children whilst doing something very important is teaching them about the environment. Explain to them how people throw too much away, point to the amount of rubbish you have and maybe show them pictures from the internet about rubbish dumps (show them the one in Rio that is absolutely massive) and explain that the rubbish has to go somewhere and doesn't just disappear. Explain that people have to go through all of the rubbish and it's not safe or nice for them to do this. Tell them that there are ways of using things again instead of throwing them out. Glass jars can become storage containers things they find in the forest for example. Show them how you recycle and get them to help you sort it out. When you go food shopping get them to help you choose something that doesn't need any packaging.

Talk about water use and that in some countries it doesn't rain very often and people don't have enough water to drink. Explain that all water is precious so that turning on taps too often is not good and having long showers or deep baths is a real waste.

Let your children know that many animals are endangered because of being poached or because we are using too much land for wood and for farming. Teach them that many people are starving in the world because they have no food. These people need help from people like us to improve their lives. Talk to them about organic farming and how food should be grown without chemicals. Get them to help their neighbour or grandma by doing something thoughtful and kind. Explain that the world needs more caring people and that there is a big job to do with sorting all the world's problems out.

Tell them about Clinton Hill, the boy who started *Kids For Saving Earth*. Clinton tragically died from cancer at age 11 but before he did, he started a kids club dedicated to helping the environment. His parents explained to him what was happening to the planet, that toxins and chemicals were destroying our health and harming the environment and that we were also being very cruel to animals with certain ways we farm them. Clinton wanted to do something and something that would make a real difference. Thousands of kids from all over the world have now joined his group and the parents (and a whole team of people) run the not for profit organisation in his memory. Clinton's mission was to educate and inspire kids to protect the environment. Kids from the organisation have even given moving speeches at the United Nations. Teachers from around the world have used the materials from *Kid For Saving Earth* in their classrooms. Newsletters are sent out bi-monthly to all members and teachers. You can buy books, posters, stickers, certificates, non- toxic materials, and all sorts of other eco-friendly things.

All sorts of memberships are offered. You can join as family, as an individual and as a group/parent. There is even a free membership for an individual. Prices for all of the other types of memberships are very reasonable. They all come with certificates so that you can put your child's name on it so that they can make a contract with the planet to be better to it. What an amazing little guy Clinton Hill was. Explain to your children that Clint is the perfect example of what anyone can do if they have a vision and to stick their mind to it. You can check out Clinton's organisation and there are other websites below to help kids become more earth conscious too. I've already signed Lola and myself up.

- ✓ kidsforsavingearth.org
- ✓ earthsaversclubforkids.com
- ✓ inchinapinch.com
- ✓ savetheearthforkids.com
- ✓ cehn.org

There is a wonderful international movement called 'Forest Schools' which is a program implemented by schools who take their children to nature as often as they can, so that they can play and learn outdoors in a natural environment. They take children out in all sorts of weather conditions so that they can experience nature in all of it's seasons. There have been many studies done on the effects of learning in nature and how it benefits all sorts of children, and their conditions such as learning and attention disabilities. Even many schools in inner London, which is quite far from any greenery have joined up to this inititiave after teachers realised that many children, depending on where they live (i.e. lower socioeconomic housing estates) would not visit nature at all if it wasn't for these programs. If you have children at school who don't have a lot of outdoor area to play at it might be worthwhile mentioning this scheme to them. The website below offers teachers programs.

✓ forestschools.com

Many families are now homeschooling their children because they realize that the typical school systems are not offering enough of a creative outlet like they wish their children to have. I will be discussing the problems with education today in the next chapter as well as offering alternative school systems.

Below are some helpful websites which may give you ideas on how to enhance your child's creativity.

✓ imagineproject.org
✓ kidscreative.org
✓ creativekids.org.uk
✓ creativekids.info
✓ creativekidssask.ca
✓ mycreativekids.com
✓ eastside.org.uk
✓ edenproject.com

Chapter 42

Education Today and How It's Failing Our Children

A new child is an open book and we are damaging the pages of learning because of a lack of knowledge within ourselves, and reluctance to change our outlook or even consider, for once, that we don't know it all! ... Those responsible for the education of our children owe it to themselves, as well as those in their charge, to be open-minded enough to consider new and less restrictive avenues of teaching for young minds.

Josephine Sellers, *Parallel Worlds*

This brings me to another very important subject that truly concerns me, and that is *education*. This entire system is in a complete mess, and it's actually the Western countries like USA, UK and Australia (who ironically have the most resources) that are really suffering, or should I say, where the *children* are suffering. They are leaving school without really knowing the basics, and the way they are being taught is so regimented with hardly any emphasis on allowing children to think for themselves, all the while squashing their own natural creativity and instincts.

Not many of us give much thought to how long ago the education system that we still follow today was introduced and why the structure is the way it is. And not many question how it needs to change with the times – and why hasn't it?

In the late 19th century, most of Western, Central, and parts of Eastern Europe began to provide elementary education in reading, writing, and arithmetic, partly because politicians believed that education was needed for orderly behavior. As more people became able to read, they realized that most secondary education was only open to those who could afford it. After governments had created primary education, most students were then able to go on to secondary school, with most schools becoming free. Before the 1900s, it was only the wealthy who could send their children to school.

Today, school is free for all in most Western countries, so children are being educated, but not many are actually *learning* anything of value. This typical mainstream system really only seems to work for a very small amount of children, with a certain type of intelligence, and the majority are left feeling like they hardly learnt anything at school. They leave school uninspired, unsure and unmotivated because they do not know where their own passions and talents lie. School simply does not cater to exploring all the different types of intelligence. Sir Ken Robinson shares the following in his book, *The Element*:

> Harvard psychologist Howard Gardner has argued to wide acclaim that we have not one but multiple intelligences. They include linguistic, musical, mathematical, spatial, kinesthetic, intra-personal (knowledge and understanding of the self) intelligence. He argues that these types of intelligence are more or less independent of each other, and none is more important, though some might be 'dominant' while others are 'dormant'. He says that we all have different strengths in different intelligences and that education should treat them equally so that all children receive opportunities to develop their individual abilities.[192]

We are *all* born with gifts, but if we do not have a chance to discover what these are, then what hope do we have for being truly happy? In regards to myself, I only discovered at the age of 32 that I really loved to write, so for all those years (15 in total!) since finishing school I wandered through life unsure of my own desires and talents. I felt lost, and had low self-esteem as I felt I couldn't offer anything to the world. How many 'me's are out there right now, who feel the same? They completed school, but are not *any* closer to finding out what they want to do and love?

Some state (public) schools are full of such bored and uninspired kids that the amount of crime that goes on at school requires metal detectors to keep kids from bringing in weapons to school. Sounds very far-fetched I know, but it's *much* more common than you think. Even the school I went to in Australia way back in the 1980s (which was in a smallish country town) now has to deal with kids bringing knives to school as well as trying to handle the bullying that goes on. Sure, in this case, it's not just the school making kids resort to crime – their home life more than likely is not good either – but if what they were learning was fun and right for them, they would at least find their days away from home a good thing and their behavior would show it.

Parents, who used to be able to breathe a sigh of relief when children were sent off to school, are now beginning to worry that the time spent at school is *not* doing what it's supposed to do. The children are simply not learning enough, nor in the right way. And because of the amount of bullying that goes in secondary schools, parents are now very worried about how tough these years will be for their children. What will it do to them long term?

Even the schools that were formally known as 'outstanding' are now losing their status because more and more children are leaving without good grades, said to be mainly due to lack of high-quality teaching. Governments are now admitting that the schools are failing our children, but the worrying response from them is that they think children should spend longer in school and have fewer holidays. This is possibly one of the *worst* things we could do. If anything, children need *less* school time (but we should *increase* the quality) and more time to think for themselves, rather than being told what to do all day. John Taylor-Gatto, author of *Dumbing Us Down*, puts it brilliantly:

Right now we are taking from our children all the time they need to develop self-knowledge. That has to stop. We have to invent school experiences that give a lot of time back. We need to trust children from a very early age with independent study, perhaps arranged in school, but which takes place *away* from the institutional setting. We need to invent curricula where each kid has a chance to develop private uniqueness and self-reliance.[193]

What is very alarming is the lack of 'life studies' that are taught in schools. Don't we think that kids could do with being taught about what the *real* world is like, the harsh reality of what will be expected when away from their parents' care? Why don't we teach our children how to respect money? Why don't we teach them about health and the importance of good food? Why don't we teach them about relationships and how difficult they can be, and offer them solutions? Why don't we talk to them about the pressures in society to look a certain way? Let's teach them about being kind, volunteering their services, and connecting with their community. Or let's teach them how to grow their own food. And how about this – let's teach them how to develop good self-esteem!

Can you *imagine* how much better off kids would be learning all of these things? And how much more of a *benefit* to society these children would be if they learnt all of these highly important skills from a young age?

So *why* do these things not get taught in schools? For many, the answer to this is: it's not taught for many reasons – one probably being about money. If children knew how to respect money then they would not become addicted to buying things like they are these days. They would not become so obsessed with their looks and themselves, if they learnt from a young age that all of this stuff is to distract them from what's important. This is the problem with following a system that is well in need of a huge overhaul. But to change a schooling system that has been in place for decades would be almost impossible and would cost a heck of a lot of money. And I just don't think the governments want to do this. It's too big a problem.

For the world to progress we need to make sure our children grow up happy, healthy and confident individuals, and education, yes, plays a *massive* role in this. But it's *what* and *how* we educate them that *really* matters. The majority of schools have no idea (nor the allowance or time) how to discover what the best way is to bring out children's talents. It's simply not important for them to do this. We are teaching a curriculum that has not changed much at all since the system was put in place, many decades ago. And sadly, because we now have such a strict schooling system implemented in many countries with very long hours, we now also have way too many children in the classes, so the teachers really do not have time to help each individual. So, many children's needs fall right between the cracks, impacting on the rest of their lives. Many children who become bored and unmotivated absolutely despise going to school and, when older, may often completely stop paying attention or start not going to school at all, which of course means not much hope for a good future.

From an early age, we are told, 'School allows you to learn all of the things you need so you can go to college or university so you can get a very good job.' But now, with an ever-growing population and not enough jobs, many school leavers who take up extra study complete their courses to find that they *cannot* get a job. Then they are left with a *huge* amount of debt and no way to pay it back. So in their 20s, they are now *jobless* and also owe a heck of a lot of money, as well as more than likely having low self-esteem with a piece of paper that means absolutely nothing. To have spent such a large part of early life in school and college, and now be in this type of situation, is just heartbreaking.

Another tragic element to add to this subject is the amount of children who are diagnosed with 'learning disabilities'. The numbers of children on medication is absolutely staggering and I believe that drugging them is *not* the best way to treat these children at all. Dr Joseph Mercola explains:

As of 2006, at least 4.5 million American children under the age of 18 were diagnosed with ADHD, according to CDC statistics. The study above, published in the *Journal of Health Economics* in June, determined that about 20 percent of these children have likely been misdiagnosed. That's nearly one million children in the US alone. The study found that many of the youngest children in any given grade level are perceived as exhibiting 'symptoms' of ADHD, such as fidgeting and inability to concentrate, simply because they're compared to more mature classmates.

In 2006 I was diagnosed myself with ADHD (Attention Deficit Disorder) by several doctors. I had a very busy office job where I was just making so many mistakes; I had too much to do and could not handle the multi-tasking. I was put on the recommended medication but quickly came off it due to the horrible side effects – it was like being on hard drugs! I realized that instead of medicating myself to be able to keep a job that I did not want to do, I was going to set off on my own journey of finding something I was good at. I knew it was out there; I just did not know at the time what that was. And, now realizing what I *am* capable of doing, after detoxing my body, it's madness to think that the doctors wanted to put me on toxic drugs!

We must remember that *everyone* has a special talent (or many for some) and, for most people, that will only be discovered through creative outlets and with the nurturing and encouragement that is needed to allow that to flourish. And in regards to the majority of children *not* receiving *quality* education, this leads to a whole host of *other* problems such as unemployment, which drains the government (and taxpayer) funds, and it can also lead to other things which are much more serious, like kids getting involved in gangs, drugs, drinking and crime. They become so bored, have no sense of belonging and no future that seems in their reach. So they give up and get involved in lifestyles that give them a false sense of happiness and belonging. But mostly what is so tragic is the damage done to their self-esteem. They are lost without any direction whatsoever, and this can affect the rest of their lives, which will also affect their own children. And as we have discovered, parenting well is a very tough job indeed. You have to have strong emotional intelligence yourself to treat children in the way they need.

For children to *thrive* and become well-adjusted adults, they must find out what their own talents are, through other methods rather than just regimented schooling. Many children dream of having a career around music, the arts or the performance world but because of the pressure to become doctors or lawyers or other highly thought-of professions, these dreams tend to get pushed under the carpet.

Society doesn't help at all with this either, due to the influences of media and television; people tend to believe they need lots of money to live in this world and that you are *only* successful if you become *wealthy*. They are simply not taught about what really matters.

How often do we hear from people that their dreams were squashed by parents or even teachers when younger because they were told, 'There isn't any money in being a musician' or 'So many people are trying to be artists, authors, as well as you'. So, their dream is put aside and the possible incredible talent has gone to waste due to needing to please our elders and to fit into society as well. They then go on to choose a career to please others, and finally get to the ripe old age of 65 and realize that their whole life was spent doing something they did not want to do, for people (their parents!) that probably aren't even alive still! Isn't this tragic?

To achieve success for ourselves, we *must* follow our hopes and dreams, no matter what anyone says. We need to have this *nurtured* and *encouraged*, not shot to bits, ignored and put down. A good school system will recognize that *each* child is gifted and that even though one child's gift may differ from another's, they are no more or less important.

If everyone had given up on their dreams, we would all behave like robots; there would be no musicians, no artists, no inventors and the world would be a pretty bleak place. People that have gone after their dreams, despite being put down or told that they won't get anywhere, have really been able to achieve such wonderful things in the world which we all couldn't live without. Even some of the most famous people who have come from nowhere had dreams and many were told not to bother trying to achieve them. If they had listened, their lives would be very different.

After falling pregnant myself, and after discovering how much of a concern schooling is today, I have looked into many different methods and have discovered three that really stand out.

Steiner Waldorf schools

Steiner schools are really popular all over the world due to their humanistic approach to teaching based upon the philosophy of the famous Austrian philosopher Rudolf Steiner. At a Steiner school learning is focused on integrating practical, creative and conceptual elements. The approach emphasizes the role of the profound importance of the use of imagination in learning, developing thinking that includes a creative as well as an analytic component. The educational philosophy's goals are to provide young people the basis on which to develop into free morally responsible and integrated individuals, and to help every child fulfill his or her unique destiny. Schools and teachers are given considerable freedom to define curriculum within peer structures.

Steiner is unique because it:

- Works for all children irrespective of academic ability, class, ethnicity or religion
- Takes account of the needs of the whole child – academic, physical, emotional and spiritual
- Is based on an understanding of the relevance of the *different* phases of child development
- Develops a love of learning and an enthusiasm for school

- Sees artistic activity and the development of the imagination as integral to learning
- Is tried and tested and is part of state-funded, mainstream provision in most European countries
- Is respected worldwide for its ability to produce very able young people who have a strong sense of self and diverse capacities that enable them to become socially and economically responsible citizens.

Steiner identified three main phases of development of children

- *The first seven years* the child is developing their physical body and is primarily living in their will. During this period, learning is primarily through physical actions and imitation.
- *From the ages 7 to 13* the child becomes increasingly aware of a wider world outside of the family and begins to develop a sense of self. This period is one of strong feelings, and effective teaching involves engaging the child's imagination pictorially rather than through analysis.
- *The period from 14 to 21* marks the transition from childhood to adulthood and is characterized by the development of thinking. The role of the teacher and curriculum in this period is to guide the student's use of critical thinking into constructive ends, and to help them to develop self-direction and independent judgement.

After reading about the Steiner schools, and having the experience of visiting one in the UK, it is evident to see just how much fun these school children have. They learn organic farming, study one subject at a time till everyone understands and 'gets it', and spend a large percentage of school hours being immersed in creative activities. For each subject they include painting, music and even poetry, to learn in different ways. The students stay with the same teacher through the lower school years and also have another teacher throughout their entire high school years. This creates a special bond among the students and the teachers.

At Steiner schools, there is also a huge community atmosphere with the parents being encouraged to join in on school activities such as fairs and markets. Instead of these schools having the typical cold atmosphere, Steiner schools exude happiness, fun and health. Even the quality of food that they serve is of high organic standards and parents are instructed not to fill their child's lunch box with junk foods. If I could go back in time again and go through school, this is exactly how I would want to be taught. Lola is enrolled at a Steiner school.

Check to see if a Steiner school is near you. In some countries there are government-funded Steiner schools.

✓ steinerwaldorf.org

We consider Steiner education the best decision we ever made

by Sarah Best

My husband and I both went to conventional schools – mine a state school and his a private school. Neither of us has happy memories of our school days, as neither of these schools met our needs as individuals. Conventional education is simply not designed to do that, and after our son was born we both knew that we wanted something different for him.

To cut a long story short, when he started school at age 5 we enrolled him into a Steiner school. He's 10 now and we consider it the best decision we ever made. Here's why:

- The Steiner educational system is designed to work in harmony with the different phases of the child's development. So in the early years, rather than trying to force academic, left-brain learning (which the child is not ready for at this time) the focus is on learning through play, creative activities and the development of the imagination.

- Even when the children are older, Steiner education is not just about academic learning; equal weight is given to each pupil's physical, emotional and spiritual needs.
- Steiner education fosters in children an appreciation of nature and natural whole foods. From age 9 they begin learning how to grow organic vegetables. Junk foods are not allowed in school. Thanks to a recognition of how sensitive children's brains and entire systems are to synthetic foods, not only are crisps and chocolate bars expressly disallowed; all packaged foods are discouraged. In a similar vein, whereas in most schools, unvaccinated children are in the minority, here they are the norm.

Our son loves school and is thriving. We never imagined that the shy little boy who started in the kindergarten at age 5 would be so confident and assured by age 10. In addition, because of the Steiner system's respect for the stages of childhood, he retains a joyful innocence that many children have sadly lost by his age. Of course, no system of education is perfect but we couldn't be happier with our choice.

Sarah Best is an investigative journalist and was an editor of Get Fresh Magazine *for five years. She has her own website where she writes many articles related to health and well being.*

✓ sarahbesthealth.com

Montessori pre-schools

Montessori education is characterized by an emphasis on independence, freedom within limits, and respect for a child's natural psychological development, as well as technological advancements in society. Although a range of practices exists under the name 'Montessori', the Association Montessori Internationale (AMI) and the American Montessori Society (AMS) cite these elements as essential:

- Mixed-age classrooms, with classrooms for children aged 2½ or 3 to 6 years old by far the most common
- Student choice of activity from within a prescribed range of options
- Uninterrupted blocks of work time
- A theory of knowledge or 'discovery' model, where students learn concepts from working with materials, rather than by direct instruction
- Specialized educational materials developed by Maria Montessori and her collaborators

In addition, many Montessori schools design their programs with reference to Montessori's model of human development from her published works, and use lessons and materials introduced in teacher training derived from courses presented by Montessori during her lifetime.

✓ www.montessori.org/

These schools, of course, are generally not free (although are still usually cheaper than private schools) so I do understand that while many parents would love to send their children to either of these schools, they may not be able to afford to. Some do offer financial assistance though so it is always worth looking into by contacting the schools and asking about their programs.

What I can recommend, however, is looking into the system that you would prefer and reading about how they teach their students. On the weekends and on school holidays, you could adapt some of their methods to your children's free time. Many kids who go to these schools do not ever say that they dislike going; in fact, it's often hard for the parents to get them to leave! So, do not feel that you are being too pushy by trying to introduce some of the curriculum to their lives. Concentrate on the fun and creative activities and your child is sure to bloom and fall in love with learning. Or, try and find a school that is not so big; smaller schools are able to offer children better education generally, simply due to having fewer students.

My take on Montessori

by Victoria Leith – mother to Maya

When I walked into Maidford Montessori, a school based on a farm with acres of beautiful land in Northamptonshire, I was instantly presented with the atmosphere in the room where 20 or so young people (3 or 4 years old) were getting on with various tasks and activities, helping each other out, bringing their work to tables, interacting with the materials, exploring them then packing them neatly away. One of the boys came up to Maya and showed her how. She joined in like she had been going for years. The owner of the school came up to Maya, got down to her level and spoke to her. I was so impressed by how she interacted with my daughter – as if Maya was her equal and not just a little child standing before her. What I heard in the voice was respect, courtesy and actually ... love for the child! Being part of the Baha'i community where we learn and practice daily to acquire such attributes and virtues, I was not only impressed, I was hooked!

I graduated in 1998 with a BEd Honors teaching degree and started my first post in a middle school in Northamptonshire. I always knew I would be there for two years and then leave to set up a performing arts collective, which I subsequently did and went into schools leading creative dance, singing and drama workshops for six years. During the course of our entire degree, I don't remember us covering the life or times or philosophies of Maria Montessori. We certainly didn't study her principles and now that I have had first-hand experience working in the 'mainstream' system and also as a volunteer in a Montessori for two years, I really don't understand why it is not the pivotal learning ground for all teachers who want to work with children.

When I became pregnant with my daughter Maya, I looked into Montessori schools. I had learned about Maria Montessori from a good friend and reading in magazines and was interested to know more. The further I read about Montessori schools, I knew that I had to find one for my daughter, at least for two years from ages 3 to 5 years (part-time). It's not that Montessori schools are 'better than other schools' – any school out there can employ and undertake the teachings of Montessori – any school can treat children with love and respect and value their input. Many schools, however, do not and I truly believe that a great part of this has to do with the initial training that teachers receive. Schools are seldom about virtues and values (although of course many schools do have a 'good ethos' but more about targets and attainment). With Montessori training, you are learning not just about the physical and academic development of the child but the spiritual development. And how, with your facilitation, you can assist the child to unearth the gems that already lie latent within themselves.

Education is so important in our world right now and every child must have access to being educated. But I have seen first hand what damage can be done to a child's self-esteem and life because the teacher, who is trained, is not seeing the child as a person, as someone who has value and who has a voice. This to me is the greatest difference I saw within the Montessori setting. But the good news is, anyone can adopt these methods. Any teacher who wants to work with children, in my opinion, simply must love and respect children. I know my own mother works with children every day, is not Montessori trained but has all the values of a very wonderful teacher indeed, who loves all the children she works with. But that is her personality and she chose the right job. I would invite every educational professional to at least look into the teachings and ideas of Maria Montessori and bring them into their own current practice. And also encourage some people to at least into teaching – if you feel you might irreparably damage a child's psyche or development, go into another profession instead.

My daughter now attends a school which is not Montessori but which I feel encourages that same independence, encourages them to find their light and to shine, to work hard together as a team, to work on themselves daily and to enjoy education. I couldn't ask for more.

Victoria Jane Leith is an author of several books, is a singer and creator of carameliacakery.co.uk

✓ littleguru.co.uk

Homeschooling aka 'un-schooling'

Another option that is becoming so popular is homeschooling. Homeschooling or homeschool (also known as home education or home-based learning) is the education of children typically by parents but sometimes by private tutors at the home rather than in the usual formal settings of public or private schools. Historically, prior to the introduction of compulsory school attendance laws, commonly childhood education occurred within the family or in the community.

Parents say there are numerous reasons as to what motivates them to homeschool, including higher academic test results, one-on-one instruction, it helps the public system with fewer kids, offers more hands-on environments, to avoid poor public school environments, religious needs, improved character and behavior development, to avoid the expense of private education, and due to objections to what is taught locally in public schools.

Homeschooling can be a great option for families living in isolated locations, living temporarily overseas, and to allow for more time for traveling. Many young athletes and actors are taught at home. Studies have shown that when children are homeschooled, they often show they are 5 to 10 years ahead of their formally trained peers, in their ability to think for themselves.

Homeschooling takes a bit more effort, planning and preparation on the parents' part and, of course, you need to be home quite often too. I know quite a few parents that homeschool their children and report to me how happy and creative their children are, yet they have still learnt all the other academic requirements of regular schools.

In the USA alone, there are said to be approximately 2 million children being homeschooled, with a huge movement also underway in the UK. If the education system is letting our children down then homeschooling may be the best thing to take control of what our kids learn instead. It's certainly something I will be considering in the future.

Kate Magic's story of how homeschooling has worked for her family

I have homeschooled all three of my boys, and I have to say, it's one of the best things I've ever done.

I was sure I didn't want to put them through state education, which I didn't feel would encourage their creativity and self-expression adequately. The current education system was created in Victorian times, and the world will live in now is so different, I don't feel that it's still relevant. The way we live is changing so fast, and we cannot imagine what our lifestyles will be like when our children are the age we are now. Most of them will be doing jobs that haven't even been created yet! I feel the best I can do for them is to give them the tools to know who they are, and have the strength and awareness to successfully be a person of integrity in the world.

We tried Steiner education, but I still felt it was too prescriptive. Although the curriculum is beautifully crafted and the level of care much more holistic than that of our current state system, it didn't allow my children enough freedom to explore who they are. It was still about having them sit behind a desk and be told what to think about that day. So I didn't exactly choose home education, I just felt it was the best option for us, but it has turned out to be the most wonderful experience, for many different reasons.

Firstly, I love the mornings; we all wake up naturally together, no alarm clocks, no stressing. Schoolwork is not the focus of our day, but instead, at the pre-GCSE age, I feel it's more important that they have life skills such as being able to tidy their bedrooms, do the shopping, help with jobs around the house. They all know how to make their own meals and clear up after themselves.

We spend just a few hours a day doing academic work, which I have to admit isn't anyone's favorite part of the day! But when children are given the right foods to make them happy and healthy, and are raised in a supportive, loving environment, they are naturally keen to learn. They don't need to be forced to sit behind a desk all day in order to think. The day is filled with learning opportunities, and they naturally gravitate towards the subjects they are interested in. So while we cover the obvious English and maths, we can also look at a special topic that comes up in conversation, or that they might be curious about anything from volcanoes, to blood, to Picasso. They all learn instruments, and do a lot of physical activities such as swimming, yoga and skateboarding. We get to travel when it suits us and not just in school holidays. They all have different strengths, so we spend extra time on those: Reuben is writing a sci-fi novel; Ethan creates amazing digital art.

Reuben is now in his GCSE year, and this is the period that I thought might be challenging for homeschoolers, but actually I'm finding again that our way of doing things has many benefits over the conventional system. Reuben is only taking five subjects, and he is spacing them out over the year, so he can focus on one or two at a time. All his tutor groups are very small so he is getting excellent personal tuition that he would never get in a classroom. And he is used to motivating himself to get on with his subjects, so not finding the extra workload too challenging.

Everyone imagines that home education is difficult but to me it is the easiest option available. If it's something you are considering, I would highly recommend trying it for a while and seeing how you find it. I think you might be surprised at how straightforward and fun it is. I easily fit in my own work around them, before they get up, while they are out at groups and classes, and after they go to bed. I also have an excellent child-minder who takes them for two afternoons a week.

I always say that my children are my greatest teachers, and by home educating them, I have had the greatest learning experience myself. It is enriching, fulfilling, and rewarding, and I'm confident that it's giving them the best foundation I can offer them to have the most wonderful lives. Yes, it has been a sacrifice in terms of time and income lost, but I feel sacrifice is what good parenting demands, however we choose to raise our children. We live in such a profoundly selfish culture, it is in fact gratifyingly self-improving to give some of that up for such a great cause – the next generation. The benefits to our day-to-day lifestyle far outweigh the disadvantages we have encountered, and the investment I have put into their future is immeasurable.

Kate Magic is one of the UK's leading raw food experts, and she has authored four books.

✓ Find more about Kate at: katesmagicbubble.com

* * *

Another school that is becoming much talked about is the 'Green School', set among the rice paddies in Bali, Indonesia. Made entirely out of bamboo, this sustainable international school has a waiting list a mile long with parents wanting their children to learn while being as close to Nature as possible.

✓ greenschool.org

Chapter 43

A Tragic Problem with Parenting
– Quality Time

Another epidemic in our current society is the poor *emotional state* of many children. They are growing up feeling very unloved and desperately unhappy and many can often end up using drugs and/or getting involved with the wrong crowd, and on a more serious note, even end up in jail. Some children (like me) can go through many years of very troublesome times, and eventually straighten themselves out, but sadly, some do not ever know how to do this, nor have any reason to.

While we cannot always say it's the parents' fault, evidence does show that *how* children are brought up, literally from birth, does shape how they are going to feel and behave for their entire lives. We only have to take a walk outside on the streets and see how most children are today. Swearing, smoking and hanging out with bad peers, dressing way too maturely, seems to be more normal compared to seeing well-adjusted, happy and polite children.

With so many parents striving to provide a decent lifestyle (and let's not deny, it is *very* tough – living costs are so high these days), many children are left alone at home to fend for themselves. In a recent focus group spanning across three countries, 250 children were asked what they really wanted in life. More than the nicest house or best toys and games, they 'just wanted Mum and Dad to be at home and to behave like a normal family, having dinner together and spending quality time on the weekends'. Many children felt like their parents were often 'buying' them off, by giving them computer games when all that they wanted was to know that Mum and Dad were always there for them. A large percentage of the children commented that they were deeply unhappy that their mum and or dad was always too tired after work to talk or play with them.

Isn't this so *tragic?* And many parents are having to parent on their own, as they have either divorced or perhaps never married in the first place.

We now also have many teenage parents who are still way too young themselves and the statistics get higher and higher each year. More than likely due to the constant over-sexualization that is blasted over the TV, in movies and in magazines. It is a very real worry what will happen to society when these children of generally immature teenagers grow up themselves. What will they be like, how will they find their place in the world? Will they be able to develop well? How will they fit into society? How will they treat their own children?

There are many reasons why children grow up to be unhappy and unruly, and many reasons why they don't. I would need to write another book about that to explain them all, as it's so in-depth, but I want to suggest what you can do for your own children so that they do not grow up feeling unloved. Reading and understanding childhood development is something I really recommend any parent doing. This will teach you what influences a child's growth and development, emotionally and spiritually. It will give you the tools to allow you to nurture your children in a way they understand and respond well to.

No parent ever gets it 100% right, despite all the best intentions, but I do believe we can do a lot of learning *before* we are blessed with a child. Our job is to nourish and guide them, instilling good values, but not to own and dictate to. We do not have children so that we can mold them into what we 'wished we were', or what we hope they will be. We are their guides in life, not their rulers. We should allow our children to embrace their uniqueness and their opinions, however different they may be to ours.

You can still make a child feel special even if you don't have much time. Dedicate a certain amount every day to just be with them, even if it's only 15–20 minutes. In that time, *really* be there, don't get distracted, make it fun and make sure you tell your child how much you love them.

Chapter 44

Teach Your Children the Value of Money

Another huge problem, yet a barely talked-about subject, is money. We are a world that *does not know how to spend their money wisely or how to save*. If this was not true, there wouldn't be as much credit card debt as there is today, or a huge amount of people living from pay to pay or, even worse, below the poverty line!

At school we learn so much about reading, science, maths and writing, yet children do not really learn about how important it is to *value* money or how to save and that it should not be spent so carelessly. No one ever tells us that money, and how much we have, will make or break us later in life.

When there is lack of respect and understanding about how to handle money, there are big repercussions for what happens to that child's life. We only have to look at the current financial market where problems with money have affected millions and millions of people (and not just from childhood either); we see how society and the media have conditioned us to desire so many 'things' to make us happier. We have not been taught that many times simple living is quite often the best and most fulfilling way. We have been manipulated to 'keep up with the Joneses' while getting ourselves further and further into debt. We can blame the banks most certainly for acting so dishonorably, but at the same time, due to individual senseless actions, we have allowed ourselves to get into massive debt too. It never ceases to surprise me that when all of these mortgages were handed out, why didn't people think, 'What if something goes wrong – what if we can't pay it back, what will it mean?'

Children learn from a very young age that they too love 'stuff'. New, bright shiny things they see in shops and on TV make them become addicted to things really early on so that they just want as much stuff as possible! And when they go to school, it is usually even worse because other kids bring new things to show their friends and everyone now wants the same thing. This love of being accepted and cool because of the things we have stays with someone perhaps for their entire lives.

I too had a big problem with money, for my whole life really, that has only recently been rectified. I had my first credit card straight out of school and spent the entire amount, $2000 in the space of one weekend, on clothes and makeup; I do not have any of it still in my possession today. In fact, I can't even remember what I bought, only that it took *forever* to pay off. Not only did it literally take me years to get rid of the debt (and of course with an extra enormous amount of interest added to the bill), I also had to get my parents to help me out. And it wasn't the last time. I was *always* running to them for help, needing my rent paid or my phone or electricity bill.

I had developed this bad habit of seeing money as something that was either there or it wasn't, and if it was there, it was meant to be spent due to the fact that I had a really big obsession and addiction with shopping. And if it wasn't there, someone would help me out by giving me the money. I know, what a very bad attitude!

I grew up not having a clue how to save and that money really did not grow on trees. I was lucky to live in a lovely house, with plenty of food and nice things and to be spoilt at Christmas time with many gifts. I saw money all around me, but did not appreciate the hard work it took my parents to get it. My father, who is a very caring but workaholic doctor, was hardly ever home and would often work 14-hour days. My mum pretty much had to bring up three children on her own, look after the house and also my dad's busy medical practice, leaving little time for herself. Now that I realize just how hard they *both* have had to work to provide for us kids, it makes me feel very ashamed that I disrespected their hard-earned money so much.

When I was younger, I did the typical childhood chores to earn pocket money; my mum would usually have to bribe me with money to do things to help around the house. Helping out never came naturally to me; it was always 'Well, what will *I* get for helping *you*?' I also had a job in the local pizza restaurant after school when I was about 16, but I still did not get how money was something I needed to be careful with. As soon as I got paid, I spent it. And before I even got paid, I had plans for what to buy next. And that kind of mentality carried right on through to just recently – living from pay to pay etc.

I saw my parents sometimes worry about money, but at the same time we always had so much food in the house and everything we needed, had the bills paid off and regularly went shopping together. Perhaps it was this that made me think money really did grow on trees, or that I would always be fine no matter what, as I had never really seen what happens when there is truly no money. I now know that I simply *never* learnt to *respect* money. And this started from a very young age.

I thought to myself: how will we educate our kids, then, to appreciate money? In the *New York Times* best-selling book *The First National Bank of Dad*, author David Owen has developed a very unique and simple way of teaching children to respect money, which if implemented correctly, tends to last with them all through their lives.

Basically, David instructs parents to 'act' as their children's 'bank'. The parents literally take care of the money the kids save up (including creating professional-looking bank records and statements), all the while using the typical banking structure so the children's money accrues interest (which you decide according to the child's age at the time, and what your household can afford).

The kids soon learn that when they are given money this way, if they keep it in the 'bank' and do not spend it willy-nilly, their money will grow in time, with interest. The 'bank' (that's the parents) does not question what the child wants to do with the money (like a real bank does not ask why we want to draw out money, although wouldn't it be funny if they did e.g. 'Do you really need another new pair of black heels?'); this gives the *responsibility* to the child, and eventual young adult, that they must decide how to *wisely* spend their money. Of course, the parents must keep an eye on what the children are spending it on, but most of the time, whatever the child wants to get is totally up to them. If they go through a stage of buying useless things, they will soon learn that indeed it was a waste of money and will start to value items better in the future.

Parents are often advised to teach the value of money to a child from a young age, by opening them a savings account during the first few years of school. But because the young child is told they can't have their savings until they leave school, this is probably one of the *worst* things to do. Right from the start, children do not see saving as something that they want to do as there is nothing for them to have in the near future. To them, waiting 15+ years for a return on their investment seems about 450 years, so they immediately become disinterested in this saving game.

To respect money, kids need to learn right from the start how money works in the real world when they are adults. And of course, it would be sensible to tell your children that even though you will take care of them through school, one day they will have to fend for themselves which means making their own money and learning how to never run out!

This mature, responsible and sensible approach to money has such a high success rate with children (because it's fun to see how their savings grow) that they learn very quickly not to waste their money on rubbish and things they don't really want. If a child is to spend your hard-earned money, then the purchases might not be so cautious.

It's not just kids that are having problems; we as a society are too. Debt has truly gotten out of hand and many families are in financial ruin. Even people who are 'high income earners' can often be in so much debt and don't have any type of steps in place to protect it. It's because none of us really get how money can work if you know the tools.

Helpful Money Saving Websites for Kids And Adults

✓ suzygreaves.com

✓ financial-coaching.co.uk

✓ managingmymoney.com

✓ bettermoneyskills.com

✓ suzeorman.com

✓ deniseduffieldthomas.com

✓ moneycrashers.com

✓ kidmoney.about.com

✓ kidswealth.com

Chapter 45

How to Discipline without Damaging Self-Esteem and Emotional Development

When people hear the word 'discipline', quite often they think that it must mean some kind of a physical method to get a child to conform. Not so; *discipline* means encouraging children how to behave – learning right and wrong, and setting boundaries. No one wants a bratty rude child in their household and most parents intentions are to make sure their child does not turn out like that. Children certainly need *boundaries*, but the question is, how do we set those boundaries so that they do understand right from wrong, without harming the vital formation of their self-esteem?

Most of us have grown up disappointing our parents (for me, it was a lot because I was very naughty!) and can often remember just how that felt. We can remember the words that were told to us after we acted in a certain way. Yet, looking back, we know that we didn't mean to behave that way. We were young and were trying to find our way in the world. Making mistakes was simply our way of learning.

The problem with disciplining our children is mainly that we forget to see the world through *their* eyes. We may even discipline our children in the way that we were disciplined, which might not always be the best way. If we sit and look back at how we were spoken to by our own parents, we may think, 'Actually, what they said to me really hurt and I was just so resentful of it.' So with this clarity we more than likely really need to rethink how we are going to speak to our children.

We also, more often than not, do not know what our children can and cannot understand at that particular stage in their life, so we end up getting cross and frustrated with them, and they don't understand why we are mad. Communication is always what makes any relationship positive or negative and we (parent and child) both need to be communicating on the same level, without anger and with lots of patience and understanding.

Learning about child development is therefore *highly important* so that you know how to direct and speak to your child appropriately for the stage that they are at. It's a huge subject and I can't recommend enough to take the time to study this subject in more depth.

What's also very important is knowing when and what they can understand and then tailoring your own behavior and speech and direction around the child's stage that they are in. You can do many things to avoid upset and stressful situations by making sure your house is very safe with things far away from where a child can reach it. Even in your garden, you must childproof it and think, 'What would I do here if I was young – what would I like to touch or pull apart?'

Children are naturally inquisitive (we would have reason to be worried if they were not!) and will therefore want to touch everything they see. Life is like a game to them when young and they just want to explore as much as they can.

Think about this common situation: If you left a mug on the edge of the coffee table and your child grabbed it and caused it to fall over, whose fault do you really think it is? Yours, of course, yet who will probably get the blame? More often than not, the *child* does because it has messed up the carpet and now you have to clean it up – and if you are not in the best mood to begin with then you aren't likely to take it very well. This situation can leave you angry and your child in tears.

The child does not understand what has just happened as he (or she) doesn't know his boundaries. He saw the mug there; it was in reach so he wanted to touch it. Even with the scolding, the child does not understand what just happened – only that it did something 'bad' which upset Mum or Dad. When you have to take something that could be dangerous away from a child, try and replace it with something else that they can look at and feel.

It is also important to mention that parenting of course brings much stress and tiredness. If you are looking after another person 24/7, without having any 'you' time, then you are going to be more likely to suffer with fatigue and low energy which can lead to having a 'short fuse', lack of patience, and means you may inevitably take it out on the child. This is when you must try and ask for help so that you can spend some time on yourself each week, where you can do something that you enjoy or is your way of relaxing. This will help you manage your energy better and also your behavior towards the child.

It must be said that being tired as a parent makes it so much more important to work on your own health, eat well, exercise when you can and to keep on top of dealing with your own toxic exposure. When you *don't* take care of yourself, your health and energy are bound to suffer, which makes parenting so much harder.

I have included a brilliant list of books at the end of this book for you to look at to help with understanding childhood development and there is a section on boosting your own energy naturally.

The book *The Manual* by Dr Faye Snyder will give you lots of help in this area I really think if I had to choose which book every parent should have, it's this one!

Chapter 46

What's Your Child's Love Language? How to Love Your Child in the Way They Want

Just like adults, children need to be loved in the way that makes them feel secure and confident. Until recently, I had no idea that there were different ways to show love! I thought it was always just the same thing, but there are in fact *many* ways to express love to someone. And just like adults have different ways of needing love, there are different ways that children crave to be loved too.

Yet, how do we know what sort of love is what they want? They are too young to tell us and we often cannot understand enough through their cries to know exactly what they are needing. But what if we do not love them in the way they need? Are we already setting them up to have problems later in life? Yes, it seems so. Children who grow up unfulfilled often turn into adults that have addictions, ill health and depression because they feel like something is missing inside of them, but do not know what that is. If you show them your own way of being loved, and it's not what they need, then more than likely they aren't going to recognize your efforts. It's like if you really, really wanted a pair of shoes for Christmas and were always trying to hint to someone you wanted those shoes, yet you were given, instead, something you were totally not interested in. That present would go unnoticed and you would feel very unfulfilled and disappointed because someone didn't pay any attention to what you were crying out for.

Well, it's the same with feeling loved.

If you start learning to figure out how to love your child in the way they need, and giving it to them, when your child is very young, this effect could remain with them for their entire lives. To grow up knowing that he/she was truly loved and that nothing was missing can only help a child grow up into a well-adjusted, healthy and kind human being.

When we feel like we have lacked something so important at a young age, subconsciously we may grow up trying to find it, but unfortunately in all of the wrong places. With the rate of addictions so high these days, not receiving the love that people needed when younger could well and truly be one of the main reasons why. So, it makes sense to try and avoid this from learning, right from the word go, how your child responds to different love methods.

Gary Chapman, who wrote the *Five Love Languages* (which we discussed in the chapter 'Happy Loving Relationships'), had such great success with it that he wrote one purely for children and teenagers which is a must-read. The same methods for adults apply here for children as well.

Physical Touch – does your child give you signals they need lots of affection?

Your child will respond very well to being hugged and kissed as often as possible. Even though we tend to hold babies all the time when young, when the children become older, sometimes the affection really stops, to the point that a parent may only hug their child a few times a day. If the child was used to so much affection and all of a sudden it stops, they may withdraw, become irritable, sad and may even throw tantrums. If you think your child may crave more affection, give it a try and see if they respond well to it. If not, then there may be something else missing.

Words of Affirmation – does your child need to be given lots of words of encouragement?

This is a very common need for children these days, as many adults that I have spoken to say they have low self-esteem and were always disappointing their parents. They only ever heard the 'bad' things they did, and rarely or never at all were they told about the things they did well. This leads to adults feeling like they are worthless and are failures. It's important not to praise children's actions all the time, but instead, praise them for their whole being; say things like 'I really enjoy being around you', 'You're a wonderful boy/girl', 'You have so many special talents/abilities', 'I am always proud of you'. If you are always saying how good a certain *action* is, the child may start to crave needing praise all the time – almost like an addiction. They need to know that their *whole being* and character is loved by you.

Quality Time – does your child need you to spend quality time with them?

Sadly, this one of the biggest problems parents have these days. Life is so expensive, and getting more so, and the pressure is on more than ever before for parents to provide for their children. But this can often mean lonely times for the child when they just wish that they could spend some time with Mum or Dad or both. If you work full time and come home tired all the time (which is not surprising), this can impact on your behavior towards your child. They sense that you don't want to be around them and this can often lead to deep sadness. One way of working around this is to try putting aside 15 minutes (during a work week) every day (*without* fail) to read a story or just to talk and do something with your child. Even this short amount of time will be seen as your own special time and can help to create a strong bond. The key is to give your *undivided* attention. It's very sad hearing adults remember that they were regularly told to go away and leave their parents alone, and sometimes even their grandparents would ask them to go away. This is very hurtful for the child and they are not able to understand that you are stressed or tired.

On the weekends it's very important to put aside much more time and even arrange 'family evenings' where you all do something fun together. When kids see their parents working all the time, they tend to not understand *why* you have to work so hard and just take it that you don't want to spend time with them. It's not until much older that they realize you were just trying to do the right thing by providing for them, but when younger, they just feel hurt and sadness. If you suffer with low energy problems then it's vital that you really try and work on them; your child needs you to have the energy to deal with them.

I remember a friend telling me about a family she knew who really got the true meaning of quality time with their children. Each year, one of the children was able to plan something very special with one of the parents (the other would stay behind and look after the other siblings) and got to go away somewhere, overnight or even for a weekend. They would organize trips to the zoo, fun museums with dinner somewhere after, trips to the beach, or even camping. The children (when it was their turn) would be excited all year about their trip, and when they were on it, they had complete undivided attention from the parent. It also created lasting happy memories that they have to this day and an inner knowledge of knowing they were truly loved by their parents. And for the parents, it gave them the chance to see their children's nature and character away from the other children.

Gifts – does your child need you to show you care by thoughtful gifts?

It's important to note here that this does not mean 'buying off' your children. If you are always working too hard, giving them gifts rather than spending meaningful time with them will be seen as 'paying off'. This is one of the Love Languages that definitely needs to go hand in hand with another one. You do not want your child growing up to just want 'things'. However, gift giving can work really well if you make the gifts sporadic and special.

Just say you work away from home a lot; well, it can be a lovely gesture to buy a gift such as a teddy bear from somewhere special and tell your child that you saw it in the window and thought of them and knew you would love it. These types of gifts, with also words of encouragement, affection and other signs of love, can create lasting memories where that toy becomes something very special to the child. It is a symbol of your love, when given in the right way. In fact gifts like this can be respected and cared for by the child.

Remember though – do not use gifts as bribery for getting your child to do homework or jobs around the house; this is not the way you use gifts as a sign of your love.

Acts of Service - does your child need you to do things for them to show you care?

Even though bringing up a small child, and for many years too, is about doing lots for them and giving lots to them, which can be very draining for a parent, it's important to realize that you may need to continue doing this for your child to still see that you love them. Acts of Service can mean: cooking with your child, helping them with their homework, painting with them, making costumes, reading, having play time, singing and dancing, and other things like that where you can include your little one. But it must be in a way that's not stressful and where you are not scolding them for not doing it the right way. Otherwise they may fear this time together and will miss out on getting their emotional tank filled.

Although your child will respond the best to one of these Love Languages or maybe will need a high amount of two, I do believe that it's still best to give them a bit of all of these things combined, with the majority of time and effort spent on the main one that works so well with your child. You will know you have got it right when your child is very happy, secure and also well-behaved. In my opinion, when a child feels satisfied, assured and loved, the rate of tantrums would more than likely dramatically drop!

Gary Chapman's book also teaches you to deal with children when they hit the teen years. For much more advice on this subject, I cannot recommend owning a copy of Gary Chapman's and Ross

Campbell's book *The Five Love Languages for Children.*

You can also check out Gary's website and his other brilliant books here:

✓ garychapman.org

And Man created the plastic bag and the tin and aluminum can and the cellophane wrapper and the paper plate, and this was good because Man could then take his automobile and buy all his food in one place and he could save that which was good to eat in the refrigerator and throw away that which had no further use. And soon the earth was covered with plastic bags and aluminum cans and paper plates and disposable bottles and there was nowhere to sit down or walk, and Man shook his head and cried: 'Look at this Godawful mess.'

~ Art Buchwald, 1970

PART 4

LIVING GREEN IN OUR TOXIC WORLD

Chapter 47

When Will We Wake Up?

It's no secret that there are many problems with how the earth and its inhabitants (us!) are today. Most of us are aware of climate change concerns and that we are creating too much waste. But is it really sinking in? For the vast majority, the answer is no. You only have to take a walk through a busy shopping area or mall to see just how many people have absolutely no concern for what they are buying, what they are eating, what they are wearing and what they desire for their future. The small number that is left over (people like us) are desperately trying to make them aware that they too must change, and quickly, to help the entire planet.

Despite all of us playing a part in what is happening to the environment, you and I aren't to blame as such. It's governments and industries that cause the most damage. They are the ones who can really make a huge difference by stopping or changing what they are doing. Even though I do want to urge you to change your ways of doing certain things, I am not that naive and neither should you be, to think that the world will change overnight just because of us. It's got to be the governments and corporations that change their ways. We can, however, try and urge them to do it through sending in letters to our local Congress and Members of Parliament. We can also talk to our friends and family about it all too.

I recently watched a brilliant movie called The Island President which is about the possible future extinction of the beautiful islands of the Maldives. These 2000+ islands are home to some of the most luxurious and exotic resorts in the world which the rich and famous, honeymooners and holiday makers visit all year round. These islands are also in a state of environmental emergency, for the waters are rising (from global warming) at such a huge rate that they are starting to lose massive chunks of their land. Environmental scientists predicted years ago how fast this erosion would happen, but sadly, they underestimated the amount; it's happening at pretty much almost twice the rate of what they predicted. If the world does not reduce its carbon emissions to the amount of about 350, the Maldives will be completely under water, which would mean that hundreds and thousands of Maldivian people would require environmental refugee rehoming and an entire culture would be lost, not to mention probably deaths of people left behind.

The now ex-president (sadly he resigned in February 2012 because of a coup), of a country once ruled by a dictatorship, was partly responsible for creating a democracy in the Maldives after a 30-year rule under a president, Maumoon Abdul Gayoom, who was not exactly a nice guy. People were not free to vote or free to speak their minds. They lived in terror for many years and if anyone spoke out against the president, they were sent to jail and tortured and some were even killed.

Mohamed 'Anni' Nasheed, himself, even spent 18 months in solitary confinement in a jail on one of the islands. This did not destroy him, and in fact, spurred him on to set so many wrongs right. He is one of those very rare world leaders who actually truly cares about his country and its people. He spent the entire time as president traveling the world, meeting with other world leaders to bring awareness to the issue of global warming, and explaining that what could happen to the Maldives could happen to other parts of the world, such as New York city because it is situated above sea level equal to that of the Maldives. During his term as president, he also vowed to make the Maldives the first carbon-neutral country and quickly began building energy-saving features into his country's capital, Male.

What affected me the most in this movie was knowing that so many see this beautiful country and its jewel-like islands as something to use and abuse. They use it for when they want to go on a beautiful relaxing holiday yet when it came down to changing their own country to help impact the environmental health of the

Maldives, many simply did not care. There was a climate change summit in Copenhagen a few years ago where countries were to sign a document that agreed to certain terms. It was very shocking to see that the countries hugely responsible for such terrible emissions would not sign the document.

The future of the Maldives, and therefore the world, is an example to the rest of us that we must care about this small country, and change our ways, because if we do not, then it will pave the way for many other countries to disappear in the future also.

The facts are undeniable: the sea level is rising and very, very fast. But there are some things we can do individually to help make at least a small difference.

Chapter 48

Environmentally Kind Tips for Daily Living

Because every little bit adds up to create something big, it makes sense that we can all individually do something to limit our effect on the environment. Some people feel very helpless. 'The problem with our environment is so enormous,' they say, 'yet *what* can we do that will make even a scrap of difference?' While yes, what you do may seem to be a small drop in the ocean, just doing something may even help others. Just say you have people over for dinner and they see what you have purchased to clean your house with, or they see how well you recycle and the sort of food you buy – this can influence *them* to change their own ways. Then *they* may change someone else's, so you making these little steps can become like a domino effect which means quite a big change. It's also a good idea to change your mentality, to 'We can all make a difference' rather than feeling defeat.

We really must pressure our governments to put pressure on the big industrial and chemical corporations, for they are harming the environment in a massive way. Individuals like you and me can help by protesting about what these corporations are doing.

There are *so* many things we can do to help the environment, with many I have listed throughout the book. Changing your beauty and cleaning products is one of the best things you can do (not only for your health) because it means that whatever goes down the drain is not going to add to the pollution in our already pretty dismal waterways. It's also even more important to use 'green' cleaning products because regular products do more harm to the environment than any other forms of polluting. What you can do in your home can make a difference, no matter how small it seems. There are really about a million tips to be more environmentally friendly at home but I have included the most user-friendly ones I have discovered, which are realistic in terms of all of us being able to do them.

- Recycle as much as you can – check what your local council recycles and if they want items washed.
- Cut down on eating meat, chicken and fish.
- Use your food scraps for compost.
- Purchase energy-saving light switches, heating enhancers and water savers.
- Conserve power by switching things off, and you can even insulate your homes in colder climates so that you do not have to rely on central heating so much.
- Use recycled goods (buy recycled aluminum, plastic bags, bin liners, bottles) that have already been recycled previously.
- Keep glass bottles and reuse them.
- If you receive phone books that you never use, call up the company and have them stopped. Or recycle the ones that get delivered.
- When washing your laundry, try not to use hot water always and use quick cold and warm cycles.
- If you live in a cold country and have a water heater, purchase an insulating blanket which is placed directly over the unit. This will help to retain the warmth – and saves you money too.
- Buy fewer electrical goods as much as possible; many of the materials (precious metals) come from Third World countries that are involved in slave labor and armed conflict. Rethink getting the latest mobile phone.
- Buy organic food as much as you can.
- Don't keep the fridge door open for too long; lots of energy is wasted this way when people open the fridge and decide what to eat. It also costs you more money too.
- Turn off the tap when brushing your teeth, and do the same when you are in the kitchen wiping a bench down. Turn on the

taps only when you need to.

- Cancel your junk mail (who reads it anyway?!) – put a sign on the letterbox saying 'no junk mail'.
- Source locally produced food (preferably organic too).
- Use safe and no-chemical products in your garden.
- Purchase pre-loved furniture rather than always buying brand new.
- Buy organic fabrics when you can – clothing, linen and towels etc. Just buy when something needs to be replaced.
- Think about buying environmentally friendly items (such as toilet paper, washing detergent products, food items) in bulk; this saves you money and also helps with energy consumption – and with excess packaging as the items are in one big box instead of several smaller ones.
- Purchase safe cleaning and beauty products – preferably biodegradable.
- Only use your dishwasher when it's full, and don't do a prewash cycle either. If food is on the dishes etc., fill up one sink's worth of water and let them soak – then place in the machine.
- Buy far less stuff.
- Use Ebay, Amazon and other online websites which sell pre-loved items.

Parents, please be much more conscious about what nappies you use. If you live in a country with a regular supply of water, then maybe look into using bamboo or organic cotton washable nappies (these can be used on more than one child, by the way) or if you decide to use the throwaway ones, then you can purchase biodegradable ones. Regular mainstream nappies take *forever* to degrade (decades – some say 400 years) and end up in landfill, often in Third World countries, where they are shipped from the West. Bear in mind that even in biodegradable ones, usually only approximately half of the material is the type that will decompose more quickly; the rest will still take about 400 years.

By the time a toddler is 2, a parent will have thrown out about 3000–4000 nappies. And of course the more kids you have, the more that adds up as well. If you saw 3000+ nappies in a room at once, you would fall over in shock. Can you imagine the amount from every single baby who has ever used throwaway nappies?

For a great brand of nappies, I recommend Attitude (especially when baby is a newborn) as they are biodegradable, vegetable-based, CO_2 neutral, fragrance free and chlorine free. You can purchase them in many countries all over the world. Beaming Baby is also another good brand.

- ✓ cleanattitude.com
- ✓ beamingbaby.co.uk

Light bulbs

One product that I really want you to *avoid* buying, which have also been a big fat con, are energy-saving light bulbs. While we have been led to believe that they are wonderful for the environment and a real breakthrough in eco design, they are in fact *highly toxic* and also give off a high level of electromagnetic frequencies (EMFs), which as we have covered previously are harmful for human health and, in particular, infants.

Here is a comparison of EMF output:

- Energy-saving light bulb – 26,740 Hz
- Incandescent – 350 Hz
- LED – 230 Hz

Pretty shocking difference in the levels, isn't there?

The inside of these so-called green bulbs also contains mercury, and if they smash or explode, you are at *big* risk of poisoning. When people throw out these light bulbs, they end up in landfill, which means they can harm the people who work in the garbage dumps and they will also leach the dangerous heavy metals into the ground, contaminating other things.

What you can buy instead of energy-saving light bulbs is LED light bulbs. These are much safer for the environment and last a much longer time too. I recently had my whole house decked out with LED lights from LEDhut.co.uk. They say that you can save up to 90% off your lighting costs. We are looking forward to having a much cheaper electricity bill this coming year.

If you want to purchase LED lights for your home, please google them to see where you can buy from.

Chapter 49

Water Preservation

Fresh water only covers 3% of the Earth's surface – the rest is sea water and, tragically, only 20% of the world's population has access to this 3% of fresh water. Over *1 billion* people do not have any access to clean fresh water. Quite alarming, isn't it? And, by 2025, to cope with the booming population, we will need to increase the water supply by as much as 22%. Goodness knows *how* we are going to do this. When we see how much water is wasted in Western countries (even flushing our toilets wastes so much water – up to 40% of our water we have in our homes goes down the toilet), it just seems completely crazy that we have access to so much water, and waste it, yet in Third World countries they have no access to water at all and many will die because of it.

Water is already running out on the planet, and some countries are in a complete drought state. Certain areas such as Las Vegas (and other popular tourist places in hot countries) are very abusive because they use precious water to water the lawns on the golf courses and luxury hotels – for all of the rich and famous people who visit on their holidays!

When you use water, try and conserve it as much as possible. Use a short wash cycle when using the washing machine and don't bath or shower for long periods. A great tip for conserving water in the house is to not actually flush the toilet each time you go. I know that sounds gross but if you are super-cautious with how much flushing you do then this can make a big difference. If you have your own bathroom then this is going to be very easy as you have the privacy to not worry about anyone seeing it.

If this really doesn't appeal to you (and I certainly understand if it doesn't) then try and put a brick in the toilet's cistern to make less water flush. I share my bathroom with my husband so it's easy for me to do this, but I understand if you share it with others they might not exactly like what you are doing. In this case, the brick will at least help.

I actually think that we bathe ourselves far too much (I used to have up to three showers each day back in Australia) and it's far better for our skin and the environment to wash only every few days. I know, that sounds a bit off if you are used to bathing every day, but it doesn't mean if you have fewer showers that you can't be clean. If you live in a cold country then you won't really sweat too much. To clean yourself, you can fill a sink full of warm/hot water and use a soft flannel to wash yourself, rather than using a huge amount of water every day. In countries like Morocco where water is scarce, they use a special clay that they mix with a tiny bit of water, apply to the skin and leave to dry. Then they remove it with a wet cloth and find their skin clean, and softer than a baby's behind. Smart people. We can learn a lot from cultures which are used to surviving on not much. One day soon, that might be all of us.

I come from Australia where it is so hot that we needed to get cool, but over here in the UK we don't really sweat much, so we don't really get dirty underneath our winter coats.

After Lola was born, we did not (and still don't) bathe her every day. I do of course clean her backside, face and hands. To bathe newborns and infants every 2–3 days will be much better for their skin in the long run. Water is particularly drying on anyone's skin (especially if it's not been filtered in any way) and babies' skins are so delicate that less washing, really is better for them.

In the future, I hope that it becomes very common that in places like the UK we harvest our rainwater. It absolutely baffles me that we are not already doing this. It's easy to install a tank on the side of houses and attach a UV filter to it so that it cleans our water, yet the water companies are not telling us to do this. Why? Because they want our money to pay them for using their water. I know when I build my dream house, I am going to be using natural rainwater as much as we can, instead of paying a water company which puts chemicals such as the deadly fluoride in it and then charges us a high price for it.

Chapter 50

Waste Is Such a Waste!

I watched a movie called *Wasteland* recently which I encourage you to check out. You won't believe your eyes. It's about the rubbish dump in Rio de Janeiro which actually is bigger than a small city. It shows the shocking amount of rubbish that is dealt with in just one day, how it gets sorted and how much gets recycled, and also the type of people whose job it is to sort it all out. It is absolutely *horrifying* how much waste we create. Even with my small family of my husband, Lola and I, the amount of rubbish we throw out is so much, and we even purchase quite differently (more consciously) than the average family.

If we all had to keep our rubbish at our houses, instead of getting the garbage trucks to pick it up for us, it would be a different story. We would bring home hardly anything, eat all of our food and therefore not waste anything, and we would be super-conscious about what we bought in the first place. Yet we live in an illusion because we have our rubbish removed weekly, which means 'out of sight, out of mind'. I get sent so much stuff to review which arrives in cardboard boxes and, quite often, I have to write to the company and say, 'Can you please make sure you decrease your packaging next time?' I often receive small products in quite big boxes, filled with packing material (despite the fact that the product is unbreakable), which is just madness.

The richest 20% of the world's population consume 88% of the world's goods and services, while the poorest consume only 3.3%.
UN Human Development Report, 2003

It probably makes sense that the next thing I am going to mention is, please buy less *stuff*! Try and make a conscious decision to ask yourself, when you are out shopping, 'Do I *really* need this or is it a want?' Is there a more environmentally friendly alternative? Something with less packaging perhaps?

When we lived in London, I ordered our organic food from Able and Cole. It was delivered in recycled cardboard boxes which I returned the next week to the delivery driver so that they were used again. The fruits and vegetables were placed in the box without much or any plastic. It was a great way to order food and to limit waste.

We moved out of London in January 2012 to an area which is surrounded by organic and bio-dynamic farms. We are now buying food that couldn't be any more locally sourced. We are drinking water collected free from the local spring. We don't need to use much plastic as we can carry everything in canvas bags or in our roller trolley. It's also much cheaper to purchase the produce from these farms directly. In fact, we have discovered we are saving money by buying the best-quality food which is actually cheaper than buying non-organic food from the supermarket. Not to mention we now have our own garden where we can start to grow produce as well. Not everyone can move out of the city like we have, but further on in this section of the book I share some tips about how to grow produce indoors. The key to sustainability on this planet is for us as individuals and families to grow as much food as we can in our homes.

In the resource section you will also find listings of organic companies which home-deliver food, and you can try and source locally grown food through farmers' markets. It's a great way to meet local farmers. You may need to use Google to find out what is near you.

Chapter 51

Shopping Wisely

Most people do not realize the power we all have when it comes to purchasing. When you think about it, it's entirely because of *us* that many companies now have amassed great fortunes and *power* which, in most cases, is being completely and shamefully abused. This happens because *we* are naive about the manipulation behind their clever advertising – which we are bombarded with everywhere we go. This brainwashing (starting from literally just a few years old when the brain registers certain information) means that we have all bought many things which we probably *really* don't need – because we have been led to believe that, without them, we cannot be happy.

Due to our massive addiction to shopping, many industries have now caused much environmental destruction, and slave labor of men, women and children, in countries which stretch over the entire globe. Even in Western countries, slavery goes on every day, in a way that's very hidden, but more so of course in the Third World countries where it is out in the open and governments seem to care even less about their own people. China, for example, has made so much money purely around slave-labor industries. They seem to think it's OK to make their people (often very young women) work for 18 hours a day and pay them next to nothing. What is really shocking is that wages in China are actually *worse* now than they were 10 years ago. Due to the demand for cheaper products, the companies have slashed the workers' wages even more to meet the Western countries' needs.

Child labor has always been a huge industry in the world, but the actual statistics of how many children are involved is highly disgusting and almost unbelievable. It is reported that there are *170 million* children involved in industries that expose them to hazardous and dangerous situations. In the silk trade, for example, many children are forced into working in dark, cramped and poorly ventilated factories and made to handle the dead worms which can cause them to catch an infection. Often they will have to stand for 12–16 hours a day with hardly any breaks. They also breathe in the vapors, not only from boiling the cocoons of the silk worms, but from the diesel engines that are also used in production. This exposure, day after day, to the chemicals often causes their growth development and neurological function to be impaired. And there is no such thing as health insurance for these kinds of people. They simply get sicker and sicker with no medical help.

This is only *one* example of the child slave labor industry. There are many other stories which would bring tears to your eyes. And even more alarming is knowing that there are about *8 million* children involved in much more serious working conditions which expose them to prostitution, armed conflict, illegal activities and, the most disturbing of all, pornography. We are very much shielded from the reality of what is going on every day in far corners of the earth that affect precious children. And when we choose a product, we hardly ever think, 'Where did it come from? Who made it and what is their life like?'

Sometimes it's hard to know how to make a truly ethical choice. It's difficult because nothing seems to be *100%* ethical. Just say you are deciding between buying a product grown locally but is not organic (but has low transport costs) or a fair trade certified organic product that has been brought in from overseas. Which one is the most environmentally friendly? Some would say the product that has been purchased nearby due to the minimal carbon footprint, yet some would say, no way – it has also been grown with chemicals which go directly into the environment and also harm our health. Or some would say, the fair trade product is better, as it means that the people who produced the product were treated well and paid a decent wage. But the big negative with the fair trade product is, it has been flown halfway around the world, which adds to more pollution in our skies. So buying ethically is not always easy to decide. But both choices are always better than buying from big companies which do not have any ethical codes of conduct incorporated into their workplace. You just have to decide what feels right to you.

So is fair trade fair, or is it a farce?

The 'Fair Trade' label has gained much popularity over the years and is now a very recognized symbol and people are tending to buy more of it, especially among the younger generation who seem to be much more naturally compassionate. It is great seeing big chains like Starbucks start to use fair trade products such as coffee. But, like all labels, sometimes they are not always legitimate. You have to really know your product and to be sure that the label is not 'green washing' (pretending to be green when really it is not). Like most things, anything that is popular ends up getting abused, so unfortunately, we really have to investigate if it's really what it says it is. When we hear of something being 'Fair Trade' we often think that the entire product is fairly traded but the truth is, with some of the new regulations, as little as 10% of a product may be actually fair trade. So in a bar of chocolate, for example, maybe only two ingredients are fairly traded and the rest isn't, yet the bar says 'Fair Trade Chocolate'. Still, buying this chocolate compared to another brand that has no fairly traded ingredients is better, but it's very disheartening that we still have to have be dubious of claims in the 'ethical' world. Some fair trade products are really ethical; it's just very difficult to find the proof of what is.

The websites below may help you to choose an ethical purchase.

✓ fairtrade.net
✓ fairtradeusa.org

Chapter 52

Climate Change – Fact or Fiction?

Another subject people can't seem to see eye to eye on is climate change – and if it really is being caused by humans. So many scientists say yes and a smaller amount say no – that this temperature change is part of the earth's natural cycle. While yes, ice ages have happened before (and things like floods and hurricanes), the difference with now is that back then there was no severe polluting like there is today. All of these toxic chemicals simply had not been created then.

In my opinion, it *doesn't matter* if we keep trying to argue the point of whether climate change is a natural environmental change or it isn't – the point is, pollution and raping the earth is *not* going to help it to get any better and we *do* have to change our ways. I sometimes think people use the excuse of saying, 'Oh, this is happening naturally' so that they don't have to make any positive changes; it means they can continue doing exactly what they are doing – which is taking *zero* responsibility for environmental concerns.

Also, the earth does not have nearly as many trees as it did thousands of years ago. Trees, as we have covered before, act as 'lungs' – absorbing toxins and putting out healthy oxygen back into the environment. So the more they are cut down, the less they will be able to do their job, which means that more toxins and gasses will be in our environment – waiting for us to breathe them in, which means more death and sickness.

I feel we need to plant lots more *trees*, and quick smart, to help balance out these pollutants. And we need to stop wasting time arguing about whether or not climate change is real, and just use our brains; we 100% need to change *our* ways as individuals, as cities, as companies, as governments, as entire countries – by producing less stuff, and pumping out far fewer industrial chemicals. We need to use better types of energy, farm in more effective ways and use bio-fuel instead of fossil fuels. Doesn't this all make sense?

Many countries are now jumping on the 'Carbon Tax' bandwagon and charging a ridiculous fortune, and making some countries even more broke than they already are — yet the money does not seem to be going back into *helping* the environment. Governments, yet again, are manipulating us and using serious issues for their own good.

Chapter 53

How the World Is Changing in a Positive Way – Housing and Gardening Ideas

I have discussed some pretty alarming information in this book, haven't I, and it might be making you think, 'Oh dear, what *hope* have we got for the future? Isn't the world in too much of a mess?' Well, let me assure you that the world is *still* a very beautiful place, and actually, never before in our history has there been a more amazing time for seeing mankind come together to create a better world. People's consciousness is changing rapidly and many are starting to sit up and care much more about the world, their impact and the people around them.

Yes, some are abusing the 'green' movement and are not as green as they want you to believe; unfortunately no industry is always full of decent and ethical people and it saddens me to know this, but for every negative story there are dozens more positive and inspiring stories. I love reading about what people are creating, designing and supporting. It gives us hope, as it should, because hope *and* action is now all we have to make our futures much brighter. I want to share with you some great things that are happening around the world, proving what can be done when like-minded, caring people join together.

Community eco villages

As we have learnt, normal houses are quite toxic chemically and the majority also use precious wood and other materials that come from Nature. This means that quite a bit of environmental damage is being caused and the general housing market is far removed from being sustainable. More and more people are becoming aware of this and desire to live somewhere that is an example of how they want the world to be. Less damaging to the earth, less reliant on fossil fuels, yet still beautiful.

Many citizens have also lost faith in their governments (with darn good reason) and are not enjoying living their lives in big polluted cities. They are craving a sense of real community, where they know their neighbors who share similar views of creating a healthier and kinder world. They are also concerned about their children, growing up in such a tough and unhealthy society. They want to get away from using gas-guzzling vehicles and expensive fuels and want to become more 'off the grid'.

Cropping up all over the world are 'eco villages'. These are usually in the countryside, where a huge piece of land has been purchased so that it can be divided up and people can have their own environmentally friendly and energy-efficient houses, but still be fairly close to everyone else that lives there. There is usually a main building where people can meet and discuss what needs to be done. Organic food is grown on the property and renewable energy sources are put into place. The villages are usually run by a democratic system, where people vote for changes and everyone gets their say. Houses are usually much more inexpensive than they would be in the 'real' world and, for some people, this really is a wonderful way to achieve their dream life.

There are many eco villages being built at the moment and one that I really love is Mahalaya, which is an organization that plans to create many villages all over the world. The first one is being built in Hawaii and sounds absolutely amazing. This state-of-the-art village is offering people a sustainable lifestyle that truly is one in a million, but without costing that much! The architecture is incredible, and the people who are organizing it are highly talented and successful business people (some own Fortune 500 companies) in their own right. Mahalaya is certainly not going to be reminiscent of anything like a hippy commune! This is the sort of place where you will be offered everything you need plus more. A true visionary for the future.

Mahlaya Communities will provide its members with (i) sustainable housing, (ii) fresh nutritious organic foods and phyto-medicines, (iii) renewable energy, (iv) new paradigm economic opportunities, (v) whole-person wellness center and healthcare, (vi) applied and interactive education, (vii) conscious childcare, (viii) clean transportation, (ix) technology, science and innovation centers, (x) creative centers for art, music and media, (xi) and entrepreneurial centers to help community members start their own businesses – all for significantly less money, time and effort than is the norm in our current socio-politico-economic structure. Mahalaya Communities are currently concentrating its efforts of land acquisition in Hawaii, Colorado, Arkansas, North Carolina, New Zealand and Latin America. Mahalaya's flagship development is currently focused in Hawaii and New Zealand.

Some eco communities fail because they have not had the right management, but Mahalaya is one that I am sure is going to be renowned for being one of the most successful and legitimate.

✓ mahalayacommunities.com

The Village

In Ireland, the Village is setting the way for communities that are very close to being in total action. As of November 2011 there are about 30 finished houses with 25 more being built. Each house is being built with the environment in mind. The Village is set within Cloughjordan, which is in the middle of Ireland. It is surrounded by 50 acres of stunning woodland and is perfect for growing food. They have a renewable energy centre which provides the heat and hot water for the homes. There is also an 'Eco Hostel' which is already open for business. The Village has lots more plans in the pipeline such as a 'green enterprise centre' and many more community buildings. They will have an education centre in place as well as sharing transport to reduce costs and save on greenhouse emissions. They offer permaculture courses and home buyers can become involved in the actual building of their property. There is already a huge community organic farm in place (since 2008) which feeds up to 80 families. This place truly is going to be incredible and, if you live in the UK, it just might be worth thinking about!

✓ thevillage.ie

✓ You may also like to check out findhorn.org for another eco community up and running (since the 1960s) in the UK.

Earthship homes

If living near others in a community doesn't really appeal to you but you do have a dream of having an environmentally friendly home, and also living 'off the grid', then an Earthship may be right up your street! An Earthship is a type of solar house made entirely of natural and recycled materials. The homes are mainly constructed to work as autonomous buildings and are generally made of earth-filled tyres, and use thermal mass construction to naturally regulate indoor temperature. They also usually have their own special natural ventilation system. Earthships are generally also known as off-the-grid homes, reducing their reliance on public utilities and fossil fuels – which means saving you a *huge* amount of money. Earthships are built to make use of the available resources, especially energy from the sun. For example, their windows on sun-facing walls admit lighting and heating, and the buildings are often horseshoe-shaped to use as much natural light as possible and solar-gain power during winter months. The thick, inner walls provide a thermal mass that naturally regulates the interior temperature during both cold and hot outside temperatures. Internal, non-load-bearing walls are often made of a honeycomb of recycled cans joined by concrete and are referred to as 'tin can walls'. These walls are usually thickly plastered with stucco. The roof of an Earthship is heavily insulated – often made with earth for added energy efficiency.

These Biotecture homes were the brain child of the incredibly talented architect Michael Reynolds. They range in price according to your budget and even the least expensive are still pretty spectacular. A family of four can live here for a long time without needing to pay any bills or to visit a shop for food!

Benefits of an Earthship

- No heating bills
- No water bills
- No energy bills
- Minimum food bills
- Beautiful to look at
- Built-in greenhouse
- Built using sacred geometric patterns
- Built using the thermal mass to help the environment and keep the temperature cool in summer and warm in winter

Not only are they one of the most environmentally friendly homes, they are absolutely unique in their design. All are one of a kind and look straight out of a fairy tale. You can even learn how to make your own Earthship by attending a special workshop. You can also visit some of the homes already constructed and stay overnight to test them out. Earthships have been constructed all over the world. Living like this is the way of the future. My husband and I plan to hope to build one in the years to come.

- ✓ earthship.com
- ✓ groundhouse.com
- ✓ brightonpermaculture.org.uk

Bamboo houses

Wood has been chopped down at such a fast rate that we have little rainforest left these days. What's been done to the Amazon, and continues to this day, is a hideous crime against Nature. Some of the woods that are used in building houses and furniture can take up to 100 years to grow (such as mahogany) so when they get cut down, it means that it will take an *entire* century to grow back. We need to get away from using natural materials that are simply not sustainable. We need trees to help the planet breathe, so another option must be found.

Thankfully, there is an option 100 times better than wood. Bamboo is one of the *most* sustainable building materials there is on the planet. It grows super-fast and is also super-strong. According to Green by Design, in the right conditions bamboo grows at an astonishing rate of *2 inches an hour*! And conservative estimates place its growth rate at around 24 inches a day – pretty amazing, right? It is also as strong as steel but far lighter. It's so tough that you can place solar and hot-water panels on the roof. Another great benefit is that bamboo is not liked by termites, so you don't have to worry about treating it with chemicals (like you do wood) to keep those damaging critters at bay.

One would also think, due to the lightness of the bamboo, that it would blow over in a hurricane, but in actual fact bamboo will bend, rather than snap, in windy weather, which means that it will more than likely still be standing after even the most powerful storm. Back in April 1991, 20 bamboo houses were built for the National Bamboo Foundation in Costa Rica. Each and every house did not suffer any structural damage after a 7.5 Richter scale earthquake hit the area. And what is even more remarkable is that the houses were directly over the epicenter.

Using bamboo to build your house with is also very good for the air quality inside. It is resistant to mold and mildew.

Architecturally, bamboo houses are some of the most beautifully designed I have ever seen. Bamboo has a very 'zen'-like feel to it and has a wonderful energy. Bamboo is not just for the exterior; you can use it for the floors, walls, and ceilings. These houses are being built all over the world and with good reason: they are stunning, strong *and* sustainable.

✓ bambooliving.com

Shipping container homes

When I was in Costa Rica in 2011, I stayed at a yoga retreat in Dominical. What was unique about the accommodation was that the building was actually a renovated shipping container. This style of housing is another booming industry. People are able to buy them very cheaply but can fit them out in the most amazing and often quite luxurious ways. You can fit several or even lots more together to create a much larger space, ideal for families, or they can be turned into unique offices. Some clever designers also put grass on the top so that you can grow plants and flowers and have a rooftop terrace to sit out in the sun and watch the world go by.

So many people are craving much less space these days, wanting a more simple life, and for anyone with not much spare funds the shipping container option is really very appealing. You can still design an incredible home but for much less than what you would think. They are pretty safe in all types of weather as well. Shipping containers often get dumped and this is a great way to make good use of them.

✓ containerhome.info
✓ containercabins.com.au

Cuba – the unlikely country leading the way in sustainability

When you think of the country Cuba, I bet you think of the 'Cuban Missile Crisis' and that's pretty much about it in terms of what Cuba is all about. Not many people know that Cuba is one of the most sustainable countries in the world. When the USA declared an embargo against Cuba back in the 1960s and again in 1992, this at first looked like being a very bad thing for the country and its people, but today there is proof that it was actually a very good thing. Pesticides, oil and other chemicals were not traded as they were previously to Cuba, so the people had to step up and change their ways pretty much overnight. Their lives depended on this quick action. They turned their regular chemical agriculture into organic farming, they began to use solar and wind energy to power their homes, schools and medical centers, and began to use bikes instead of cars for transport. Or if people did have cars, they would car pool and share with friends and family. People began sharing their homegrown produce with their neighbors, and city dwellers also used any bit of land that they could find (land that may have been previously used as a rubbish dump) to grow their own food. They stopped using tractors to farm with and instead used old-fashioned oxen and, because of these traditional farming methods, noticed a huge improvement in the quality of the soil. They began to go *with* Nature, instead of against it.

The country also has many more doctors per thousand people than the USA. There are also about 50 universities in Cuba, which is very impressive for a country of its size. Despite it still being governed by a dictatorship, the people are not complaining and still live a fairly free and healthy life. Quite ironic when you look at Western democratic countries whose people do have the 'freedom' to vote yet do not have any real say in what happens to their country and are being led by governments which use and abuse our tax-paying dollars and pounds for things that we don't really agree with. Not to mention a large amount of that money gets spent on things we don't even know about!

Because of the Cuban embargo, the country has had no choice but to become as sustainable as possible, which has created more jobs and an economy that really only needs to rely on itself. And guess what? The entire population have their own homes and 85% of people actually own these homes! And it gets even more impressive: Cuba has free healthcare for every citizen in the country and has done so since the 1950s. So to say this country is 'Third World' or a developing country is a bit ironic when you compare the state of its environment and healthcare system to that of the USA.

Cuba, to me, shows what can happen when we have no choice but to find other ways. Many people are very fearful of a 'world collapse', which does indeed seem fairly imminent. It can be a terrifying thought to think, 'What will happen when the oil runs out? What will we eat, how will we travel, how will we power our homes?' Yet, we can look at Cuba as they are doing just fine.

What I really want to drive home to people reading this book is that we can do things right now, to help us make this possible transition from life the way it is now (which is a very wasteful and greedy culture) to living with a lot less. That is the only way forward, to buy fewer things, change the way we produce our food, become more in sync with Nature, and stop relying on fossil fuels.

We can all do something and that is to be as sustainable and self-sufficient as possible. And it is possible. Whether you live on a farm, or live in a city, we can all grow things in our homes, no matter how small the space is. And we can all become part of a community.

The gardening boom

Something that has taken the world by storm is homegrown gardening! In the last few years, people have started to desire to produce their own food from home. In the UK, community shared gardens have always been around but they have now become so popular that there are waiting lists for garden space. No matter how big or small your property is, there are ways of growing things in or outside your home. You can grow potatoes in garbage bins, herbs in small pots, things like tomatoes and cucumbers also in pots – any container can grow a variety of things. All that you need is some soil. And as long as you have a window with regular sunlight, you don't always have to grow things outside. Many people in New York live in warehouse-type apartments with no outside space. This hasn't stopped them from growing lettuces, herbs and other types of produce. Limited space just means using your creativity a little bit more. You could use shelving (like that of a bookcase) to grow things on each ledge. If you do have space outside (say a terraced area) you can use raised beds if you don't have any actual grassy areas. Growing anything is always very cathartic, and to have the ability to eat the food that you have grown is a wonderful way to connect with

Nature. Not to mention it makes eating much cheaper and more satisfying as well! It's also a *great* way to get your children interested in eating healthy food because if they help you garden, they are more likely to want to try what they have helped you grow.

Lots of us desire to start gardening, but don't know where to start; if you are one of those people there are plenty of websites which can steer you in the right direction.

✓ thegardeningwebsite.co.uk

✓ gardenorganic.org.uk

✓ smilinggardener.com

✓ organicgardening.com

✓ landshare.net

If you want to purchase trees and plants already pre-grown, you may find the following website really great. The wonderful website Spalding Plant and Bulb Company sell fruit trees that are delivered to your house already half grown. If left in the pot provided, these beautiful tiny trees will remain small and something that you can grow inside your house or in the patio. They will be able to be harvested at the appropriate time, meaning you can pick fruit straight from your tree. You won't need to actually plant these in the ground if you don't have any garden space. You can purchase pear, apple, blackberry, cherry, fig, raspberry, gooseberry, nectarine, plus many other types of trees.

Prices are very inexpensive. I also purchase inexpensive healthy-air plants from this great site.

✓ spaldingbulb.co.uk

Aquaponics

It seems that in the very near future, most of our food may be grown by an Aquaponic system. This is a sustainable food production system which combines aquaculture (the raising of aquatic animals such as snails, fish or prawns in tanks) with hydroponics (the cultivation of plants in water). These two systems are brought together so that they work in harmony. The byproducts of aquaculture, such as bacteria, are broken down by nitrogen-fixing bacteria which is then filtered out by the plants as nutrients. Basically the fish feed the plants, and the plants clean the fish water. The bacteria in the grow beds convert fish waste into plant food.

Some say this clever system is far better than organic food farming because it requires no soil, no weed pulling and uses very little water. It certainly seems like an incredible way to produce food and if you have the space at home and interest in growing your own food, then you might want to look into aquaponics. There is a video on the website listed below explaining how it all works and there is even an online course you can do. The site owner has also written a book, called *Aquaponic Gardening*. Aquaponics is really exciting stuff.

✓ Read more at theaquaponicsource.com

Shared produce

With food prices going up, yet so much food still being wasted, many people are opting to get to know their community members so that they can share their produce. Sometimes gardening produces such a lot that you simply won't be able to eat it all, and there is only so much pickling you can do, and only a certain amount of room in your freezer. You might be growing some things that other community members aren't, so you could do a 'swap' with them. They grow tomatoes, you don't, so why not swap your pumpkins with them? All that you need to do is get to know your neighbours and just ask what they are growing. This is another industry that's catching on fast, and one that just makes so much sense.

✓ ampleharvest.org
✓ localharvest.org
✓ locavore365.org
✓ growington.com (UK)

Community sharing in action

A very interesting story I came across in one of the papers is about a town in the UK called Todmorden which is in West Yorkshire. They are aiming to be the first self-sufficient town in the world by 2018, meaning they will grow all of their own food for the *entire* town. They are already growing things near police stations, car parks, train stations – in total at the moment there are 70 garden beds around the town where they are growing raspberries, carrots, apricots, blackcurrants, apples, strawberries, beans, peas and all sorts of herbs. They are also trying to promote home gardening too so that the townsfolk start to get more interested in growing things themselves.

What is so special about this town is that the food is actually free for the community. And because the people are so conscious-minded, no one actually takes more than they need.

Similar schemes are now being implemented in about 21 other towns in the UK, and other countries such as Spain, Germany, Hong Kong and Canada are showing interest. A truly exciting development and one that I hope catches on in even more cities and towns.

Please check out their website below if you want to know more.

✓ incredible-edible-todmorden.co.uk

Community-supported agriculture

In the USA, CSA has become a very popular way to become involved in supporting local farmers and to eat healthier foods. This is how it works: a customer signs up to a membership-type scheme where they will pay a certain price to a farm and receive a 'share' in the farmer's business. The customer will receive a veggie/fruit box in return. This helps the farmer in a few ways: 1) they receive regular money, 2) they have an opportunity to get to know their customers, 3) they get to spend time on marketing before they have to spend all their waking minutes on the farm.

Customers benefit in these ways: 1) they get to eat the best fresh food direct from the growers, 2) they can often be exposed to new types of vegetables and learn new ways to cook them, 3) they can visit the farm if they wish to, 4) kids tend to love the food that is grown at the farm they visit, 5) they can develop a relationship with the farmer and learn more about how their food is grown.

✓ localharvest.org/csa/

Growing food indoors

No matter where we live, most of us have at least some space to grow food. It might not be like a conventional back garden, but many creative people are figuring out ways to grow food indoors. As long as there is light in your house or flat, you can grow food. And even if you didn't have natural light coming through, you can grow things hydroponically. While sunlight is the best for growing food, hydro-ponics (and aquaponics) can still offer highly nutritious foods.

The most exciting invention I have seen in a while for growing food at home is the Hyundai Kitchen Nano Garden. This looks like a big fridge but has clear glass doors and trays as shelves, so allows you to grow many different herbs and greens on each level. You will not need any kind of spray to keep bugs away either, so the produce will be as fresh and as pure as can be. If you use the best-quality water, it will only add to the nutrient level of these hydroponically grown organic foods. It's not out in stores yet at time of writing, but keep an eye out for it soon!

Another incredible invention for growing produce indoors was developed by an American company called Window Farms, which wanted to discover if it was possible to grow food without soil. A Window Farm is a vertical hydroponic growing platform which needs to be put somewhere near natural sunlight. They can easily be built by yourself and the website gives you instructions to do this or you can buy one from them already built. The produce grows due to being watered with liquid nutrients that goes up outside of the plants then down into the top part of the vertical platform and then trickles through each plant, over its root section, and gets all of the nutrition it needs to grow. The reservoir at the bottom of the platform is where the liquid nutrients are kept (and need to be refilled from time to time) and where the water comes from. Kits can be shipped all over the world.

For more info check out:

✓ windowfarms.org

Other short-of-space growing ideas

As long as you have an imagination, there is really no lack of creative ideas for growing things indoors or in a small outside area. You can use large deep bins to grow things like potatoes and other root vegetables, and grow tomatoes in a medium-sized flower pot. I have also seen people grow things on a bookcase or hanging off a wall in their apartment. Again, as long as there is natural light coming in, or you can set up an artificial light, you can grow so many things. I think it's also beautiful to surround yourself with living things in your home environment, and it will also help to create better air quality if you are growing fruit trees.

A really great book to help you discover simple yet effective ways of growing your own food is *Apartment Gardening: Plants, Projects, and Recipes for Growing Food in Your Urban Home* by Amy Pennington. Another one is *Growing Tasty Tropical Plants in Any Home, Anywhere: 60 Tasty Tropical House Plants You Can Grow No Matter Where You Live* by Laurelynn and Byron Martin.

The following websites can help you grow things from your home, no matter how small.

✓ urbanorganicgardener.com
✓ capitalgrowth.org
✓ amy-pennington.com

Shared purchasing

Another innovative and exciting industry that is growing super-fast is shared purchasing. Let's face it, we already have enough 'stuff' to look after everyone in the world and so much of it goes to waste Some conscious owners are now willing to share with others so that you can not only share in the costs, but also share in the use, which makes it more environmentally friendly. For those that don't really want a simple life and desire to have luxury items, you can share in big expensive things like houses, planes and super-yachts or even much smaller planes. You can meet like-minded people who want to buy the same thing and make that purchase together and share all of the costs and upgrades. If you are having money problems with something you already own but do not want to part with it, you can also put up a certain percentage for selling. This means that you will still be able to use the item but you can get some money back.

You can also share items such as lawnmowers, tents, power tools and other useful things that only get used occasionally. The website below will show you what people are open to sharing.

- ✓ goshared.com
- ✓ ecomodo.com
- ✓ thingloop.com

A really great book which is all about the future in regard to sharing, and lists many sites which are all about sharing (from cars to office space to baby items), is called *What's Mine Is Yours* by Rachel Botsman and Roo Rogers.

Sharing with your neighbors

People are also starting to share items with their neighbors or those in the immediate area. Just say you needed to do some electrical work but didn't own the right piece of equipment. Instead of going to the shops to buy something you may only need to use once a year, you could log on to the website and see who has what you need, nearby to you. Isn't this a great idea? And really, we should have started doing this a *long* time ago. This is what community means – caring and sharing with others. If we get to know our neighbors more, sharing things will be so much more acceptable and easier and financially better for all!

Environmentally friendly holidays

Going on holiday can be another way to help the environment. So many resorts and hotels are really harming the planet, by using *massive* amounts of energy from the lighting to the air conditioning and heating, food (and lots goes to waste as people on holidays tend to expect to eat so much food!), water, and using toxic chemicals to build and clean the buildings with. Luckily, another green trend to start sweeping the globe is environmentally friendly resorts and hotels..

When I visited Costa Rica back in April 2011, I went there to check out why the country is renowned for its green travel. Costa Rica is undoubtedly one of the most diverse and stunning countries on earth. But without people caring as much as they do for this beautiful country, it could easily be spoilt. And sadly, some of it has been, but as a whole, it is leading the way for being a shining example of preserving the natural surroundings yet still encouraging people to visit the country.

About 20 years ago, Finca Rosa Blanca was built in a valley near San Jose, the country's capital. The owners, Glenn Jampool and his wife (who also had an organic coffee farm) opened up the country's first ever Certified Sustainable Tourism eco hotel (certified by the CST organization) where their mission was to create the least amount of impact to the surrounding environment. These are the practices they have put in place:

- Underground electrical systems that do not interfere with surrounding wildlife or endanger the coffee workers
- Solar panels to heat water coupled with energy-saving auxiliary on-demand heating systems
- Their own organic shade-grown certified coffee in menu offerings, to share with the guests and spa treatments
- Recycling of the coffee 'pulp' to be used as fertilizer
- Copper/silver ionization system to clean swimming pool water
- Recycled materials throughout the grounds such as roof tiles and waste receptacles

- 1 gallon flush toilets are used throughout the inn
- Philanthropic donation programs to help the schools and our community
- All of the employees are from the local area so we can 'recycle' our earnings back into our community
- Education of employees, guests and neighbors about good practices
- Linens made from bamboo fiber (a very sustainable product)
- An advanced vermiculture-based compost system (worm beds) to recycle organic waste
- A greenhouse where organic vegetables and herbs are grown for our restaurant. The soil comes from composted material prepared in our recycling area.

Not only were they the first sustainable hotel, the owner Glenn Jampool has been instrumental in encouraging other hotels and resorts to incorporate green practices. So passionate is he about the environment that he became president of CANECO which is an organization that supports sustainable tourism and corporate responsibility aimed at environmental protection and management. CANECO promotes community development and preservation of its attractions. As of the end of 2010, there are now approximately 210 hotels and 15 tour operators, which are certified by the CST. In a small country such as Costa Rica this amount is very impressive and a shining example as to what can be done to preserve precious land.
    ✓ fincarosablanca.com

When organizing your travel, check out your hotel or resort's sustainability practices to see if they are doing anything to help the environment. If not, consider staying somewhere else that does, or have a chat with management to encourage them to become greener. In the resource section of this book you can find some websites which can help you choose green places to stay

Chapter 54

DIY – How to Make Your Own Inexpensive Organic Cleaning & Beauty Products

If you want to be truly environmentally friendly, then you can make your own cleaning products. I have actually just recently discovered the joys of cleaning with vinegar, lemon juice, salt, hydrogen peroxide and baking soda. These ingredients are so inexpensive but really do work! My house looks and smells so clean and I love that it's also hygienic as well, but without the use of chemicals. With the following simple recipes you will be able to clean your entire house without needing to resort to buying any mainstream toxic products. And you will save money too because the items you need to make these mixtures hardly cost anything at all. Who would have thought that such simple ingredients could rival some of the most heavy-duty products!

I clean my entire bathroom and kitchen (sink, table tops, table, furniture, stove, fridge, bin, floors) and all the other places in my house with these recipes below.

Cleansing scrub for cleaning kitchen and bathroom

Mix equal parts of white vinegar + salt – store in a glass jar or a Tupperware container. Use on table tops, bath, sinks, shower recess, kitchen worktops. The salt acts as a scrub to help remove any stubborn stains, and the vinegar also helps to make this more effective as well as being a disinfectant. Very inexpensive, and very easy to make.

Glass cleaner

Take ¼ cup of white vinegar + 1 tablespoon of corn starch + 1.2 liters of water. Pour this mixture into a spray bottle and use on any glass, windows, and shower screen. Remove with a soft damp or dry cloth.

All-purpose cleaner

Here is a really great tip – take 1–2 tablespoons of Dr. Bronners 18-1 Liquid Castile Soap and add to a spray bottle, filling the rest of it with water. Give it a shake and then use this on any surface. This mixture is effective to use in the kitchen, bathroom, and even on furniture as the olive oil and other oils that are in Dr. Bronners will only add to the beauty of the furniture. If you have a scented Dr. Bronners, then you will find that the spray smells lovely! I love to use the rose soap in my mixture.

Anti-mold spray

I used to think that I had to use chemicals to keep mold at bay, but luckily there is another safe option! Take 2 drops of tea tree oil and add 1 cup of water into a spray bottle. Shake and use anywhere mold is normally a problem. Let it soak on the area and remove with a scrubbing brush and cloth. This mixture is not only very effective but has no nasty toxic smells!

Cleaning silver

I have memories of seeing my mum clean all our silver and the smell of the cleaner didn't exactly smell safe. I have since told her that there is another way to clean her items that is effective and kinder to her and the planet. Take a stainless steel bowl and add some aluminum foil in the bottom. Fill up the bowl with warm water and pour in some baking soda (about 50 grams), then put in the silver item and let it soak for 15 minutes – remove and then polish the item with a soft cloth.

Clear blocked drains

Again, this is something I thought would always need harsh chemicals as it seemed like such a tough problem to fix. You can actually use baking soda and vinegar which chemically creates a foam-type consistency. Take 2 tablespoons of baking soda and put in a small tub, pour in apple cider vinegar and watch it foam up. Pour this down the drain/plug hole and wait for 15 minutes. Then run water through it and you will see it's unblocked. Brilliant! Much kinder for our waterways. You can also use this exact same mixture in the bath. To help your skin feel super-soft and to also help it detoxify, add it to your bath mixture and soak for 15 minutes. Not only will you be clean, the bath will be clean too.

Floor cleaner

Use equal parts of white vinegar and really hot water + a few drops of essential oil (Dr. Bronners could work well too). Mop over your floors and they will not only look clean but will be hygienically clean too – far safer for pets and small children.

Whiten your whites

Take 1 cup of hydrogen 3% peroxide to add to your laundry when you want to whiten them but without bleach.

To clean your dishwasher

Add ¼ cup of hydrogen 3% peroxide to the rinse aid compartment, then put it on a normal washing cycle.

Washing fruit and vegetables

Using hydrogen peroxide will also help to remove chemicals from fruits and veggies. Add salt in addition to ¼ cup 3% hydrogen peroxide to a sink full of cold water. Rinse and dry.

To remove red wine stains

You can also use hydrogen peroxide to remove red wine stains, even from a white carpet! Pour on undiluted hydrogen peroxide, and let it sit for a few minutes to get right into the carpet. Take a spray bottle with equal parts water and equal parts carpet cleaner. Mist the stain, then remove excess with a cloth. Vodka also works too!

Refresh fabric furniture

If your couch is looking a bit dull you can use vodka to give it a bit of a lift. Take a spray bottle and fill it with straight vodka. Mist over the fabric. Completely safe for the environment, and your furniture. You could even use this spray on your hands to kill any germs – much better than using a chemical-based hand sanitizer.

Help keep moths away naturally

* You can use the following dried herbs mixed together:

- Mint
- Lavender
- Cedar (this is a wood)
- Rosemary
- Thyme
- Lemon

* Here are some fun and easy recipes you can follow:

- 50/50 rosemary and mint
- 1 part dried lavender, 1 part rosemary, ½ part dried lemon peel, 1 tablespoom cloves
- 1 part whole cloves, 1 part whole peppercorns, 2–4 cinnamon sticks broken in pieces
- 1 part dried lavender, 1 part dried lemon peel, 1 broken cinnamon stick
- 1 part cedar shavings, 1 part thyme
- 1 part peppermint, 1 part spearmint, 1 part rosemary, ½ part thyme

You can mix and match your own recipes, or just use 100% of one ingredient if you like.

* Recipes sourced from tipnut.com

Natural beauty tips and homemade recipes

Having a bathroom stocked with many different beauty products can be expensive. But if you make your own, you can not only have fun, but save money too!

Here are some inexpensive ways to make your beauty routine safe and effective:

- Throw away chemical-based exfoliants and use a bristle brush to keep the skin on your body super-soft. This is also very stimulating for the entire body, and if you use long strokes towards the heart, it will help push lymph along, helping your body to keep you toxin-free. Try to do it every day in the morning for best effect. Your skin will feel amazing after regular use.

- Organic bicarbonate of soda as a facial exfoliant is incredible. It is so simple yet one of the best I have ever come across. Makes the skin so baby-soft and is dirt cheap to purchase.

- Make your own tooth cleaner. Take a small pot and add baking soda as well as essential oils. Dip your wet toothbrush into the mixture and apply to the teeth and gums. Brush gently. Baking soda whitens teeth too.

- To keep your toothbrush clean, soak the head in peroxide to kill any bacteria.

- You can make your own invigorating body scrub with sugar (brown or white sugars) or fine salt and mix it with olive oil or something similar, such as almond oil. Add a few drops of essential oils to make it smell how you like it. Very inexpensive to do and will cost only a few pounds or dollars. Don't use a salt mixture after shaving though, as it may sting.

- Make your own deodorant by using ¼ cup of cornstarch or arrowroot powder, ¼ cup of aluminum-free baking soda, 10 drops of tea tree oil, 10 drops of lavender or another oil of your liking. Mix this all together with some coconut oil, then pour the mixture into an empty deodorant stick container and keep it in the fridge. Once it's set after a few hours, you can use it as often as you like.

- Another recipe for a very effective deodorant is this: take a small empty spray bottle (holds 20 mls), squeeze one lemon and one lime, remove the seeds and add to the liquid 5 drops of Pure Body zeolites and 4 drops of organic essential oil. I love using peppermint but you could use anything you like. Add a teaspoon of bicarbonate of soda, the aluminum-free kind. Shake together and it's now ready use. It's absolutely brilliant, and really masks any unwanted underarm smell. Its the best natural one I have ever used

- Instead of spending lots of money on a body lotion, use organic coconut oil or raw shea butter. Both are absolutely amazing on the skin: very healing, moisturizing and they smell great.

- Purchase a soft organic muslin cloth to remove makeup. It even acts as an exfoliant; these cloths are long lasting and can be machine-washed again and again.

- Use raw honey as a facial mask – take a teaspoon of honey and smooth it over a cleansed face and neck. Leave on for 15 minutes then remove with a warm, damp soft cloth.

- Mash up some avocado and either use it as a face mask or in your hair as a treatment. You can add some lemon juice to the mixture as the acid in the lemon will help slough away dead skin. Used in the hair it will help to lighten any blond pieces of hair you have but without the damage of nasty bleach.

- For an itchy scalp, instead of reaching for toxic anti-dandruff shampoos, use some organic apple cider vinegar. This not only soothes the scalp (feels instantly cooling and calming) but stops the flakes from coming back. Apple cider vinegar is also a great way to make your hair look shiny. Pour straight onto the scalp or mix with some warm water to dilute. Use as a final rinse after you have shampooed your hair.

- Moroccan Argan Oil is now in a lot of hair serums these days, but unfortunately they also add other ingredients too which aren't so natural. Using pure oil on your skin or in your hair does a wonderful job of repairing and softening. You can also use coconut oil too for a hair treatment! Just don't use too much as it can be hard to wash out.

- For sensitive and dry skin, mash up a banana till creamy and smooth. Apply all over the face and around the eyes too. Leave for 10 minutes and remove with a soft cloth.

- To clear impurities from your skin, take a large glass bowl and pour in hot water – being very careful to not spill it - and a few drops of lemon essential oil. Place the bowl on a table with a towel over your head and bowl, and let the hot water steam your skin. Remember, be very careful you don't spill the water on yourself.

- Epsom salts are not only great to use in a bath but they can be used on your face as well. Mix a teaspoon of the salts into a milky cleanser and gently exfoliate your face and neck using circular movements. You can also use bicarbonate of soda to exfoliate the skin with too – it's cheap and brilliant.

- Instead of using typical perfumes, take some organic essential oil such as jasmine and dab it on your neck, elbows and wrists. Smells amazing, and is much less expensive and long lasting.

- For cellulite you can make your own invigorating oil by using jojoba oil and mix in some mandarin and grapefruit essential oils. These two combined will help to break down fatty deposits and help to push the toxins away. Massage in vigorously twice a day for best results. Cellulite is hard to get rid of but massage really is something that does help.

For other ideas on how to make your own natural and homemade beauty products you can read *The Holistic Beauty Book* by Star Khechara.

We become part of the change by becoming part of the solution. As ethical consumers we have great power to change the world economy from a power-over institution to one which supports local community, local produce, the life enhancing production of goods, fairly traded goods, cooperatives, recycled products, food which is free of harmful chemicals, pesticides or genetic modification, and products that do not harm the Earth.

~ Glennie Kindred, *Earth Wisdom*

Afterword

Well, here we are now – well done for making it the whole way through. Even though this book has now come to an end, I hope that it's actually just the *beginning* for you, on your own journey to becoming healthier and happier. If this information inspires you to change things for yourself, and your family then I have achieved my goal. Despite this being a very big book, I've really only told you a small amount about these very important subjects. There is *so* much more information to be found out there, and I do hope this sets you off on a path to discovering much more.

Are you in a bit of shock right now with all of the information I have shared with you? Perhaps most of all, in regards to toxicity and the dangerous effects its having on our health? I don't blame you at all for being a wee bit freaked out. I was when I first looked into all of this; in fact, I couldn't really sleep well for a week or so, as I felt I had known nothing about the real world and what *really* affects us.

Most of this stuff is mainly kept hidden from us by mainstream media, it's not explained at all in schools, and really, many industries *don't* actually want us to be more conscious and healthier – they just want us to keep spending our money on all the things they make and to keep believing the lies and half truths they tell us.

I genuinely believe you can get a lot out of this book which can help you a great deal, but I am also aware that it doesn't have all the answers to everything – no one does. The world is so complex, so are it's people - but I feel very strongly this book can set you off on a much brighter, happier path when you embrace and implement what you have learnt.

If you are a bit overwhelmed, please do not *fear*; you can start today to change in a healthy and positive way. Just begin with little things if you find it too difficult to do lots at once. It's not about becoming scared to live your life (as fear = stress = health problems) but just learning the reality as to what we are all being affected by, and what we can do to actually stop it from happening.

I want to tell you, though, that living consciously is *not* about you having to always be perfect. We must never make ourselves feel that we have to be perfect every single day as this sets us up for feeling like a failure if we do something that we perhaps should not. I know I am definitely not always perfect! I won't always eat the right things (at times I will have a slight chocolate or cake binge!) and sometimes I won't be in the happiest mood 24/7, nor will I exercise nearly as much as I should. Sometimes I won't be the most patient mother, I certainly haven't yet sorted out all my issues from childhood, and I don't have a house full of enough plants. Nor is my wardrobe full of only organic clothes, but that's alright – I am only human. I'm going to spending the rest of my life improving on all of these things.

If we can just do the *best* we can, as often as we can, then that will make a huge difference to our life.

The power is in your hands; you now have a lot of knowledge, with a fair amount of serious warnings thrown in, so I *really* hope you do take advantage of what you have just learnt.

And take it from me, I am living proof of what happens when you *do not* look after yourself, eat terrible foods, suffer from a lot of stress and unhappiness, and take lots of medicines. I know what it's like to be clinically depressed, to feel sick every single day, have absolutely no energy, and to feel like I was actually slowly... wasting away. Although I may have been an extreme case, what happened to me in my early life is more likely going to happen in later life, to so many people if they do not change what they are doing to themselves now.

When you *do* look after yourself, by detoxing, eating well and changing habits for the better - you really *can* turn your health and life around, even when you get told you can't!

If you are a young person reading this, or are pregnant, or have young kids, please take this stuff *seriously* and know that you can change your future starting right now. It's even more important if you have children. We have to help them no matter what. If you have been ignoring your health and happiness for far too long, I will tell you something - it's never, ever too late to change.

No matter if you are 23 or 93.

Your body craves to be healthy, for that is how it's *meant* to be, and it's actually trying every day to survive, no matter what it is facing. It is a beautiful machine when given the right fuel and attention. But why not let it thrive, instead of just allowing it to survive?

It's also very important to remember, despite all of the horrors that we face, the world is still so beautiful, and life truly is a precious gift. We just need to keep it, and ourselves in balance, and that means becoming as healthy and as happy as possible.

I wish you much happiness and greater health!

Anna Rodgers

Please feel free to leave a review on Amazon and I do hope you will visit my website:

✓ www.missecoglam.com

Resources – Suggested Reading, Watching and Learning Materials

Over the years, I have read many life-changing books, viewed lots of inspiring movies and also stumbled across some wonderful websites that have really helped me with my knowledge of health, happiness and in finding my spirit. I think they may help you too.

Recipe books

Raw Magic – Kate Magic

Raw Living – Kate Magic

Super Foods for Super People – Kate Magic

Ani's Raw Food Kitchen – Ani Phyo

Ani's Raw Food Desserts: 85 Easy, Delectable Sweets and Treats: 85 Easy, Delectable Living Foods Desserts – Ani Phyo

Ani's Raw Food Essentials – Ani Phyo

The Mystic Cook Fire: The Sacred Art of Creating Food to Nurture Friends and Family – Veronika Sophia Robinson

Honestly Healthy – Natasha Corrett and Vicki Edgson

Crazy Sexy Kitchen – Kris Carr and Chad Sarno

Hungry for Change: Ditch the Diets, Conquer the Cravings and Eat Your Way to Lifelong Health – James Colqhoun, Laurentine Ten Bosch, Mark Hyman

Forks Over Knives: The Cook Book – Del Sroufe

Clean Start: Inspiring You to Eat Clean and Live Well with 100 New Clean Food Recipes – Terry Walters

A Nourishing Kitchen – Amy Crawford

I quit sugar – Sarah Wilson

I quit sugar cookbook – Sarah Wilson

Nourishing Traditions - Sally Fallon

Real Food Fermentation: Preserving Whole Fresh Food with Live Cultures in Your Home Kitchen – Alex Lewin

How to Make Probiotic Drinks for a Raw Food Diet: Kefir, Kombucha,

Ginger Beer, and Naturally Fermented Ciders, Sodas, and Smoothies – RJ Ruppenthal

More Than Hummus - Classic Hummus Recipes And So Much More - Katherine Canning

How to Make Kefir - A Beginners Guide Patricia Robertson

The Everything Coconut Diet Cookbook: The Delicious and Natural Way To, Lose Weight Fast, Boost Energy, Improve Digestion, Reduce Inflammation and Get Healthy for Life (Everything Series) - Anji Sandage

Delicious food websites/blogs

earthsprout.com

theholisticingredient.com

mouthwateringvegan.com

thefaceliftdiet.com

sweetlyraw.com

carameliacakery.co.uk

fruitforbeauty.com

purelytwins.com

carmellassunnyrawkitchen.com

healinggourmet.com

thenourishinghome.com

sproutedkitchen.com

macrobioticmeals.com

fragrantvanillacake.blogspot.co.uk

mostlyeating.com

simplycooked.blogspot.co.uk

celeryandcupcakes.com

keepinghealthygettingstylish.com

Health supplies and food websites

red23.co.uk

rawliving.eu

aggressivehealthshop.com

greenpolkadotbox.com

sprouts.com

thegoodapple.com

vitacost.com

store.naturalnews.com

detoxyourworld.com

Law of Attraction books

The Secret – Rhonda Byrne

Tip Top Spiritual Lessons – Frank Arrigazzi

Lucky Bitch – Denise Duffield-Thomas

Get Rich, Lucky Bitch – Denise Duffield-Thomas

The Law Of Attraction: The Basics of the Teachings of Abraham by Esther and Jerry Hicks

The Key To Living The Law of attraction: The Secret to Creating the Life Of Your Dreams by Jack Canfield

Levraging the Universe: 7 Steps To Engaging Life's Magic, Mike Dooley

Infinite Possibilities: the Art of Living Your Dreams, Mike Dooley

Change Your Words, Change Your World, Andrea Gardner

I Believe: When What You Believe Matters! Eldon Taylor

Parenting

The Continuum Concept – Jean Liedloff

Attachment Parenting – Dr. William Sears and Martha Sears

The Breastfeeding Book – Dr. William Sears and Martha Sears

The Successful Child – Dr. William Sears and Martha Sears

The Discipline Book – Dr. Sears and Martha Sears

The Magical Child – Joseph Chilton Pearce

The First National Bank of Dad – David Owen

The Five Love Languages of Children – Chapman and Campbell

Child Development: A First Course – Sylva and Lunt

Dumbing Us Down: The Hidden Curriculum of Compulsory Schooling – John Gatto

The Wonder Weeks – Hetty van de Rijt PhD and Frans Plooij PhD

Child Sense – Priscilla Dunstan

How to Talk So Kids Will Listen and Listen So Kids Will Talk – Adele Faber and Elaine Mazlish

The Honest Life – Jessica Alba

The Manual – Dr Faye Snyder

Spontaneous Creation – Jock Doubleday

The Drinks are On Me: Every Thing Your Mother Never Told You About Breast Feeding – Veronika Sophia Robinson

The Birth Keepers: Reclaiming an Ancient Tradition – Veronika Sophia Robinson

Children's health

Your Healthy Child with Homeopathy – Tricia Allen

How to Raise a Healthy Child in Spite of Your Doctor – Dr. Robert S. Mendelssohn

Creating Healthy Children – *Through Attachment Parenting and Raw Foods* – Karen Ranzi MA, CC-SLP

Happy Healthy Children – Ian White

Is This Your Child?: Discovering and Treating Unrecognized Allergies – Doris J Rapp

Is this Your Child's World? : How You can Fix the Schools and Homes That Are Making Your Children Sick,- Doris J Rapp

Health websites

nurturewithlove.com

knowthecause.com

mercola.com

naturalnews.com

greenmedinfo.com

naturalsociety.com

wddty.com

joyoushealth.ca

drgreene.com

organicauthority.com

homesteadsurvival.blogspot.co.uk
hugginsappliedhealing.com
drweil.com
drsircus.com
naturaldoc.co.uk
drrapp.com
naturalhealth365.com
westonaprice.org
russellblaylockmd.com
ashleysgreenlife.blogspot.co.uk

Health books

Cellular Awakening – Barbara Wren
You Can Heal Your Life – Louise Hay
Hot, Healthy, Happy – Dr. Christy Fergusson
Aggressive Health – Mike Nash
The Toxic Consumer – Karen Ashton and Elizabeth Salter Green
The Holistic Beauty Book – Star Khechara
The Invisible Killers – Rik Dietich
The Organic Pharmacy Guide – Margo Marrone
The Vitamin D Solution – Michael F. Holick
Official Stories – Liam Scheff
Raw Food Controversies: How to Avoid Common Mistakes That May Sabotage Your Health - Frederic Patenaude
Supplements Exposed: The Truth They Don't Want You to Know About Vitamins, Minerals, and Their Effects on Your Health – Brian Clement
The Hundred-Year Lie: How to Protect Yourself from the Chemicals That Are Destroying Your Health – Randall Fitzgerald
This Is Your Brain on Joy: A Revolutionary Program for Balancing Mood, Restoring Brain Health, and Nurturing Spiritual Growth – Earl Henslin and Dr. Daniel Amen
Change Your Brain, Change Your Life: The Breakthrough Programme for Conquering Anger, Anxiety and Depression – Daniel G. Amen

Magnificent Mind at Any Age: Natural Ways to Maximize Your Brain's Health and Potential – Dr. Daniel G. Amen

Toxic Metal Syndrome: How Metal Poisonings Can Affect Your Brain – Dr. Richard Casdorph and Dr. Morton Walker

It's All in Your Head: The Link Between Mercury Amalgams and Illness – Dr. Hal A Huggins

Conquer Your PCOS Naturally – Dr Rebecca Harwin

The Business of baby – Jennifer Marqulis

Silent Spring – Rachel Carson

Homeopathy websites

joettecalabrese.com

homeopathyhelpline.com

naturopathiccentre.co.uk

Organic beauty websites

nourishedlife.com.au

biggreensmile.com

lucyrose.biz

pravera.co.uk

lovelula.com

greenpolkadotbox.com

Inspiring & life changing books

The Buddha, Geoff and Me – Edward Canfor-Dumas

Anastasia and the Ringing Cedars Series - Vladimir Megré and Leonid Sharashkin

Finding Your Spirit – Sonia Choquette

The Conversations with God series – Neale Donald Walsch

Sassy – Lisa Clarke

Tip Top Spiritual Lessons – Frank Arrigazzi

Am I Being Kind? – Michael J. Chase

Waking from Sleep – Steve Taylor

Amish Peace: Simple Wisdom for a Complicated World - Suzanne Woods

Fisher

Low Cost Living: Live Better, Spend Less – John Harrison

The Self-Sufficiency Bible: From Window Boxes to Smallholdings – Hundreds of Ways To Become Self-Sufficent – Simon Dawson

Frugillionaire: 500 Fabulous Ways To Live Richly and Save A fortune – Francine Jay

Miss Minimalist: Inspiration to Downsize, Declutter, and Simplify – Francine Jay

Vaccination books

The Vaccination Bible – edited by Lynne McTaggart

Evidence of Harm – David Kirby

The Truth about Vaccines – Dr Richard Halvorsen

Vaccine Illusion - Tetyana Obukhanych

Into the Labyrinth – Jock Doubleday

VACCeptable Injuries - Markus Heinze

Vaccination is Not Immunization - Dr. Tim O'Shea

Vaccine Free: 111 Stories of Unvaccinated Children - Andreas Bachmair

Helens Story: A Routine Vaccination Ruined My Daughters Life Forever. This Is The Inspiring Story Of How I took on the Government And Won - Rosemary Fox

Vaccination And Immunisation: Dangers, Delusions and Alternatives (What Every Parent Should Know) - Leon Chaitow

Calling the Shots: Childhod Vaccination - One Family's Journey - Mary Alexander

Vaccine information websites

vaccineresistancemovement.org

vaccinationcouncil.org

vaccineriskawareness.com

vaxtruth.org

vaxtruth.com

vaccinesafety.edu

nvic.org
vaccinesuncensored.org
medalerts.org

Pharmaceutical industry books

Bad Pharma – Ben Goldacre

The Eden Prescription – Ethan Evers

Anatomy of an Epidemic: Magic Bullets, Psychiatric Drugs, and the Astonishing Rise of Mental Illness in America – Robert Whitaker

The Truth about the Drug Companies: How They Deceive Us and What to Do about It – Marcia Angell

Let Them Eat Prozac: The Unhealthy Relationship between the Pharmaceutical Industry and Depression (Medicine, Culture, and History) – David Healy

Your Drug May Be Your Problem, Revised Edition: *How and Why to Stop Taking Psychiatric Medications* – David Cohen and Peter Breggin

Unhinged: The Trouble with Psychiatry: A Doctor's Revelations about a Profession in Crisis – Daniel Carlat

Big Pharma – Jacky Law

Magazines

The Mother Mag

The Green Parent

Yoga Magazine

Coco Eco Magazine

Juno Magazine

Prediction Magazine

Peppermint Magazine

Eco Egg Magazine

Ethical Consumer Magazine

Movies

Home

Sweet Misery

Killer at Large

Fast Food Nation

The Green Beautiful

The Future of Food

Food Inc

Thrive: The Movie

Shots in the Dark: Silence on Vaccine

The Greater Good

Vaccine Nation

Autism Made in the USA

Food Matters

Tapped

Wasteland

Babies: The Business of Being Born

Forks Over Knives

Fat, Sick and Nearly Dead

War On Health

The Cancer Sell

An Inconvenient Tooth

The Weight of the Nation

Fast Food, Fat Profits: Obesity in America

Fast Food Baby

Selective Hearing: Brian Deer and the GMC

Burzynski: Cancer Is Serious Business

Dying to Have Known

Pill Poppers

Vegucated

House of Numbers

The Marketing of Madness: Are We All Insane?

Hoxsey: How Healing Becomes a Crime

Prescription for Disaster

Modern Meat
The Drugging of Our Children
Big Bucks, Big Pharma: Marketing Disease and Pushing Drugs
Poison in the Mouth
Statin Nation
The Moo Man

Many of these films can be viewed for free at:

topdocumentaryfilms.com or documentarywire.com – also check out YouTube, or help the documentary makers by purchasing a copy.

Organic baby food brands

so-baby.co.uk
ellaskitchen.co.uk
babyorganic.com
greenpolkadotbox.com
holle.ch
sproutbabyfood.com
plumorganics.com
hipp.co.uk
organix.com
heavenlytastyorganics.com
organicbubs.com
bellamysorganic.com.au
littleorganics.com.au

Organic baby skincare

Akamuti.co.uk
greenpolkadotbox.com
Sheamooti.co.uk
Greenpeople.co.uk
weleda.co.uk
organicmonkey.co.uk

honest.com

Biodegradeable Nappies, Nappy Bags & Wipes

naty.com

beamingbaby.co.uk

eenee.com

honest.com

earthsbest.com

whole food's 365 everyday diapers

ecofriendlybabies.com

seventhgeneration.com

Tushies

Broody Chick 100% Natural Fully Compostable Diapers

Bambo

Attitude

Thirsties

Nature Babycare

Reuseable Nappies

gnappies.com

lizziesrealnappies.co.uk

goreal.org.uk

bumgenius.com

bambinomio.com

babipur.co.uk

pure rest organics

kushies

littlelambnappies.com

babykind.co.uk

FuzziBunz

Eco paints

ecodecorators.org

ecospaints.com

ecospaints.net
earthbornpaints.co.uk
littlegreene.com
ecolour.com.au
livos.com.au
house-paint.com.au
coloursbynature.com.au
ecoathome.com.au
benjaminmoore.com
aurousa.com
milkpaint.com
timberprocoatings.com
weatherbos.com
medimports.net
greendepot.com

Eco baby websites

organic-baby-resource.com
thelittlegreensheep.co.uk
Abacaorganics.co.uk
Honest.com
ecobaby.ie
ecobabygear.com
purerest.com
eco-baby.com.au
ecobabybuys.com
ecobabyco.co.za
ecobaby.dk
ecochild.com.au
babyearth.com

Organic toys & supplies

otoys.co.uk
babipur.co.uk

theorganicbabycompany.co.uk
shop.ecokidsusa.com/product/eco-paint
ecotoys.com.au
magiccabin.com
ecotoystore.co.uk
greentoys.com
downtoearthtoys.com
ecofabulous.com
bigjigstoys.co.uk

Websites to help you find trustworthy organic food, products and companies

organicconsumers.org/btc/BuyingGuide.cfm
green-patriot.com/greenconsumer.html
naturalfoodnet.com
simplesteps.org/eat-local

Organic food delivery in the UK

ableandcole.co.uk
farmaround.co.uk
riverford.co.uk
organicdeliverycompany.co.uk
realfoods.co.uk/organic
farmaround.co.uk
hankhamorganics.co.uk
organicfreshfoodcompany.co.uk
graigfarm.co.uk
thelocalfoodcompany.co.uk
woodlandsfarm.co.uk
eversfieldorganic.co.uk
organicfood.co.uk
avidorganics.co.uk
planetorganic.com

Organic food delivery in the USA

greenpolkadotbox.com

naturalorganic.biz

farmfreshtoyou.com

organicslive.com

organiclifestyle.com

offthevine.org

boxedgreens.com

organicdirect.com

puresprouts.com

doortodoororganics.com

planetorganics.com

Wild & Ethical Meat, Seafood and Dairy Sources

honoredprairie.com

shop.mercola.com

wildmeat.co.uk

eatwild.com

smgfoods.com

wildmeats.co.za

hillsfoods.com

rothervalleyorganics.com

brokenarrowranch.com

fishonline.org

sustainableseafood.org.au

seachoice.org

davidsuzuki.org

realmilk.com

Organic food delivery in Australia

organicoz.com.au

victoriaorganicdelivery.com.au

goodness.com.au

lettucedeliver.com.au

aussiefarmers.com.au

foodiesorganic.com.au

organicdeliverysydney.com.au

santostrading.com.au

organicangels.com

ceresfairfood.org.au

theorganicgrocer.com.au

ripenraworganics.com.au

freshline.com.au

organicfooddirectory.com.au

freshorganics.com.au

cairnsonlineorganics.com.au

babybistro.com.au

organicfeast.com.au

Organic Food Delivery in Canada

organicfooddelivery.com

greenearthorganics.com

mamaearth.ca

frontdoororganics.com

planborganicfarms.ca

wanigan.com

claviersbaroques.com

zephyrorganics.com

wheelbarrowfarm.com

lovegan.com

foodshare.net

Sustainable and Eco places to stay in Costa Rica

Farm of Life – farmoflifecr.com

Latitude 10 – latitude10resort.com

Playa Nicuesa – nicuesalodge.com

Arenas Del Mar – arenasdelmar.com

El Silencio – elsilenciolodge.com

Hotel Punta Islita – hotelpuntaislita.com

Eco hotels in the UK
The Scarlet in Cornwall – scarlethotel.co.uk
Hotel Rafayel in London – hotelrafayel.com

The websites below are for finding holiday places worldwide, which offer guests organic food, and many locations usually offer other eco elements as well
organicplacestostay.co.uk

itstaygreen.org

responsibletravel.com

ecotravel.org.uk

ecoluxury.com

ecotourdirectory.com

ecotourism.org

Green websites – be educated, get involved, become inspired
EWG.org

EPA.gov

nigelsecostore.com

ethicalsuperstore.com

inhabitat.com

treehugger.com

liftshare.com/uk

uk.freecycle.org

worldchanging.com

realclimate.org

greenpolkadotbox.com

biggreensmile.com

grist.org

seat61.com

recyclenow.com

planetark.com

adili.com

ecorazzi.com

idealbite.com

blogactionday.org

ecogeek.org

breathingearth.net

wgrnradio.com

rootroots.com

shiftyourhabit.com

bethechangeinc.org

thedailygreen.com

waterkeeper.org

takepart.com

earth911.com

beyondpesticides.org

nrdc.org

panna.org

greencleancertified.com

greenpeace.org

cat.org.uk

earthday.org

foe.co.uk

recyclenow.com

anniebbond.com

care2.com

Eco Friendly Phone Apps

Dirty Dozen

PaperKarma

Seafood Watch

iRecycle

JouleBug

GoodGuide

Recyclebank
Farmers Market Finder
Waterprint
ecoFootprint
Treehugger
EWG Sunscreen Buyer's Guide
Go Green
Ocean Wise
iGreenpeace
iGrowit

Homesteading and Living Off The Land Websites and Blogs
modernhomesteading.ca
twolanelivin.com
veganslivingofftheland.blogspot.co.uk/
off-grid-living.com/
community.theurbanfarmingguys.com
homestead.orghomesteadingtoday.com
motherearthnews.com
homesteadersupply.com
themorristribe.com

Organic and GMO-Free Seed Companies
seedtoplate.co.uk
seedsofchange.com
organicseedfinder.org
realseeds.co.uk
sustainableseedco.com
seedsavers.org
terraedibles.ca
cottagegardener.com

References

Chapter 1

1. Bryson, B., 2004: *A Short History of Nearly Everything*. Transworld Publishers, 687 pp.

Chapter 2

2. Pain Relief Health and Wellness.com, cited 2011: Detoxing Chemicals and Pollutants for Optimal Health – available online at http://www.harryfriedmando.com/articles/detoxing.html

3. Environmental Working Group, cited 2012: A benchmark investigation of industrial chemicals, pollutants and pesticides in umbilical cord blood. Available online at http://www.ewg.org/reports/bodyburden2/execsumm.php

4. Mellowship, D, 2009: Toxic Beauty. Octopus Publishing Group Ltd, 303 pp.

5. Enviro Health Policy, cited 2011: Is childhood cancer increasing? Available online at http://www.envirohealthpolicy.net/kidstest/Cancer%20Pages/IncreasingChildhoodCancer.htm

6. Center for Disease Control, cited 2013: Why Are Autism Spectrum Disorders Increasing? Available online at http://www.cdc.gov/Features/AutismPrevalence/

Chapter 3

7. Mercola, Dr. J., cited 2011: New Studies Reveal Alarming Hidden Cause of Breast Cancer http://articles.mercola.com/sites/articles/archive/2011/03/18/vaccines-increase-cancer-risk.aspx

8. Casdorph, Dr. H., Walker, Dr. M.: Toxic Metal Syndrome. Avery Publishing Group, 413 pp.

9. Huggins, Dr. Hal, 1993: It's All in Your Head. Avery Publishing Group, 193 pp.

10. Huggins, Dr. Hal, 1993: It's All in Your Head. Avery Publishing Group, 193 pp.

11. Adventures in Autism, cited 2011: Beginning at the Beginning. Available online at http://adventuresinautism.blogspot.co.uk/2005/08/beginning-at-beginning.html

12. Vaccine Safety cited 2012: Thimerosal Content in Some US Licensed Vaccinations. Available online at http://www.vaccine-safety.edu/thi-table.htm

13. Mercola, Dr. J., cited 2011: The Hidden Risks in This Heavily Promoted Seasonal Routine. Available online at http://articles.mercola.com/sites/articles/archive/2011/10/31/flu-vaccination-epa-safety-limit-for-mercury.aspx

14. Casdorph, Dr. H, Walker, Dr. M.: Toxic Metal Syndrome. Avery Publishing Group, 413 pp.

Chapter 4

15. Mellowship, D., 2009: Toxic Beauty. Octopus Publishing Group Ltd, 303 pp.

16. Live Strong.com cited 2011: Chemicals in Sanitary Pads. Available online at http://www.livestrong.com/article/108477-chemicals-sanitary-pads/

17. Organic Consumers Association, cited 2011: Fact Sheet on US Cotton Subsidies and Cotton Production. Available online at http://www.organicconsumers.org/clothes/224subsidies.cfm

18. EJF Foundation, cited 2011: What's Your Poison? Available online at http://ejfoundation.org/sites/default/files/public/whats_your_poison_0.pdf

19. Mercola, Dr. J., cited 2011: Are Aluminum Containing Antiperspirants Contributing to Breast Cancer in Women? Available online at http://articles.mercola.com/sites/articles/archive/2011/10/17/aluminum-containing-antiperspirants-contribute-breast-cancer.aspx

20. Mercola, Dr. J., cited 2012: The Reckless Self-Interest of the Fragrance Industry – available online at http://articles.mercola

.com/sites/articles/archive/2010/07/22/the-reckless-selfinterest-of-the-fragrance-industry.aspx

Chapter 7

21. Environmental Protection Agency, cited 2011: An Introduction to Air Quality. Available online at http://www.epa.gov/iaq/ia-intro.html

22. Islam, Z., Harkema, J.R., Pestka, J.J., Mercola.com cited 2011: Satratoxin G from the black mold Stachybotrys chartarum evokes olfactory sensory neuron loss and inflammation in the murine nose and brain. Available online at http://articles .mercola.com/sites/articles/archive/2011/09/03/molds-making-you-ill.aspx

23. B.C., Wolverton, Nasa Technical Reports Server, cited 2012: Interior Landscape Plants for Indoor Air Pollution Abatement. Available online at http://ntrs.nasa.gov/archive/nasa/casi.ntrs. nasa.gov/19930073077_1993073077.pdf

24. Extracted from NEXUS Magazine, Volume 2, #25 (April–May '95). Mercola.com cited 2011: The Proven Dangers of Microwaving. Available online at http://www.mercola .com/article/microwave/hazards2.htm#hanshertel

25. Mercola, Dr. J., Mercola.com cited 2011: Why Did the Russians Ban an Appliance Found in 90% of American Homes? Available online at http://articles.mercola.com/sites/articles/archive/ 2010/05/18/microwave-hazards.aspx

26. Seattle Organic Restaurants.com cited 2013: Dark History of Dupont. Available online at http://www.seattleorganicrestau-rants.com/vegan-whole-foods/dupont-history/

27. useless information.com cited 2013 Teflon – If nothing sticks to it how do they get it to stick to the pan? Available online at http://www.uselessinformation.org/teflon/index.html

28. Environmental Working Group cited 2013: EWG Finds Heated Teflon Pans Can Turn Toxic Faster than Dupont Claims. Available online at http://www.ewg.org/reports/toxicteflon

29. Environmental Work Group cited 2013: Cleaning Chemicals 'Reach' Baby. Available online at http://www.ewg.org /news/cleaning-chemicals-reach-baby

30. Organic Consumers Association cited 2013 How Toxic Are Your Household Cleaning Supplies. Available online at http://www.organicconsumers.org/articles/article_279.cfm

31. Gosselin, Smith and Hodge, cited 2013. Clinical Toxicology of Commercial Products. Academic Press, 921pp.

32. National Toxicology Program cited 2013: Report on Carcinogens – Tetrachloroethylene. Available online at http://ntp.niehs.nih.gov/ntp/roc/twelfth/profiles/Tetrachloroet hylene.pdf

Chapter 8
33. Walsh, P. cited 2013: Does This Clutter Make My Butt Look Fat? Free Press, 244 pp.

Chapter 9
34. Batmanghelidj, Dr. F. Water Cure.com cited 2012: Biography of F. Batmanghelidj MD. Available online at http://www. watercure.com/about_dr_b.html

35. Hattersley, Joseph G. Orthomolecular.org cited 2013: The Negative Health Effects of Chlorine. Available online at http://orthomolecular.org/library/jom/2000/articles/2000-v15n02-p089.shtml

36. Frazier, Wade. A Healed Planet.net cited 2013: Fluoridation: A Horror Story. Available online at http://www. ahealedplanet.net/fluoride.htm

37. Harvard School of Public Health, cited 2013: Impact of Fluoride on Neurological Development in Children. Available online at http://www.hsph.harvard.edu/news/features/features/fluoride -childrens-health-grandjean-choi.html

38. Mercola, J. Dr., Mercola.com cited 2013: Harvard Study Confirms Fluoride Reduces Children's IQ. Available online at

http://articles.mercola.com/sites/articles/archive/2012/08/14/flu
oride-effects-in-children.aspx

39. Rense.com cited 2013: The Use of Fluoridation for Mass Mind Control. Available online at http://rense.com/general 79/hd3.htm

40. Fluoride Alert.org cited 2012: Dental Fluorosis available online at http://www.fluoridealert.org/issues/fluorosis/

41. Harvard School of Public Health, cited 2013: Impact of Fluoride on Neurological Development in Children. Available online at http://www.hsph.harvard.edu/news/features/features/fluoride-childrens-health-grandjean-choi.html

42. Fluroide Alert.org cited 2013: Letter to the Food and Drug Administration from the Department of Health, Education and Welfare dated August 15, 1963. Available online at http://www.fluoridealert.org/uploads/fda-1963.pdf

43. New Scientist.com cited 2013: Top 11 Compounds in US Drinking Water. Available online at http://www.newscientist.com/article/dn16397-top-11-compounds-in-us-drinking-water.html

44. Environmental Working Group, cited 2012: Dupont to Pay $8.3 Million. Available online at http://www.ewg.org/release/dupont-pay-83-million

Chapter 10

45. Woolf, Marie. Martin Frost, cited 2012: Junk Food Nation available online at http://www.martinfrost.ws/htmlfiles/may 2007/junkfood_nation.html

46. Health.howstuffworks.com cited 2013: The Dangers of Monosodium Glutamate. Available online at http://health.howstuffworks.com/wellness/food-nutrition/facts/the-dangers-of-monosodium-glutamate.htm

47. Huffington Post.com cited 2012: High Fructose Corn Syrup Consumption Linked With Type 2 Diabetes Prevalence. Available online at http://www.huffingtonpost.com/2012/

11/27/high-fructose-corn-syrup-diabetes-hfcs-type-2_n_
2194173.html

48. Black, Richard, BBC.co.uk cited 2013: Pesticides Hit Queen Bee
Numbers. Available online at http://www.bbc.co.uk/
news/science-environment-17535769

49. Forbes.com cited 2013: Five Reasons to Eat Organic Apples:
Pesticides, Healthy Communities, and You. Available online at
http://www.forbes.com/sites/bethhoffman/2012/04/23/five-
reasons-to-eat-organic-apples-pesticides-healthy-commu-
nities-and-you/

50. Environmental Protection Agency, cited 2013: Nitrates and
Nitrites TEACH Chemical Summary. Available online at
http://www.epa.gov/teach/chem_summ/Nitrates_summary.pdf

51. Journals.lww.com cited 2013: Ingestion of Nitrate and Nitrite
and Risk of Stomach Cancer in the NIH-AARP Diet and Health
Study. Available online at http://journals.lww.com/epidem
/Fulltext/2011/01001/Ingestion_of_Nitrate_and_Nitrite_and_Ri
sk_of.305.aspx

52. Sweet Poison.com cited 2012: Aspartame Symptoms Submitted
to the FDA. Available online at http://www.sweetpoison.com/
articles/0706/aspartame_symptoms_submit.html

53. Guardian.co.uk cited 2013: Study linking GM maize to cancer
must be taken seriously by regulators. Available online at
http://www.guardian.co.uk/environment/2012/sep/28/study-
gm-maize-cancer

54. Forbes.com cited 2013: Obama's Science Commitment, FDA
Face Ethics Scrutiny in Wake of GMO Salmon Fiasco. Available
online at http://www.forbes.com/sites/jonentine/2012/12/28
/obamas-science-commitment-fda-face-ethics-scrutiny-in-
wake-of-gmo-salmon-fiasco/

55. Natural Food Finder.co.uk cited 2013: Michelle Obama –
Organic Victory Garden. Available online at http://www.
naturalfoodfinder.co.uk/michelle-obama-organic-victory-
garden

56. Grassfedgirl.com cited 2013 Suicide by Sandwich 12 Reasons to Banish Bread. Available online at http://www.grassfedgirl .com/suicide-by-sandwich-12-reasons-to-banish-bread/

57. Mercola.com cited 2013: The Problems with Radiated Food: What the Research Says. Available online at http://www. mercola.com/article/irradiated/irradiated_research.htm

58. Natural Resources Defense Council – nrdc.org cited 2013: Mercury Contamination in Fish – a guide to staying healthy and fighting back. Available online at http://www.nrdc .org/health/effects/mercury/protect.asp

59. Treehugger.com cited 2012: Latin American Farmers Sue over Pesticides. Available online at http://www.treehugger .com/green-food/latin-american-banana-farmers-sue-over-pesticides.html

Chapter 11

60. Mercola, Dr. J. cited 2012: Movie Death by Medicine. Available online at http://www.mercola.com

61. Well Assembled.com cited 2013 Drugs and Devices That Might Change Your Practice. Available online at http://www. wellassembled.com

62. The Student Room.co.uk cited 2013: Paracetamol overdose – the consequences. Available online at http://www.thestuden-troom.co.uk/showthread.php?t=549759

63. webmd.com cited 2013: Most New Drugs Tapped from Nature – 70% in last 25 years were derived from or inspired by Nature. Available online at http://www.webmd.com/news/2007 0316/most-new-drugs-tapped-from-nature

64. Naturalnews.com cited 2012: Tamiflu Vaccine Linked with Convulsions, Delirium and Bizarre Deaths. Available online at http://www.naturalnews.com/023324_Tamiflu_convulsions_de ath.html#ixzz1lbGfdC4d

65. mercola.com cited 2013: The 6 Types of Pills Big Pharma Wants You Hooked On for Life. Available online at http://articles

.mercola.com/sites/articles/archive/2012/05/14/mercks-adhd-drugs-unsafe.aspx

Chapter 12

66. Casdorph, Dr. H., Walker, Dr. M.: Toxic Metal Syndrome. Avery Publishing Group, 413 pp.
67. Organic Wine Journal.com cited 2012: Pesticide Residues Found in Conventional European Wines. Available online at http://www.organicwinejournal.com/index.php/2008/03/pestic ide-residues-found-in-conventional-european-wines/
68. Stop Smoking Programs.org. cited 2012: Chemicals in Cigarettes. Available online at http://www.stop-smoking-programs.org/chemicals-in-cigarettes.html
69. Sears, Dr. Al., Alsearsmd.com cited 2012: First Your Smile, Then the Rest of You. Available online at http://www.alsearsmd.com/first-your-smile-then-the-rest-of-you/

Chapter 13

70. Ray, Dr. Timothy. Naturallygood.eu cited 2012: Investigating The Secret. Available online at http://naturallygood.eu/investi-gating/
71. Natural Health Information Centre.com cited 2013: Codex Alimentarious – The Sinister Truth behind Operation Cure-All. Available online at http://www.natural-health-information-centre.com/codex-alimentarius.html
72. Momotaj, Dr. H., Hussain, Dr. A.Z.M. cited 2013: Presentation 'Arsenic in Drinking Water: An International Conference at Columbia University, New York, November 26–27, 2001'. Available online at http://www.bvsde.paho.org/bvsacd/arsenico/spirulina.pdf
73. Pubmed.gov. cited 2012: Clinotoptilite Studies. Available online at http://www.ncbi.nlm.nih.gov/pubmed?term=clinop-tilolite

Chapter 15

74. Amen, Dr Daniel. Cited 2013: Documentary 'Doctored' Submarine Deluxe Directed by Bobby Sheehan.

75. CNN.com cited 2013: Columbine Shooter Was Prescribed Antidepressant. Available online at http://articles.cnn.com/1999-04-29/health/9904_29_luvox.explainer_1_antidepressant-ssris-drugs?_s=PM:HEALTH

76. Telegraph.co.uk cited 2103: Felicia Boots: Postnatal depression led to 'fixation' children would be taken from her. Available online http://www.telegraph.co.uk/news/uknews/crime/9643536/Felicia-Boots-Post-natal-depression-led-to-fixation-children-would-be-taken-from-her.html

77. Next Generation Pharma.com cited 2012: Psychiatric Drugs: A Booming Business. Available online at http://www.ngpharma.com/article/psychiatric-drugs-a-booming-business/

78. SSRIstories.com cited 2013: SSRI Stories Antidepressant Nightmares. Available online at http://ssristories.com/

79. Natural News.com cited 2013: Psychiatry Goes Insane: Every Human Emotion Now Classified as a Mental Disorder in New Psychiatric Manual DSM-5. Available online at http://www.naturalnews.com/038322_dsm-5_psychiatry_false_diagnosis.html

80. The Wall Street Journal cited 2012: Are ADHD Medications Overprescribed? Available online at http://online.wsj.com/article/SB10000872396390444301704577631591596516110.html

81. drugwatch.com cited 2012: Prescription Drug Deaths on the Rise. Available online at http://www.drugwatch.com/2012/01/18/prescription-drug-deaths/

82. Business.highbeam.com cited 2013: Antidepressant drug trials: fast track to over prescription? Available online at http://business.highbeam.com/136989/article-1G1-91752194/antidepressant-drug-trials-fast-track-overprescription

Chapter 16

83. Weil, Dr. A., Foreword cited 2013: The Vitamin D Solution: A 3 Step Strategy to Cure Our Most Common Health Problems. Hudson Street Press.

84. Hollick, Dr. M. F., cited 2012: The Vitamin D Solution: A 3 Step Strategy to Cure Our Most Common Health Problems. Hudson Street Press.

85. Moritz, Andreas. Cited 2012: Heal Yourself with Sunlight. Ener Chi Wellness Press, 68 pp.

86. Mercola, Dr. J., Mercola.com cited 2012: The Surprising Cause of Melanoma (And No, It's Not Too Much Sun). Available online at http://articles.mercola.com/sites/articles/archive/2011/11/20/deadly-melanoma-not-due-vitamin-d-deficiency.aspx

87. Hollick, Dr. M. F., cited 2012: The Vitamin D Solution: A 3 Step Strategy to Cure Our Most Common Health Problems. Hudson Street Press.

88. CNN.com cited 2012: Avoid Sunscreens with Potentially Harmful Ingredients, group warns. Available online at http://www.cnn.co.uk/2012/05/16/health/sunscreen-report/index.html

89. Breakingnews.ewg.org/2012sunscreen cited 2012: EWG's Skin Deep Sunscreens 2012. Available online at http://breakingnews.ewg.org/2012sunscreen/

90. Huffington Post.com cited 2013: The Toxic Truth of Sunscreen. Available online at http://www.huffingtonpost.com/2010/05/26/the-toxic-truth-of-sunscr_n_590516.html#s93626&title=Increased_Risk_Of

91. BMJ.com cited 2013: Sunscreens and Melanoma – Letter to the Editor. Available online at http://www.bmj.com/rapid-response/2011/10/30/sunscreens-and-melanoma

92. CBS.com cited 2013: Man Catches Fire after Applying Spray-On Sunscreen before Grilling. Available online at http://www.cbsnews.com/8301-504763_162-57447309-10391704/man-

catches-fire-after-applying-spray-on-sunscreen-before-grilling/

93. AOLnews.com cited 2013: Study: Many Sunscreens May Be Accelerating Cancer. Available online at http://www. aolnews.com/2010/05/24/study-many-sunscreens-may-be-accelerating-cancer/

94. Moritz, Andreas. Cited 2012: Heal Yourself With Sunlight. Ener Chi Wellness Press, 68 pp.

95. Moritz, Andreas. Cited 2012: Heal Yourself With Sunlight. Ener Chi Wellness Press, 68 pp.

96. sunlightandvitamind.com cited 2011: Some D Deficiency or Insufficiency Linked Conditions. Available online at http://www.sunlightandvitamind.com/#Deficiency

97. Evers, Ethan. Naturalnews.com cited 2011: Vitamin D: How to Maintain Healthy Levels during Winter http://www.natura news.com/037631_vitamin_d_winter_months_deficiency.html

Chapter 17

98. Tompkins, P., Bird, C., cited 2011: The Secret Life of Plants. Penguin Publishers, 340 pp.

99. Silverstone, M., cited 2011: Blinded by Science. Lloyds World Publishing, 357 pp.

100. Ober, C., Zucker, M., Sinatra, S., cited: 2011: Earthing? The Most Important Healthy Discovery Ever? Basic Health Publications, 259 pp.

101. EMFields.com cited 2013: Mobile Phone Masts Hurt Birds. Available online at http://www.emfields.org/news/20120113-mobile-phone-masts-hurt-birds.asp

102. Wantchinatimes.com cited 2013: Nanjing Air Like Smoking 15 Packs of Cigarettes, say experts. Available online at http://www.wantchinatimes.com/news-subclass-cnt.aspx?id=20120614000068&cid=1105

Chapter 18

103. Mercola, Dr. J., cited 2011: If You Can't Beat Depression, This

Could Be Why. Available online at http://articles.mercola.com
/sites/articles/archive/2011/04/12/beware—bacteria-growing-
in-your-gut-can-influence-your-behavior.aspx

104. Mercola, Dr. J., cited 2013: Audio Interview with Caroline
Barringer. Available online http://articles.mercola.com
/sites/articles/archive/2012/03/18/mcbride-and-barringer-
interview.aspx

Chapter 19

105. Wikipedia.com cited 2013: Miso – Nutrition and Health.
Available online at http://en.wikipedia.org/wiki/Miso

Chapter 20

106. Naturalnews.com cited 2013: Exercise Your Cells by
Rebounding. Available online at http://www.naturalnews
.com/031213_rebounding_exercise.html

107. Anderson, Lynne. webmd.com cited 2012: Kettlebells: A Smart
Replacement for Dumbells? Available online at http://
www.webmd.com/fitness-exercise/features/kettlebells-smart-
smart-replacement-dumbbells

108. Livestrong.com cited 2013: Scientific Benefits of Kettle Bell
Training. Available online at http://www.livestrong.com
/article/157017-scientific-benefits-of-kettlebell-training/

109. Mercola, Dr. J., Mercola.com cited 2012: This Exercise Can
Cause a 7-Fold Surge of Heart Problems. Available online at
http://fitness.mercola.com/sites/fitness/archive/2012/06/01/lon
g-cardio-workout-dangers.aspx

110. Bestlife.com cited 2012: Some Surprising Benefits of Exercise.
Available online at http://www.thebestlife.com/

Chapter 21

111. Kindred, G., cited 2012: Earth Wisdom. Hay House Publishers,
275 pp.

112. Wilcock, D., Falling Into Easy – Help For Those That Can't

Meditate. John Hunt Publishing

Chapter 22

113. Chase, M. J., cited 2011: Am I Being Kind? Hay House Publishers, 279 pp.

Chapter 23

114. Amishnews.com cited 2011: Amish Forgiveness at Nickel Mines. Available online at http://www.amishnews.com/amish-forgiveness.html

115. Jones, C. M., Personalityresearch.org cited 2011: Genetic and Environmental Influences on Criminal Behavior. Available online at http://personalityresearch.org/papers/jones.html

116. Prisonreformtrust.org.uk cited 2013: Report No One Knows – Offenders with Learning Difficulties and Learning Disabilities. Available online at http://www.prisonreformtrust.org.uk/uploads/documents/NOKNL.pdf

Chapter 24

117. livescience.com cited 2013: Happiest Nations on Earth Revealed. Available online at http://www.livescience.com/25713-happiest-countries-happiness-gallup.html

Chapter 26

118. Chapman, G., cited 2012: The Five Love Languages: The Secret to Love That Lasts. Northfield Publishing, 203 pp.

Chapter 28

119. O'shea, T. Dr., cited 2013: The Doctor Within. Available online at http://www.thedoctorwithin.com/

120. Hyman, M. Dr., cited 2013: The Five Problems with Vitamin Supplements. Available online at http://www.touchstoneessentials.com/the-five-problems-with-vitamin-supplements/

121. Livestrong.com cited 2013: When Your Body Does Not Absorb

Vitamins? Available online at http://www.livestrong.com /article/400246-when-does-your-body-not-absorb-vitamins/

Chapter 32

122. Sylva K., Lunt I., cited 2012: Sigmund Freud – Childhood Development – A First Course. Blackwell Publishers, 262 pp.

123. Sears, W., Sears, Martha, cited 2012: The Attachment Parenting Book. Hachette Book Group.

124. Dr Momma.org cited 2013: The Dangers of Your Baby Crying It Out. Available online at http://www.drmomma.org/ 2009/12/dangers-of-your-baby-crying-it-out.html

125. Who.int cited 2012: Infant and Young Child Feeding. Available online at http://www.who.int/mediacentre/factsheets/fs342/en/

126. Askdrsears.com cited 2012: Scientific Benefits of Co-Sleeping. Available online at http://www.askdrsears.com/topics/sleep-problems/scientific-benefits-co-sleeping

127. Jackson, D. cited 2012: Three in a Bed: The Benefits of Sleeping with Your Baby. Bloomsbury Publishing Place, 312 pp.

Chapter 33

128. Folden, Dr. L., cited 2012: The Baby Bond. Lucky Press. 409 pp.

129. Theecologist.org cited 2013: Breast milk VS Formula. Available online at http://www.theecologist.org/trial_investigations/ 268337/breastmilk_vs_formula_food.html

130. beyondconformity.org.nz cited 2012: Breastmilk Stem Cells. Available online at http://www.beyondconformity.org.nz/_blog /Hilary%27s_Desk/post/Breastmilk_stem_cells/

131. Dummies.com cited 2012: Comparing Formula and Breast Milk. Available online at http://www.dummies.com/how-to/content/comparing-formula-and-breast-milk.html

132. Naturalnews.com cited 2013: Toxic Amounts of Aluminum Found in Infant Formulas. Available online at http://www .naturalnews.com/038220_aluminum_infant_formulas_toxicity .html

133. Folden, Dr L cited 2013: Formula Feeding Doubles Infant Deaths in America. Available online at http://thebaby bond.com/InfantDeaths.html

134. Dummies.com cited 2012: Comparing Formula and Breast Milk. Available online at http://www.dummies.com/how-to/content/comparing-formula-and-breast-milk.html

135. Prentice, A.M., Paul, A., Prentice, A., Black, A., Cole, T., & Whitehead, R. cited 2012: Cross-cultural differences in lactational performance. In Maternal Environmental Factors in Human Lactation. Human Lactation 2, pp. 13 = 44 [Hamosh, M., & Goldman, A.S. (eds). New York: Plenum Press].

136. Oprah.com cited 2012: One Woman's Mission to Save Babies. Available online at http://www.oprah.com/omagazine/Milk-Banks-Donating-Breast-Milk-to-Save-Babies/4

137. Spangler, A. babygooroo.com cited 2012: Soy Formula Linked to Fibroid Tumors. Available online at http://babygooroo.com/2010/02/soy-formula-linked-to-fibroid-tumors/

138. Mercola, Dr J. Mercola.com cited 2012: The Popular Food You Should Never, Ever Give Your Baby http://articles.mercola.com/sites/articles/archive/2011/04/02/soy-formula-linked-to-fibroid-tumors.aspx

139. FDA.gov cited 2013: Questions and Answers for Consumer Concerns Regarding Formula. Available online at http://www.fda.gov/Food/FoodSafety/Product-SpecificInformation/InfantFormula/ConsumerInformationAboutInfantFormula/ucm108079.htm

140. Telegraph.co.uk cited 2013: Baby Formula Recall in China after Infant Death. Available online at http://www.telegraph.co.uk/news/worldnews/asia/china/2827362/Baby-formula-recall-in-China-after-infant-death.html

141. mcspotlight.org cited 2012: McSpotlight on The Baby Milk Industry. Available online at http://www.mcspotlight.org/beyond/nestle.html

Chapter 34

142. Bennett, D. health101.org cited 2013: Food and Behavior Book Review. Available online at http://www.health101.org/art _behavior.htm

143. Naturalsociety.com cited 2013: What's in Your Milk? 20 + Painkillers, Antibiotics, and More. Available online at http://naturalsociety.com/the-cocktail-of-up-to-20-chemicals-in -a-glass-of-milk/

144. Robbins, J cited 2013: Diet for a New America. Stillpoint Publishing, 425 pp.

145. Veracity, D. Naturalnews.com cited 2012: Asthma explained by common allergy to milk and dairy products. Available online at http://www.naturalnews.com/010443_cows_milk_asthma.html #ixzz2Hla5a0fa

146. Robbins. J Foodmatters.tv cited 2012: The Truth about Calcium and Osteoporosis. Available online at http://foodmatters. tv/articles-1/the-truth-about-calcium-and-osteoporosis

147. Naturalnews.com cited 2012: CDC Admits Not a Single Person Has Died from Consuming Raw Milk Products in 11 Years. Available online at http://www.naturalnews.com/034169 _CDC_raw_milk.html#ixzz2HlhEm1fl

148. Naturalnews.com cited 2012: Raw Milk: Good enough for Queen Elizabeth but prohibited for ordinary Canadians. Available online at http://www.naturalnews.com/034747_raw _milk_Queen_Elizabeth_Canada.html

149. Ibisworld.com cited 2013: Dairy Farms in the US: Market Research Report. Available online at http://www.ibis world.com/industry/default.aspx?indid=49

150. Best, S. Sarahbesthealth.com cited 2013: Shocking Facts about Sugar. Available online at http://www.sarahbesthealth .com/shocking-facts-about-sugar/

Chapter 35

151. Boyles, S., WebMD.com cited 2012: Report: Toxins Common in

Baby Products. Available online at http://www.webmd.com /parenting/baby/news/20090312/report-toxins-common-in-baby-products

152. Nytimes.com cited 2013: Johnson and Johnson to Remove Formaldehyde from Products. Available online at http://www.nytimes.com/2012/08/16/business/johnson-johnson-to-remove-formaldehyde-from-products.html?_r=0

153. Greenhealthwatch.com cited 2013: Chemicals in Disposable Nappies Hazardous to Babies. Available online at http://www.greenhealthwatch.com/newsstories/newschildren/t oxicnappies.html

154. Mellowship, D., cited 2012: study by Ikezuki, Y. Dertimination of bisphenol A concentrations in human biological fluids reveals significant early prenatal exposure, Human Reproduction – Toxic Beauty – How Hidden Chemicals In Cosmetics Harm You. Octopus Publishing Group, 303 pp.

Chapter 36

155. Halvorsen, Dr. R., cited 2012: The Truth about Vaccines: How We Are Used As Guinea Pigs without Knowing It. Gibson Square, 312 pp.

156. Mercola, Dr. J., Mercola.com cited 2013: This Revolting Practice Targets Poor Unsuspecting People First – And You Are Next http://articles.mercola.com/sites/articles/archive/2012/02/19/dr ug-company-lies-and-uses-human-as-guinea-pigs.aspx

157. vaclib.org cited 2013: Graphical Evidence Shows Vaccines Didn't Save Us. Available online at http://www.vaclib. org/sites/debate/web1.html

158. Doubleday, J., cited 2012: Into the Labyrinth. Available online at https://www.facebook.com/photo.php?fbid=405830396138935& l=c6cdca3812

159. whale.to The Urabe Atrocity. Available online at http://www. whale.to/vaccine/mmr15.html

160. Bollinger, Ty, cited 2011: Cancer – Step Outside the Box.

161. Tomlijenovic, L. PhD ecomed.org.uk cited 2012: The vaccination policy and the Code of Practice of the Joint Committee on Vaccination and Immunisation (JCVI): are they at odds? http://www.ecomed.org.uk/wp-content/uploads/2011/09/3-tomljenovic.pdf

162. Pharma Marketing Blog cited 2013: Resurgence of Pharma Lobbying Spending. Available online at http://pharmamkting.blogspot.co.uk/2012/04/resurgence-of-pharma-lobbying-spending.html

163. Sears, Dr. R. askdrsears.com cited: 2013: Do Doctors Have a Financial Incentive to Get Their Patients Fully Vaccinated? Available online at http://www.askdrsears.com/topics/vaccines/do-doctors-have-financial-incentive-get-their-patients-fully-vaccinated

164. Drmomma.org cited 2012: CDC Mandatory Vaccine Schedule: 1983 vs 2012. Available online at http://www.drmomma.org/2011/01/cdc-mandatory-vaccine-schedule-1983-vs.html

165. Mercola, Dr. J. Mercola.com cited 2012: Flu Vaccines Part 2. Available online at http://articles.mercola.com/sites/articles/archive/2004/05/22/flu-vaccines-part-two.aspx

166. England, C. Vactruth.com cited 2012: Baby Dies after 9 Vaccines in One Day. Available online at http://vactruth.com/2012/01/19/baby-dies-after-first-shots/

167. Autisable.com cited 2013: Vaccines Far Exceed FDA Limits on Aluminum Exposure. Could this = cancer risk? Available online at http://www.autisable.com/743892431/vaccines-far-exceed-fda-limits-on-aluminum-exposure-could-this—cancer-risk/

168. Sears, Dr. R. cited 2012: The Vaccine Book. Little Brown Books.

169. mercola.com cited 2011: Vaccine Fillers and Ingredients. Available online at articles.mercola.com/sites/articles/archive/2001/03/07/vaccine-ingredients.aspx

170. Neetu Vashishut, Jacob Puliyel. Indian Journal of Medical Ethics Vol. iX No 2 April–June 2012.

171. CDC.gov. cited 2012: Measles Outbreak among Vaccinated High School Students – Illinois. Available online at http://www.cdc.gov/mmwr/preview/mmwrhtml/00000359.htm

172. England, C. Vactruth.com Minimum 40 Children Paralyzed after New Meningitis Vaccine. Available online at http://vactruth.com/2013/01/06/paralyzed-after-meningitis-vaccine/

173. Gaia-Health.com cited 2013: 1 in 100 Students Felled by Chronic Fatigue Syndrome: More Vaccine Victims? http://gaia-health.com/gaia-blog/2011-12-14/1-in-100-students-felled-by-chronic-fatigue-syndrome-more-vaccine-victims/

174. Independent.co.uk cited 2012: Jailed for a crime you didn't commit: Landmark case could be costly for UK http://www.independent.co.uk/news/uk/crime/jailed-for-a-crime-you-didnt-commit-landmark-case-could-be-costly-for-uk-8303850.html

175. Mercola, Dr. J., Mercola.com cited 2012: Warning to Parents: This Vaccine Linked to Sudden Infant Death. Available online at http://articles.mercola.com/sites/articles/archive/2011/05/19/us-government-concedes-hep-b-vaccine-causes-systemic-lupus-erythematosus.aspx

176. whale.to cited 2012: Alan Yurko. Available online at http://www.whale.to/m/yurko.html

177. vactruth.com. cited 2012: Brainwashed Police Prosecute Parents to Protect Vaccines. Available online at http://vactruth.com/2012/11/08/brainwashed-police-ignore-vaccine-injuries/

178. Mercola, Dr. J. Mercola.com cited 2012: Harvard takes it back and says that Swine Flu was oversold http://articles.mercola.com/sites/articles/archive/2010/01/02/Harvard-Takes-it-Back-and-Says-Swine-Flu-was-Oversold.aspx

Chapter 37

179. Mendelssohn, Dr. R., cited 2012: How to Raise a Healthy Child In Spite of Your Doctor. Ballentine Books, 283 pp.

180. Dailymail.co.uk cited 2012: Cut down the Calpol: New guide-

lines instruct parents to slash children's paracetamol by up to half. Available online at http://www.dailymail.co.uk /health/article-2063812/Cut-Calpol-New-guidelines-instruct-parents-slash-childrens-paracetamol-doses-half.html

181. dailymail.co.uk cited 2012: Babies given Calpol and other forms of paracetamol more likely to develop asthma. Available online at http://www.dailymail.co.uk/health/article-223 1833/Babies-given-Calpol-forms-paracetamol-likely-develop-asthma.html

182. dailymail.co.uk cited 2012: Babies given Calpol and other forms of paracetamol more likely to develop asthma. Available online at http://www.dailymail.co.uk/health/article-2231 833/Babies-given-Calpol-forms-paracetamol-likely-develop-asthma.html

183. Hiro Watanabe, PhD. The Magic of Miso. Wise Traditions Conference, November 2006. Available online at http:// www.fleetwoodonsite.com/index.php?manufacturers_id=11& osCsid=710d1e5b3567d83b3ec429eb228bb160

Chapter 38

184. chem-tox.com cited 2013: Bed and Mattress Illness Report Page available online at http://www.chem-tox.com/guest/guest book.html

185. midwiferytoday.com cited 2013: Baby's bedding: Is It Creating Toxic Nerve Gases? Available online at http://www.midwifery-today.com/articles/bedding.asp

186. greenpainters.org.au cited 2013: Paint Toxicity available online at http://www.greenpainters.org.au/Consumer-Information /Paint-Toxicity.htm

187. Michigantoday.umich.edu cited 2012: Study Suggests that Being Too Clean Can Make People Sick. Available online at http://michigantoday.umich.edu/2011/01/story.php?id=7915#.U PHv8omLK4Q

Chapter 39

188. huffingtonpost.com cited 2103: Suicides Now America's Leading Cause of Death by Injury: Study. Available online at http://www.huffingtonpost.com/2012/09/24/suicide-leading-cause-death-us_n_1909772.html

189. Sears, W., MD, Sears, M. RN, cited 2011: The Discipline Book: Everything You Need to Know to Have a Better Behaved Child from Birth to Age Ten. Little Brown Books, 316 pp.

Chapter 40

190. wikipedia.com cited 2011: E. O. Wilson. Available online at http://en.wikipedia.org/wiki/Edward_Osborne_Wilson

191. Faber Taylor, A., Kuo, F.E., & Sullivan, W.C. (2001). Coping with ADD: The surprising connection to green play settings. Environment & Behavior, 33(1), 54-77.

Chapter 42

192. Robinson, K., cited 2011: The Element: How Finding Your Passion Changes Everything. Penguin Books, 275pp.

193. Gatto, J. T., cited 2011: Dumbing Us Down: The Hidden Curriculum of Compulsory Schooling. New Society Publishers, 108 pp.

The world is a dangerous place, not because of those who do evil, but because of those who look on and do nothing.
~ Albert Einstien

About the Author

Anna Rodgers is an Australian model and journalist now living in the UK. She started her website Miss Eco Glam in 2009 and has gained a following for being honest and passionate about issues such as natural parenting, improving relationships, vaccinations, environmental, eco travel and natural health issues. Anna contributes travel articles to *Get Fresh* and *Yoga Magazine* as well as writes blogs on her website. Anna was the face of St Erasmus Ethical Couture Jewelry for three seasons. She is currently writing her next book, a health and well-being guide for teenagers.

Anna lives in East Sussex, United Kingdom with her husband Nathan and daughter Lola.

Soul Rocks is a fresh list that takes the search for soul and spirit mainstream. Chick-lit, young adult, cult, fashionable fiction & non-fiction with a fierce twist